D0914308

The Electrical Engineering Handbook
Third Edition

Sensors, Nanoscience, Biomedical Engineering, and Instruments

The Electrical Engineering Handbook Series

Series Editor
Richard C. Dorf
University of California, Davis

Titles Included in the Series

The Handbook of Ad Hoc Wireless Networks, Mohammad Ilyas
The Avionics Handbook, Cary R. Spitzer
The Biomedical Engineering Handbook, Third Edition, Joseph D. Bronzino
The Circuits and Filters Handbook, Second Edition, Wai-Kai Chen
The Communications Handbook, Second Edition, Jerry Gibson
The Computer Engineering Handbook, Vojin G. Oklobdzija
The Control Handbook, William S. Levine
The CRC Handbook of Engineering Tables, Richard C. Dorf
The Digital Signal Processing Handbook, Vijay K. Madisetti and Douglas Williams
The Electrical Engineering Handbook, Third Edition, Richard C. Dorf
The Electric Power Engineering Handbook, Leo L. Grigsby
The Electronics Handbook, Second Edition, Jerry C. Whitaker
The Engineering Handbook, Third Edition, Richard C. Dorf
The Handbook of Formulas and Tables for Signal Processing, Alexander D. Poularikas
The Handbook of Nanoscience, Engineering, and Technology, William A. Goddard, III, Donald W. Brenner, Sergey E. Lyshevski, and Gerald J. Iafrate
The Handbook of Optical Communication Networks, Mohammad Ilyas and Hussein T. Mouftah
The Industrial Electronics Handbook, J. David Irwin
The Measurement, Instrumentation, and Sensors Handbook, John G. Webster
The Mechanical Systems Design Handbook, Osita D.I. Nwokah and Yidirim Hurmuzlu
The Mechatronics Handbook, Robert H. Bishop
The Mobile Communications Handbook, Second Edition, Jerry D. Gibson
The Ocean Engineering Handbook, Ferial El-Hawary
The RF and Microwave Handbook, Mike Golio
The Technology Management Handbook, Richard C. Dorf
The Transforms and Applications Handbook, Second Edition, Alexander D. Poularikas
The VLSI Handbook, Wai-Kai Chen

The Electrical Engineering Handbook
Third Edition

Edited by
Richard C. Dorf

Circuits, Signals, and Speech and Image Processing

Electronics, Power Electronics, Optoelectronics, Microwaves, Electromagnetics, and Radar

Sensors, Nanoscience, Biomedical Engineering, and Instruments

Broadcasting and Optical Communication Technology

Computers, Software Engineering, and Digital Devices

Systems, Controls, Embedded Systems, Energy, and Machines

The Electrical Engineering Handbook
Third Edition

Sensors, Nanoscience, Biomedical Engineering, and Instruments

Edited by
Richard C. Dorf
University of California
Davis, California, U.S.A.

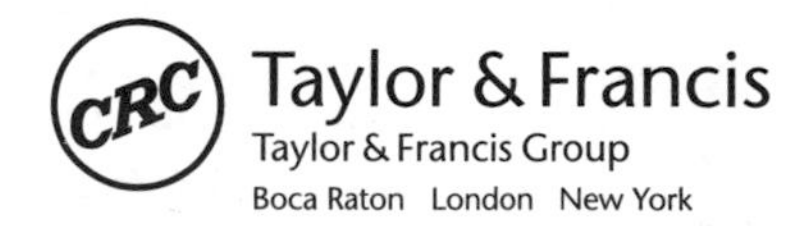

A CRC title, part of the Taylor & Francis imprint, a member of the Taylor & Francis Group, the academic division of T&F Informa plc.

Published in 2006 by
CRC Press
Taylor & Francis Group
6000 Broken Sound Parkway NW, Suite 300
Boca Raton, FL 33487-2742

Printed in the United States of America on acid-free paper
10 9 8 7 6 5 4 3 2 1

International Standard Book Number-10: 0-8493-7346-8 (Hardcover)
International Standard Book Number-13: 978-0-8493-7346-6 (Hardcover)
Library of Congress Card Number 2005054343

Library of Congress Cataloging-in-Publication Data

Sensors, nanoscience, biomedical engineering and instruments / edited by Richard C. Dorf.
p. cm.
Includes bibliographical references and index.
ISBN 0-8493-7346-8 (alk. paper)
1. Biosensors. 2. Medical electronics. 3. Biomedical engineering. I. Dorf, Richard C. II. Title.

R857.B54S4555 2005
610.28--dc22 2005054343

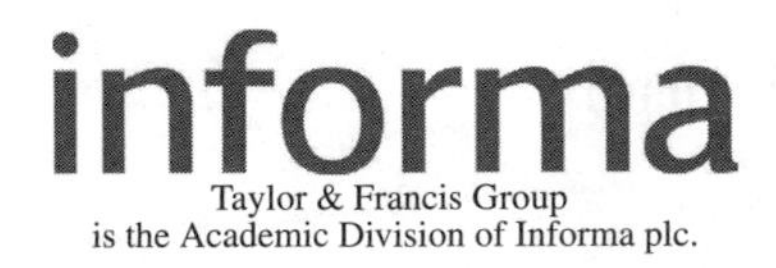

Visit the Taylor & Francis Web site at
http://www.taylorandfrancis.com

and the CRC Press Web site at
http://www.crcpress.com

Preface

Purpose

The purpose of *The Electrical Engineering Handbook, 3rd Edition* is to provide a ready reference for the practicing engineer in industry, government, and academia, as well as aid students of engineering. The third edition has a new look and comprises six volumes including:

Circuits, Signals, and Speech and Image Processing
Electronics, Power Electronics, Optoelectronics, Microwaves, Electromagnetics, and Radar
Sensors, Nanoscience, Biomedical Engineering, and Instruments
Broadcasting and Optical Communication Technology
Computers, Software Engineering, and Digital Devices
Systems, Controls, Embedded Systems, Energy, and Machines

Each volume is edited by Richard C. Dorf, and is a comprehensive format that encompasses the many aspects of electrical engineering with articles from internationally recognized contributors. The goal is to provide the most up-to-date information in the classical fields of circuits, signal processing, electronics, electromagnetic fields, energy devices, systems, and electrical effects and devices, while covering the emerging fields of communications, nanotechnology, biometrics, digital devices, computer engineering, systems, and biomedical engineering. In addition, a complete compendium of information regarding physical, chemical, and materials data, as well as widely inclusive information on mathematics is included in each volume. Many articles from this volume and the other five volumes have been completely revised or updated to fit the needs of today and many new chapters have been added.

The purpose of this volume (*Sensors, Nanoscience, Biomedical Engineering, and Instruments)* is to provide a ready reference to subjects in the fields of sensors, materials and nanoscience, instruments and measurements, and biomedical systems and devices. Here we provide the basic information for understanding these fields. We also provide information about the emerging fields of sensors, nanotechnologies, and biological effects.

Organization

The information is organized into three sections. The first two sections encompass 10 chapters and the last section summarizes the applicable mathematics, symbols, and physical constants.

Most articles include three important and useful categories: defining terms, references, and further information. *Defining terms* are key definitions and the first occurrence of each term defined is indicated in boldface in the text. The definitions of these terms are summarized as a list at the end of each chapter or article. The *references* provide a list of useful books and articles for follow-up reading. Finally, *further information* provides some general and useful sources of additional information on the topic.

Locating Your Topic

Numerous avenues of access to information are provided. A complete table of contents is presented at the front of the book. In addition, an individual table of contents precedes each section. Finally, each chapter begins with its own table of contents. The reader should look over these tables of contents to become familiar with the structure, organization, and content of the book. For example, see Section II: Biomedical Systems, then Chapter 7: Bioelectricity, and then Chapter 7.2: Bioelectric Events. This tree-and-branch table of contents enables the reader to move up the tree to locate information on the topic of interest.

Two indexes have been compiled to provide multiple means of accessing information: subject index and index of contributing authors. The subject index can also be used to locate key definitions. The page on which the definition appears for each key (defining) term is clearly identified in the subject index.

The Electrical Engineering Handbook, 3rd Edition is designed to provide answers to most inquiries and direct the inquirer to further sources and references. We hope that this handbook will be referred to often and that informational requirements will be satisfied effectively.

Acknowledgments

This handbook is testimony to the dedication of the Board of Advisors, the publishers, and my editorial associates. I particularly wish to acknowledge at Taylor & Francis Nora Konopka, Publisher; Helena Redshaw, Editorial Project Development Manager; and Susan Fox, Project Editor. Finally, I am indebted to the support of Elizabeth Spangenberger, Editorial Assistant.

Richard C. Dorf
Editor-in-Chief

Editor-in-Chief

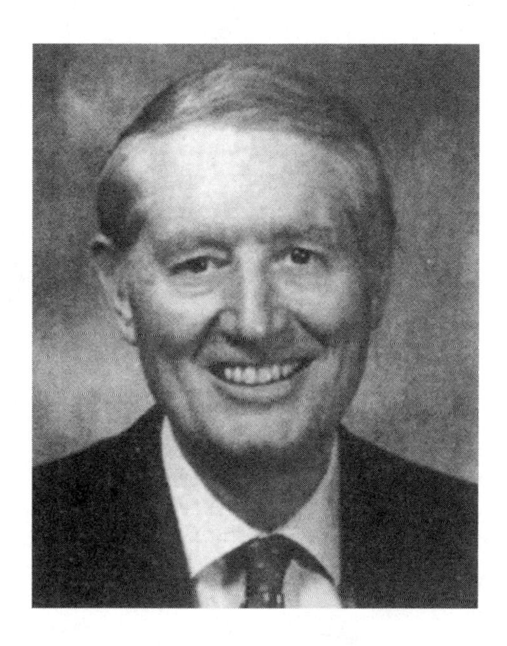

Richard C. Dorf, Professor of Electrical and Computer Engineering at the University of California, Davis, teaches graduate and undergraduate courses in electrical engineering in the fields of circuits and control systems. He earned a Ph.D. in electrical engineering from the U.S. Naval Postgraduate School, an M.S. from the University of Colorado, and a B.S. from Clarkson University. Highly concerned with the discipline of electrical engineering and its wide value to social and economic needs, he has written and lectured internationally on the contributions and advances in electrical engineering.

Professor Dorf has extensive experience with education and industry and is professionally active in the fields of robotics, automation, electric circuits, and communications. He has served as a visiting professor at the University of Edinburgh, Scotland; the Massachusetts Institute of Technology; Stanford University; and the University of California, Berkeley.

Professor Dorf is a Fellow of The Institute of Electrical and Electronics Engineers and a Fellow of the American Society for Engineering Education. Dr. Dorf is widely known to the profession for his *Modern Control Systems, 10th Edition* (Addison-Wesley, 2004) and *The International Encyclopedia of Robotics* (Wiley, 1988). Dr. Dorf is also the co-author of *Circuits, Devices and Systems* (with Ralph Smith), *5th Edition* (Wiley, 1992), and *Electric Circuits, 7th Edition* (Wiley, 2006). He is also the author of *Technology Ventures* (McGraw-Hill, 2005) and *The Engineering Handbook, 2nd Edition* (CRC Press, 2005).

Advisory Board

Contributors

Ronald Arif
Lehigh University
Bethlehem, Pennsylvania

Frank Barnes
University of Colorado
Boulder, Colorado

R.C. Barr
Duke University
Durham, North Carolina

Edward J. Berbari
Indiana University/Purdue University
Indianapolis, Indiana

Robert A. Bond
MIT Lincoln Laboratory
Lexington, Massachusetts

Joseph D. Bronzino
Trinity College
Hartford, Connecticut

B.S. Dhillon
University of Ottawa
Ottawa, Ontario, Canada

Alan D. Dorval II
Boston University
Boston, Massachusetts

Halit Eren
Curtin University of Technology
Bentley, Western Australia, Australia

Martin D. Fox
University of Connecticut
Storrs, Connecticut

L.A. Geddes
Purdue University
Lafayette, Indiana

Victor Giurgiutiu
University of South Carolina
Columbia, South Carolina

David L. Hall
The Pennsylvania State University
University Park, Pennsylvania

Bryan Stewart Hobbs
City Technology Limited
Portsmouth, England

Zhian Jin
Lehigh University
Bethlehem, Pennsylvania

Sam S. Khalilieh
Tyco Infrastructure Services
Grand Rapids, Michigan

James Llinas
State University of New York at Buffalo
Williamsville, New York

Sergey Edward Lyshevski
Rochester Institute of Technology
Rochester, New York

David R. Martinez
MIT Lincoln Laboratory
Lexington, Massachusetts

M. Meyyappan
NASA Ames Research Center
Moffett Field, California

Michael R. Neuman
Michigan Technological University
Houghton, Michigan

John Pelesko
University of Delaware
Newark, Delaware

Yuan Pu
University of California
Irvine, California

Christopher G. Relf
National Instruments Certified LabVIEW Developer
New South Wales, Australia

Bonnie Keillor Slaten
University of Colorado
Boulder, Colorado

Rosemary L. Smith
University of Maine
Orono, Maine

Ronald J. Tallarida
Temple University
Philadelphia, Pennsylvania

Nelson Tansu
Lehigh University
Bethlehem, Pennsylvania

Charles W. Therrien
Naval Postgraduate School
Monterey, California

M. Michael Vai
MIT Lincoln Laboratory
Lexington, Massachusetts

Joseph Watson
University of Wales
Swansea, United Kingdom

John A. White
Boston University
Boston, Massachusetts

David Young
Rockwell Semiconductor Systems
Newport Beach, California

Contents

SECTION I Sensors, Nanoscience, and Instruments

1 Sensors

1.1 Introduction *Rosemary L. Smith* 1-1

1.2 Electrochemical Sensors *Bryan Stewart Hobbs* 1-11

1.3 The Stannic Oxide Semiconductor Gas Sensor *Joseph Watson* 1-18

2 An Introduction to Multi-Sensor Data Fusion *David L. Hall and James Llinas* 2-1

3 Magneto-optics *David Young and Yuan Pu* 3-1

4 Materials and Nanoscience

4.1 Carbon Nanotubes *M. Meyyappan* 4-1

4.2 Modeling MEMS and NEMS *John Pelesko* 4-9

4.3 Micromechatronics *Victor Giurgiutiu and Sergey Edward Lyshevski* 4-20

4.4 Nanocomputers, Nano-Architectronics, and Nano-ICs *Sergey Edward Lyshevski* 4-42

4.5 Semiconductor Nano-Electronics and Nano-Optoelectronics *Nelson Tansu, Ronald Arif, and Zhian Jin* 4-68

5 Instruments and Measurements

5.1 Electrical Equipment in Hazardous Areas *Sam S. Khalilieh* 5-1

5.2 Portable Instruments and Systems *Halit Eren* 5-27

5.3 G (LabVIEW™) Software Engineering *Christopher G. Relf* 5-36

6 Reliability Engineering *B.S. Dhillon* 6-1

SECTION II Biomedical Systems

7 Bioelectricity

7.1 Neuroelectric Principles *John A. White and Alan D. Dorval II* 7-1

7.2 Bioelectric Events *L.A. Geddes (revised by R.C. Barr)* 7-13

7.3 Biological Effects and Electromagnetic Fields *Bonnie Keillor Slaten and Frank Barnes* 7-33

7.4 Embedded Signal Processing *David R. Martinez, Robert A. Bond, and M. Michael Vai* 7-55

8 Biomedical Sensors *Michael R. Neuman* 8-1

9 Bioelectronics and Instruments
9.1 The Electro-encephalogram *Joseph D. Bronzino* 9-1
9.2 The Electrocardiograph *Edward J. Berbari* 9-14

10 Tomography *Martin D. Fox* 10-1

SECTION III Mathematics, Symbols, and Physical Constants

Introduction *Ronald J. Tallarida* III-1

Greek Alphabet III-3
International System of Units (SI) III-3
Conversion Constants and Multipliers III-6
Physical Constants III-8
Symbols and Terminology for Physical and Chemical Quantities III-9
Credits III-13
Probability for Electrical and Computer Engineers *Charles W. Therrien* III-14

Indexes

Author Index A-1

Subject Index S-1

I

Sensors, Nanoscience, and Instruments

1 **Sensors** *R.L. Smith, B.S. Hobbs, J. Watson* 1-1
Introduction • Electrochemical Sensors • The Stannic Oxide Semiconductor Gas Sensor

2 **An Introduction to Multi-Sensor Data Fusion** *D.L. Hall, J. Llinas* 2-1
Introduction • Data Fusion Techniques • Applications of Data Fusion • Process Models for Data Fusion • Limitations of Data Fusion Systems • Summary

3 **Magneto-optics** *D. Young, Y. Pu* 3-1
Introduction • Classification of Magneto-optic Effects • Applications of Magneto-optic Effects

4 **Materials and Nanoscience** *M. Meyyappan, J. Pelesko, V. Giurgiutiu, S.E. Lyshevski, N. Tansu, R. Arif, Z. Jin* 4-1
Carbon Nanotubes • Modeling MEMS and NEMS • Micromechatronics • Nanocomputers, Nano-Architectronics, and Nano-ICs • Semiconductor Nano-Electronics and Nano-Optoelectronics

5 **Instruments and Measurements** *S.S. Khalilieh, H. Eren, C.G. Relf* 5-1
Electrical Equipment in Hazardous Areas • Portable Instruments and Systems • G (LabVIEW™) Software Engineering

6 **Reliability Engineering** *B.S. Dhillon* 6-1
Introduction • Terms and Definitions • Bathtub Hazard-Rate Concept • Important Formulas • Reliability Networks • Reliability Evaluation Methods • Human Reliability • Robot Reliability

1

Sensors

Rosemary L. Smith
University of Maine

Bryan Stewart Hobbs
City Technology Limited

Joseph Watson
University of Wales

1.1 Introduction 1-1
Physical Sensors • Chemical Sensors • Biosensors • Microsensors
1.2 Electrochemical Sensors.. 1-11
Introduction • Potentiometric Sensors • Amperometric Sensors
1.3 The Stannic Oxide Semiconductor Gas Sensor 1-18
Introduction • Basic Electrical Parameters and Operation • Operating Temperature • Substrate Materials • Electrical Operating Parameters • Future Developments

1.1 Introduction

Rosemary L. Smith

Sensors are critical components in all measurement and control systems. The need for sensors that generate an electronic signal closely followed the advent of the microprocessor and computers. Together with the ever-present need for sensors in science and medicine, the demand for sensors in automated manufacturing and environmental monitoring is rapidly growing. In addition, small, inexpensive sensors are finding their way into all sorts of consumer products, from children's toys to dishwashers to automobiles. Because of the vast variety of useful things to be sensed and sensor applications, sensor engineering is a multidisciplinary and interdisciplinary field of endeavor. This chapter introduces some basic definitions, concepts, and features of sensors, and illustrates them with several examples. The reader is directed to the references and the sources listed under Further Information for more details and examples.

There are many terms which are often used synonymously for sensor, including transducer, meter, detector, and gage. Defining the term *sensor* is not an easy task; however, the most widely used definition is that which has been applied to electrical transducers by the Instrument Society of America (ANSI MC6.1, 1975): "Transducer—A device which provides a usable output in response to a specified measurand." A transducer is more generally defined as a device which converts energy from one form to another. Usable output can be an optical, electrical, chemical, or mechanical signal. In the context of electrical engineering, however, a usable output is usually an electrical signal. The measurand is a physical, chemical, or biological property or condition to be measured.

Most but not all sensors are transducers, employing one or more transduction mechanisms to produce an electrical output signal. Sometimes sensors are classified as direct or indirect sensors, according to how many transduction mechanisms are used. For example, a mercury thermometer produces a change in volume of mercury in response to a temperature change via thermal expansion. The output signal is the change in height of the mercury column. Here, thermal energy is converted into mechanical movement and we read the change in mercury height using our eyes as a second transducing element. However, in order to use the thermometer output in a control circuit or to log temperature data in a computer, the height of the mercury column must first be converted into an electrical signal. This can be accomplished by several means, but there are more direct temperature sensing methods, i.e., where an electrical output is produced in response to a change in temperature. An example is given in the next section on physical sensors. Figure 1.1 depicts a sensor block

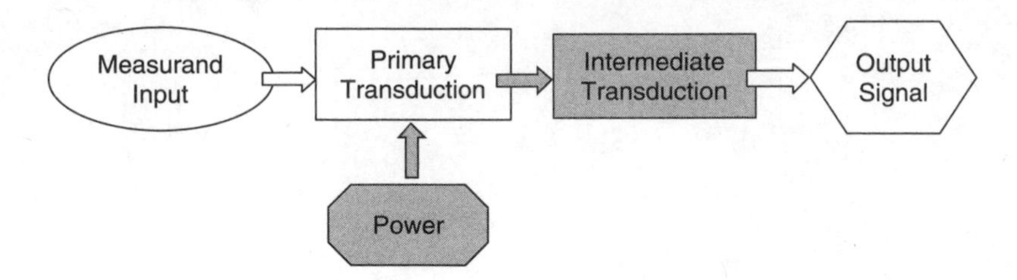

FIGURE 1.1 Sensor block diagram. Many sensors employ multiple transduction mechanisms in order to produce an electronic output in response to the measurand. Passive transduction mechanisms require input power in order to produce a usable output signal.

diagram, indicating the measurand and associated input signal, the primary and intermediate transduction mechanisms, and the electronic output signal. Some transducers are auto-generators or active, where a usable output signal, often electronic, is created directly in response to the measurand. However, many other types of transducers are modulators or passive, where an auxiliary energy source is used to transform the generated response to an electronic output signal. For example, the piezoresistor is a passive sensor. It is a resistor that changes its resistance value when it is mechanically deformed or strained. In order to measure this change, it is necessary to attach a voltage or current source. Table 1.1 is a six-by-six matrix of some of the more commonly employed physical and chemical transduction mechanisms for sensing. Many of the effects listed are described in more detail elsewhere in this handbook.

Today, sensors are most often classified by the type of measurand, i.e., physical, chemical, or biological. This is a much simpler means of classification than by transduction mechanism or output signal (e.g., digital or analog), since many sensors use multiple transduction mechanisms and the output signal can always be processed, conditioned, or converted by a circuit so as to cloud the definition of output. A description of each class and examples are given in the following sections. The last section introduces microsensors and some examples.

In choosing a particular sensor for a given application, there are many factors to be considered. These factors or specifications can be divided into three major categories: environmental factors, economic factors, and sensor characteristics. The most commonly encountered factors are listed in Table 1.2, although not all of them may be pertinent to a particular application. Most of the environmental factors determine the packaging of the sensor, meaning the encapsulation and insulation required to protect or isolate components from the environment, the input/output leads, connectors, and cabling. The economic factors determine the manufacturing method and type of materials used to make the sensor and to some extent the quality of the materials. For example, a very expensive sensor may be cost effective if it is used repeatedly or for very long periods of time. However, a disposable sensor like that used for early pregnancy testing should be inexpensive and may only need to function accurately for a few minutes. The sensor characteristics of the sensor are usually the specifications of primary concern. The most important parameters are sensitivity, stability, and repeatability. Normally, a sensor is only useful if all three of these parameters are tightly specified for a given range of measurand values and time of operation. For example, a highly sensitive device is not useful if its output signal drifts greatly during the measurement time and the data obtained may not be reliable if the measurement is not repeatable. Other sensor characteristics, such as selectivity and linearity, can often be compensated for by using additional, independent sensors or by signal conditioning circuits. For example, most sensors will respond to temperature in addition to their primary measurand, since most transduction mechanisms are temperature dependent. Therefore, temperature compensation is usually required if the sensor is to be used in an environment where temperature is not controlled.

Physical Sensors

Physical measurands include temperature, strain, force, pressure, displacement, position, velocity, acceleration, optical radiation, sound, flow rate, viscosity, and electromagnetic fields. Referring to Table 1.1, all but those

TABLE 1.1 Physical and Chemical Transduction Principles

	Secondary Signal					
Primary Signal	Mechanical	Thermal	Electrical	Magnetic	Radiant	Chemical
Mechanical	(Fluid) mechanical and acoustic effects (e.g., diaphragm, gravity balance, echo sounder)	Friction effects (e.g., friction calorimeter) Cooling effects (e.g., thermal flow meters)	Piezoelectricity Piezoresistivity Resistive, capacitive, and inductive effects	Magneto-mechanical effects (e.g., piezo-magnetic effect)	Photoelastic systems (stress-induced birefringence) Interferometers Sagnac effect Doppler effect	—
Thermal	Thermal expansion (bimetal strip, liquid-in-glass and gas thermometers, resonant frequency) Radiometer effect (light mill)	—	Seebeck effect Thermoresistance Pyroelectricity Thermal (Johnson) noise	—	Thermo-optical effects (e.g., liquid crystals) Radiant emission	Reaction activation (e.g., thermal dissociation)
Electrical	Electrokinetic and electro-mechanical effects (e.g., piezoelectricity, electro-meter, Ampere's law)	Joule (resistive) heating Peltier effect	Charge collectors Langmuir probe	Biot–Savart's law	Electro-optical effects (e.g., Kerr effect) Pockel's effect Electroluminescence	Electrolysis Electromigration
Magnetic	Magnetomechanical effects (e.g., magnetorestriction, magnetometer)	Thermomagnetic effects (e.g., Righi–Leduc effect) Galvanomagnetic effects (e.g., Ettingshausen effect)	Thermomagnetic effects (e.g., Ettingshausen–Nernst effect) Galvanomagnetic effects (e.g., Hall effect, magnetoresistance)	—	Magneto-optical effects (e.g., Faraday effect) Cotton–Mouton effect	—
Radiant	Radiation pressure	Bolometer thermopile	Photoelectric effects (e.g., photovoltaic effect, photoconductive effect)	—	Photorefractive effects Optical bistability	Photosynthesis, dissociation
Chemical	Hygrometer Electrodeposition cell Photoacoustic effect	Calorimeter Thermal conductivity cell	Potentiometry Conductiometry Amperometry Flame ionization Volta effect Gas-sensitive field effect	Nuclear magnetic resonance	(Emission and absorption) spectroscopy Chemiluminiscence	—

Source: T. Grandke and J. Hesse, *Introduction, Vol. 1: Fundamentals and General Aspects, Sensors: A Comprehensive Survey*, W. Gopel, J. Hesse, and J.H. Zemel, Eds., Weinheim, Germany: VCH, 1989. With permission.

TABLE 1.2

Environmental Factors	Economic Factors	Sensor Characteristics
Temperature range	Cost	Sensitivity
Humidity effects	Availability	Range
Corrosion	Lifetime	Stability
Size	—	Repeatability
Over range protection	—	Linearity
Susceptibility to EM interferences	—	Accuracy
Ruggedness	—	Response time
Power consumption	—	Frequency response
Self-test capability	—	—

transduction mechanisms listed in the chemical column are used in the design of physical sensors. Clearly, they comprise a very large proportion of all sensors. It is impossible to illustrate all of them, but three measurands stand out in terms of their widespread application: temperature, displacement (or associated force), and optical radiation.

Temperature Sensors

Temperature is an important parameter in many control systems, most familiarly in environmental control systems. Several distinctly different transduction mechanisms have been employed to measure temperature. The mercury thermometer was mentioned in the Introduction as a temperature sensor which produced a nonelectronic output signal. The most commonly used electrical signal generating temperature sensors are thermocouples, thermistors, and resistance thermometers. Thermocouples employ the Seebeck effect, which occurs at the junction of two dissimilar conductors. A voltage difference is generated between the hot and cold ends of the two conductors due to the differences in the energy distribution of electrons at the two temperatures. The voltage magnitude generated depends on the properties of the conductor, e.g., conductivity and work function, such that a difference voltage will be measured between the cool ends of two different conductors. The voltage changes fairly linearly with temperature over a given range, depending on the choice of conductors. To minimize measurement error, the cool end of the couple must be kept at a constant temperature and the voltmeter must have a high input impedance. A commonly used thermocouple is made of copper and constantan wires. A thermocouple is an "auto-generator," i.e., it produces a usable output signal, in this case electronic, directly in response to the measurand without the need for auxiliary power.

The resistance thermometer relies on the increase in resistance of a metal wire with increasing temperature. As the electrons in the metal gain thermal energy, they move about more rapidly and undergo more frequent collisions with each other and the atomic nuclei. These scattering events reduce the mobility of the electrons, and since resistance is inversely proportional to mobility, the resistance increases. Resistance thermometers typically consist of a coil of fine metal wire. Platinum wire gives the largest linear range of operation. The resistance thermometer is a "modulator" or passive transducer. In order to determine the resistance change, a constant current is supplied and the corresponding voltage is measured (or vice versa). Another means of making this measurement can be done by placing the resistor in the sensing arm of a Wheatstone bridge and adjusting the opposing resistor to "balance" the bridge producing a null output. A measure of the sensitivity of a resistance thermometer is its temperature coefficient of resistance, TCR $= (\delta R/R)(1/\delta T)$ in units of percent resistance per degree of temperature.

Thermistors are resistive elements made of semiconductor materials and have a negative temperature coefficient of resistance. The mechanism governing the resistance change of a thermistor is the increase in the number of conducting electrons with increasing temperature, due to thermal generation, i.e., the electrons that are the least tightly bound to the nucleus (valence electrons) gain sufficient thermal energy to break away (enter the conduction band) and become influenced by external fields. Thermistors are measured in the same manner as resistance thermometers, but thermistors have up to 100 times higher TCR values.

Displacement and Force Sensors

Many types of forces can be sensed by the displacements they create. For example, the force due to acceleration of a mass at the end of a spring will cause the spring to stretch and the mass to move. Its displacement from the zero acceleration position is governed by the force generated by the acceleration ($F = m \cdot a$) and by the restoring force of the spring. Another example is the displacement of the center of a deformable membrane due to a difference in pressure across it. Both of these examples require multiple transduction mechanisms to produce an electronic output: a primary mechanism which converts force to displacement (mechanical to mechanical) and then an intermediate mechanism to convert displacement to an electrical signal (mechanical to electrical). Displacement can be measured by an associated capacitance. For example, the capacitance associated with a gap which is changing in length is given by $C =$ area $\times$ dielectric constant/gap length. The gap must be very small compared to the surface area of the capacitor, since most dielectric constants are of the order of 1×10^{-13} farads/cm and with present methods, capacitance is readily resolvable to only about 10^{-12} farads. This is because measurement leads and contacts create parasitic capacitances that are of the same order of magnitude. If the capacitance is measured at the generated site by an integrated circuit, capacitances as small as 10^{-15} farads can be measured. Displacement is also commonly measured by the movement of a ferromagnetic core inside an inductor coil. The displacement produces a change in inductance which can be measured by placing the inductor in an oscillator circuit and measuring the change in frequency of oscillation.

The most commonly used force sensor is the strain gage. It consists of metal wires which are stretched in response to a force. The resistance of the wire changes as it undergoes strain, i.e., a change in length, since the resistance of a wire is $R =$ resistivity $\times$ length/cross-sectional area. The wire's resistivity is a bulk property of the metal which is a constant for constant temperature. A strain gage can be used to measure the force due to acceleration by attaching both ends of the wire to a cantilever beam (diving board), with one end of the wire at the attached beam end and the other at the free end. The free end of the cantilever beam moves in response to acceleration, producing strain in the wire and a subsequent change in resistance. The sensitivity of a strain gage is described by the unitless gage factor, $G = (\delta R/R)/(\delta L/L)$. For metal wires, gage factors typically range from 2 to 3. Semiconductors exhibit piezoresistivity, which is a change in resistivity in response to strain. Piezoresistors have gage factors as high as 130. Piezoresistive strain gages are frequently used in microsensors, as described later.

Optical Radiation

The intensity and frequency of optical radiation are parameters of great interest and utility in consumer products such as the video camera and home security systems and in optical communications systems. Consequently, the technology for optical sensing is highly developed. The conversion of optical energy to electronic signals can be accomplished by several mechanisms (see radiant to electronic transduction in Table 1.1); however, the most commonly used is the photogeneration of carriers in semiconductors. The most often-used device to convert photogeneration to an electrical output is the pn-junction photodiode. The construction of this device is very similar to the diodes used in electronic circuits as rectifiers. The photodiode is operated in reverse bias, where very little current normally flows. When light shines on the structure and is absorbed in the semiconductor, energetic electrons are produced. These electrons flow in response to the electric field sustained internally across the junction, producing an externally measurable current (and autogenerator). The current magnitude is proportional to the light intensity and also depends on the frequency of the light. Figure 1.2 shows the effects of light intensity on the terminal current vs. voltage behavior of a pn-junction photodiode. Note that for zero applied voltage, a net negative current flows when the junction is illuminated. This device can therefore also be used as a source of power (a solar cell). Photodiodes can be made sensitive to specific wavelengths of light by the choice of semiconductor material and by coating the device with thin film materials which act as optical filters.

Chemical Sensors

Chemical measurands include ion concentration, atomic mass, rate of reactions, reduction-oxidation potentials, and gas concentration. The last column of Table 1.1 lists some of the transduction mechanisms that

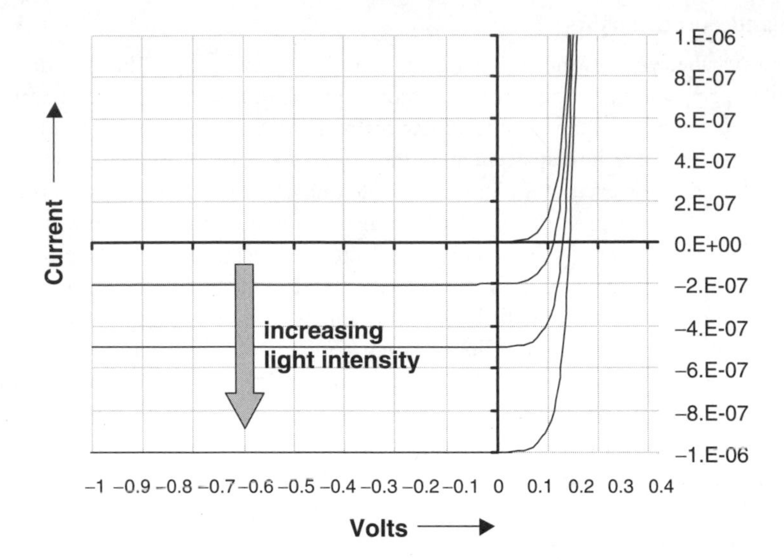

FIGURE 1.2 The current vs. voltage characteristics of a semiconductor, pn-junction, photodiode with incident light intensity.

have been or could be employed in chemical sensing. Two examples of chemical sensors are described here: the ion-selective electrode (ISE) and the gas chromatograph. They were chosen because of their general use and availability, and because they illustrate the use of a primary (ISE) vs. a primary plus intermediate (gas chromatograph) transduction mechanism.

Ion-Selective Electrode (ISE)

As the name implies, ISEs are used to measure the concentration of a specific ion concentration in a solution of many ions. To accomplish this, a membrane material is used that selectively generates a potential which is dependent on the concentration of the ion of interest. The generated potential is usually an equilibrium potential, called the Nernst potential, and it develops across the interface of the membrane with the solution. This potential is generated by the initial net flux of ions (charge) across the membrane in response to a concentration gradient, which generates an electric field that opposes further diffusion. Thenceforth the diffusional force is balanced by the electric force and equilibrium is established until a change in solution ion concentration occurs. This equilibrium potential is very similar to the so-called built-in potential of a pn-junction diode. The ion-selective membrane acts in such a way as to ensure that the generated potential is dependent mostly on the ion of interest and negligibly on any other ions in solution. This is done by enhancing the exchange rate of the ion of interest across the membrane, so that it is the fastest moving and, therefore, the species which generates and maintains the potential.

The most familiar ISE is the pH glass electrode. In this device the membrane is a sodium glass which possesses a high exchange rate for H^+. The generated Nernst potential, E, is given by the expression: $E = E_0 + (RT/F)\ \ln\ [H^+]$, where E_0 is a constant for constant temperature, R is the gas constant, F is the Faraday constant, and $[H^+]$ represents the hydrogen ion concentration. The pH is defined as the negative of the $\log[H^+]$; therefore, $\mathrm{pH} = (E_0 - E)(\log e)(F/RT)$. One pH unit change corresponds to a tenfold change in the molar concentration of H^+ and a 59 mV change in the Nernst potential at room temperature. There are many other ISEs that are commercially available. They have the same type of response, but are sensitive to a different ion, depending on the membrane material. Some ISEs employ ionophores trapped inside a polymeric membrane to achieve selectivity. An ionophore is a molecule that selectively and reversibly binds with an ion and thereby creates a high exchange rate across the membrane that contains it for that particular ion.

The typical ISE consists of a glass or plastic tube with the ion-selective membrane closing that end of the tube which is immersed into the solution to be measured. The Nernst potential is measured by making electrical contact to either side of the membrane. This is done by placing a fixed concentration of conductive filling solution inside the tube and placing a wire into the solution. The other side of the membrane is contacted by a reference electrode placed inside the same solution under test. The reference electrode is constructed in the same manner as the ISE but it has a porous membrane which creates a liquid junction between its inner filling solution and the test solution. The liquid junction is designed to have a potential which is invariant with changes in concentration of any ion in the test solution. The reference electrode, solution under test, and the ISE form an electrochemical cell. The reference electrode potential acts like the ground reference in electric circuits, and the ISE potential is measured between the two wires emerging from the respective two electrodes. The details of the mechanisms of transduction in ISEs are beyond the scope of this chapter. The reader is referred to the texts by Bard and Faulkner (1980) and Janata (1989).

Gas Chromatograph

Molecules in gases have thermal conductivities which are dependent on their masses; therefore, a pure gas can be identified by its thermal conductivity. One way to determine the composition of a gas is to first separate it into its components and then measure the thermal conductivity of each. A gas chromatograph does exactly that. In a gas-solid chromatograph, the gas flows through a long narrow column which is packed with an adsorbant solid wherein the gases are separated according to the retentive properties of the packing material for each gas. As the individual gases exit the end of the tube one at a time, they flow over a heated wire. The amount of heat transferred to the gas depends on its thermal conductivity. The gas temperature is measured at a short distance downstream and compared to a known gas flowing in a separate sensing tube. The temperature of the gas is related to the amount of heat transferred and can be used to derive the thermal conductivity according to thermodynamic theory and empirical data. This sensor requires two transduction steps: a chemical to thermal energy transduction followed by a thermal to electrical energy transduction to produce an electrical output signal.

Biosensors

Biological measurands are biologically produced substances, such as antibodies, glucose, hormones, and enzymes. Biosensors are not the same as biomedical sensors, which are any sensors used in biomedical applications, such as blood pressure sensors or electrocardiogram electrodes. Hence, although many biosensors are biomedical sensors, not all biomedical sensors are biosensors. Table 1.1 does not include biological signals as a primary signal because they can be generally classified as either biochemical or physical in nature. Biosensors are of special interest because of the very high selectivity of biological reactions and binding. However, the detection of that reaction or binding is often elusive. A very familiar commercial biosensor is the in-home, early pregnancy test, which detects the presence of human growth factor in urine. That device is a nonelectrical sensor since the output is a color change which our eye senses. In fact, most biosensors require multiple transduction mechanisms to arrive at an electrical output signal. Two examples as given below are an immunosensor and an enzyme sensor. Rather than examining a specific species, the examples describe a general type of sensor and transduction mechanism, since the same principles can be applied to a very large number of biological species of the same type.

Immunosensor

Commercial techniques for detecting antibody–antigen binding generally utilize optical or x-radiation detection. An optically fluorescent molecule or radioisotope is nonspecifically attached to the species of interest in solution. The complementary binding species is chemically attached to a substrate or beads which are packed into a column. The tagged solution containing the species of interest, say the antibody, is passed over the antigen-coated surface, where the two selectively bind. After the specific binding occurs, the unbound fluorescent molecules or radioisotopes are washed away, and the antibody concentration is determined by fluorescence spectroscopy or with a scintillation counter, respectively. These sensing techniques can be quite costly and bulky, and therefore other biosensing mechanisms are rapidly being developed. One experimental technique uses the change in the mechanical properties of the bound antibody–antigen complex in comparison to an unbound surface layer of antigen. It uses a shear mode, surface acoustic wave (SAW) device (see Ballentine et al., 1997) to sense this change as a change in the propagation time of the wave between the generating electrodes and the pick-up electrodes some distance away on the same piezoelectric substrate. The substrate surface is coated with the antigen and it is theorized that upon selectively binding with the antibody, this layer stiffens, changing the mechanical properties of the interface and therefore the velocity of the wave. The advantages of this device are that the SAW device produces an electrical signal (a change in oscillation frequency when the device is used in the feedback loop of an oscillator circuit) which is dependent on the amount of bound antibody; it requires only a very small amount of the antigen which can be very costly; the entire device is small, robust and portable; and the detection and readout methods are inexpensive. However, there are numerous problems which currently preclude its widespread, commercial use, specifically a large temperature sensitivity and responses to nonspecific adsorption, i.e., by species other than the desired antibody.

Enzyme Sensor

Enzymes selectively react with a chemical substance to modify it, usually as the first step in a chain of reactions to release energy (metabolism). A well-known example is the selective reaction of glucose oxidase (enzyme) with glucose to produce gluconic acid and peroxide, according to

$$C_6H_{12}O_6 + O_2 \xrightarrow{\text{glucose oxidase}} \text{gluconic acid} + H_2O_2 + 80 \text{ kilojoules heat}$$

An enzymatic reaction can be sensed by measuring the rise in temperature associated with the heat of reaction or by the detection and measurement of reaction by-products. In the glucose example, the reaction can be sensed by measuring the local dissolved peroxide concentration. This is done via an electrochemical analysis technique called amperometry (Bard and Faulkner, 1980). In this method, a potential is placed across two inert metal wire electrodes immersed in the test solution and the current which is generated by the reduction/oxidation reaction of the species of interest is measured. The current is proportional to the concentration of the reducing/oxidizing species. A selective response is obtained if no other available species has a lower redox potential. Because the selectivity of peroxide over oxygen is poor, some glucose sensing schemes employ a second enzyme called catalase which converts peroxide to oxygen and hydroxyl ions. The latter produces a change in the local pH. As described earlier, an ISE can then be used to convert the pH to a measurable voltage. In this latter example, glucose sensing involves two chemical-to-chemical transductions followed by a chemical-to-electrical transduction mechanism.

Microsensors

Microsensors are sensors that are manufactured using integrated circuit fabrication technologies and/or micromachining. Integrated circuits are fabricated using a series of process steps which are done in batch fashion meaning that thousands of circuits are processed together at the same time in the same way. The patterns which define the components of the circuit are photolithographically transferred from a template to a semiconducting substrate using a photosensitive organic coating, called photoresist. The photoresist pattern is then transferred into the substrate or into a solidstate thin film coating through an etching or deposition process. Each template, called a photomask, can contain thousands of identical sets of patterns, with each set representing a circuit. This "batch" method of manufacturing is what makes integrated circuits so reproducible and inexpensive. In addition, photoreduction enables one to make extremely small features, of the order of microns, which is why this collection of process steps is referred to as microfabrication (Madou, 1997). The resulting integrated circuit is contained in only the top few microns of the semiconductor substrate and the submicron thin films on its surface. Hence, integrated circuit technology is said to consist of a set of planar, microfabrication processes. Micromachining refers to the set of processes which produce three-dimensional microstructures using the same photolithographic techniques and batch processing as for integrated circuits. Here, the third dimension refers to the height above the substrate of the deposited layer or the depth into the substrate of an etched structure. Micromachining can produce structures with a third dimension in the range of 1 to 500 microns. The use of microfabrication to manufacture sensors produces the same benefits as it does for circuits: low cost per sensor, small size, and highly reproducible features. It also enables the integration of signal conditioning or compensation circuits and actuators, i.e., entire sensing and control systems, which can dramatically improve sensor performance for very little increase in cost. For these reasons, there has been a great deal of research and development activity in microsensors over the past 30 years.

The first microsensors were integrated circuit components, such as semiconductor resistors and pn-junction diodes. The piezoresistivity of semiconductors and optical sensing by photodiodes were discussed in earlier sections of this chapter. Junction diodes are also used as temperature sensors. When forward-biased with a constant diode current, the resulting diode voltage increases approximately linearly with increasing temperature. The first micromachined microsensor to be commercially produced was the silicon pressure sensor. It was invented in the mid to late 1950s at Bell Labs and commercialized in the 1960s. This device contains a thin, square, silicon diaphragm ($\approx$10 microns thick), which is produced by crystal orientation dependent, chemical etching. The thin diaphragm deforms in response to a pressure difference across it (Figure 1.3). The deformation produces two effects: a position-dependent displacement, which is maximum at the diaphragm center, and position-dependent strain, which is maximum near the diaphragm edge. Both of these effects have been used in microsensors to produce an electrical output which is proportional to differential pressure. The membrane displacement can be sensed capacitively as previously described. Alternatively, the strain can be sensed by placing a piezoresistor, fabricated within the silicon diaphragm, along its edge. This latter type of sensor is called a piezoresistive pressure sensor and is the commercially more common type of pressure microsensor. Engineering of the design and placement of piezoresistors for optimal signal generation in response to pressure is highly developed. Because of their opposite TCRs, both n and p type materials for the piezoresistors are sometimes utilized to achieve temperature compensation of the response. In Figure 1.3, four piezoresistors are shown, one at each edge, which can be connected together in series to create a Wheatstone bridge on-chip.

Pressure microsensors constituted about 5% of the total U.S. consumption of pressure sensors in 1991. Most of them are used in the medical industry as disposables, or in automotive applications, due to their low cost and small, rugged construction. Many other types of microsensors are commercially under development, including accelerometers, mass flow rate sensors, and biosensors.

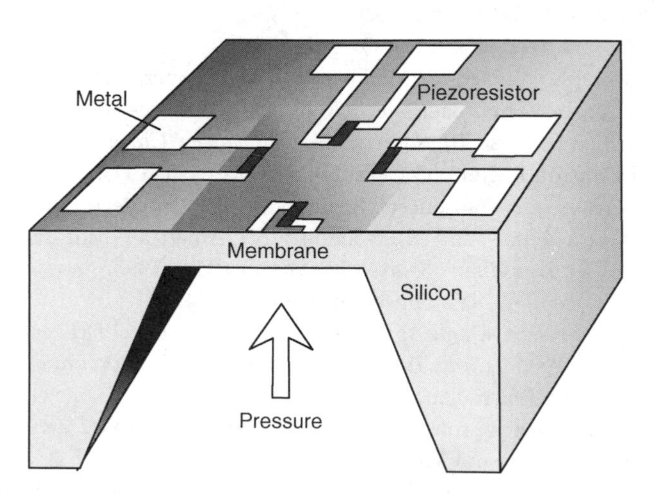

FIGURE 1.3 Schematic cross section of a silicon piezoresistive pressure sensor. A differential pressure deforms the silicon diaphragm, producing strain in the integrated piezoresistors.

Defining Terms

Micromachining: The set of processes that produces three-dimensional microstructures using sequential photolithographic pattern transfer and etching or deposition in a batch processing method.

Microsensor: A sensor that is fabricated using integrated circuit and micromachining technologies.

Repeatability: The ability of a sensor to reproduce output readings for the same value of measurand when applied consecutively and under the same conditions.

Sensitivity: The ratio of the change in sensor output to a change in the value of the measurand.

Sensor: A device that produces a usable output in response to a specified measurand.

Stability: The ability of a sensor to retain its characteristics over a relatively long period of time.

References

ANSI, "Electrical transducer nomenclature and terminology," ANSI Standard MC6.1–1975 (ISA S37.1), Research Triangle Park, NC: Instrument Society of America, 1975.

D.S. Ballentine, Jr. et al., *Acoustic Wave Sensors: Theory, Design, and Physico-Chemical Applications*, San Diego, CA: Academic Press, 1997.

A.J. Bard and L.R. Faulkner, *Electrochemical Methods: Fundamentals and Applications*, New York: John Wiley & Sons, 1980.

R.S.C. Cobbold, *Transducers for Biomedical Measurements: Principles and Applications*, New York: John Wiley & Sons, 1974.

W.Göpel, J. Hesse, and J.N. Zemel, "Sensors: a comprehensive survey," in *Fundamentals and General Aspects*, vol. 1, T. Grandke and W.H. Ko, Eds., Weinheim, Germany: VCH, 1989.

J. Janata, *Principles of Chemical Sensors*, New York: Plenum Press, 1989.

M. Madou, *Fundamentals of Microfabrication*, Boca Raton, FL: CRC Press, 1997.

Further Information

Sensors: W. Gopel, J. Hesse, and J.N. Zemel, Eds., *A Comprehensive Survey*, Weinheim, Germany: VCH, 1989–1994.

Vol. 1: Fundamentals and General Aspects, T. Grandke and W.H. Ko, Eds.

Vol. 2, 3, pt. 1–2: Chemical and Biochemical Sensors, W. Gopel et al., Eds.

Vol. 4: Thermal Sensors, T. Ricolfi and J. Scholz, Eds.

Vol. 5: Magnetic Sensors, R. Boll and K.J. Overshott, Eds.

Vol. 6: Optical Sensors, E. Wagner, R. Dandliker, and K. Spenner, Eds.

Vol. 7: Mechanical Sensors, H.H. Bau, N.F. deRooij, and B. Kloeck, Eds.

J. Carr, *Sensors and Circuits: Sensors, Transducers, and Supporting Circuits for Electronic Instrumentation, Measurement*, and Control, Englewood Cliffs, NJ: Prentice-Hall, 1993.

J.R. Carstens, Electrical Sensors and Transducers, Englewood Cliffs, NJ: Regents/Prentice-Hall, 1993.

J. Fraden, *Handbook of Modern Sensors*, 2nd ed., Woodbury, NY: American Institute of Physics Press, 1996.

G.T.A. Kovacs, *Micromachined Transducers Sourcebook*, McGraw Hill, 1998.

S.M. Sze, Ed., *Semiconductor Sensors*, NY: John Wiley & Sons, 1994.

D. Tandeske, *Pressure Sensors: Selection and Application*, New York: Marcel Dekker, 1991.

M.J. Usher and D.A. Keating, *Sensors and Transducers: Characteristics, Applications, Instrumentation, Interfacing*, 2nd ed., New York: Macmillan, 1996.

Sensors and Actuators is a technical journal, published bimonthly by Elsevier Press in two volumes: Vol. A: *Physical Sensors and Actuators*, and Vol. B: *Chemical Sensors*.

The International Conference on Solid-State Sensors and Actuators is held every two years, hosted in rotation by the U.S., Japan, and Europe. It is sponsored in part by IEEE in the U.S. and a digest of technical papers is published and available through IEEE.

1.2 Electrochemical Sensors

Bryan Stewart Hobbs

Introduction

Electrochemical sensors possess many attractive features which have led to their adoption over a wide range of applications for detecting and monitoring chemical species, "analytes," in both the gas and liquid phases. They are generally available as small, compact, relatively low cost devices, mechanically robust, simple, and reliable in operation.

A great advantage of electrochemical sensors is that they can operate in ambient temperatures between about $-50°C$ and $+50°C$, without the need for any external heating. Consequently, their power requirements can be extremely low; some are completely self-powered, additional power only being required for such extra-sensor functions as alarms, data recording, and transmission, etc. In this respect, electrochemical sensors are ideally suited to portable instruments where battery power, size, and cost are important considerations. Only where it is not possible to obtain a satisfactory electrochemical response are cheaper, solid-state, semiconductor or pellistor devices used instead, for example, in hydrocarbon gas detection.

In fixed instrument applications, where power requirements are a less important criterion, electrochemical sensors occupy an intermediate position between the comparatively cheaper, but less selective and repeatable, semiconductor devices and the more sophisticated and complex analytical techniques of optical and mass spectrometry, chromatography, etc.

Electrochemical sensors divide into two broad categories: "potentiometric" types, producing a voltage response to an analyte, and "amperometric" sensors, which give an electrical current response. Both sensor types comprise at least two electrodes, separated by an intervening body of an ionically conducting liquid or solid electrolyte.

In the majority of electrochemical sensors, the electrolytes used are aqueous solutions of salts, acids, or bases, and operate at room temperature. However, some specialized products utilize nonaqueous electrolytes and/or are operated at elevated temperatures. Examples of the latter include solid ceramic electrolyte sensors based on zirconia which work in environments of several hundreds of degrees centigrade, such as automotive exhausts and combustion stacks [1]. When operated in normal ambient temperatures, these sensors require heating via external power supplies, as do semiconductor devices such as the stannic oxide gas sensor.

Potentiometric Sensors

In its simplest form, a potentiometric sensor comprises two electrodes, separated by an electrolyte. The analyte interacts with one electrode, "the sensing electrode," so as to establish an "equilibrium potential" at the interface between the sensing electrode surface and the electrolyte [2]. A second, "reference electrode," which is unresponsive to the analyte, establishes a fixed potential with respect to the electrolyte, enabling the sensing electrode potential to be measured by means of an external voltmeter [3]. Potentiometric measurements are made under conditions where practically no current flows and voltage measuring circuitry of very high input impedance is used [4,5].

The voltage output of a potentiometric sensor varies logarithmically with the analyte concentration according to the so-called Nernst equation [6] which has the general form:

$$E = E^{\circ} + \text{constant} \ln [C] \tag{1.1}$$

where E is the measured voltage from the sensor, E^{o} is the cell voltage under standard conditions [7], and C is the analyte concentration.

For gases, either in the dissolved or gaseous states, the C term in Equation (1.1) becomes the partial pressure of the gas.

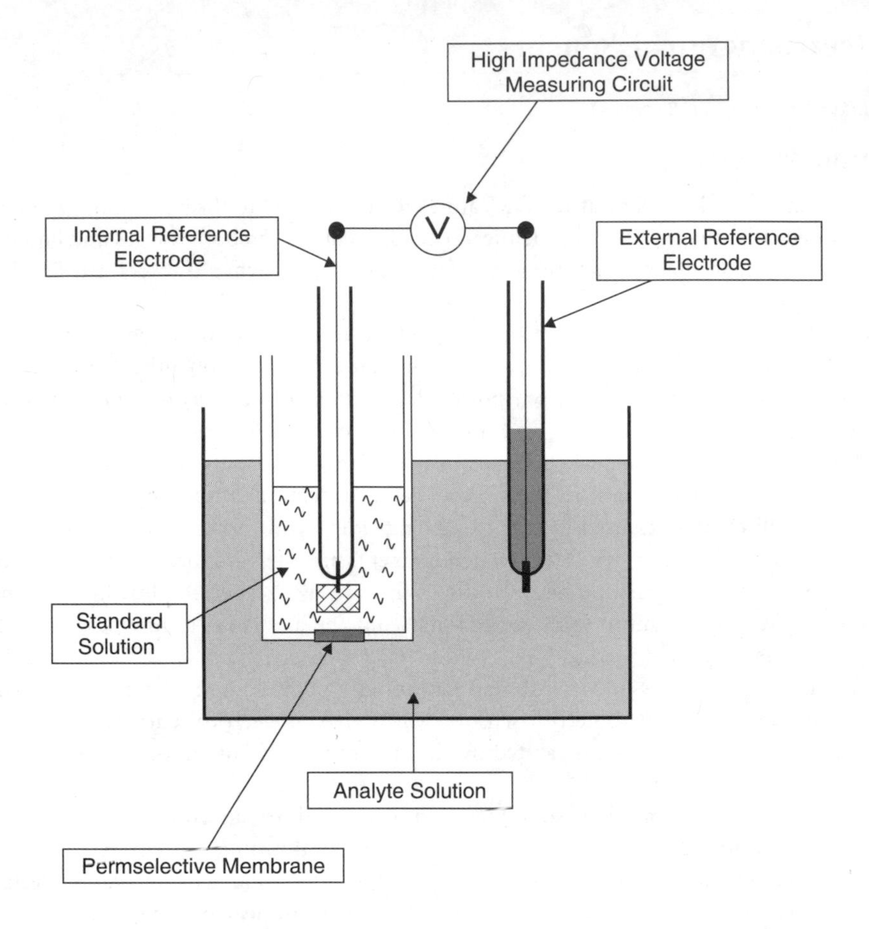

FIGURE 1.4 Schematic representation of the basic construction of an ion-specific electrode arrangement.

Sensing electrodes take a variety of forms; some comprise simple metallic surfaces such as a noble metal (e.g., Pt) wire or foil. A common feature in present day sensors is the use of a perm-selective membrane, located between the sensing and reference electrodes [8–10]. The membrane exchanges ions with the analyte to form a potential, the Donnan potential, which is related to the analyte concentration in much the same way as other electrode potentials. The specific ion incorporated by the membrane, and thereby measured, depends on the nature of the membrane material which can take many forms, for example, glasses, polymers, ion-exchange resins, and suchlike. A schematic representation of the basic construction of an ion-specific electrode (ISE) is depicted in Figure 1.4.

One of the earliest, and probably the most familiar, membrane electrode is the glass electrode, used to measure pH [11]. The Severinghaus electrode, based on the glass electrode is used to measure carbon dioxide in blood and other biological fluids [12]. Membrane sensors find particular application in measuring biological analytes [10,13,14] for which a greater variety of material choice exists.

Potentiometric sensors are ideally suited to liquid phase measurements; with suitable design and choice of materials, they can be highly specific to the analyte. However, their reliance on the establishment of reversible potentials from electrochemical reactions in equilibrium renders them unsuitable for sensing chemical species which react irreversibly, for example, oxygen and carbon monoxide. At elevated temperatures the reaction kinetics of these analytes can become fast enough to produce a reversible electrode potential and for example, oxygen is routinely measured potentiometrically with high temperature devices, based on zirconia electrolyte [1]. Generally, however, amperometric sensors are employed for species which react irreversibly.

Amperometric Sensors

The amperometric principle can be described in terms of an oxygen sensor by way of example. The cell's basic elements comprise at least two electrodes with an intervening body of electrolyte, as for potentiometric devices. The sensing electrode is made from materials (electrocatalysts) that support the electrochemical reduction of oxygen, represented by the equation:

$$O_2 + 2H_2O + 4e = 4OH^- \tag{1.2}$$

Typical materials would be silver, gold, or platinized graphite on a porous PTFE membrane, either as metallized films or in hydrophobic, gas diffusion, fuel cell electrodes.

The standard reversible potential of this reaction (E°) is 1.229 V at 20°C on the hydrogen scale. However, due to the irreversible nature of this reaction, even on very active catalysts such as platinum, observed rest potentials of oxygen electrodes are generally nearer to a volt. Any attempt to draw current from these electrodes results in sharp polarization of the measured electrode potential, resulting in even lower values.

The counter electrode comprises an anode of a readily corrodible metal such as lead. Lead reacts with hydroxyl ions (OH^-) migrating from the oxygen cathode reaction through the electrolyte and releases electrons which flow through the external circuit to feed the oxygen reaction:

$$2Pb + 4OH^- = 2PbO + 2H_2O + 4e \tag{1.3}$$

The overall reaction of this metal–air battery cell is given by

$$2Pb + O_2 = PbO + \text{current} \tag{1.4}$$

A large anode surface area, relative to the oxygen cathode, coupled with a low impedance external electrical circuit connecting the two electrodes, ensures that the lead remains essentially unpolarized and "holds" the cathode at the lead potential where the oxygen reduction reaction takes place at a high rate.

This electrochemical power source is converted to a sensor by the inclusion of a diffusion barrier between the sensing electrode and its access to the external environment. The barrier restriction is designed to ensure that the cell operates in the "diffusion controlled, limiting current condition" [15] as illustrated in Figure 1.5 and Figure 1.6.

Operated in this condition, all the oxygen diffusing to the sensing electrode from the external environment reacts as it arrives at the cathode. The oxygen partial pressure at the cathode will be near zero and the concentration gradient across the barrier will be equal to the external oxygen partial pressure p_{O2}. From Fick's first law of diffusion, it follows that the measured limiting current from the cell, I_L will be directly proportional to the oxygen partial pressure in the external environment [15]:

$$I_L = \text{constant}(p_{O2}) \tag{1.5}$$

The nature of the diffusion barrier exerts considerable influence on the sensor characteristics. Early examples of oxygen sensor, developed by Clark [16,17], employed metallized solid polymer membranes (typically, PTFE). The gas transport mechanism through these membranes, involving a process of gas dissolution and diffusion in the solid state, has an inherently high exponential temperature coefficient of about 2% to 3% per °C and temperature compensation is essential. Sensor outputs with these membranes are linear with p_{O2}.

Tantram et al. [15] developed an oxygen sensor based on a porous diffusion barrier, the simplest form consisting of a single capillary orifice. The gas transport mechanism through porous barriers involves the physical process of gas-phase diffusion which results in a cell limiting current governed by the following form

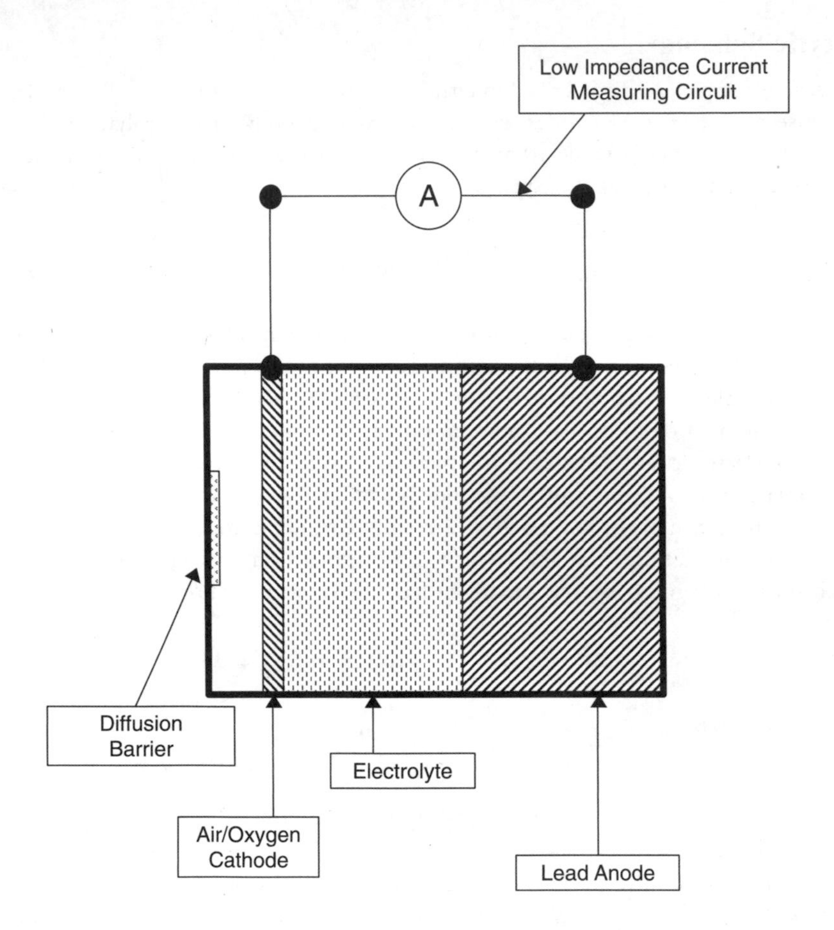

FIGURE 1.5 Schematic diagram of an oxygen–lead electrochemical sensor.

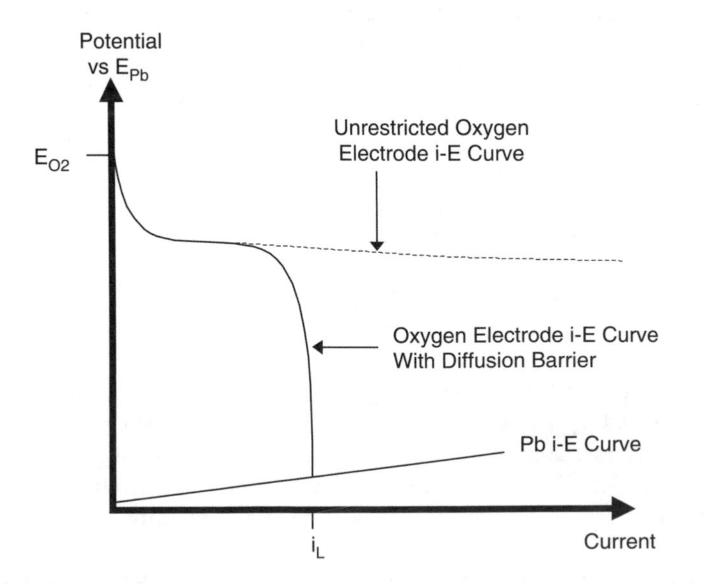

FIGURE 1.6 Schematic depiction of oxygen cathode and lead anode current–potential curves, with and without diffusion barrier.

of equation

$$I_L = \text{constant}.(T^{0.5}).P^{-1}.p_{O2} \tag{1.6}$$

where T is the absolute temperature (K) and P is the total pressure.

The square-root temperature dependence gives coefficient values of about 0.2% per °C, about one tenth that of solid membranes, which considerably reduces the compensation requirements.

The current output is a function of p_{O2}/P, the volume fraction of the gas, rather than the partial pressure. This provides a signal which is essentially independent of ambient barometric pressure, which is a preferred characteristic with most gas-phase measurement applications.

Because of bulk flow effects, porous barriers become increasingly nonlinear with increasing gas concentration [18]. Up to about 20% oxygen, a small secondary correction may be applied to linearize the output and below a few percent gas analyte, the output is essentially linear.

Sensor life, regardless of diffusion barrier type, will ultimately be determined by the current and the amount of lead used in these Pb/O_2cells. Commercially available cells are capable of two or more years of life in air (21% oxygen), weigh only a few grams and are about the size of a small alkaline battery cell.

The basic amperometric principle described for oxygen has been adapted to provide sensors for measuring the concentrations of a range of toxic gases such as CO, H_2S, NO, NO_2, SO_2, and Cl_2 [19]. Many of these gases undergo an electrochemical oxidation at the sensing electrode and an oxygen reducing counter electrode is used; for example, the electrode reactions for a CO sensor are as follows:

$$\text{sensing electrode (CO oxidation)} \quad 2CO + 2H_2O = 2CO_2 + 4H^+ + 4e \tag{1.7}$$

$$\text{counter electrode (O}_2\text{ reduction)} \quad O_2 + 4H^+ + 4e = 2H_2O \tag{1.8}$$

$$\text{cell reaction} \quad 2CO + O_2 = 2CO_2 + \text{current} \tag{1.9}$$

The oxygen supply comes from the external environment and such cells operate as self-powered fuel cells. There are no life-limiting, consumable elements in these toxic gas sensors, in contrast to lead anode in the Pb/O_2 oxygen sensor.

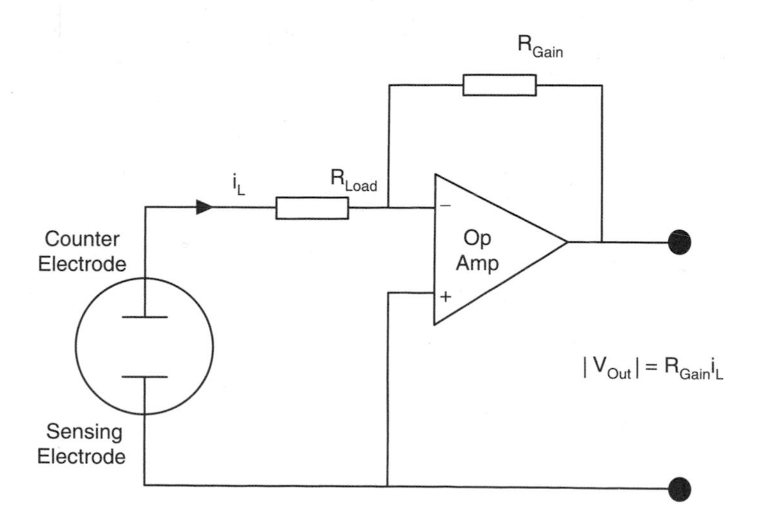

FIGURE 1.7 Two-electrode circuit for an amperometric gas sensor.

Measurement of the current from a two-electrode amperometric sensor can be accomplished by simply measuring the voltage across a low value resistor connecting the electrodes. Alternatively, a potentiostatic circuit can be used, which consumes very little external power and enables the cell to run at an effectively zero load resistance [4,20] (Figure 1.7). This circuit yields a faster response and reduces polarization effects from the oxygen counter electrode in toxic gas sensors which tend to destabilize the signal.

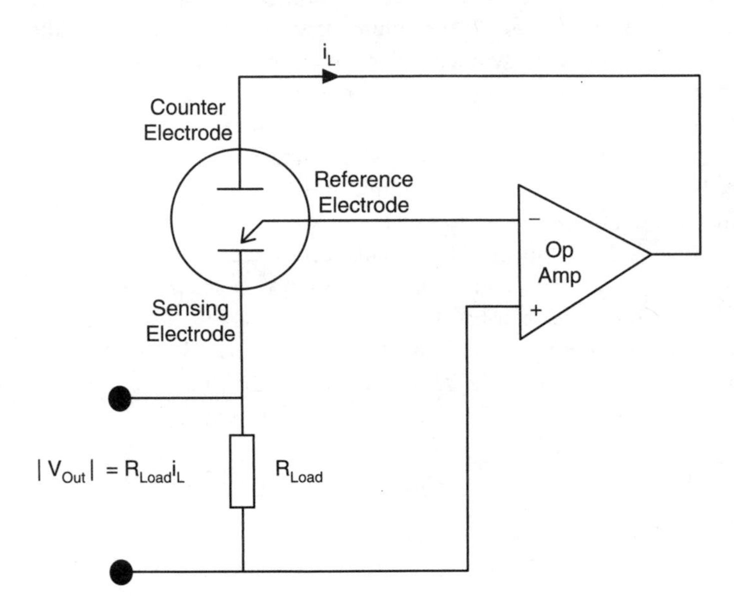

FIGURE 1.8 Three-electrode circuit/zero bias.

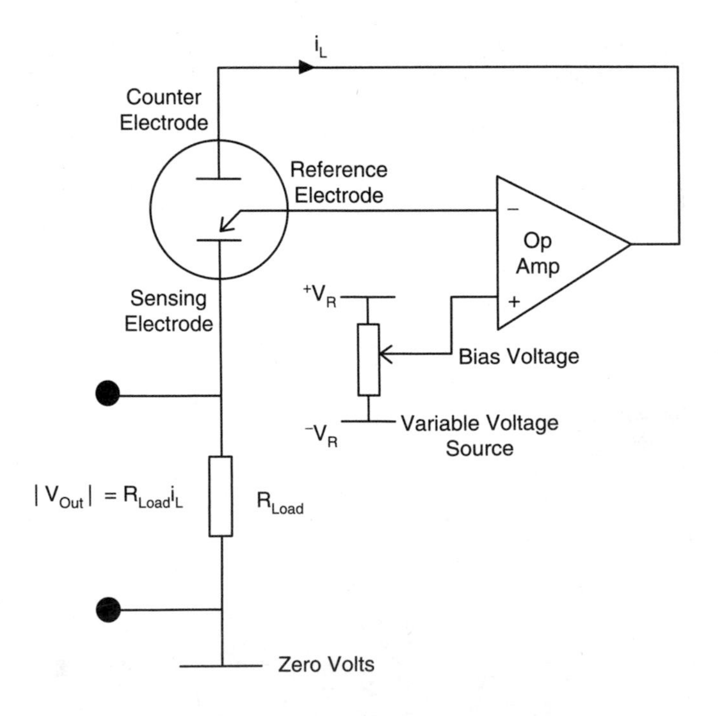

FIGURE 1.9 Biased three-electrode circuit.

Most toxic sensors are operated with a third, reference electrode and an external three-electrode potentiostatic circuit (Figure 1.8). The reference electrode is normally formed by an additional, oxygen-responsive counter electrode from which no current is drawn. The potentiostat in Figure 1.8 operates to "hold" the sensing electrode at the reference electrode potential. The cell current, passing between counter and sensing electrodes, is measured in the amplifier feedback loop to eliminate completely all polarization effects within the cell [4,5,20].

Three-electrode circuits also allow the possibility of "biasing" the sensing electrode operating potential with respect to the reference electrode as depicted in Figure 1.9, thus giving more flexibility in choosing optimal operating potentials for the analyte and/or suppressing cross interfering gas reactions [20].

References

1. W.C. Maskell, *Techniques and Mechanisms in Gas Sensing*, P.T. Moseley, J.O.W. Norris, D.E. Williams, Eds., IOP Publishing, 1991, pp. 1–42.
2. C.W. Davies and A.M. James, *A Dictionary of Electrochemistry*, New York: Macmillan Press, 1976, pp. 86–89 (see also pp. 92–96).
3. D.J.G. Ives and G.J. Janz, *Reference Electrodes, Theory and Practice*, London: Academic Press, 1961.
4. D.T. Sawyer and J.L. Roberts, *Experimental Electrochemistry for Chemists*, New York: Wiley, 1974, Chap. 5.
5. M.J.D. Brand and B. Fleet, "Operational amplifiers in chemical instrumentation," *Chem. Br.*, vol. 5, no. 12, pp. 557–562, 1969.
6. C.W. Davies and A.M. James, *A Dictionary of Electrochemistry*, New York: Macmillan Press, 1976, p. 168.
7. C.W. Davies and A.M. James, *A Dictionary of Electrochemistry*, New York: Macmillan Press, 1976, p. 87.
8. C.W. Davies and A.M. James, *A Dictionary of Electrochemistry*, New York: Macmillan Press, 1976, pp. 150–153.
9. M.J. Madou and S.R. Morrison, *Chemical Sensing with Solid State Devices*, London: Academic Press, 1989, Chap. 6.
10. D.J.G. Ives and G.J. Janz, *Reference Electrodes, Theory and Practice*, London: Academic Press, 1961, Chap. 9.
11. D.J.G. Ives and G.J. Janz, *Reference Electrodes, Theory and Practice*, London: Academic Press, 1961, Chap. 5.
12. D.J.G. Ives and G.J. Janz, *Reference Electrodes, Theory and Practice*, London: Academic Press, 1961, pp. 497–501.
13. D.J.G. Ives and G.J. Janz, *Reference Electrodes, Theory and Practice*, London: Academic Press, 1961, Chap. 11.
14. A.P.F. Turner, I. Karube and G.S. Wilson, Eds., *Biosensors, Fundamentals and Applications*, Oxford: Oxford University Press, 1987.
15. A.D.S. Tantram, M.J. Kent, and A.G. Palmer, U.K. Patent 1571282, 1977.
16. D.T. Sawyer and J.L. Roberts, *Experimental Electrochemistry for Chemists*, New York: Wiley, 1974, pp. 383–384.
17. L.C. Clark Jr., *Trans. Am. Soc. Artif. Intern. Organs*, 2, 41, 1956.
18. B.S. Hobbs, A.D.S. Tantram, and R. Chan-Henry, *Techniques and Mechanisms in Gas Sensing*, P.T. Moseley, J.O.W. Norris, and D.E. Williams, Eds., IOP Publishing, 1991, pp. 171–172.
19. A.D.S. Tantram, J.R. Finbow, Y.S. Chan, and B.S. Hobbs, U.K. Patent 2094005, 1982.
20. B.S. Hobbs, A.D.S. Tantram, and R. Chan-Henry; *Techniques and Mechanisms in Gas Sensing*, P.T. Moseley, J.O.W. Norris, and D.E. Williams, Eds., IOP Publishing, 1991, pp. 180–183.

1.3 The Stannic Oxide Semiconductor Gas Sensor

Joseph Watson

Introduction

There are numerous different methods of gas detection using transduction methods from mechanical through chemical to optical. For example, in the very common case of carbon dioxide detection, infrared optical techniques remain the most satisfactory because of the comparative nonreactivity of that gas. There are also complex methods such as gas chromatography for the measurement of very low gas concentrations. However, for more reactive gases in concentrations from one to several thousand parts per million, simpler methods are widespread, and electrochemical and solid-state techniques are the two most commonly employed. Crudely put, electrochemical sensors tend to provide better selectivity and repeatability, thus making them suitable as monitoring instruments, while solid-state devices are cheaper, long-lived, and thus better suited to alarm systems. However, for portable applications, solid-state devices have limited application because they require heating, which sometimes involves unacceptable battery drain.

There are actually many types of gas sensors that can be described as "solid-state", the smaller and apparently simpler of which include the catalytic Pellistor and the various polymer sensors found largely in some "electronic nose" instruments. However, the stannic oxide (i.e., tin dioxide, or SnO_2) sensor has become the most common by far, and its chemistry is reasonably well established [1], though the actual mechanisms by which dopants (implying the inclusion of centres of catalysis) operate are less clear. Furthermore, the electrical performance of the sensors is markedly affected by their physical configurations and operating conditions and indeed by the nature of the substrates upon which the active material is deposited.

The basic SnO_2 gas sensor is deceptively simple and consists essentially of an insulating substrate with a pair of electrode metalizations on one side and a heater on the other. Gas-sensitive stannic oxide in its hard ceramic form is deposited across the electrodes and is heated via the substrate to a temperature appropriate for operation, at which its resistance reaches an equilibrium value. A fall in this resistance occurs on the arrival of any reducing gas and is measured by an associated electronic circuit, subsequently operating an alarm or displaying the concentration of that gas. There are many variations on this constructional theme, including the tubular configuration and housing adopted by Figaro Inc. of Japan, as shown in Figure 1.10. More recent sensors are on very small substrates that allow the heater to be deposited on the same side of the substrate without severe degradation in the temperature gradient across the substrate chip.

The actual chemical and physical principles underlying the change in resistance of the sensor have been elucidated over many decades and here it will suffice to say that the basic mechanism involves the adsorption of oxygen ion species from the atmosphere until equilibrium is reached at a given temperature. Then, in the presence of a reducing gas, some of the adsorbed oxygen ions combine with that gas, thus releasing electrons that become available for conduction, which lowers the resistance. Though this is a simplistic explanation, it is adequate as background information in the present context.

Basic Electrical Parameters and Operation

If the resistance of a typical tin dioxide gas sensor is plotted against gas concentration, it follows the form of the curve shown in Figure 1.11. The slope of this curve at any point defines the *incremental sensitivity*, $\Delta R_S/\Delta C_G$, which is clearly greatest at low concentrations, and is markedly different from the chord sensitivity $(R_a\text{-}R_S)/C_G$, where R_a is the sensor resistance in clean air. This being so, and considering the shape of the curve, it is more subjectively acceptable to display the sensor conductance, which approaches a straight line over a considerable concentration range. That is, the incremental sensitivity is not so different from the chord sensitivity, as shown in Figure 1.12. Furthermore, only a very simple operational amplifier circuit is needed to perform this measurement, as shown in Figure 1.13. Here, a constant voltage is applied across the active material and the amplifier acts as a current-to-voltage converter, the output voltage being proportional to

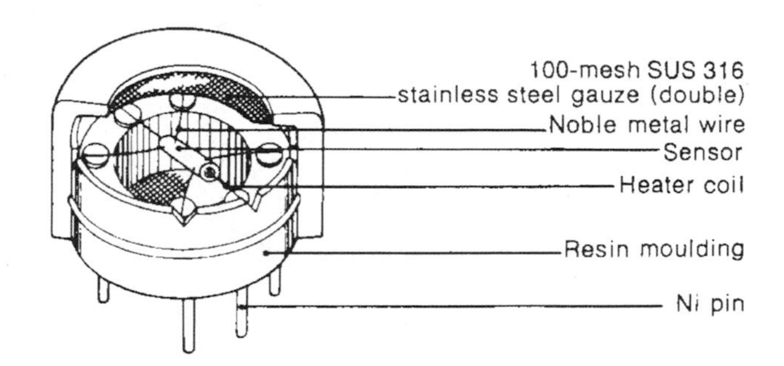

FIGURE 1.10 Figaro gas sensor configuration.

the conductance of the material [2] as follows:

$$V_{out} = -I_F R_F = I_S R_F$$
$$\text{where } I_S = V_S/R_S = V_S G_S$$
$$\text{giving } G_S = V_{out}/V_S R_F$$

However, in current practice, the foregoing fundamental definitions of sensitivity tend not to be used. Instead, a figure-of-merit, also called "sensitivity", has become common. This is actually the resistance ratio R_S/R_a, which obviously has a value of unity in clean air and falls with gas concentration. Furthermore, this "sensitivity" may be defined not only with reference to R_a but also with reference to a particular gas concentration, R_0. For example, the "sensitivity" of a particular sensor may be defined as R_S/R_0 where a comparison of the sensor resistance at "C_G" ppm is compared with that at C_0 ppm of the same gas. Usually, logarithmic plots of such resistance ratios against logarithmic plots of gas concentration are provided by

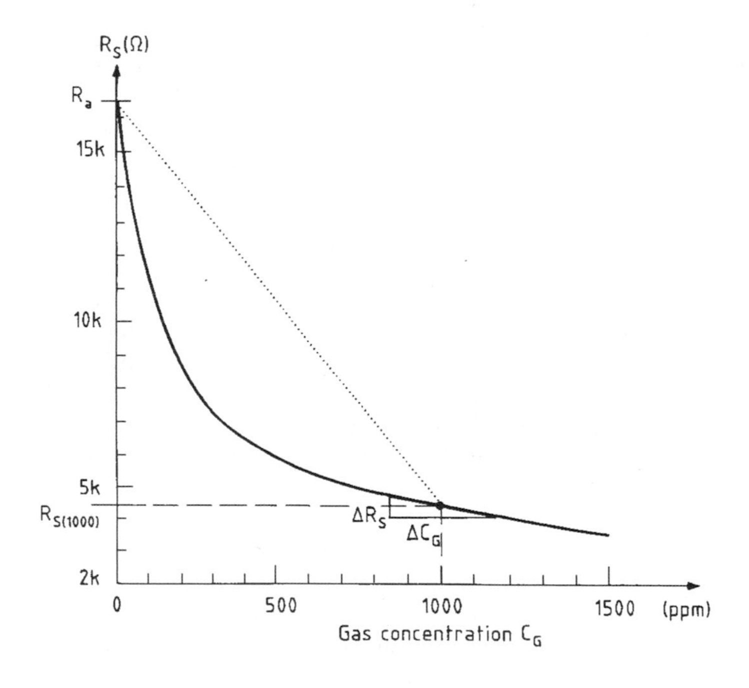

FIGURE 1.11 A typical sensor resistance (R_s) plot vs. gas concentration (C_G).

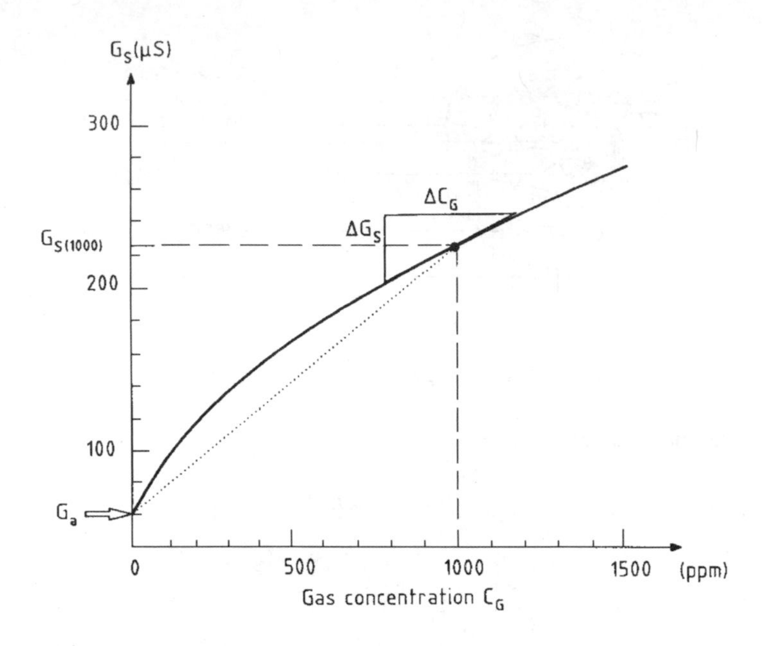

FIGURE 1.12 A typical sensor conductance (G_S) plot vs. gas concentration (C_G).

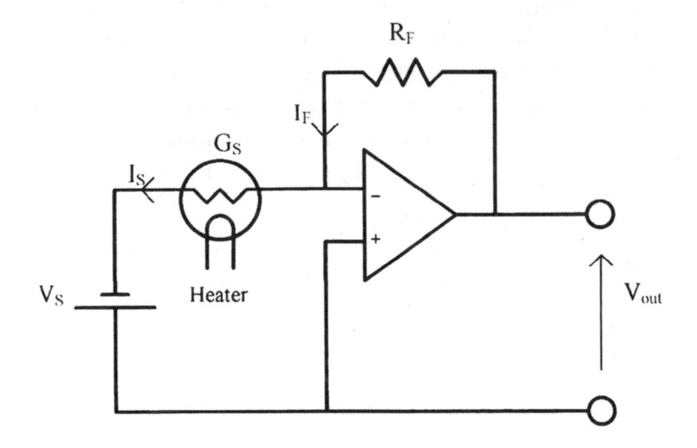

FIGURE 1.13 Circuit for measurement of sensor conductance.

manufacturers and result in fairly straight, downward-sloping lines as exemplified by Figure 1.14. Here, R_0 is the resistance at 250 ppm of carbon monoxide, so that R_S/Rx_0 at that concentration is unity.

This figure shows that the device is sensitive also to hydrogen, though not to methane, as shown by the crosses. In fact, all stannic oxide sensors are sensitive to very many gases, though the carefully monitored inclusion of dopants can succeed in tailoring their responses to achieve considerable degrees of selectivity. In this context, perhaps the most common "nuisance gas" is water vapor and though again there are techniques to minimize this, it remains a major problem for this form of gas sensor.

The circuit shown is the basis of most instruments which utilize the stannic oxide sensor for measurement purposes, though a much simpler configuration can be used for alarm systems. This would consist of a load resistor in series with the sensor so that any change in the resistance of the sensor due to the presence of a detectable gas would change the proportion of the supply voltage appearing across each. This can be detected as an alarm signal. Furthermore, the same supply voltage can be used to energize the heater, thus making for an extremely cheap network.

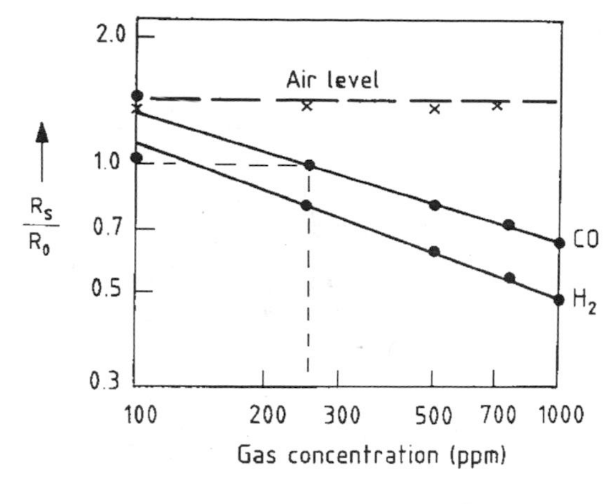

FIGURE 1.14 Resistance ratio plot for a typical sensor.

Operating Temperature

The operating temperature is determined by the heater structure, which consists typically of a metalization pattern on one side of the substrate through which an appropriate current is passed in the manner of a filament lamp. Thus, if a constant voltage is applied, the positive resistance/temperature coefficient typical of metals ensures that the temperature will stabilize, except for any excess rise due to exothermal reactions at the active material surface. (This latter effect actually describes the operation of the purely catalytic Pellistor-type sensor, which involves the measurement of the small resistance change in the heater filament via a bridge circuit, which necessitates an identical, but passive sensor.) Although this mode of operation is adequate for most purposes, negative feedback may be applied via an electronic heater circuit for more stringent operating requirements.

The heater itself poses several problems. First, recognizing that the active material is usually sintered in situ during manufacture, the heater must tolerate the sintering temperatures involved, which can exceed 800°C for some materials. Platinum is the best material to cope with such temperatures, but inevitably incurs high costs. The second problem is that a uniform temperature across the substrate and hence the active material is difficult to achieve with a patterned heater metalization. Considerable work has been performed in this area and, as is seen in Figure 1.10, Figaro Engineering Inc. has developed a tubular structure with a heater filament in the center and the active material deposited on the outside. This is an example of good geometric design leading to a low temperature gradient. Both Figaro and Capteur Sensors and Analysers Ltd. (now City Technology Ltd.) of the U.K. have also used thick-film ruthenium dioxide heaters, which can give rise to very flat temperature gradients using small alumina tile topology.

The need for uniform temperature is illustrated by Figure 1.15, which is a plot from a seminal paper by Firth et al. [3] showing sensitivity (in this case measured as R_a/R_{1000}) vs. temperature for two gases. Here, the sensitivity is clearly a marked function of the sensor operating temperature, which means that unless this temperature is held within narrow limits, the sensitivity will vary considerably. Furthermore, unless the temperature gradient is small, different parts of the active material will exhibit different sensitivities, which raises a second point. If some degree of selectivity is desired, for example a measurement of CO concentration in the presence of CH_4, this can clearly be achieved by maintaining the operating temperature at a point shown by the vertical dashed line, that is, at about 300°C. Here, the sensitivity to CH_4 is negligible, but should the operating temperature vary across the active material, parts of that material may be at temperatures where the sensitivity to CH_4 is significant, so that the desired level of selectivity is lost.

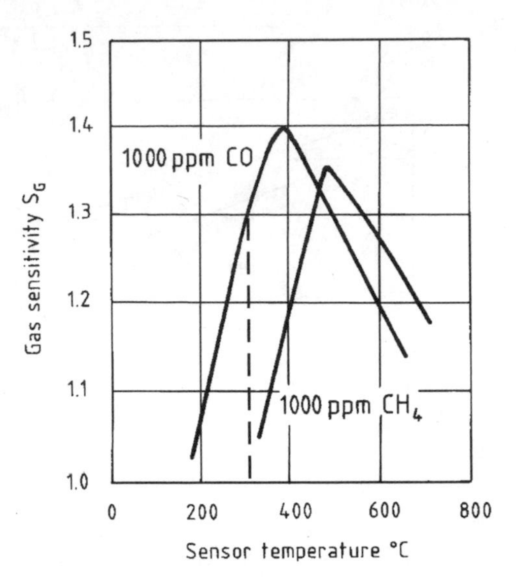

FIGURE 1.15 The effect of sensor temperature on the gas sensitivity of a tin dioxide sensor. (After Firth et al. [3].)

Substrate Materials

Alumina in ceramic form is very heat stable and is an electrical insulator, which are good reasons for its use as a substrate. However, it is also a good thermal insulator, which is unfortunate in that it helps to maintain the undesirable thermal gradients described above. A better material would exhibit the same electrically insulating properties but would also be a good thermal conductor, which would help to minimize temperature variations. Several such materials exist [4], the best being beryllia (Be_2O_3). Although the processing of beryllia requires specialist procedures, beryllium being highly toxic, firms such as CBL Ceramics Ltd. in the U.K. already produce beryllia forms for many other purposes and have engaged in work on gas sensor substrates, for which patents have been filed.

In addition to the maintenance of a constant operating temperature and a flat temperature gradient, the question of heater power consumption arises, especially where battery operation is desired [5]; this suggests that the size of the sensor should be reduced and, concomitantly, the heat loss. However, this implies that the thermal capacity will also be small, which in turn means that even low-velocity air flows will cool the sensor significantly unless quite sophisticated electronics are used to maintain the proper operating temperature. Such problems have been addressed and, for example, in addition to their tubular structure, Figaro Engineering Inc. has produced a range of substrates little more than 1 mm^2 carrying very small active material depositions and using ruthenium dioxide thick-film heater structures insulated from the active material proper. Although an alumina substrate is used, its small size and the thick-film ruthenium dioxide heater make for a very uniform temperature distribution. When this sensor is operated using a pulse-train technique (described below), the total power consumption can be less than 60 mW. Interestingly, the major source of heat loss from small structures like this occurs via the electrical leads rather than from convection or radiation.

A radical departure from traditional substrate materials is found in the use of micromachined silicon [6,7], and though considerable work has been performed on this technique, commercial sensors have yet to achieve acceptance. Here, the active element is deposited on a silicon dioxide layer, which itself is deposited on a silicon membrane, the latter being small and thin to minimize heat loss via conduction. The heater can be amorphous silicon embedded inside the SiO_2 layer so that its life is not compromised by evaporation. The concatenation of somewhat mutually exclusive fabrication techniques has so far precluded mass production at prices competitive with alumina-substrate-based sensors.

Electrical Operating Parameters

In addition to new departures in substrate materials and geometry, there are various methods of electrical control and measurement, usually involving pulsed as opposed to continuous operation [8]. There are several reasons for this, as follows.

The first is a requirement for low power consumption, thereby making battery operation more feasible. If a sensor is sufficiently small — that is, it has a very low thermal capacity — it may be driven up to its optimum operating temperature within a few milliseconds. So, keeping in mind that contaminant gas concentrations do not change significantly in so short a time, the sensor can be operated intermittently instead of continuously. A case in point is that of the Figaro type 2440, which has a very small structure. This sensor is operated by applying a 5 V heater supply for 14 msec followed by a "resting" period of 236 msec that is, a duty cycle of nearly 1:18. This results in an average power consumption lower than 60 mW. During every fourth "resting" period, the active material is interrogated by a 5 V pulse lasting some 5 msec. That is, the read-out is updated on a one-second basis, which is much less than the time taken for an atmospheric carbon monoxide concentration to change significantly.

Second, if the optimum operating temperature of a sensor is low — typically about 100°C for CO-selective types — water vapor and trace concentrations of pollutant gases in the atmosphere can temporarily poison that sensor. However, if the temperature is increased to well above the operating level, such contaminants can usually be removed — a process known as "purging". So, one method of operation is to sequentially heat the sensor to a high temperature for this purpose, allow it to cool to its optimum operating temperature, then to make an electrical measurement. The Figaro TGS 2440 again affords an example of this. The 14 msec heating pulse is actually long enough to bring the temperature to more than 300°C and this falls to the optimum measuring temperature some 150 msec later, which is when the interrogation pulse arrives. It should be noted that for this mode of operation, materials must be selected very carefully for the various parts of the sensor structure because the whole assembly must withstand a continuing sequence of thermal shocks over many years without damage.

Third, a comparatively new *modus operandi* involves the measurement of conductance rise-times upon application of the polarizing voltage across the active material. In this method, the sensor is maintained at the optimum operating temperature and a fast rise-time polarizing voltage is applied. The resulting active material conductance change has been shown to be dependent upon the gas concentration. Furthermore, there is evidence that the rise-times may also provide gas recognition information [9].

Future Developments

Considerable progress in the chemistry and physics of the active material is currently ongoing. A good illustration is the use of nano-particles along with pulsed-operation techniques [10]. The use of stannic oxide sensors in arrays with each member having different characteristics has also received attention in the context of "electronic nose" technology [11,12]. Here, sophisticated computer techniques have been used to derive both qualitative and quantitative information about mixtures of gases using sensors that have overlapping selectivity and sensitivity characteristics. It has therefore become clear that although the stannic oxide gas sensor has achieved prominence in mass-produced and inexpensive devices such as domestic gas alarms, it is a viable sensor for measurement and monitoring instruments and has by no means reached the limit of its capabilities.

References

1. K. Ihokura and J. Watson, *The Stannic Oxide Gas Sensor*, Boca Raton, FL: CRC Press, 1994.
2. J. Watson, "A note on the characterisation of gas sensors," *Sens. Actuators*, B8, 173–177, 1992.
3. J.G. Firth, A. Jones, and T.A. Jones, "Solid-state detectors for carbon monoxide," *Ann. Occup. Hyg.* 18, 63–68, 1975.
4. M.P. Elwin, G.S.V. Coles, and J. Watson, "New substrates for thick and thin film gas sensors," *Sens. Appl. Conf. VII*, 37–42, 1996.

5. D.M. Wilson, S. Hoyt, J. Janata, K. Booksh, and L. Ohando, "Chemical sensors for portable handheld instruments," *IEEE Sens. J.*, vol. 1, no. 4, pp. 256–273, 2001.
6. D. Mutschall, C. Scheibe and E. Obermeier, "Basic micromodule for chemical sensors with on-chip heater and buried sensor structure," *8th Int. Conf. Solid-state Sens. Actuators Eurosensors IX*, Stockholm, 1995.
7. G.G. Mandayo, E. Castano and F.J. Gracia, "Carbon monoxide detector fabricated on the basis of a tin oxide novel doping method," *IEEE Sens. J.*, vol. 2, no. 4, pp. 322–328, 2002.
8. T. Amamoto, Tamaguchi, Y. Matsuura and Y. Kajiyama, "Development of pulse-drive semiconductor gas sensor," *Sens. Actuators*, B13/14, 587–588, 1993.
9. E. Llobet, X. Vilanova, J. Brezmes, J.E. Sueiras, and X. Correig, "Transient response of thick film tin oxide gas sensors to multicomponent gas mixtures," *Sens. Actuators B*, vol. 47, no. 1-3, pp. 104–112, 1998.
10. T.K.H. Starke and G.S.V. Coles, "Reduced response times using adsorption kinetics and pulsed-mode operation for the detection of oxides of nitrogen with nanocrystalline SnO_2 sensors," *IEEE Sens. J.*, vol. 3, no. 4, pp. 447–453, 2003.
11. I. Sagayo, Md. C. Horvillo, S. Baluk, M. Alexandre, M.J. Fernandez, L. Ares, M. Garcia, J.P. Santos, and J. Gutierrez, "Detection of toxic gases by a tin oxide multisensor," *IEEE Sens. J.*, vol. 2, no. 5, pp. 387–393, 2002.
12. D.S. Lee, D.D. Lee, S.W. Ban, M.H. Lee, and Y.T. Kim, "SnO_2 gas sensing array for combustible and explosive gas leakage recognition," *IEEE Sens. J.* vol. 2, no. 3, pp. 140–149, 2002.

2

An Introduction to Multi-Sensor Data Fusion[1]

David L. Hall
The Pennsylvania State University

James Llinas
State University of New York at Buffalo

2.1 Introduction 2-1
2.2 Data Fusion Techniques 2-3
2.3 Applications of Data Fusion 2-5
2.4 Process Models for Data Fusion 2-7
2.5 Limitations of Data Fusion Systems 2-12
2.6 Summary 2-13

2.1 Introduction

Multi-sensor data fusion involves combining information and data from multiple sources to obtain the most accurate and specific assessment of an observed environment or situation [1–6]. Examples of data fusion applications include monitoring the health of a complex machine [7], use of multiple sources to improve medical diagnosis [8], automated target recognition for military applications [9], and environmental monitoring [10]. Automated data fusion systems seek to emulate the ability of humans and animals to improve their assessment of the external world by integrating information from multiple senses. Techniques for automated data fusion range from signal processing and image processing techniques, to statistical based estimation (e.g., Kalman filters), pattern recognition methods (cluster algorithms and adaptive neural networks), voting, Bayesian and Dempster–Shafer methods, to automated reasoning techniques such as expert systems, fuzzy logic, blackboard systems, and intelligent agents. An overview of these methods is provided by Hall and McMullen [1] and Waltz and Llinas [2]. This chapter provides an introduction to multi-sensor data fusion including the basic concepts, models, and processing architectures, algorithms and techniques, and applications. A brief discussion of the state of the art of data fusion is provided at the end of the chapter.

Data fusion mimics the human cognitive process involving integrating sensory data to understand the external world. Humans receive and process sensory data (sights, sounds, smells, tastes, and touch) that are assessed to draw conclusions about the environment and what it means. The development of data

[1]Note: While this is original material, it is based on a previous introduction to multi-sensor data fusion provided by Hall and Llinas [6] and by Hall and McMullen [1].

fusion techniques is a natural extension to the historical development of sensors to improve our ability to observe the environment. The invention of telescopes, microscopes, acoustic sensors, and other sensor technologies extends our human senses beyond the immediate to the microscopic, macroscopic, and beyond the relatively narrow bandwidth of human vision and hearing. For example, rapid advances in micro-electrical mechanical systems (MEMS) provide the ability to create micro-scale sensors that can be distributed throughout the environment for applications such as smart buildings, surveillance, and monitoring of complex systems [11, 12]. Such technology is being applied to improve human senses, such as the introduction of advanced signal processing in hearing aids [13]. Similarly, data fusion technology extends our ability to *make sense of* the environment. Many of the techniques developed for data fusion seek to emulate the ability of humans (or animals) to perform fusion.

The concept of extended sensing and multisensor data fusion is illustrated in Figure 2.1. Multiple sensors are used to provide surveillance of the Earth (e.g., to monitor crops, weather, or the environment), and these data are input to a fusion system along with information from models, textual data (e.g., reports from databases and human observers), computer-based model information, and semantic information such as syntactical information. The sensor data may include signal data, images, scalar, and vector information. This information is combined using techniques such as signal or image processing, feature extraction and pattern recognition, statistical estimation techniques, and automated reasoning to result in a fused assessment of the observed situation or environment.

The actual techniques by which the fusion may be performed are discussed in the next section of this chapter. A special challenge of data fusion systems is to combine information from heterogeneous sources (e.g., processing signal data, images, and scalar and vector data along with text-based information). In essence, the data fusion system seeks to combine diverse data and to transform that data into knowledge suitable for use by a human-in-the-loop decision maker. Because of this heterogeneity of input data, in general a single algorithm is unable to perform the functions desired. A number of different techniques are required from diverse disciplines such as signal and image processing, pattern recognition, statistical estimation, optimization, and automated reasoning/artificial intelligence. Continuing challenges in data fusion are to determine which algorithms are suitable for a given set of data, how to use these algorithms in concert for effective information fusion, and how to represent and propagate the uncertainty associated with the information sources.

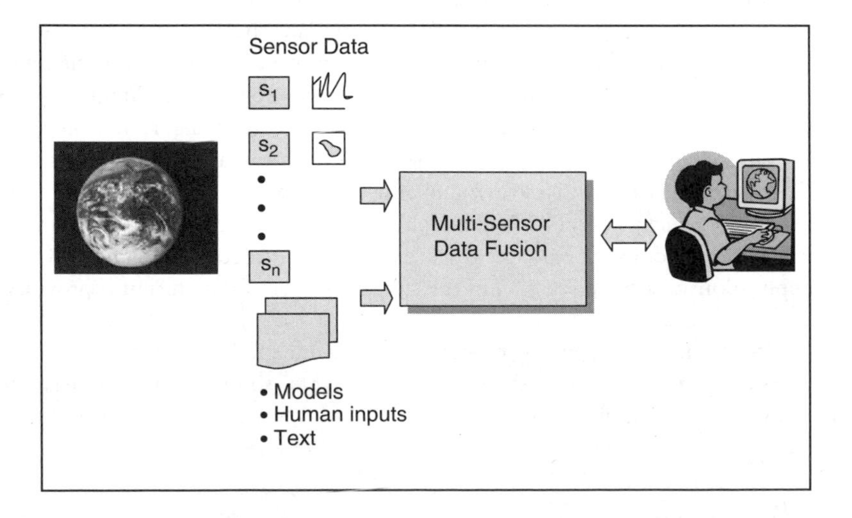

FIGURE 2.1 A conceptual view of ubiquitous sensing and information fusion.

2.2 Data Fusion Techniques

How is the actual fusion of data and information performed? There is no simple answer to this question because there are multiple techniques that can be utilized to perform the fusion. General discussions of these issues are provided by Hall and Linn [14], Bowman and Steinberg [15], Waltz and Hall [16], and Hall and Linn [17]. A discussion of the selection of algorithms specifically for correlation and association of data is provided by Hall et al. [18]. The appropriate selection of algorithms depends upon a number of issues. A brief description of these issues is provided here.

The Nature and Heterogeneity of the Input Data—Ideally, all data could be fused directly at the data level. For example, if the data consisted of two images, these images could be combined on a pixel-by-pixel basis using statistical estimation techniques, assuming that the data could be correctly aligned and associated so that the (i, j) pixel in image A matched the corresponding (m, n) pixel in image B. If the input data are homogeneous (viz., if the input sensors are measuring the same physical phenomena) then data level fusion may be performed using a variety of estimation techniques. In general, however, data from different types of sensors cannot be fused directly (e.g., fusing image information directly with scalar or vector information). In such cases, the data are characterized by a representative feature vector and fusion proceeds based on the feature vectors. Alternatively, the raw data or feature vectors from each sensor or source are processed independently to produce state vectors or (single-source) decisions regarding the observed situation. Subsequently these decisions or state vectors are fused using decision-level processes.

An example of a decision-level fusion process is shown in Figure 2.2. The heterogeneous sensor data may consist of images, signals, vectors, or scalars. The process shown in Figure 2.2 includes:

- *Data alignment and conditioning*: Alignment of the data from each sensor to reference a common set of units and coordinate frame; conditioning of the data via signal or image processing to maximize the amount of extractable information.
- *Feature extraction*: Representation of the signal or image data via a representative vector (e.g., coefficients of a Fourier or wavelet transform, autoregressive moving average coefficients, etc.) to characterize the data.
- *Pattern recognition*: Application of a pattern recognition algorithm such as a neural net or cluster algorithm to transform the feature vector into a declaration of identity or state (e.g., declaration of target identification or condition such as a fault condition in a mechanical system).
- *Correlation and association*: Correlation and association of the feature vectors to insure that a specified set of feature vectors or data refer to a common observed entity, event, or activity (e.g., data to track association, or track-to-track correlation for systems observing moving objects).
- *Decision-level fusion*: Combination and fusion of the decisions made by individual sensors to produce a joint declaration of identity; techniques include voting, Bayesian belief networks, and Dempster–Shafer's method.

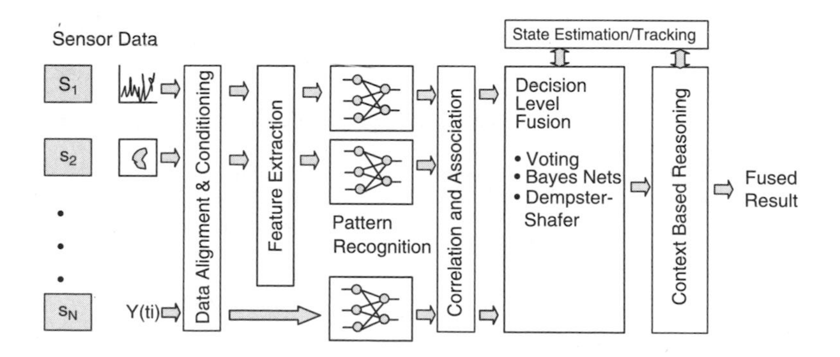

FIGURE 2.2 Example of decision-level fusion.

TABLE 2.1 Techniques for Data Fusion

Function	Description	Example Techniques	References
Data alignment	Alignment of data from different sensors to be processed in a common frame of space and time	• Coordinate transformations • Adjustment of units	[53] [2] [58] [60]
Data/object correlation and association	Grouping data together to insure that the data all refer to a common entity, target, event or activity	• Gating methods • Multiple hypothesis association; probabilistic data association • Figures of merit • Nearest neighbor	[55] [56] [57] [59] [61] [62]
Signal conditioning	Techniques to process input signal or image data to improve subsequent fusion processing	• A very wide variety of signal and image processing methods exist; sec the general references provided	[63]
Feature extraction	Characterization of signal and image data via vector representations	• Time domain/time series representations • Time-frequency representations • Higher order spectral methods • Wavelet methods	[106] [107] [108] [96] [97]
Pattern recognition	Recognition of patterns in data; transformation from input feature vector to declaration of target identity, classification of phenomena, activity or event detection	• Physical models • Cluster algorithms • Neural networks • Syntactic models • Hybrid reasoning models	[63] [64] [65] [66] [67] [68] [69] [70] [71] [72] [73]
Decision-level fusion	Fusion of reports or declarations of target or entity identity; fusion of reports for joint declarations	• Rule-based systems • Bayes networks • Fuzzy logic systems • Intelligent agents • Blackboard systems • Case-based reasoning	[74] [75] [76] [77] [78] [79] [80] [81] [82] [83] [84] [85] [86] [87]
State estimation and tracking	Estimation of the state vector or system state based on observations and/or feature vectors; tracking the evolution of parameters in time and/or space	• State estimators • Kalman filters • Particle trackers • Multiple hypothesis trackers (MHT) • Probabalistic data association (PDA) • Interacting multiple models (IMM)	[55] [56] [88] [89] [90] [91] [92] [93] [94] [95]

(Continued on next page)

TABLE 2.1 (Continued)

Function	Description	Example Techniques	References
Context-based reasoning	Automated reasoning about the context of the observed situation; interpretation of the meaning of activities, events, association among tracked or identified entities; understanding the relationship of the observed entities with respect to the environment	• Knowledge-based systems • Rule-based expert systems • Fuzzy logic logical templating • Neural networks • Case-based reasoning • Intelligent agent systems	[74] [75] [76] [77] [78] [79] [80] [83] [84] [98]
Process control and resource allocation	Allocate use of sensor or observing resources; refinement of the on-going fusion process for improved inferences	• Multi-objective optimization • Utility theory • E-commerce auction methods • Genetic algorithms	[99] [100] [101] [102] [103]

Source: Adapted from D.L. Hall and J. Llinas, "An introduction to multisensor data fusion," *Proc. IEEE*, vol. 85, no. 1, pp. 6–23, 1997.

- Estimation and tracking: Estimation of the state vector(s) in time to produce a target or feature vector track; this allows prediction of the state of the system in time.
- Context-based reasoning: Application of automated reasoning techniques to interpret the meaning of the fused data (e.g., relationships among objects or targets, understanding the meaning of the environment, etc.).

Note that this process flow is intended to be conceptual only. An actual implemented data fusion system would combine and interleave some of the functions identified in the figure. For example, in Figure 2.2 the state estimation function (viz., the utilization of an estimator such as a Kalman filter to estimate a state vector such as the position and velocity of an observed target) is shown as being separate from the identity level decision fusion. However, in a real fusion system, these functions might be combined via a multiple hypothesis tracking algorithm. A summary of types of algorithms corresponding to the functions in Figure 2.2 are listed in Table 2.2.

The A Priori Knowledge about the Input Data and Estimation Processes – Different techniques require different levels of knowledge about the nature of the input data and the observation process. For example, probabilistic methods such as Bayes method require *a priori* knowledge about the accuracy of the sensing process and the state estimation process. For target tracking, extensive probability models may be developed related to the sensing process, nature of the observed targets, the target tracking estimation process, etc. [55]. If such information is not available, then less restrictive models such as least-squares methods or voting techniques must be used. The selection of fusion algorithms must consider what can realistically be assumed or known about the observation and estimation process.

The Overall Data Fusion Architecture – A third factor that affects the selection of algorithms is the physical and logical architecture for the sensing/fusion system. Are the sensors and processors geographically distributed? Can all data be sent to a centralized processor for fusion or is processing performed at individual sensor nodes? Methods for allocating data fusion processes among system processing nodes and corresponding selection of algorithms are discussed by Hall and Llinas [5]. The rapid evolution of smart sensors and wireless communications systems [104] has increasingly led to distributed data fusion systems. Architectures for distributed fusion systems are described by Liggins and Chong [103].

2.3 Applications of Data Fusion

There are numerous evolving applications of data fusion. A summary of several emerging areas is provided in Table 2.2 and summarized below.

TABLE 2.2 Summary of Emerging Applications

Application	Focus	Types of Inferences	References
Condition-based monitoring of complex systems	Monitoring the health and status of complex mechanical systems; e.g., helicopters	• Status of machinery • Identification of evidence of impending failure conditions • Classification of fault conditions • Prediction of time to failure	[7] [19] [20] [21]
Environmental monitoring	Observing and understanding the physical environment, e.g. monitoring weather, crop phenomena	• Condition of environmental phenomena (e.g., weather, terrain) • Condition of crops • Spread of dust, flooding, etc.	[32] [33]
Medical applications	Utilization of multiple sensors and sources to determine the health and condition of human or animal bodies	• Identification of medical conditions • Medical diagnosis • Characterization of tumors or biological phenomena	[22] [23] [24] [31]
Nondestructive evaluation (NDE)	Determining the condition and constituency of materials or products without using destructive testing	• Product testing • Evaluation of material condition (e.g., search for flaws or weaknesses)	[25] [26] [27] [29]
Military applications	Utilization of multiple sensors and sources for improved understanding of a battle-space environment	• Automatic target recognition • Target tracking • Threat identification • Situation assessment	[28] [2] [3] [9] [30]

- *Condition-Based Monitoring (CBM) of Complex Systems* – The ability to instrument complex systems such as aircraft mechanical systems using MEMS sensors provides the opportunity to create intelligent health monitoring systems [19–21]. Such systems monitor the current health and state of a mechanical system, identify precursors to failure conditions, classify and identify faults, and seek to predict time to failure (under assumed operating demands). The motivation for CBM is driven by a combination of concern for safety and for reduced maintenance costs. In military systems, for example, the total ownership cost of a large-scale platform such as a ship, submarine, or airplane is driven by maintenance costs. Over 40% of the life-cycle cost of such a system involves maintenance. Currently, maintenance is performed using a time-based or use-based approach (viz., perform maintenance after so many hours or miles of operation). Time- or use-based maintenance is unduly expensive since it is performed in anticipation of potential failures. Perfectly good equipment may have preventive maintenance performed on it. In addition to the cost of unnecessary maintenance, the very act of maintenance can induce errors or problems, even when such maintenance is performed correctly. Thus, there is extensive research related to application of fusion for determining the condition and time to failure for complex mechanical systems [34–37].
- *Environmental Monitoring* – Environmental monitoring is another potential application for multi-sensor data fusion [32, 33]. The need to determine the condition of crops, water supplies, soil conditions, weather conditions, and the potential for environmental contamination (due to natural or man-made disasters) requires multiple types of sensors such as infrared, visible, temperature, humidity, and other types of sensors. Data fusion provides the opportunity to improve knowledge and assessment of an area of interest by combining these diverse types of data. Observing platforms may include satellites, airborne reconnaissance, ground-based sensors, and human observers. Advances in environmental monitoring include the use of hyper-spectral image sensors and unattended ground based sensors. Exciting research is ongoing to utilize insects and plants as sensing devices. An example of a data fusion system for environmental monitoring is shown in Figure 2.3.

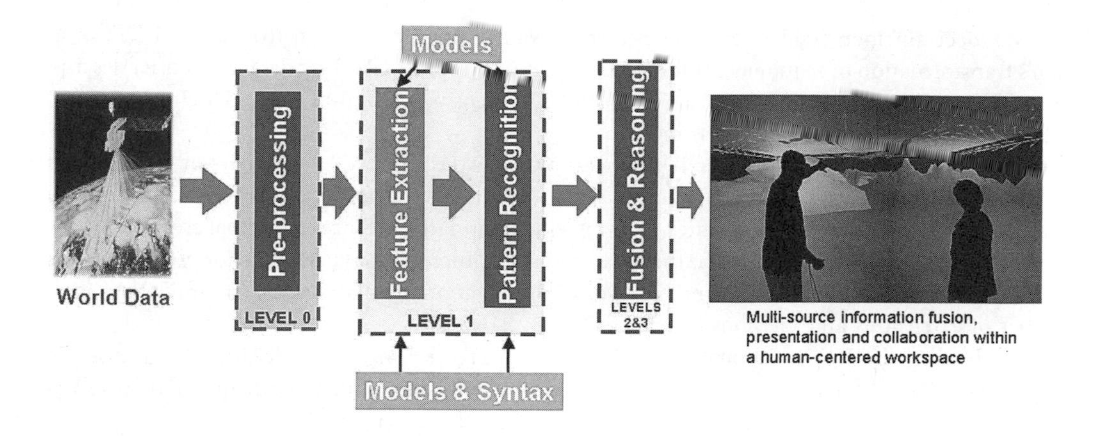

FIGURE 2.3 Data fusion system for NASA environmental data.

- *Medical Applications* – Medical applications of data fusion include medical diagnosis, intensive care monitoring, and characterization of biological systems [22–24, 31]. Medical applications involve fusion of image sensors (e.g., x-ray, MRI imaging, acoustic based imaging), as well as biological testing and self-reports from the human subject being diagnosed. Research to date has focused primarily on fusion of image data. However, early research in automated medical diagnosis contributed to the development of technology for expert reasoning systems and resulted in famous expert systems such as MYCIN [38].
- *Nondestructive evaluation (NDE)* – An application related to condition monitoring of complex systems is NDE. NDE seeks to determine the quality or state of a product, materials, or structures without performing tests that would adversely affect the observed product or material [25–27, 29]. Sensors such as x-ray imaging, acoustic imaging, visual inspection, and other techniques may be combined to determine the state of the observed product or material. Gros[25,26] describes the application of data fusion for this area.
- *Military applications*—The majority of funding and research related to advancement of multi-sensor data fusion concepts, algorithms, systems engineering guidelines, and systems have been provided in support of Department of Defense (DoD) applications. Surveys of DoD related data fusion systems have been performed by Hall et al. [30] and by Nichols [9]. Emerging military concepts of network centric warfare, Joint Vision 2020 (http://www.dtic.mil/jointvision/) and related visions recognize that the rapid evolution of smart sensors, wide-band communications, and increasingly capable computers provide the opportunity for ubiquitous sensing and understanding of the environment or situation. The DoD legacy from this extensive research and system prototyping includes process models [39–42], taxonomies of algorithms [1, 14], a data fusion lexicon [43], engineering guidelines for system design and development [15–17], software tools [44, 45], prototype systems [9] and test beds (see Center) (http://www.rl.af.mil/programs/fic/Fusion_web_main.html).

2.4 Process Models for Data Fusion

Several views can be developed to represent the data fusion process. A functional model can illustrate the primary functions, relevant databases, and interconnectivity to perform data fusion; an architectural model can specify hardware and software components, associated data flows, and external interfaces; and a mathematical model can describe algorithms and logical processes. This section provides an introduction to several process models that have been described in the data fusion literature. These include (1) the Joint Directors of Laboratories (JDL) data fusion process model [39, 40], (2) Dasarathy's functional model [42],

(3) Boyd's decision loop model [48], (4) Bedworth and O'Brien's omnibus process model [41], and (5) Fabian's transformation of requirements for the information process (TRIP) model [46]. A brief description of these models is provided in this section. Because of its extensive utilization in the DoD community, more details are provided on the JDL process model.

JDL Data Fusion Process Model – The JDL process model was developed by members of the Joint Directors of Laboratories Data Fusion Subcommittee to assist system developers and researchers in communicating about data fusion algorithms, architectures, and implementation issues. Since its original creation in 1991 [39], the model has been widely referenced in the data fusion literature, used as a baseline for government requests for proposals and cited on web sites. Since its original presentation, the JDL data fusion model has undergone a number of extensions and revisions (see Refs. [40, 51, 52]).

The top level of the JDL functional model is shown in Figure 2.4. The model includes a series of high-level processes (labeled level 1 to level 5) that constitute the main functions required to fuse data and information. A brief description of the inputs, outputs, and functions within the JDL model are shown in Table 2.3. Note that the complete hierarchical model has two additional layers. For each function (e.g., level one, level two, etc.), there have been defined a set of subfunctions and ultimately algorithms to accomplish those functions. Details of these subfunctions and algorithms are described by Hall and McMullen [1].

On the left side of Figure 2.4, the model shows input data received from multiple sensors and types of sensors. Information such as environmental data, *a priori* data, and human guidance/inferences may also be input to the illustrated fusion system. Major functions include preliminary filtering, collection management, level 1 processing, level 2 processing, level 3 processing, a database management system, and creation and maintenance of situation and support databases. External interfaces provide for a man–machine interface and continuous or offline evaluation of system performance. These functions are summarized below.

Preliminary filtering of input data provides an automatic means of controlling the flow of data into a fusion system. Typically, any fusion system can be computationally overwhelmed by data from multiple sensors. The sensor data rates frequently exceed the computational ability of a fusion system. Thus, preliminary filtering can be performed to sort data according to observation time, reported location, data or sensor type, and identity or signature information. Filtering may also utilize environmental or sensor quality information (e.g., signal-to-noise ratio, reported quality indicators, covariance error estimates, etc.). This information provides a means to associate data into general categories and prioritize data for subsequent processing.

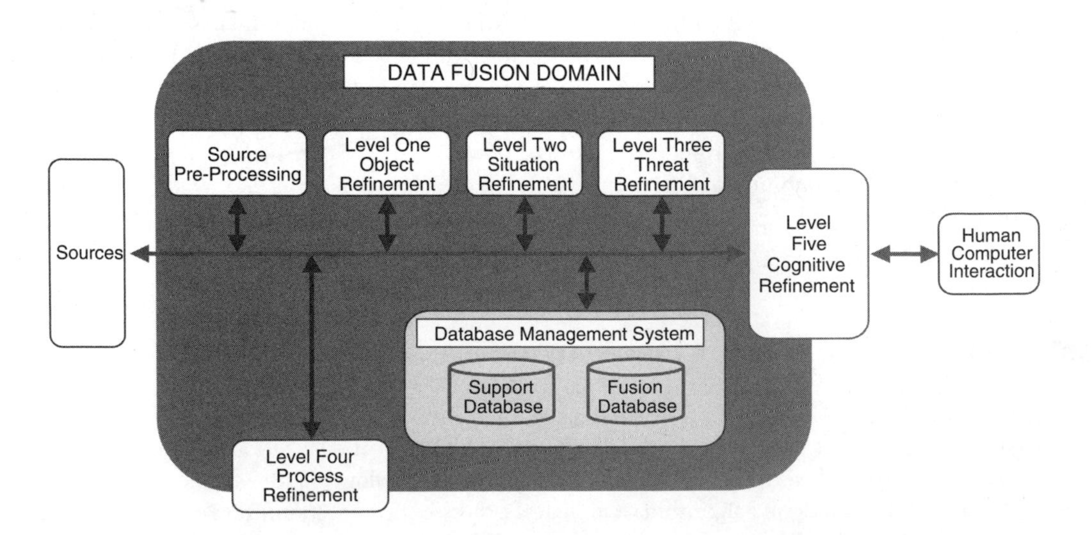

FIGURE 2.4 The Joint Directors of Laboratories (JDL) data fusion process model.

TABLE 2.3 Summary of JDL Data Fusion Model Components

JDL Model Component	Description	Example Functions
Level 0 Processing: Source preprocessing	Preprocessing of data from sensors and databases to correct biases, standardize inputs and extract key information	• Signal processing and conditioning • Image processing • Platform corrections • Bias corrections • Unit conversions • Feature extraction
Level 1 Processing: Object refinement	Combination of data and information to obtain estimates of an entity's location, motion, attributes, characteristics and identity	• Data alignment • Association and correlation • Position, kinematic and attribute estimation • Identity estimation
Level 2 Processing: Situation refinement	Interpretation of an evolving situation based on assessment of relationships among entities and their relationship to the environment	• Object aggregation • Event, activity detection and aggregation • Context-based interpretation • Multi-perspective reasoning
Level 3 Processing: Impact assessment	Projection of the current situation into the future to assess inferences about alternative futures or hypotheses concerning the current situation; assessment of threats, risks, and impacts	• Estimate consequences of current situation • Predict system evolution • Identify possible threats, risks, failure conditions • Multi-perspective assessment
Level 4 Processing: Process refinement and resource management	Monitoring the ongoing data fusion process to optimize the utilization of sensors or information sources to achieve the most useful set of information	• Predict sensor measurements • Compute measures of performance • Optimization of resource utilization • Sensor and resource tasking
Level 5 Processing: Cognitive refinement	Monitoring the ongoing interaction between the data fusion system and a human decision-maker; optimization of displays and focus of attention	• Focus of attention management • Cognitive aids • Search engines • Human–computer interaction control

Source: Adapted from D.L. Hall and J. Llinas, "An introduction to multisensor data fusion," *Proc. IEEE*, vol. 85, no. 1, pp. 6–23, 1997.

Data from individual sensors or sources may be processed to correct biases, translate raw data into other representations, and address individual characteristics of the sensors or sources.

Three levels of processing are shown in the center of Figure 2.4. Level 1 processing fuses data to establish the position, velocity, and identity of low-level entities or activities. The term *entity* refers here to a target, platform, emitter, or geographically (location) distinct object observed by multiple sensors. Level 1 processing combines positional and identity data from multiple sensors to establish a database of identified entities, target tracks, and uncorrelated raw data. Level 1 processing may be partitioned into four functions: (1) data alignment, (2) association, (3) tracking, and (4) identification.

Data alignment functions transform data received from multiple sensors into a common spatial and temporal reference frame. Specific alignment functions include coordinate transformation (e.g., from topocentric noninertial coordinates to geocentric inertial coordinates), time transformations (e.g., mapping from reported observation times to actual physical events), and unit conversions. Alignment may also require significant computational efforts. For example, transforming from image coordinates for an infrared sensor to an absolute direction in space may involve integral deconvolution transformations.

Data association and correlation address the problem of sorting or correlating observations from multiple sensors into groups, with each group of representing data related to a single distinct entity. In a dense tracking environment in which many targets of unknown identity are in close physical proximity, this problem requires multiple strategies. Association and correlation thus compare observation pairs (i.e., observation N vs. observation N-l, N-2, etc.) and determine which observations "belong" together as being from the same entity, object, event, or activity. Association and correlation also seek to determine which, if any, new observations belong to an observation or group of observations already contained in the fusion database. Clearly, this problem scales as N^2, where N is the current number of observations or tracks in the database. The term *association* is generally used to describe the process of measuring the "closeness" between observation pairs (or observations to tracks), while the term *correlation* is used to describe the decision process of actually assigning observations to observations, observations to tracks, or tracks to tracks.

Tracking refers to a process in which multiple observations of positional data are combined to determine an estimate of the target/entities position and velocity. A common tracking problem involves direction finding, in which multiple angular observations (e.g., lines of bearing) are combined to estimate the location of a nonmoving target. Another common tracking problem involves the use of observations from radar to establish the track of an aircraft. Tracking algorithms begin with an *a priori* estimate of an object's location and velocity (viz., either an initial estimate based on a minimum data set, or an *a priori* track established in the database) and update the estimated position to the time of a new observation. The new observation is utilized to refine the position estimate to account for the new data. Tracking algorithms are closely coupled to association strategies, particularly in a dense tracking environment.

Identification completes the category of level 1 processing functions. Identification methods seek to combine identity information, analogous to the estimation of position utilizing positional data. Identity fusion combines data related to identity (i.e., either actual declarations of identity from sensors, or parametric data that can be related to identity). Identity fusion techniques include cluster methods, adaptive neural networks, templating methods, and Dempster–Shaffer and Bayesian inference methods.

Level 2 processing or situation assessment seeks a higher level of inference above level 1 processing. Thus, for example, while level 1 processing results in an order of battle (e.g., location and identity of low level entities such as emitters or platforms), level 2 processing aims to assess the meaning or patterns in the order of battle data. To obtain an assessment of the situation, the data are assessed with respect to the environment, relationships among entities, and patterns in time and space.

Level 3 processing (for military or intelligence fusion systems) performs threat assessment. The purpose of threat assessment is to determine the meaning of the fused data from an adversarial view. Threat assessment functions include determination of lethality of friendly and enemy forces, assessment of friendly ("blue force") and enemy ("red force") compositions, estimate of danger, evaluation of indications and warnings of impending events, targeting calculations, and weapon assessment calculations. Level 3 processing is an inferential process to assess the enemy's threat or future implication of the current situation.

In order to manage the ongoing data fusion process, a level 4 meta-process is often used. This is a process that monitors the data collection and the fusion processing to optimize the collection and processing of data to achieve accurate and useful inferences. The level 4 process is deliberately shown as being partly inside and partly outside the data fusion process. The reason is that actions could be taken by the level 4 process (e.g., use active sensors) that could impede an operational mission. Hence, level 4 processing must be cognizant of mission needs and constraints. Within level 4 processing, the collections management function manages or controls the data collection assets (sensors) available to a fusion system. Specific functions involve determining the availability of sensors, tasking sensors to perform collections, prioritization of tasking, and monitoring sensor health/status in a feedback loop. Sensor tasking, in particular, requires predicting the future location of dynamic objects to be observed, computing the pointing angles for a sensor (viz., from the predicted position of an object and location of the sensor it computes the directions, ranges, etc., required for a sensor to point to a target), computing the controls for sensor pointing scheduling the sensor's observations, and optimizing the use of sensor resources (e.g., power requirements or movement from one target to another). For a large sensor network, the collection management function can be extremely challenging. Ideally, the collection management function should work in concert with other data fusion functions to optimize the rate and accuracy of inferences output from the fusion system.

Finally, a fifth level of processing was proposed by Hall et al. [51] to recognize the importance of addressing human in the loop decision processes. Level 5 processing involves functions such as human–computer interaction, cognitive aides to reduce human biases, adaptation of information needs and system control to individual user preferences and constraints, automated interpretation of data using multiple human sensory mechanisms, and tools such as search engines. The purpose of the level 5 processing is to help adapt the fusion system to the human-in-the-loop decision maker and to improve the effectiveness of the fusion system for supporting a human operation such as crisis management or situation assessment.

Functions in a fusion system include database management, man–machine interface, and evaluation functions. These functions may actually comprise a major portion of a fusion system.

Dasarathy's Functional Model – Dasarathy [42] defined a categorization of data fusion functions based on types of data, the information to be processed, and the types of information that result from the fusion process. The input is partitioned among data (e.g., signals and images), features (feature vectors), or objects (decision-level reports related to objects or identity declarations). The output data are partitioned in the same way as data, features, or object information. Dasarathy describes processes for each of the nine combinations of input/output characteristics (e.g., data input/data output, data input/features output, features input/object information output, etc.). For each of these categories, Dasarathy's model identifies types of algorithms which are suitable for processing. Steinberg and Bowman [47] have developed an expanded view of this model and have linked Dasarathy's view to the JDL model levels.

Boyd's Decision Loop Model – Col. John Boyd [48, 49] articulated the concept of an Observe, Orient, Decide, and Act (OODA) loop for effective tactical command and control in a military situation. This common sense but effective method for addressing dynamic decision-making situations has been applied to a variety of domains including driver's education, library science, and crisis management. The process entails systematic mindfulness of four key steps:

- *Observe* – Gather information via human senses, sensing devices, and other information sources
- *Orient* – Perform a situation assessment to understand the observed data and information
- *Decide* – Consider the likelihood of alternate hypotheses and their consequences and select the best alternative
- *Act* – Perform the indicated actions including possible collection of additional data

Development of tools and techniques to automate or support these steps is one way to view information fusion processing.

Bedworth and O'Brien's Omnibus Model – Bedworth and O'Brien [41] reviewed a number of different data fusion models and synthesized an omnibus model. The model is similar to Boyd's decision loop model but incorporates or maps levels of the JDL model to the decision loop as well as linking aspects of the systems engineering waterfall model and general components of the intelligence (disseminate, evaluate, collate, and collect) cycle. The Omnibus model associates key fusion functions to the OODA loop functions. For example, pattern matching and feature extraction are linked to the orient OODA step. Similarly, signal processing and sensing are linked to the observe OODA step.

Transformation of Requirements to Information Processing (TRIP) Model – A team led by William Fabien [50], under contract to the Defense Advanced Research Projects Agency (DARPA), developed a model called the TRIP model. This model seeks to define the transformation of information needs by a tactical commander to the specific tasking of sensors and information sources. Kessler and Fabien [50] suggest that the model has four basic purposes:

- To describe the process for formulating collection tasks based on information needs or requirements
- To understand the interaction and relationships between collection management and the situation estimation process
- To understand how the human-in-the-loop decision maker interacts with the ongoing collection management process and the situation assessment/fusion process
- To understand how internal and external drivers affect the intelligence, surveillance, and reconnaissance (ISR) process

The TRIP model is quite detailed and has been used to develop a hierarchy of functions, processes, and the inputs and outputs. The TRIP model is focused primarily on tactical military applications, but could be useful for other applications due to its level of detail.

2.5 Limitations of Data Fusion Systems

It is only fair in this introduction to data fusion to identify some limitations of data fusion systems. Hall and Steinberg [105] have discussed these limitations and identified a number of issues or "dirty secrets" in data fusion systems. These are summarized below. A summary of the state of the art in data fusion, based on the JDL model, is provided in Table 2.4.

TABLE 2.4 Summary of the State of the Art in Data Fusion

JDL Process	Current Practices	Limitations and Challenges
Level 1: Object refinement	• Sensor preprocessing using standard signal and image processing methods • Explicit separation of correlation and estimation problem • Multiple target tracking using multiple hypothesis tracking (MHT). • Use of *ad hoc* maneuver models • Object identification dominated by feature based methods • Pattern recognition using neural networks • Emerging guidelines for selection of correlation algorithms	• Dense target environments • Rapidly maneuvering targets • Complex signal propagation • Co-dependent sensor observations • Background clutter • Context-based reasoning • Integration of identity and kinematic data • Lack of available training data (for target identification) • No true fusion of image and non-image data (at the data level)
Level 2: Situation refinement	• Numerous prototype systems • Dominance of rule-based knowledge-based systems (KBS) • Variations include blackboard systems, logical templating, and case-based reasoning • Emerging use of fuzzy-logic and agent-based systems	• Limited operational systems • No experience in *scaling up* prototypes to operational systems • Very limited cognitive models • Perfunctory test and evaluation against *toy* problems • No proven technique for knowledge engineering
Level 3: Threat refinement	• Same as Level 2 processing • Limited advisory status • Limited deployment experience • Dominated by *ad hoc* methods • Doctrine-specific, fragile implementations • Very limited ability to predict the evolution of phenomena (e.g., failure phenomena) • Emerging use of hybrid reasoning involving implicit and explicit information	• Same as Level 2 • Difficulty to quantify *intent* • Models require established enemy doctrine • Difficult to model rapidly evolving situations
Level 4: Process refinement	• Robust methods for single-sensor systems • Formulations based on operations research • Limited context-based reasoning • Focus on measures of performance (MOP) versus measures of effectiveness (MOE) • Emerging use of auction-based methods from e-commerce applications • Emerging use of agents as proxies for bidding for resources	• Difficult to incorporate mission constraints • Scaling problem when many sensors (10^N) and adaptive systems • Difficult to optimally use noncommensurate sensors • Very difficult to link human information needs to sensor control
Human–computer interface (HCI)	• HCI dominated by the *technology of the week* • Focus on ergonomic versus cognitive-based design • Numerous graphics-based displays and systems • Advanced, 3D full immersion HCI available and haptic interfaces • Initial experiments with multi-modal sensory interactions • Initial experiments with agent-based cognitive aids	• Very little research has been performed to understand how human analysts process data and make accurate inferences • Creative HCI is needed to adapt to individual users and to provide mitigation of known cognitive biases and illusions

- *There is no substitute for a good sensor*: No amount of data fusion can substitute for a single accurate sensor that measures the phenomena that you want to observe. While a combination of sensors may provide robust system operation, these sensors will not necessarily observe the feature of interest. For example, in a mechanical system, conditions such as operating speed, vibration levels, and lubrication pressure may provide valuable information about a system's operation. However, these do not provide direct evidence of the system operating temperature. In this example, the introduction of an appropriate sensor such as a thermometer of a thermo-couple would obtain the desired information about the state of the system.
- *Downstream processing cannot make up for errors (or failures) in upstream processing*: Data fusion processing cannot correct for errors in processing (or lack of preprocessing) of individual sensor processing. For example, failure to identify and extract the correct features from a signal cannot be corrected by a sophisticated pattern recognition scheme. Hence, attention must be paid to every step in the data fusion processing flow.
- *Sensor fusion can result in poor performance if incorrect information about sensor performance is used*: A common problem in data fusion is to characterize the sensor performance in an *ad hoc* or convenient (but incorrect) way. Failure to accurately model sensor performance will result in a corruption of the fused results, because the sensor weights (or effects of the data from individual sensors) will be incorrect. This is especially difficult for sensors in complex observing environments (e.g., involving a difficult signal transmission media, complex interference environment, etc.).
- *There is no such thing as a magic or golden data fusion algorithm*: Despite claims to the contrary, there is no perfect algorithm that is optimal under all conditions. Real applications may not meet the underlying assumptions required by data fusion algorithms. (e.g., available prior probabilities or statistically independent sources). Thus, algorithm selection requires knowledge about the characteristics of the observing environment, sensor performance, the processing environment, and the fundamental information requirements of the candidate algorithms.
- *There will never be enough training data:* In general, there will never be sufficient training data for pattern recognition algorithms applications such as automatic target recognition. Hence, hybrid methods must be used (e.g., model-based methods, syntactical representations, or combinations of methods).
- *It is difficult to quantify the value of a data fusion system:* A challenge in data fusion systems is to quantify the utility of the system at a mission level. While measures of performance can be obtained for sensors or processing algorithms, measures of mission effectiveness are difficult to define. How does the application of data fusion algorithms assist in discovering how well a system (e.g., machine, factory, weapon system) will perform in an operational environment?
- *Fusion is not a static process:* Finally, the data fusion process in not static, but rather an iterative dynamic process that seeks to continually refine the estimates about an observed situation or threat environment. The level 4 process seeks to optimize the ongoing fusion process.

These factors should be kept in mind in studying and applying methods in data fusion.

2.6 Summary

The advent of smart micro- and nano-scale sensors, wideband communications, and rapidly evolving microprocessors enable the creation of multi-sensor data fusion systems for use in a wide variety of applications such as monitoring complex systems, environmental monitoring, medical diagnosis, or military applications. Limitations of observation capability and communications are giving away to the limitations of the ability to ingest or fuse the heterogeneous data. This chapter provided a brief introduction to the concepts of data fusion. Development of information fusion systems for increased understanding of the observed environment or situation involves understanding and utilization of a diverse set of algorithms and techniques. These range from signal and image processing to pattern recognition, statistical estimation, optimization techniques, and automated reasoning. The enormous legacy provided by DoD developments has laid the groundwork for a new generation of intelligent sensing and fusion systems.

References

1. D. Hall and S.A. McMullen, *Mathematical Techniques in Multisensor Data Fusion*, 2nd ed., Norwood, MA: Artech House, 2004.
2. E. Waltz and Llinas, J., *Multisensor Data Fusion*, Norwood, MA: Artech House, 1990.
3. E. Waltz, "C^3I: A tutorial," in *Command, Control, Communications Intelligence (C^3I)*, Palo Alto, CA: EW Communications, 1986, pp. 217–226.
4. L.A. Klein, *Sensor and Data Fusion Concepts and Applications*, New York: SPIE Optical Engineering Texts, 1993.
5. D.L. Hall and J. Llinas, Eds., *Handbook of Multisensor Data Fusion*, The Electrical and Applied Signal Processing Series, Boca Raton, FL: CRC Press, 2001.
6. D.L. Hall and J. Llinas, "An introduction to multisensor data fusion," *Proc. IEEE*, vol. 85, no. 1, pp. 6–23, 1997.
7. C.S. Byington and A.K. Garga, "Data fusion for developing predictive diagnostics for electromechanical systems," in *Handbook of Multisensor Data Fusion*, D.L. Hall and J. Llinas, Eds., The Electrical and Applied Signal Processing Series, Boca Raton, FL: CRC Press, 2001, pp 23-1–23-30.
8. J.D. Williams, "Use of biometrics and biomedical imaging in support of battlefield diagnostics," in *Fusion '98: First Int. Conf. Multi-Source, Multi-Sens. Info. Fusion*, Las Vegas, NV, 1998.
9. M.L. Nichols, "A survey of multisensor data fusion systems," in *Handbook of Multisensor Data Fusion*, D.L. Hall and J. Llinas, Eds., The Electrical and Applied Signal Processing Series, Boca Raton, FL: CRC Press, FL, 2001, pp. 22-1–22-7.
10. D.G. Goodenough, P. Bhogal, D. Charlebois, S. Matwin, and O. Niemann, "Intelligent data fusion for remote sensing," *Proc. Intl. Geosci. and Remote Sensing Symp.*, IGARSS, vol. 3, pp. 2157–2160, 1995.
11. N. Malud, *An Introduction to Microelectromechanical Systems*, Norwood, MA: Artech House, 1999.
12. D.C. Swanson, *Signal Processing for Intelligent Sensor Systems*, New York: Marcel Dekker, 2000.
13. M.A. Trenas, J.C. Rutledge, and N.A. Whitmal, "Wavelet-based noise reduction and compression for hearing aids," *Proc. IEEE 21st Int. Conf. IEEE Eng. Med. Biol. Soc.*, October 1999.
14. D. Hall and R. Linn, "A taxonomy of multisensor data fusion algorithms," *Proc. 1990 Joint Serv. Data Fusion Symp.*, Johns Hopkins University Applied Research Laboratory, Laurel, MD. vol. 1, 1990, pp. 593–610.
15. C. Bowman and A. Steinberg, "A systems engineering approach for implementing data fusion systems," in *Handbook of Multisensor Data Fusion*, D.L. Hall and J. Llinas, Eds., The Electrical and Applied Signal Processing Series, Boca Raton, FL: CRC Press, 2001, pp. 16-1–16-38.
16. E. Waltz and D. Hall, "Requirements derivation for data fusion systems," in *Handbook of Multisensor Data Fusion*, D.L. Hall and J. Llinas, Eds., The Electrical and Applied Signal Processing Series, Boca Raton, FL: CRC Press, 2001, pp. 15-1–15-8.
17. D.L. Hall and R. Linn, "Algorithm selection for data fusion systems," *Proc. 1987 Tri-Service Data Fusion Symp.*, Laurel, MD: Applied Physics Laboratory, Johns Hopkins University, vol. 1, pp. 100–110, 1987.
18. D.L. Hall, J. Llinas, B. Neuenfeldt, L. McConnell, D. Bohney, C. Bowman, L. Lochocki, and P. Applegate, "Studies and analyses within project correlation: An in-depth assessment of correlation problems and solution techniques," *Proc. Ninth Natl Symp. Sens. Fusion*, Monterey, CA: Naval Postgraduate School, 12–14 March 1996, pp. 171–188.
19. C.S. Byington and A.K. Garga, "Platform level reasoning for an SH-60B helicopter using intelligent agents," *Proc. 54th Soc. Mach. Fail. Prev. Technol.*, Virginia Beach, VA, 2000.
20. D.L. Hall, R.J. Hansen, and S.K. Kurtz, "A new approach to the challenge of machinery prognostics," *J. Eng. Gas Turb. Power, Trans. Am. Soc. Mech. Eng. (ASME)*, April 1995, pp. 320–325.
21. D.L. Hall, R.J. Hansen, and D.C. Lang, "The negative information problem in mechanical diagnostics," *Trans. ASME* 119, 370–377, 1997.

22. H. Alto et al., "Image processing: radiological and clinical information fusion in breast cancer detection," *Proc. SPIE Conf. Sens. Fusion: Architect., Algorithms Appl. IV*, Orlando, FL, 3–5 April, 2002, pp. 134–181.
23. M. Akay and A. Marsh, Eds., *Information Technologies in Medicine*, Vol. 1, Medical Simulation and Education, New York: Wiley-IEEE Computer Society, 2001.
24. J. Webster, Ed., *Minimally Invasive Medical Technology*, New York: Institute of Physics Publisher, 2001.
25. X.E. Gros, Ed., *NDT Data Fusion*, New York: Arnold, 1997.
26. X.E. Gros, Ed., *Applications of NDT Data Fusion*, New York: Kluwer Academic, 2001.
27. F. Ansari, Ed., *Condition Monitoring of Materials and Structures*, American Society of Civil Engineering Publishers, 2000.
28. R. Antony, *Principles of Data Fusion Automation*, Norwood, MA: Artech House, 1995.
29. G.W. Nickerson and D.L. Hall, "NDT: The blurring distinction between NDT and onboard diagnostics," in *Proc. 34th Annu. Br. Conf. NDT*, London, U.K., June 1995.
30. D.L. Hall, R. Linn, and J. Llinas, "A survey of data fusion systems," *Proc. SPIE Conf. Data Struct. Target Classif.*, April 1991, pp. 13–29.
31. J.M. Martin and D. Tobin, *Principles and Practice of Intensive Care*, New York: McGraw Hill, 1997.
32. J. Jahnke, *Continuous Emission Monitoring*, 2nd ed., New York: Wiley, 2000.
33. A. Camara and A.S. Da Camara, *Environmental Systems: A Multidimensional Approach*, Oxford: Oxford University Press, 2002.
34. D. Hall, A. Garga, B. Grimes, S. Kumara, I. Petrick, and S. Purao, "Intelligent preparation of the logistics battle space: The role of data fusion," *Proc. 2004 MSS Nal Symp. Sens. Data Fusion*, Johns Hopkins University Applied Physics Laboratory, June 8–10, 2004.
35. D. Hall, K. Schroyer, S.A. McMullen, and J.J. McMullen, "On the use of analog problems to address level-2 and level-3 information fusion," *Proc. 2004 MSS Natl Symp. Sens. Data Fusion*, Johns Hopkins University Applied Physics Laboratory, June 8–10, 2004.
36. J. Erdley, *Improved Fault Detection using Multisens. Data Fusion*, M.S. thesis in Electrical Engineering, The Pennsylvania State University, 1997.
37. D. Hall, "Intelligent monitoring of complex systems," in *Advances in Intelligent Systems for Defence*, L.C. Jain, N.S. Ichalkaranje, and G. Tonfoni, Eds., World Scientific Publishing Company, 2003.
38. B.G. Buchanon and E.H. Shortliffe, *Rule-Based Expert Systems: The MYCIN Experts of the Heuristic Programming Project*, Reading, MA: Addison-Wesley, 1983.
39. O. Kessler, K. Askin, N. Beck, J. Lynch, F. White, D. Buede, D. Hall, and J. Llinas, *Functional Description of the Data Fusion Process*, Technical report developed for the Data Fusion Development Strategy, Office of Naval Technology, Warminster, PA, November, 1991.
40. A.N. Steinberg, C.L. Bowman, and F.E. White, "Revisions to the JDL data fusion process model," in *Proc. SPIE AeroSense: Sens. Fusion: Architectures, Algorithms Appl. III*, B. Dasarathy and F.L. Orlando, Eds., vol. 3719, 1999, pp 430–441.
41. M. Bedworth and O'Brien, "The Omnibus model: A new model of data fusion?," in *Proc. 2nd Int. Conf. Info. Fusion*, Johns Hopkins University Applied Physics Laboratory, May 24–27, 1999 (see http://www.inforfusion.org/fusion99/cdrom.htm).
42. B. Dasarathy, *Decision Fusion*, New York: IEEE Computer Society Press, 1994.
43. D. Hall, *Lexicon of Multisensor Data Fusion Terms*, State College, PA: Tech Reach, 1997.
44. S.A. Hall and R.S. Sherry, "A survey of COTS software for multisensor data fusion: What's new since Hall and Linn?," *Proc. 2002 MSS Natl Symp. Sens. Data Fusion*, San Diego, CA, 2002.
45. D. Hall and G. Kasmala, "A visual programming toolkit for multisensor data fusion," *Proc. SPIE Aerospace 1996 Symp.: Digitization of the Battlefield*, R. Suresh and W. Langford, Eds., vol. 2764, Orlando, FL, March 1996, pp 181–187.
46. O. Kessler and B. Fabian, "Estimation and ISR Process Integration," *Def. Adv. Res. Proj. Agency (DARPA) Tech. Rep.*, Washington, DC, 2001.
47. A. Steinberg and C. Bowman, "Revisions to the JDL data fusion processing model," in *Handbook of Multisensor Data Fusion*, D. Hall and J. Llinas, Eds., Boca Raton, FL: CRC Press, 2001, Chapter 2.

48. Boyd, R. John, *A Discourse on Winning and Losing*, August 1987, Private Collections. Master copy in Library at Marine Corps University, Quantico, VA.
49. G. Hammond, *The Mind of War: John Boyd and American Security*, Washington, DC: Smithsonian Institution Press, May 2001.
50. O. Kessler and B. Fabian, *Estimation and the ISR process integration*, technical briefing prepared for the Defense Advanced Research Projects Agency (DARPA), Washington, D.C., 2001.
51. M.J. Hall, S.A. Hall, and T. Tate, "Removing the HCI bottleneck: how the human computer interface (HCI) affects the performance of data fusion systems," *Proc. 2000 MSS Natl Symp. Sens. Data Fusion*, San Diego, CA, June 2000, pp. 89–104.
52. A. Steinberg and C. Bowman, "Rethinking the JDL data fusion levels," *Proc. 2004 MSS Natl Symp. Sens. Data Fusion*, Johns Hopkins University Applied Research Laboratory, June 7–9, 2004.
53. R. Escobal, *Methods of Orbit Determination*, Melbourne, FL: Krieger, 1976.
54. E.L. Zavaleta and E.J. Smith, *Goddard Trajectory Determination System User's Guide*, Silver Spring, MD: Computer Sciences Corporation Technical Report, 1975.
55. S. Blackman, *Multiple Target Tracking with Radar Applications*, Norwood, MA: Artech House, 1986.
56. Y. Bar-Shalom and E. Tse, "Tracking in a cluttered environment with probabilistic data association," *Automatica*, 2, 451–460, 1975.
57. T.E. Fortman, Y. Bar-Shaolom, and M. Scheffe, "Multi-target tracking using joint probabilistic data association," in *Proc. 1980 IEEE Conf. Decis. Control*, December 1980, pp. 807–812.
58. J.O. Cappellari, C.E. Velez, and A.J. Fuchs, *Mathematical Theory of the Goddard Trajectory Determination System*, Technical Report, Greenbelt, MD: NASA Goddard Space Flight Center, 1976.
59. F.L. Wright, "The fusion of multi-sensor data," *Signal*, 1980, pp 39–43.
60. N.D. Sanza, M.A. McClure, and J.R. Cloutier, "Spherical target state estimators," *Proc. Am. Control Conf.*, Baltimore, MD, June 1994, pp. 1675–1679.
61. M. de Feo, A. Graziano, R. Miglioli, and A. Farina, "IMMJPDA vs MHT and Kalman filter with NN correlation: Performance comparison," *IEE Proc. Radar, Sonar Navigation*, 144, pp. 49–52, 1999.
62. D. Lerro and Y. Bar-Shalom, "Interacting multiple models tracking with target amplification feature," *IEEE Trans. Aerospace Electron. Syst.*, AES-29, 494–509, 1993.
63. K. Fukanaga, *Introduction to Statistical Pattern Recognition*, 2nd ed., New York: Academic Press, 1990.
64. M.S. Aldenderfer and R.K. Blashfield, *Cluster Analysis*, in the series: Quantitative Applications in the Social Sciences, No. 07-044, London: Sage Press, 1984.
65. R. Dubes and A. Jain, "Clustering algorithms in exploratory data analysis," *Advances in Computers*, vol. 19, 1980, pp. 113–228.
66. H. Skinner, "Dimensions and clusters: A hybrid approach to classification," *App. Psycholog. Meas.*, 3, 327–341, 1979.
67. A.J. Cole and A. Wishart, "An improved algorithm for the Jardine-Sibson method of generating clusters," *Comput. J.*, 13, 156–163, 1970.
68. R.P. Lippman, "An introduction to computing neural networks," *IEEE ASSP Mag.*, 3–4, 4–22, 1987.
69. B. Widrow and R. Winter, "Neural nets for adaptive filtering and adaptive pattern recognition," *IEEE Comput.*, 21–3, 24–40, 1988.
70. D. Mush and B. Horne, "Progress in supervised neural networks: What's new since Lippman?," *IEEE Signal Process. Mag.*, 8–39, January, 1993.
71. D. Touretzky, *Advances in Neural Information Processing Systems*, 2nd ed., Palo Alto, CA: Morgan Kauffman, 1990.
72. R.O. Duda and P.E. Hart, *Pattern Classification and Scene Analysis*, New York: Wiley, 1973.
73. D. Hall and A. Garga, "Hybrid reasoning techniques for automated fault classification," *Proc. 51st Meet. Soc. Mach. Fail. Prev.*, April, 1997.
74. R. Kurzwil, *The Age of Intelligent Machines*, Cambridge, MA: MIT Press, 1990.
75. P. Jackson, *Introduction to Expert Systems*, 3rd ed., New York: Addison-Wesley, 1998.
76. R.A. Benfer, E.E. Brent, and L. Furbee, *Expert Systems*, vol. 77, London: Sage, 1991.
77. J.C. Giarranto, *Expert Systems: Principles and Programming*, Pacific Grove, CA: Brooks/Cole, 1998.

78. R.E. Neopolitan, *Probabilistic Reasoning in Expert Systems: Theory and Algorithms*, New York: Wiley, 1990.
79. S. Post and A.P. Sage, "An overview of automated reasoning," *IEEE Trans. Syst., Man Cybernet.*, 20, 202–224, 1990.
80. K.C. Ng and B. Abramson, "Uncertainty management in expert systems," *IEEE Expert*, 1990, pp. 29–48.
81. L.A. Zadeh, "Fuzzy logic," *Computer*, 83–92, 1988.
82. J. Llinas and R. Antony, "Blackboard concepts for data fusion and command and control applications," *Proc. Int. J. Pattern Recogn. Artif. Intel.*, 1992.
83. D.F. Noble, "Template-based data fusion for situation assessment," in *Proc. 1987 Tri-Service Data Fusion Symp.*, Laurel, MD: Johns Hopkins University, Applied Physics Laboratory, 1987, pp. 226–236.
84. D.L. Hall and R.J. Linn, "Comments on the use of templating for multi-sensor data fusion," *Proc. 1989 Tri-Service Data Fusion Symp.*, Laurel, MD: Johns Hopkins University Applied Physics Laboratory, 1989, pp. 152–162.
85. F.V. Jensen, *Bayesian Networks and Decision Graphs*, New York: Springer, 2001.
86. M. Woodridge, *Introduction to Multi-Agent Systems*, New York: John Wiley and Sons, 2002.
87. J. Yen, J. Yin, T.R. Ioerger, M. Miller, D. Xu, and R.A. Volz, "CAST: Collaborating agents simulating teamwork," *Proc. Int. Joint Conf. Artif. Intel. (IJCAI 2001)*, Seattle, WA, 2001, pp. 1135–1142.
88. H.W. Sorenson, "Least squares estimation: from Gauss to Kalman," *IEEE Spectrum*, July 1970, pp. 63–68.
89. A. Gelb, *Applied Optimal Estimation*, Cambridge, MA: MIT Press, 1974.
90. A.H. Sayed and T. Kailath, "A state-space approach to adaptive RLS filtering," *IEEE Signal Process. Mag.*, 18–70, July 1994.
91. A. Poore, "Multi-dimensional assignment formulation of the data association problem arising from multi-target and multi-sensor tracking," *Comput. Optimiz. Appl.*, 3, 27–57, 1994.
92. R.L. Streit and T.E. Luginbuhl, "A probabilistic multi-hypothesis tracking algorithm without enumeration and pruning," in *Proc. 6th Joint Serv. Data Fusion Symp.*, Laurel, MD: Johns Hopkins University Applied Research Laboratory, June 1993.
93. R.L. Streit, "Maximum likelihood method for probabilistic multi-hypothesis tracking," *SPIE Proc.*, 2234-5, 394–406, 1994.
94. R. Mahler, "A unified foundation for data fusion," *Proc. 1994 Data Fusion Syst. Conf.*, Laurel, MD: Johns Hopkins University Applied Physics Laboratory, June 1987.
95. I.R. Goodman, R.S. Mahler, and H.T. Nguyen, *Mathematics of Data Fusion*, New York: Kluwer Academic, 1997.
96. Kittler, "Mathematical methods in feature selection in pattern recognition," *Int. J. Man-Mach. Stud.*, 7, 609–637, 1975.
97. C. Lee and D.A. Landgrebe, "Decision boundary feature extraction for nonparametric classification," *Trans. Syst. Man Cybernet.*, 23, 433–444, 1993.
98. M. Lenz, B. Bartsch-Spori, H. Burkhard, S. Wess, G. Goos, J. Hartmanis, and J. Van Leeuwan, *Case-Based Reasoning Technology: From Foundation to Application*, New York: Springer-Verlag, 1998.
99. G.A. McIntyre, *A Comprehensive Approach to Sensor Management and Scheduling*, Ph.D. dissertation, Department of Information Technology, George Mason University, 1998.
100. A.N. Steinberg, "Threat management systems for combat aircraft," *Proc. Tri-Serv. Data Fusion Symp.*, Laurel, MD: Johns Hopkins University, 1987, pp. 532–52.
101. P.L. Rothman and S.G. Bier, "Evaluation of sensor management systems," *Proc. 1991 Fusion Syst. Conf.*, Laurel, MD: Johns Hopkins University Applied Physics Laboratory, October 1991.
102. P.C. Fishburn, *Nonlinear Preference and Utility Theory*, Laurel, MD: Johns Hopkins University Press, 1988.
103. M.E. Liggins II and C.Y. Chong, "Distributed fusion architectures and algorithms for target tracking," *Proc. IEEE*, vol. 85, no. 1, 1997.
104. C.Y. Chong and S.P. Kumar, "Sensor networks: evolution, opportunities, and challenges," *Proc. IEEE*, vol. 91, no. 8, 2003.

105. D. Hall and A. Steinberg, "Dirty secrets in multisensor data fusion," in *Handbook of Multisensor Data Fusion*, D.L. Hall and J. Llinas, Eds., The Electrical and Applied Signal Processing Series, Boca Raton, FL: CRC Press, 2001.
106. A. Weigend and N.A. Gershenfeld, *Time Series Prediction: Forecasting the Future and Understanding the Past*, Reading, MA: Addison Wesley, 1994.
107. L. Cohen, "Time frequency distribution – a review," *Proc. IEEE*, 77, 941–981, 1989.
108. P.A. Delany and D.O. Walsh, "A bibliography of higher order spectra and cumulants," *IEEE Signal Process. Mag.*, 61–74, July 1994.

3

Magneto-optics

David Young
Rockwell Semiconductor Systems

Yuan Pu
University of California

3.1 Introduction 3-1
3.2 Classification of Magneto-optic Effects 3-2
Faraday Rotation or Magnetic Circular Birefringence • Cotton–Mouton Effect or Magnetic Linear Birefringence • Kerr Effects
3.3 Applications of Magneto-optic Effects 3-5
Optical Isolator and Circulator • MSW-Based Guided-Wave Magneto-optic Bragg Cell • Magneto-optic Recording

3.1 Introduction

When a magnetic field **H** is applied to a magnetic medium (crystal), a change in the magnetization **M** within the medium will occur as described by the constitution relation of the Maxwell equations $\mathbf{M} = \overleftrightarrow{\chi} \cdot \mathbf{H}$ where $\overleftrightarrow{\chi}$ is the magnetic susceptibility tensor of the medium. The change in magnetization can in turn induce a perturbation in the complex optical permittivity tensor $\overleftrightarrow{\varepsilon}$. This phenomenon is called the magneto-optic effect. Mathematically, the magneto-optic effect can be described by expanding the permittivity tensor as a series in increasing powers of the magnetization (Torfeh et al., 1977) as follows:

$$\overleftrightarrow{\varepsilon} = \varepsilon_0[\varepsilon_{ij}] \tag{3.1}$$

where

$$\varepsilon_{ij}(\mathbf{M}) = \varepsilon_r \delta_{ij} + j f_1 e_{ijk} M_k + f_{ijkl} M_k M_l$$

Here, j is the imaginary number. M_1, M_2, and M_3 are the magnetization components along the principal crystal axes X, Y, and Z, respectively. ε_0 is the permittivity of free space. ε_r is the relative permittivity of the medium in the paramagnetic state (i.e., $\mathbf{M} = 0$), f_1 is the first-order magneto-optic scalar factor, f_{ijkl} is the second-order magneto-optic tensor factor, δ_{ij} is the Kronecker delta, and e_{ijk} is the antisymmetric alternate index of the third order. Here we have used Einstein notation of repeated indices and have assumed that the medium is quasi-transparent so that $\overleftrightarrow{\varepsilon}$ is a Hermitian tensor. Moreover, we have also invoked the Onsager relation in thermo-dynamical statistics, i.e., $\varepsilon_{ij}(\mathbf{M}) = \varepsilon_{ji}(-M)$. The consequences of Hermiticity and Onsager relation are that the real part of the permittivity tensor is an even function of **M** whereas the imaginary part is an odd function of **M**. For a cubic crystal, such as yttrium–iron–garnet (YIG), the tensor f_{ijkl} reduces to only three independent terms. In terms of Voigt notation, they are f_{11}, f_{12}, and f_{44}. In a principal coordinate system, the tensor can be expressed as

$$f_{ijkl} = f_{12}\delta_{ij}\delta_{kl} + f_{44}(\delta_{il}\delta_{kj} + \delta_{ik}\delta_{lj}) + \Delta f\,\delta_{kl}\delta_{ij}\delta_{jk} \tag{3.2}$$

where $\Delta f = f_{11} - f_{12} - 2f_{44}$.

In the principal crystal axes [100] coordinate system, the magneto-optic permittivity reduces to the following forms:

$$\overleftrightarrow{\varepsilon} = \varepsilon_0 \begin{bmatrix} \varepsilon_{11} & \varepsilon_{12} & \varepsilon_{13} \\ \varepsilon_{12}^* & \varepsilon_{22} & \varepsilon_{23} \\ \varepsilon_{13}^* & \varepsilon_{23}^* & \varepsilon_{33} \end{bmatrix}$$

where * denotes complex conjugate operation. The elements are given by

paramagnetic state

$$\overleftrightarrow{\varepsilon} = \varepsilon_0 \begin{bmatrix} \varepsilon_r & 0 & 0 \\ 0 & \varepsilon_r & 0 \\ 0 & 0 & \varepsilon_r \end{bmatrix}$$

Faraday rotation

$$+ \varepsilon_0 \begin{bmatrix} 0 & +jf_1M_3 & -jf_1M_2 \\ -jf_1M_3 & 0 & +jf_1M_1 \\ +jf_1M_2 & -jf_1M_1 & 0 \end{bmatrix}$$

Cotton–Mouton effect

$$+ \varepsilon_0 \begin{bmatrix} f_{11}M_1^2 + f_{12}M_2^2 + f_{12}M_3^2 & 2f_{44}M_1M_2 & 2f_{44}M_1M_3 \\ 2f_{44}M_1M_2 & f_{12}M_1^2 + f_{11}M_2^2 + f_{12}M_3^2 & 2f_{44}M_2M_3 \\ 2f_{44}M_1M_3 & 2f_{44}M_2M_3 & f_{12}M_1^2 + f_{12}M_2^2 + f_{11}M_3^2 \end{bmatrix} \quad (3.3)$$

In order to keep the discussion simple, analytic complexities due to optical absorption of the magnetic medium have been ignored. Such absorption can give rise to magnetic circular dichroism (MCD) and magnetic linear dichroism (MLD). Interested readers can refer to Hellwege (1978) and Arecchi and Schulz-DuBois (1972) for more in-depth discussions on MCD and MLD.

3.2 Classification of Magneto-optic Effects

Faraday Rotation or Magnetic Circular Birefringence

The classic Faraday rotation takes place in a cubic or isotropic transparent medium where the propagation direction of transmitted light is parallel to the direction of applied magnetization within the medium. For example, if the direction of magnetization and the propagation of light is taken as Z, the permittivity tensor becomes (assuming second-order effect is insignificantly small):

$$\overleftrightarrow{\varepsilon} \cong \varepsilon_0 \begin{bmatrix} \varepsilon_r & jf_1M_3 & 0 \\ -jf_1M_3 & \varepsilon_r & 0 \\ 0 & 0 & \varepsilon_r \end{bmatrix} \quad (3.4)$$

The two eigenmodes of light propagation through the magneto-optic medium can be expressed as a right circular polarized (RCP) light wave:

$$\tilde{E}_1(Z) = \begin{bmatrix} 1 \\ j \\ 0 \end{bmatrix} \exp\left[j\left(\omega t - \frac{2\pi n_+}{\lambda_0} Z \right) \right] \tag{3.5a}$$

and a left circular polarized (LCP) light wave:

$$\tilde{E}_2(Z) = \begin{bmatrix} 1 \\ -j \\ 0 \end{bmatrix} \exp\left[j\left(\omega t - \frac{2\pi n_-}{\lambda_0} Z \right) \right] \tag{3.5b}$$

where $n_\pm{}^2 \cong \varepsilon_r \pm f_1 M_3$; ω and λ_0 are the angular frequency and the wavelength of the incident light, respectively. n_+ and n_- are the refractive indices of the RCP and LCP modes, respectively. These modes correspond to two counterrotating circularly polarized light waves. The superposition of these two waves produces a linearly polarized wave. The plane of polarization of the resultant wave rotates as one circular wave overtakes the other. The rate of rotation is given by

$$\begin{aligned} \theta_\Gamma &\cong \frac{\pi f_1 M_3}{\lambda_0 \sqrt{\varepsilon_r}} \text{ rad/m} \\ &= \frac{1.8 f_1 M_3}{\lambda_0 \sqrt{\varepsilon_r}} \text{ degree/cm} \end{aligned} \tag{3.6}$$

θ_F is known as the Faraday rotation (FR) coefficient. When the direction of the magnetization is reversed, the angle of rotation changes its sign. Since two counterrotating circular polarized optical waves are used to explain FR, the effect is thus also known as optical magnetic circular birefringence (MCB). Furthermore, since the senses of polarization rotation of forward traveling and backward traveling light waves are opposite, FR is a nonreciprocal optical effect. Optical devices such as **optical isolators** and **optical circulators** use the Faraday effect to achieve their nonreciprocal functions. For ferromagnetic and ferrimagnetic media, the FR is characterized under a magnetically saturated condition, i.e., $M_3 = M_S$, the saturation magnetization of the medium. For paramagnetic or diamagnetic materials, the magnetization is proportional to the external applied magnetic field H_0. Therefore, the FR is proportional to the external field or $\theta_F = VH_0$ where $V = \chi_0 f_1 \pi / (\lambda_0 \sqrt{\varepsilon_r})$ is called the Verdet constant and χ_0 is the magnetic susceptibility of free space.

Cotton–Mouton Effect or Magnetic Linear Birefringence

When transmitted light is propagating perpendicular to the magnetization direction, the first-order isotropic FR effect will vanish and the second-order anisotropic Cotton–Mouton (CM) effect will dominate. For example, if the direction of magnetization is along the Z axis and the light wave is propagating along the X axis, the permittivity tensor becomes

$$\overleftrightarrow{\varepsilon} = \varepsilon_0 \begin{bmatrix} \varepsilon_r + f_{12} M_3^2 & 0 & 0 \\ 0 & \varepsilon_r + f_{12} M_3^2 & 0 \\ 0 & 0 & \varepsilon_r + f_{11} M_3^2 \end{bmatrix} \tag{3.7}$$

The eigenmodes are two linearly polarized light waves polarized along and perpendicular to the magnetization direction:

$$\tilde{E}_{\|}(x) = \begin{bmatrix} 0 \\ 0 \\ 1 \end{bmatrix} \exp\left[j\left(\omega t - \frac{2\pi}{\lambda_0} n_{\|} x \right) \right] \tag{3.8a}$$

$$\tilde{E}_{\perp}(x) = \begin{bmatrix} 0 \\ 1 \\ 0 \end{bmatrix} \exp\left[j\left(\omega t - \frac{2\pi}{\lambda_0} n_{\perp} x \right) \right] \tag{3.8b}$$

with $n_{\|}^2 = \varepsilon_r + f_{11}M_3^2$ and $n_{\perp}^2 = \varepsilon_r + f_{12}M_3^2$; $n_{\|}$ and $n_{\perp}$ are the refractive indices of the parallel and perpendicular linearly polarized modes, respectively. The difference in phase velocities between these two waves gives rise to a magnetic linear birefringence (MLB) of light which is also known as the CM or Voigt effect. In this case, the light transmitted through the crystal has elliptic polarization. The degree of ellipticity depends on the difference $n_{\|} - n_{\perp}$. The phase shift or retardation can be found by the following expression:

$$\psi_{cm} \cong \frac{\pi(f_{11} - f_{12})M_3^2}{\lambda_0\sqrt{\varepsilon_r}} \text{ rad/m}$$

or (3.9)

$$\frac{1.8(f_{11} - f_{12})M_3^2}{\lambda_0\sqrt{\varepsilon_r}} \text{ degree/cm}$$

Since the sense of this phase shift is unchanged when the direction of light propagation is reversed, the CM effect is a reciprocal effect.

Kerr Effects

Kerr effects occur when a light beam is reflected from a magneto-optic medium. There are three distinct types of Kerr effects, namely, polar, longitudinal (or meridional), and transverse (or equatorial). Figure 3.1 shows the configurations of these Kerr effects. A reflectivity tensor relation between the incident light and the reflected light can be used to describe the phenomena as follows:

$$\begin{bmatrix} E_{r\perp} \\ E_{r\|} \end{bmatrix} = \begin{bmatrix} r_{11} & r_{12} \\ r_{21} & r_{22} \end{bmatrix} \begin{bmatrix} E_{i\perp} \\ E_{i\|} \end{bmatrix} \tag{3.10}$$

where r_{ij} is the reflectance matrix. $E_{i\perp}$ and $E_{i\|}$ are, respectively, the perpendicular (TE) and parallel (TM) electric field components of the incident light waves (with respect to the plane of incidence). $E_{r\perp}$ and $E_{r\|}$ are, respectively, the perpendicular and parallel electric field components of the reflected light waves.

The diagonal elements r_{11} and r_{22} can be calculated by Fresnel reflection coefficients and Snell's law. The off-diagonal elements r_{12} and r_{21} can be derived from the magneto-optic permittivity tensor,

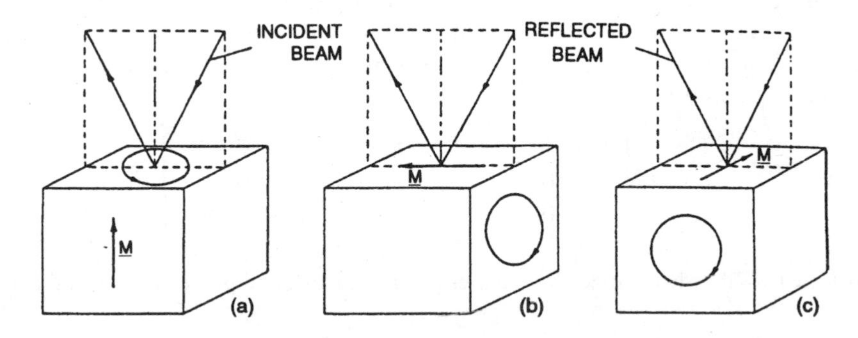

FIGURE 3.1 Kerr magneto-optic effect. The magnetization vector is represented by M while the plane of incidence is shown dotted: (a) polar; (b) longitudinal; (c) transverse. (*Source:* A.V. Sokolov, *Optical Properties of Metals,* London: Blackie, 1967. With permission.)

the applied magnetization and Maxwell equations with the use of appropriate boundary conditions (Arecchi and Schulz-DuBois, 1972). It is important to note that all the elements of the reflectance matrix r_{ij} are dependent on the angle of incidence between the incident light and the magneto-optic film surface.

Polar Kerr Effect

The polar Kerr effect takes place when the magnetization is perpendicular to the plane of the material. A pair of orthogonal linearly polarized reflected light modes will be induced and the total reflected light becomes elliptically polarized. The orientation of the major axis of the elliptic polarization of the reflected light is the same for both TE ($E_{i\perp}$) or TM ($E_{i\|}$) linearly polarized incident lights since $r_{12} = r_{21}$.

Longitudinal or Meridional Kerr Effect

The longitudinal Kerr effect takes place when the magnetization is in the plane of the material and parallel to the plane of incidence. Again, an elliptically polarized reflected light beam will be induced, but the orientation of the major axis of the elliptic polarization of the reflected light is opposite to each other for TE ($E_{i\perp}$) and TM ($E_{i\|}$) linearly polarized incident lights since $r_{12} = -r_{21}$.

Transverse or Equatorial Kerr Effect

This effect is also known as the equatorial Kerr effect. The magnetization in this case is in the plane of the material and perpendicular to the plane of incidence. The reflected light does not undergo a change in its polarization since $r_{12} = r_{21} = 0$. However, the intensity of the TM ($E_{r\|}$) reflected light will be changed if the direction of the magnetic field is suddenly reversed. For TE ($E_{r\perp}$) reflected light, this modulation effect is at least two orders of magnitude smaller and is usually ignored.

3.3 Applications of Magneto-optic Effects

Optical Isolator and Circulator

In fiber-optic-based communication systems with gigahertz bandwidth or coherent detection, it is often essential to eliminate back reflections from the fiber ends and other surfaces or discontinuities because they can cause amplitude fluctuations, frequency instabilities, limitation on modulation bandwidth, noise or even damage to the lasers. An optical isolator permits the forward transmission of light while simultaneously preventing reverse transmission with a high degree of extinction. The schematic configuration of a conventional optical isolator utilizing bulk rotator and permanent magnet (Johnson, 1966) is shown in Figure 3.2. It consists of a 45° polarization rotator which is nonreciprocal so that back-reflected light is rotated by exactly 90° and can therefore be excluded from the laser. The nonreciprocity is furnished by the Faraday effect. The basic operation principle is as follows: A Faraday isolator consists of rotator material immersed in a longitudinal magnetic field between two polarizers. Light emitted by the laser passes through

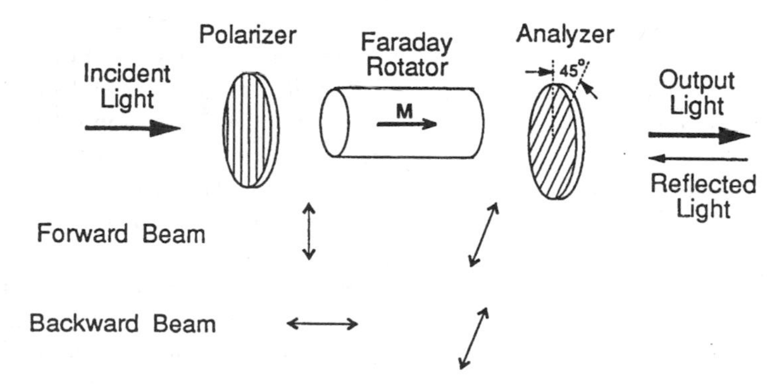

FIGURE 3.2 Schematic of an optical isolator. The polarization directions of forward and backward beams are shown below the schematic.

TABLE 3.1 Characteristics of YIG and BIG Faraday Rotators

	YIG	BIG
Verdet constant (min/cm-Gauss)		
1300 nm	10.5[a]	−806
1550 nm	9.2	−600
Saturated magneto-optic rotation (degree/mm)		
1300 nm	20.6	−136.4
1550 nm	18.5	−93.8
Thickness for 45° rotation (mm)		
1300 nm	2.14	0.33
1550 nm	2.43	0.48
Typical insertion loss (dB)	>0.4	<0.1
Typical reverse isolation (dB)	30–35	40
Required magnetic field (Gauss)	>1600	120
Magnetically tunable	No	Yes[b]

[a] Variable.
[b] Some BIG not tunable.
Source: D.K. Wilson, "Optical isolators adapt to communication needs," *Laser Focus World*, p. 175, April 1991. ©PennWell Publishing Company. With permission.

the second polarizer being oriented at 45° relative to the transmission axis of the first polarizer. Any subsequently reflected light is then returned through the second polarizer, rotated by another 45° before being extinguished by the first polarizer—thus optical isolation is achieved.

The major characteristics of an optical isolator include isolation level, insertion loss, temperature dependence, and size of the device. These characteristics are mainly determined by the material used in the rotator. Rotating materials generally fall into three categories: the paramagnetics (such as terbium-doped borosilicate glass), the diamagnetic (such as zinc selenide), and the ferromagnetic (such as rare-earth garnets). The first two kinds have small Verdet constants and mostly work in the visible or shorter optical wavelength range. Isolators for use with the InGaAsP semiconductor diode lasers ($\lambda_0 = 1100$ to 1600 nm), which serve as the essential light source in optical communication, utilize the third kind, especially the YIG crystal. A newly available ferromagnetic crystal, epitaxially grown bismuth–substituted yttrium–iron–garnet (BIG), has an order-of-magnitude stronger Faraday rotation than pure YIG, and its magnetic saturation occurs at a smaller field (Matsuda et al., 1987). The typical parameters with YIG and BIG are shown in Table 3.1. As the major user of optical isolators, fiber optic communication systems require different input-output packaging for the isolators. Table 3.2 lists the characteristics of the isolators according to specific applications (Wilson, 1991).

For the purpose of integrating the optical isolator component into the same substrate with the semiconductor laser to facilitate monolithic fabrication, integrated waveguide optical isolators become one of the most exciting areas for research and development. In a waveguide isolator, the rotation of the polarization is accomplished in a planar or channel waveguide. The waveguide is usually made of a magneto-optic thin film, such as YIG or BIG film, liquid phase epitaxially grown on a substrate, typically gadolinium–gallium–garnet (GGG) crystals. Among the many approaches in achieving the polarization rotation, such as the 45° rotation type or the unidirectional TE–TM mode converter type, the common point is the conversion or coupling process between the TE and TM modes of the waveguide. Although very good results have been obtained in some specific characteristics, for example, 60-dB isolation (Wolfe et al., 1990), the waveguide optical isolator is still very much in the research and development stage.

Usually, the precise wavelength of any given semiconductor diode is uncertain. Deviation from a specified wavelength could degrade isolator performance by 1 dB/nm, and an uncertainty of 10 nm can reduce isolation by 10 dB. Therefore, a tunable optical isolator is highly desirable. A typical approach is to simply place two isolators, tuned to different wavelengths, in tandem to provide a broadband response. Curves C and D of Figure 3.3 show that isolation and bandwidth are a function of the proximity of the wavelength peak positions. This combination of nontunable isolators has sufficiently wide spectral bandwidth to accommodate normal

TABLE 3.2 Applications of Optical Isolators

Application	Type	Wavelength Tunable	Isolation (dB)	Insertion Loss (dB)	Return Loss (dB)
Fiber to fiber	PI	Yes/no	30–40	1.0–2.0	>60
Fiber to fiber	PS	Normally no	33–42	1.0–2.0	>60
Single fiber	PS	No	38–42	Complex	Complex
Bulk optics	PS	No	38–42	0.1–0.2	

PI = polarization insensitive.
PS = polarization sensitive.
Source: D.K. Wilson, "Optical isolators adapt to communication needs," *Laser Focus World*, p. 175, April 1991. With permission.

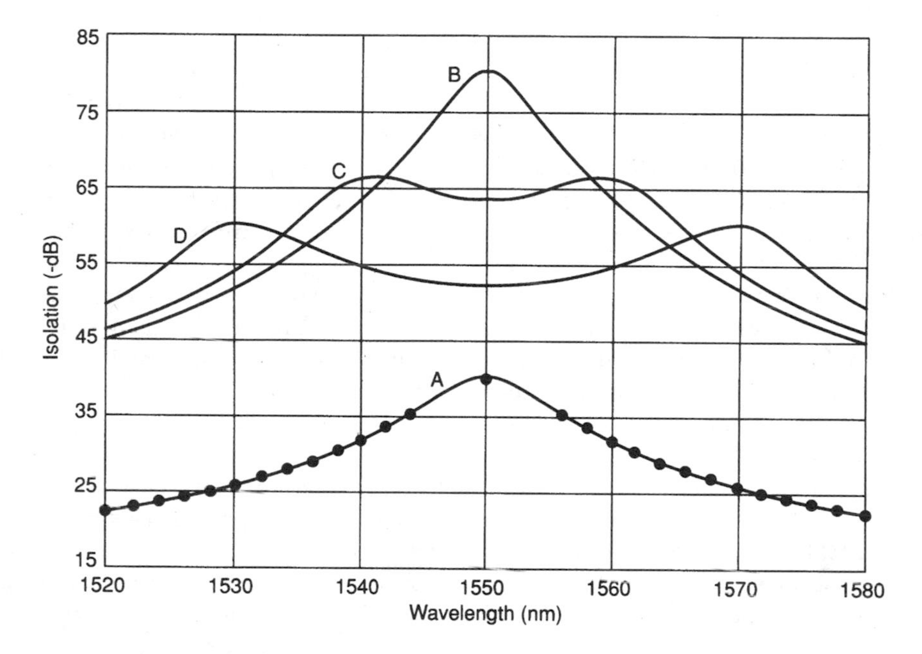

FIGURE 3.3 Isolation performance of four isolators centered around 1550 nm shows the effects of different configurations. A single-stage isolator (curve A) reaches about –40 dB isolation, and two cascaded single-wavelength isolators (curve B) hit –80 dB. Wavelength broadening (curves C and D) can be tailored by cascading isolators tuned to different wavelengths. (*Source:* D.K. Wilson, "Optical isolators adapt to communication needs," *Laser Focus World*, April 1991. With permission.)

wavelength variations found in typical diode lasers. In addition, because the laser wavelength depends on its operating temperature, this broadened spectral bandwidth widens the operating temperature range without decreasing isolation.

The factors that limit isolation are found in both the polarizers and the Faraday rotator materials. Intrinsic strain, inclusions, and surface reflections contribute to a reduction in the purity of polarization which affects isolation. About 40 dB is the average isolation for today's materials in a single-isolator stage. If two isolators are cascaded in tandem, it is possible to double the isolation value.

Finally, an optical circulator (Fletcher and Weisman, 1965) can be designed by replacing the polarizers in a conventional isolator configuration with a pair of calcite polarizing prisms. A laser beam is directed through a calcite prism, then through a Faraday rotator material which rotates the polarization plane by 45°, then through a second calcite prism set to pass polarization at 45°. Any reflection beyond this second calcite prism returns through the second prism, is rotated by another 45° through the Faraday material, and, because its polarization is now 90° from the incident beam, is deflected by the first calcite prism. The four ports of the circulator then are found as follows: (1) the incident beam, (2) the exit beam, (3) the deflected beam from the first calcite prism, and (4) the deflected beam from the second calcite prism.

MSW-Based Guided-Wave Magneto-optic Bragg Cell

When a ferrimagnet is placed in a sufficiently large externally applied dc magnetic field, H_0, the ferrimagnetic materials become magnetically saturated to produce a saturation magnetization $4\pi M_S$. Under this condition, each individual magnetic dipole will precess in resonance with frequency $f_{res} = \gamma H_0$ where γ is the gyromagnetic ratio ($\gamma = 2.8$ MHz/Oe). However, due to the dipole–dipole coupling and quantum mechanical exchange coupling, the collective interactions among neighboring magnetic dipole moments produce a continuum spectrum of precession modes or spin waves at frequency bands near f_{res}. Exchange-free spin wave spectra obtained under the magnetostatic approximation are known as magnetostatic waves (MSWs) (Ishak, 1988). In essence, MSWs are relatively slow propagating, dispersive, magnetically dominated electromagnetic (EM) waves which exist in biased ferrites at microwave frequencies (2 to 20 GHz). In a ferrimagnetic film with a finite thickness, such as a YIG thin film epitaxially grown on a nonmagnetic substrate such as GGG, MSW modes are classified into three types: magnetostatic surface wave (MSSW), magnetostatic forward volume wave (MSFVW), and magnetostatic backward volume wave (MSBVW), depending on the orientation of the dc magnetic field with respect to the film plane and the propagation direction of the MSW. At a constant dc magnetic field, each type of mode only exists in a certain frequency band. An important feature of MSW is that these frequency bands can be simply tuned by changing the dc magnetic field.

As a result of the Faraday rotation effect and Cotton–Mouton effect, the magnetization associated with MSWs will induce a perturbation in the dielectric tensor. When MSW propagates in the YIG film, it induces a moving optical grating which facilitates the diffraction of an incident guided light beam. If the so-called Bragg condition is satisfied between the incident guided light and the MSW-induced optical grating, Bragg diffraction takes place. An optical device built based on this principle is called the **magneto-optic Bragg cell** (Tsai and Young, 1990).

A typical MSFVW-based noncollinear coplanar guided-wave magneto-optic Bragg cell is schematically shown in Figure 3.4. Here a homogeneous dc bias magnetic field is applied along the Z axis to excite a Y-propagating MSFVW generated by a microstrip line transducer. With a guided lightwave coupled into the YIG waveguide and propagating along the X axis, a portion of the lightwave is Bragg-diffracted and mode-converted (TE to TM mode and vice versa). The Bragg-diffracted light is scanned in the waveguide plane as

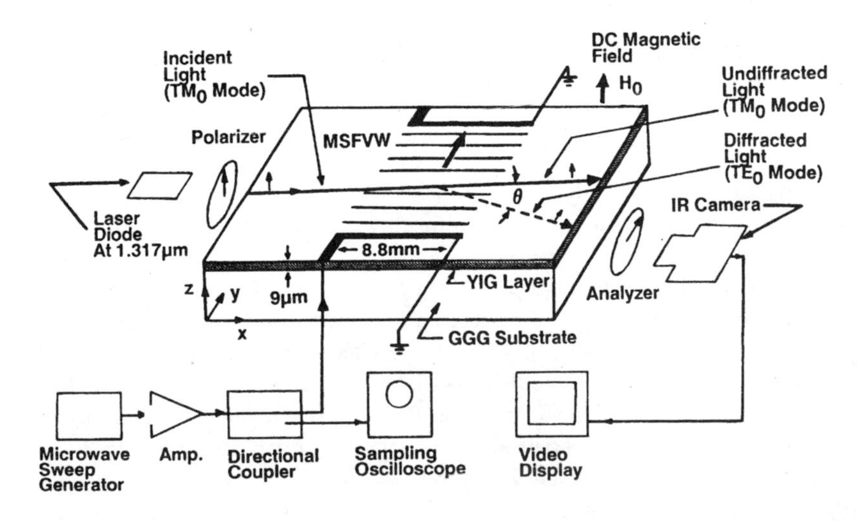

FIGURE 3.4 Experimental arrangement for scanning of guided-light beam in YIG–GGG waveguide using magnetostatic forward waves.

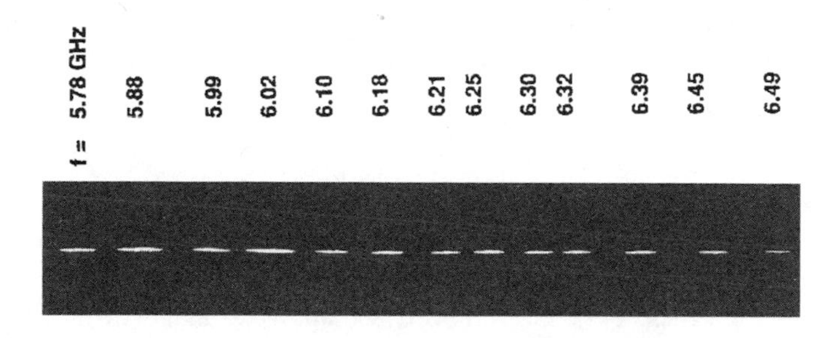

FIGURE 3.5 Deflected light spots obtained by varying the carrier frequency of MSFVW around 6 GHz.

the frequency of the MSFVW is tuned. Figure 3.5 shows the scanned light spots by tuning the frequency at a constant dc magnetic field.

MSW-based guided-wave magneto-optic Bragg cell is analogous to surface acoustic wave (SAW)-based guided-wave acousto-optic (AO) Bragg cell and has the potential to significantly enhance a wide variety of integrated optical applications which had previously been implemented with SAW. These include TE–TM mode converter, spectrum analyzer, convolvers/correlators, optical frequency shifters, tunable narrowband optical filters, and optical beam scanners/switches (Young, 1989). In comparison to their AO counterparts, the MSW-based magneto-optic Bragg cell modules may possess the following unique advantages: (1) A much larger range of tunable carrier frequencies (2 to 20 GHz, for example) may be readily obtained by varying a dc magnetic field. Such high and tunable carrier frequencies with the magneto-optic device modules allow direct processing at the carrier frequency of wide-band RF signals rather than indirect processing via frequency down-conversion, as is required with the AO device modules. (2) A large magneto-optic bandwidth may be realized by means of a simpler transducer geometry. (3) Much higher and electronically tunable modulation/switching and scanning speeds are possible as the velocity of propagation for the MSW is higher than that of SAW by one to two orders of magnitude, depending upon the dc magnetic field and the carrier frequency.

Magneto-optic Recording

The write/erase mechanism of the **magneto-optical (MO) recording system** is based on a thermomagnetic process in a perpendicularly magnetized magneto-optic film. A high-power pulsed laser is focused to heat up a small area on the magneto-optic medium. The coercive force of the MO layer at room temperature is much greater than that of a conventional non-MO magnetic recording medium. However, this coercive force is greatly reduced when the heated spot is raised to a critical temperature. Application of a bias magnetic field can then easily reverse the polarization direction of the MO layer within the heated spot. As a result, a very small magnetic domain with magnetization opposite to that of the surrounding area is generated. This opposite magnetic domain will persist when the temperature of the medium is lowered. The magnetization-reversed spot represents one bit of stored data. To erase data, the same thermal process can be applied while reversing the direction of the bias magnetic field.

To read the stored information optically, the Kerr effect is used to detect the presence of these very small magnetic domains within the MO layer. When a low-power polarized laser beam is reflected by the perpendicularly oriented MO medium, the polarization angle is twisted through a small angle θ_k, the Kerr rotation. Furthermore, the direction of this twist is either clockwise or counterclockwise, depending on the orientation of the perpendicular magnetic moment, which is either upward or downward. Therefore, as the read beam scans across an oppositely magnetized domain from the surrounding medium, there is a total change of $2\theta_k$ in the polarization directions from the reflected beam coming from the two distinct regions. Reading is done by detecting this phase difference.

The MO recording medium is one of the most important elements in a high-performance MO data-storage system. In order to achieve fast writing and erasing functions, a large Kerr rotation is required to produce an acceptable carrier-to-noise (C/N) ratio. In general, a high-speed MO layer has a read signal with a poor C/N ratio, while a good read-performance MO layer is slow in write/erase sensitivity.

Defining Terms

Cotton–Mouton effect: Second-order anisotropic reciprocal magneto-optic effect which causes a linearly polarized incident light to transmit through as an elliptically polarized output light wave when the propagation direction of the incident light is perpendicular to the direction of the applied magnetization of the magneto-optic medium. It is also known as magnetic linear birefringence (MLB).

Faraday rotation: First-order isotropic nonreciprocal magneto-optic effect which causes the polarization direction of a linearly polarized transmitted light to rotate when the propagation direction of the incident light wave is parallel to the direction of the applied magnetization of the magneto-optic medium. It is also known as magnetic circular birefringence (MCB).

Kerr effects: Reflected light from a magneto-optic medium can be described by the optical Kerr effects. There are three types of Kerr effects: polar, longitudinal, and transverse, depending on the directions of the magnetization with respect to the plane of incidence and the reflecting film surface.

Magneto-optic Bragg cell: A magnetically tunable microwave signal processing device which uses optical Bragg diffraction of light from a moving magneto-optic grating generated by the propagation of magnetostatic waves within the magnetic medium.

Magneto-optic recording system: A read/write data recording system based on a thermomagnetic process to write oppositely magnetized domains onto a magneto-optic medium by means of high-power laser heating. Magneto-optic Kerr effect is then employed to read the data by using a low-power laser as a probe beam to sense the presence of these domains.

Optical circulator: A four-port optical device that can be used to monitor or sample incident light (input port) as well as reflected light (output port) with the two other unidirectional coupling ports.

Optical isolator: A unidirectional optical device which only permits the transmission of light in the forward direction. Any reflected light from the output port is blocked by the device from returning to the input port with a very high extinction ratio.

References

F.T. Arecchi and E.O. Schulz-DuBois, *Laser Handbook*, D4, Amsterdam: North-Holland, 1972, pp. 1009–1027.

P.C. Fletcher and D.L. Weisman, "Circulators for optical radar systems," *Appl. Opt.*, 4, pp. 867–873, 1965.

K.H. Hellwege, *Landolt-Bornstein Numerical Data and Functional Relationships in Science and Technology, New Series*, vols. 4 and 12, New York: Springer, 1978.

W.S. Ishak, "Magnetostatic wave technology: a review," in *Proc. IEEE*, vol. 76, pp. 171–187, 1988.

B. Johnson, "The Faraday effect at near infrared wavelength in rare-earth garnet," *Brit. J. Appl. Phys.*, 17, 1441, 1966.

K. Matsuda, H. Minemoto, O. Kamada, and S. Isbizuka, "Bi-substituted, rare-earth iron garnet composite film with temperature independent Faraday rotation for optical isolators," *IEEE Trans. Mag.*, MAG-23, 3479, 1987.

M. Torfeh, L. Courtois, L. Smoczynski, H. Le Gall, and J.M. Desvignes, "Coupling and phase matching coefficients in a magneto-optical TE-TM mode converter," *Physica*, 89B, pp. 255–259, 1977.

C.S. Tsai and D. Young, "Magnetostatic-forward-volume-wave-based guided-waveless magneto-optic Bragg cells and applications to communications and signal processing," *IEEE Trans. Microw. Theory Technol.*, vol. MTT-38, no. 5, pp. 560–30, 1990.

D.K. Wilson, "Optical isolators adapt to communication needs," *Laser Focus World*, 175, 1991.

R. Wolfe et al., "Edge tuned ridge waveguide magneto-optic isolator," *Appl. Phys. Lett.*, 56, 426, 1990.

D. Young, "Guided wave magneto-optic Bragg cells using Yttrium Iron Garnet-Gadolinium Gallium Garnet (YIG-GGG) thin film at microwave frequencies," Ph.D. Dissertation, University of California, Irvine, CA, 1989.

Further Information

Current publications on magneto-optics can be found in the following journals: *Intermag Conference Proceedings* published by the IEEE and *International Symposium Proceedings on Magneto-Optics.*

For in-depth discussion on magnetic bubble devices, please see, for example, *Magnetic-Bubble Memory Technology* by Hsu Chang, published by Marcel Dekker, 1978.

An excellent source of information on garnet materials can be found in *Magnetic Garnet* by Gerhard Winkler, published by Friedr. Vieweg & Sohn, 1981.

Numerous excellent reviews on the subject of magneto-optics have been published over the years, for example, J.F. Dillon, Jr., "Magneto-optics and its uses," *Journal of Magnetism and Magnetic Materials*, vol. 31–34, pp. 1–9, 1983; M.J. Freiser, "A survey of magneto-optic effects," *IEEE Transactions on Magnetics*, vol. MAG-4, pp. 152–161, 1968; G. A. Smolenskii, R.V. Pisarev, and I.G. Sinii, "Birefringence of light in magnetically ordered crystals," *Sov. Phys. Usp.*, vol. 18, pp. 410–429, 1976; and A.M. Prokhorov, G.A. Smolenskii, and A.N. Ageev, "Optical phenomena in thin-film magnetic waveguides and their technical application," *Sov. Phys. Usp.*, vol. 27, pp. 339–362, 1984.

4

Materials and Nanoscience

4.1 Carbon Nanotubes 4-1
Introduction • Structure and Properties • Growth • Nano-Electronics • AFM Imaging Using CNT Probes • Sensors • Field Emission • Summary

4.2 Modeling MEMS and NEMS 4-9
Micro- and Nano-Electromechanical Systems • The Science of Scale • Modeling Approaches

4.3 Micromechatronics 4-20
Introduction to Micromechatronics Systems • Synchronous Micromachines • Fabrication Aspects • Electroactive and Magnetoactive Materials • Induced-Strain Actuators • Piezoelectric Wafer Active Sensors • Microcontrollers Sensing, Actuation, and Process Control

4.4 Nanocomputers, Nano-Architectronics, and Nano-ICs............ 4-42
Introduction • Nano-Electronics and Nanocomputer Fundamentals • Nanocomputer Architecture • Hierarchical Finite-State Machines and Their Use in Hardware and Software Design • Reconfigurable Nanocomputers • Mathematical Models for Nanocomputers • Nanocompensator Synthesis and Design Aspects

4.5 Semiconductor Nano-Electronics and Nano-Optoelectronics 4-68
Introduction to Semiconductor Nanotechnology • Fundamental Physics of Semiconductor Nanotechnology—Quantum Physics • Semiconductor Nano-Electronics—Resonant Tunneling Diode • Semiconductor Nano-Electronics—Single Electron Transistors • Semiconductor Nano-Optoelectronics • Future: Quantum Effects and Semiconductor Nanotechnology

M. Meyyappan
NASA Ames Research Center

John Pelesko
University of Delaware

Victor Giurgiutiu
University of South Carolina

Sergey Edward Lyshevski
Rochester Institute of Technology

Nelson Tansu
Lehigh University

Ronald Arif
Lehigh University

Zhian Jin
Lehigh University

4.1 Carbon Nanotubes

M. Meyyappan

Introduction

Carbon nanotubes (CNTs) were discovered in 1991 [1] by Sumio Iijima of the NEC Corporation. Since then, research activities exploring their structure, properties, and applications have exploded across the world. Carbon nanotubes exhibit unique electronic properties and extraordinary mechanical properties, and, hence, have received attention in nano-electronics, sensors, actuators, field emission devices, high strength composites and a host of other applications. A detailed discussion on properties, growth, characterization, and application development can be found in a recent textbook [2]. Here, a brief overview of these subject matters is presented.

Structure and Properties

Configurationally, a carbon nanotube can be thought of as a two-dimensional graphene sheet rolled up in the form of a tube. A single-walled carbon nanotube (SWNT) is a tubular shell made of hexagonal rings (in a sheet) of carbon atoms, with the ends of the shells capped by dome-like half-fullerene molecules. The SWNTs are classified using a nomenclature (n, m) where n and m are integer indices of two graphene unit lattice vectors corresponding to the chiral vector of a nanotube (see Figure 4.1) [3]. A multiwalled carbon nanotube (MWNT) is configurationally a stack of graphene sheets rolled up into concentric cylinders with the ends either closed with half-fullerenes or left open. Figure 4.2 shows transmission electron microscopy (TEM) images of a SWNT and a MWNT. The individual SWNTs in Figure 4.2a is about 1 nm in diameter. The MWNT has a central core with several walls with a spacing close to 0.34 nm between two successive walls (Figure 4.2b).

A SWNT can be either metallic or semiconducting depending on its chirality, i.e., the values of n and m. When $(n-m)/3$ is an integer, the nanotube is metallic; otherwise, it is semiconducting. The diameter of the nanotube is given by $d = (a_g/\pi)\ (n^2 + mn + m^2)^{0.5}$ where a_g is the lattice constant of graphite. The resistance of a metallic CNT is $h/(4e^2) \approx 6.5\, K\Omega$ where h is Planck's constant.

Growth

The earliest technique reported for producing CNTs is arc synthesis [1,4] which uses a dc arc discharge in argon created between a pair of graphite electrodes. The graphite anode has a small fraction of a transition metal such as Fe, Ni, or Co as a catalyst. The electric arc vaporizes the anode, forming nanotubes in the discharge. Later this process was mimicked in a laser ablation approach [5], wherein an argon ion laser beam vaporizes a target that consists of graphite mixed with a small amount of transition metal catalyst. Both methods produce SWNTs and MWNTs with catalyst particles and soot as common impurities. While laser ablation may not be amenable for scale up to produce large quantities, arc synthesis has been successfully used

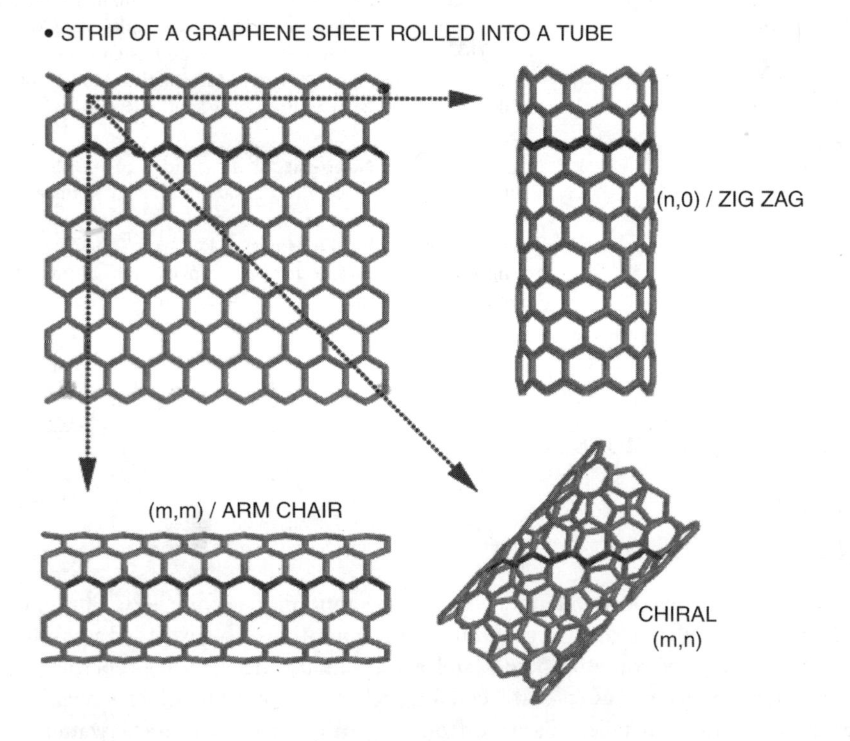

FIGURE 4.1 A strip of a graphene sheet rolled into a tube.

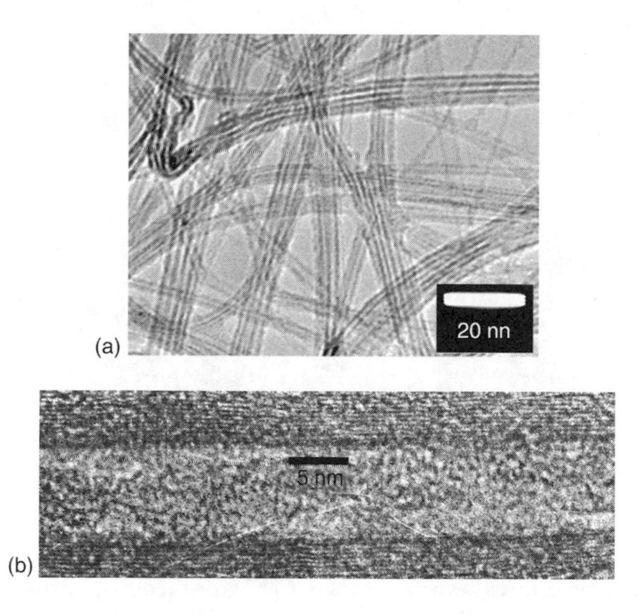

FIGURE 4.2 TEM images of (a) SWNT ropes; (b) a MWNT. (Image courtesy of Lance Delzeit.)

for high volume production of MWNTs. Moravsky et al. [6] provide an overview of arc synthesis and laser ablation for producing SWNTs and MWNTs.

Development of large-scale production techniques is critical to realize such applications as composites, catalyst support, membranes, filters, etc. However, for making nanodevices and sensors, "pick and place" from bulk samples may be too tedious to be of any value unless some bottom-up device processing schemes emerge in the future. In the meantime, growth techniques that are amenable to selectivity grow CNTs in predesigned locations and on wafers are highly desirable. In this regard, chemical vapor deposition (CVD) and its variations such as plasma enhanced CVD (PECVD) have gained much attention in the past five years [7].

CVD is well known in silicon integrated circuit (IC) manufacturing for depositing thin metallic, semi-conducting and dielectric layers. CVD of CNTs typically involves a hydrocarbon feedstock with the aid of a transition metal catalyst. Common precursors have included methane, ethylene, acetylene, and carbon monoxide, to name a few. The catalyst choices have included iron, nickel, or cobalt. These metals can be thermally evaporated as a thin film on the substrate or sputtered using ion beam sputtering or magnetron sputtering. Alternatively, the catalyst metal can be applied to the substrate, starting from the metal containing salt solution and going through a number of steps such as precipitation, mixing, evaporation, annealing, etc. The key is to obtain a particulate nature to facilitate nanotube growth. Characterization of as-deposited catalysts using TEM and atomic force microscopy [8] reveals that the particles are in the range of 1 to 10 nm in size. The catalyst may also be patterned using some form of lithography for selective growth on the wafer. The growth process proceeds at atmospheric pressure and temperatures of 550 to 1000°C with typically higher temperatures for SWNTs. Figure 4.3 shows bundles of SWNTs grown using methane with an iron catalyst prepared by ion beam sputtering. The corresponding TEM image showing the tendency of nanotubes to form bundles or ropes is shown in Figure 4.2a. Figure 4.4 shows patterned MWNT growth on a silicon substrate using an iron catalyst which appears to yield a vertical array of nanotubes. Though the ensemble looks vertical, a closer view would reveal in all cases of thermal CVD, the individual MWNT itself is not well aligned but wavy.

In contrast to thermal CVD, PECVD enables individual, freestanding, vertically aligned MWNT structures though these are disordered with a bamboo-like inner core. For that reason, they are called multi-walled carbon nanofibers (MWNFs) or simply carbon nanofibers (CNFs) [9]. PECVD is also capable of producing MWNTs, though they will be similar to the CVD material in the sense that the ensemble may appear to be vertical but not the individual nanotubes.

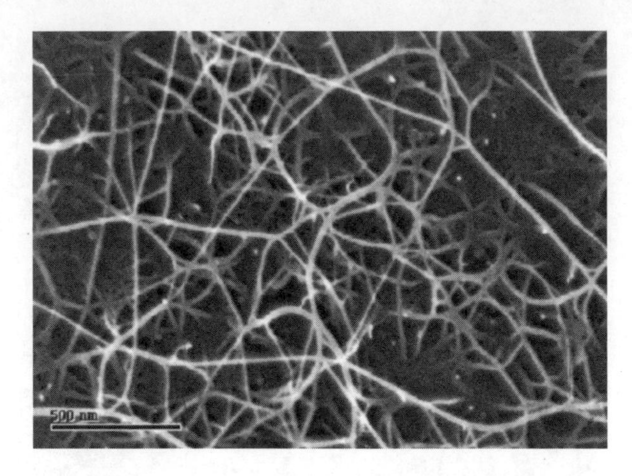

FIGURE 4.3 SEM image of single-walled nanotubes grown using CVD.

To date, a variety of plasma sources have been used in CNT growth: dc, rf, microwave, and inductive power sources [10–14]. The plasma efficiently breaks down the hydrocarbon feedstock, creating a variety of reactive radicals, which are also the source for amorphous carbon; for this reason, the feedstock is typically diluted with hydrogen, ammonia, argon, or nitrogen to keep the hydrocarbon fraction less than about 20%. Since CNT growth is catalyst activated, the growth temperature is determined by a combination of factors such as catalytic reaction on the surface and diffusion of carbon into the particle (in the so-called vapor–liquid–solid mechanism, if that is applicable). It appears from most published results that the above processes proceed at reasonable rates only at elevated temperatures, above 500°C. Though the plasma itself is capable of heating the substrate to temperatures above 500°C at moderate to high powers, the PECVD reactor for CNT growth is typically equipped with separate substrate heating. In most cases, this is in the form of a resistive heater beneath the platform holding the substrate whereas occasionally the use of a hot filament has also been reported [12]. It is entirely unlikely that such an intrusive filament would be accepted in manufacturing practice as it is a source of contamination due to the possible flaking of the filament itself.

Whereas thermal CVD of CNTs is primarily an atmospheric pressure operation, PECVD proceeds at low pressures. However, the typical 1 to 100 mTorr operation common in plasma etching and PECVD in IC

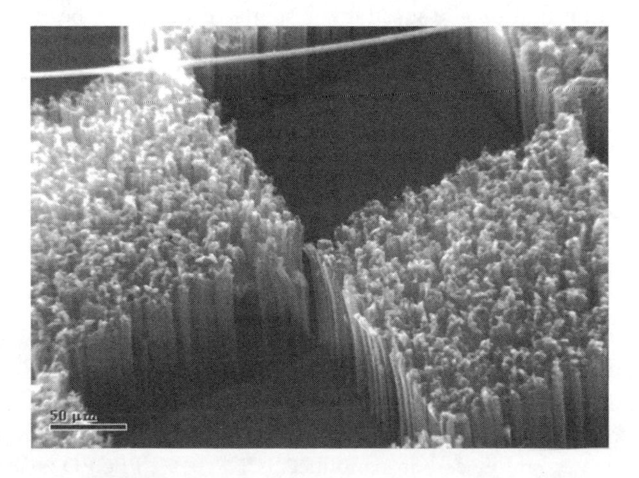

FIGURE 4.4 MWNTs grown by thermal CVD on a patterned silicon substrate using an iron catalyst (growth time = 5 min). (Image courtesy of Hou Tee Ng.)

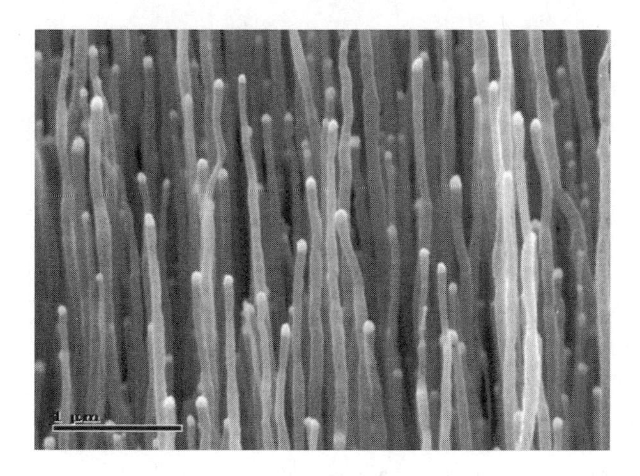

FIGURE 4.5 Vertical carbon nanofibers grown using plasma CVD. (Image courtesy of Alan Cassell.)

manufacturing has not been the case in CNT growth; mostly the growth is reported to be in the pressure range of 1 to 20 Torr. Figure 4.5 shows an SEM image of PECVD grown MWNFs wherein the individual structures are well separated and vertical. The TEM image reveals the disordered inner core and also the catalyst particle at the top. In contrast, in most cases of MWNT growth by thermal and plasma CVD, the catalyst particle is typically at the base of the nanotubes.

Nano-electronics

Silicon CMOS-based electronics has been moving forward impressively according to Moore's law with 90-nm feature scale devices currently in production and 65-nm devices in the development stage. As further miniaturization continues, a range of technological difficulties is anticipated, according to the Semiconductor Industry Association Roadmap [15]. These issues include lithography, novel dielectric materials, heat dissipation, and chip cooling issues to name a few. It was thought a few years ago that Si CMOS scaling may end around 50 nm; beyond 50 nm alternatives such as CNT electronics or molecular electronics may be needed. This is no longer true. The current wisdom is that scaling beyond 50 nm is possible, though with increased challenges. Regardless of when the need for transition to alternatives emerges, a viable alternative technology is expected to meet the following criteria.

1. The new technology must be easier and cheaper to manufacture than Si CMOS.
2. A high current drive is needed with the ability to drive capacitances of interconnects of any length.
3. A reliability factor enjoyed to date must be available (i.e., operating time > 10 years).
4. A high level of integration must be possible ($>10^{10}$ transistors/circuit).
5. A very high reproducibility is expected.
6. The technology should not be handicapped with high heat dissipation problems which are currently forecast for the silicon technology; otherwise, attractive solutions must be available to tackle the problem.

Of course, the present status of CNT electronics is too much at its infancy to evaluate how it stacks up against the goals listed above. This is due to the fact that most efforts to date [16, 17] are aimed at fabrication of single devices, such as diodes and transistors, with little effort on circuits and integration. The CNT field effect transistors are simple devices where a SWNT bridges the source and drain contacts separated by about a micron. The contacts are defined by lithography on a layer of SiO_2 grown on a silicon wafer that acts as a backgate. The *I–V* characteristics showed that the gate voltage can and does control the current flow through the nanotube. In this FET, the holes are the majority carriers and the best performance to date shows I_{on}/I_{off} ratio and transconductance values of about 10^4 and 1550 mS/mm, respectively. Attempts have been made to construct logic devices as well. Ref. [18] reports a CNT inverter by connecting *p*-type and *n*-type nanotube transistors. The inverter operated at room temperature and showed a gain greater than 1.

Carbon nanotube based flash memory has been fabricated by Choi et al. [19]. The source–drain gap was bridged with a SWNT as a conducting channel and the structure had a floating gate and a control gate. By grounding the source and applying 5 and 12 V at the drain and control gate, writing of 1 was achieved. This corresponds to the charging of the floating gate. To write 0, the source was biased at 12 V, the control gate was fixed at 0 V and the drain was allowed to float. Now the electrons on the floating gate tunneled to the source and the floating gate was discharged. To read, a voltage V_R was applied to the control gate and depending on the state of the floating gate (1 or 0), the drain current was either negligible or finite, respectively. Choi et al. [19] reported an appreciable threshold modulation for their SWNT flash memory operation. A detailed discussion of CNT electronics developments to date with operational principles can be found in Ref. [20].

AFM Imaging Using CNT Probes

Atomic force microscopy (AFM) has emerged as a powerful tool to image a wide variety of materials with high resolution. The conventional probes at the end of an AFM cantilever currently have a tip radius of curvature about 20 to 30 nm obtained by micromachining or reactive ion etching. The probes are typically silicon or Si_3N_4 and exhibit significant wear in continuous use. The worn probes can break during tapping mode or contact mode operation. Dai et al. [21] demonstrated that a MWNT tip, attached to the end of an AFM cantilever, is capable of functioning as AFM probe and provides better resolution than conventional probes. Whereas in this seminal work, the CNT was manually attached to the cantilever—which is difficult and not practical—more recently alternative schemes including *in situ* growth of the tip by CVD have been reported [22] and even large scale fabrication of probes on a 4-in. wafer using PECVD has been demonstrated [23].

Figure 4.6 shows an image of an iridium thin film collected using a SWNT probe. The nanoscale resolution is remarkable but, more importantly, the tip has been shown to be very robust and significantly slow-wearing compared to conventional probes [22]. The SWNTs with a typical diameter of 1 to 1.5 nm cannot be longer than about 75 nm for probe construction due to thermal vibration problems. The MWNTs, in contrast, can form 2- to 3-μm long probes ideal for performing profilometry in IC manufacturing.

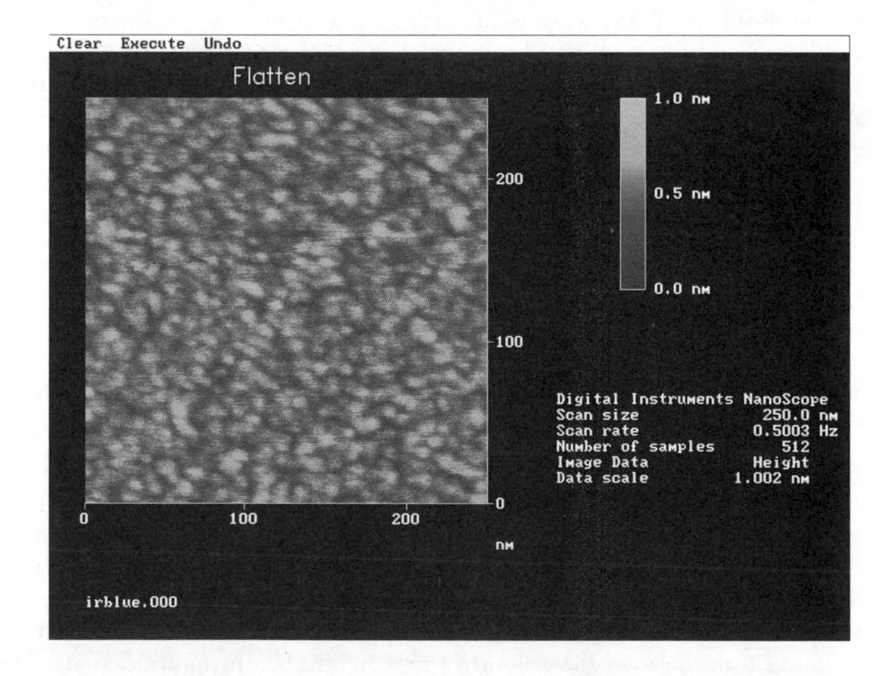

FIGURE 4.6 AFM image of an iridium thin film collected using a SWNT probe tip. (Image courtesy of Cattien Nguyen.)

It is possible to sharpen the tip of MWNTs to reach the same size as SWNTs, thus allowing construction of long probes without the thermal stability issues while yielding the resolution of SWNTs [24]. Both SWNT and sharpened MWNT probes have been used to image semiconductor, metallic, and dielectric thin films commonly encountered in IC manufacturing. In addition, imaging of biological samples such as DNA and protein has also been demonstrated. While most of the early works on imaging biological materials used dried samples, more recently imaging of DNA in aqueous environment has been reported [25]. In this case, the hydrophobic nature of the nanotube probe was altered by coating it with ethylenediamine making the probe hydrophilic to enable imaging in liquid medium.

Sensors

The interesting electronic properties and mechanical robustness, combined with the ability to attach functional chemical groups to the tip or sidewall, have made CNTs an ideal material for constructing chemical and biosensors. A SWNT with all the atoms on the surface is very sensitive to its chemical surroundings exhibited by a change in electrical conductivity due to charge transfer between the nanotube and species. This concept was first used [26] in constructing a chemical field effect transistor or CHEMFET in which a SWNT forms the conducting channel. Variations in conductivity have been measured when exposed to ammonia and NO_2. For NO_2, the charge transfer is from the CNT to the molecule which causes an enhancement of holes in the nanotube and leads to an increase in current.

The FET approach to sensing dates back to the time high temperature oxides such as tin oxide formed the channel in CHEMFET fabrication. Since the publication of Ref. [26], a much simpler device consisting of microfabricated interdigited electrodes has been fabricated which uses a bundle of SWNTs instead of a single nanotube [27]. This sensor has been shown to have a sensitivity of parts per billion (ppb) for a variety of gases and vapors such as NO_2, nitrotoluene, acetone, and benzene. The issue of selectivity has not yet been addressed in any of the conductivity-based CNT sensors.

Fabrication of biosensors takes advantage of functionalized chemical groups serving as probe molecules at the tip of the nanotube. In one approach (see Figure 4.7), nanoelectrodes are fabricated with MWNFs using microfabrication techniques [28]. First, MWNFs are grown on predetermined locations using PECVD on a patterned wafer. The separation distance between neighboring tubes is determined by the desire to avoid overlapping diffusion layers in an electrochemical approach. Also, in order to lend mechanical robustness and electrical isolation, the gap between nanotubes is filled with a dielectric such as SiO_2. This can be readily achieved by thermal CVD using TEOS followed by a chemical mechanical polishing step to provide a planar

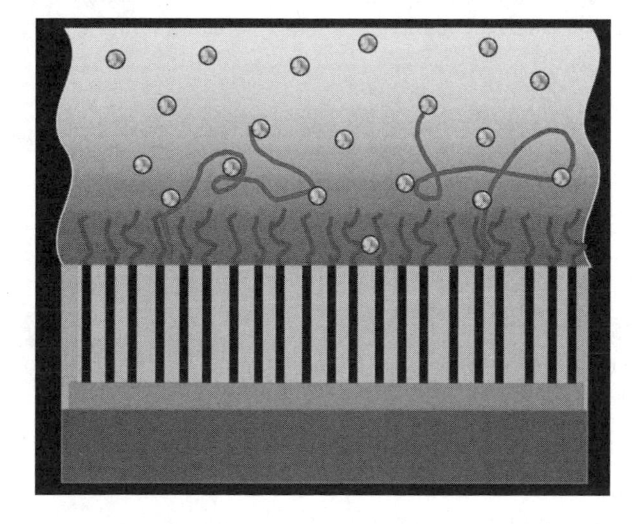

FIGURE 4.7 Schematic of carbon nanotube based biosensor. (Image courtesy of Jun Li.)

top surface with CNT ends exposed. These CNT ends can then be derivatized with DNA, PNA, or other probe molecules. Li et al. [28] performed cyclovoltammetry measurements and showed a capability of less than 1000 target molecules. This limit approaches that of laser-based fluorescence techniques and the approach offers a high degree of miniaturization and multiplex operation in molecular diagnosis. The sensor platform approach is amenable for developing handheld diagnostic devices for chemical diagnostics, biothreat detection, and similar applications.

Field Emission

CNTs have been shown to be excellent field emitters in a number of studies and a review can be found in Ref. [29]. The high aspect ratio of the CNTs and small tip radius of curvature are ideal for field emission. The emission has been observed at fields less than 1 V/μm and current densities as high as 1 A/cm^2 have been obtained. All forms of nanotubes—SWNTs, MWNTs, and MWNFs—and grown by all methods have been shown to be useful in field emission applications although emission characteristics vary with structure, preparation technique and impurity level.

Applications for CNT field emitters are broad and indeed, any application requiring an electron source is a candidate. Currently the biggest driver for the CNT field emission research is the potential to develop flat panel television displays. In a CNT-based field emission display (FED), controlled bombardment of electrons on a phosphor induces local emission, much like in a cathode ray tube (CRT). However, unlike in a CRT, the CNT–FED will have numerous electron sources, indeed one per pixel. The absence of beam scanning inherent in a CRT allows close placement of the electron source to the screen thus enabling a thin display. Currently several companies in Korea and Japan have developed prototype flat panel displays based on CNT–FED as large as 40-in. screen. Other CNT–FED applications include vacuum microelectronics, microwave amplifiers, electric propulsion, and x-ray tubes.

Summary

The interesting properties of carbon nanotubes have spurred an extraordinary amount of research activity. Much progress has been made in CNT growth by a variety of techniques, but as of now no control on the chirality of the CNTs during growth is possible. Characterization techniques to examine the grown structure have advanced rapidly and significant efforts continue across the world to measure electrical, mechanical, optical, thermal, magnetic, and other properties. Application development has been receiving the strongest attention with focus on nanoelectronics, sensors, field emission, scanning probes, actuators, gas adsorption and storage, and composites. All of these activities are in their early stages and there are no commercial products with mass market appeal in the market now. The CNT community believes that this will change in a decade.

Acknowledgment

The author gratefully acknowledges his colleagues at NASA Ames Research Center for Nanotechnology for much of the material presented in this chapter.

References

1. S. Iijima, *Nature*, 354, 56, 1991.
2. M. Meyyappan, Ed., *Carbon Nanotubes: Science and Applications*, Boca Raton, FL: CRC Press, 2004.
3. J. Han, chap. 1 in Ref. [2].
4. T. W. Ebbesen and P.M. Ajayan, *Nature*, 358, 220, 1992.
5. T. Guo et al., *Chem. Phys. Lett.*, 243, 49, 1995.
6. A.P. Moravsky, E.M. Wexler, R.O. Loutfy, chap. 3 in Ref. [2].
7. M. Meyyappan, chapter 4 in Ref. [3]; see references therein.
8. L. Delzeit et al., *Chem. Phys. Lett.*, 348, 368, 2001.

9. M. Meyyappan et al., *Plasma Sour. Sci. Technol.* 12, 205, 2003.
10. V.I. Merkulov et al., *Appl. Phys. Lett.*, 76, 3555, 2000.
11. M. Chhowalla et al., *J. Appl. Phys.*, 90, 5308, 2001.
12. Z.F. Ren et al., *Science*, 282, 1105, 1998.
13. C. Bower et al., *Appl. Phys. Lett.*, 77, 830, 2000.
14. K. Matthews et al., *J. Nanosci. Nanotech.* 2, 475, 2002.
15. *International Technology Roadmap for Semiconductors*, San Jose, CA: Semiconductor Industry Association, 2001.
16. S.J. Tans et al., *Nature*, 393, 49, 1998.
17. R. Martel et al., *Appl. Phys. Lett.*, 76, 2447, 1998.
18. X. Liu et al., *Appl. Phys. Lett.*, 79, 3329, 2001.
19. W.B. Choi et al., *Appl. Phys. Lett.*, 82, 275, 2003.
20. T. Yamada, chap. 7 in Ref. [2].
21. H. Dai et al., *Nature*, 384, 147, 1996.
22. C.V. Nguyen et al., *Nanotechnology*, 12, 363, 2001.
23. Q. Ye et al., *NanoLett.*, 2004.
24. C.V. Nguyen et al., *J. Phys. Chem. B*, 108, 2816, 2004.
25. R. Stevens et al., *IEEE Trans. Nanobio. Technol.*, 3, 56, 2004.
26. J. Kong et al., *Science*, 287, 622, 2000.
27. J. Li et al., *NanoLett.*, 3, 929, 2003.
28. J. Li et al., *NanoLett.*, 3, 597, 2003.
29. P. Sarrazin, chap. 8 in Ref. [2].

4.2 Modeling MEMS and NEMS

John Pelesko

Mathematical modeling of micro- and nano-electromechanical systems (MEMS and NEMS) is an essential part of the design and optimization process. The complexity of typical MEMS and NEMS devices often necessitates the study of coupled-domain problems. The small scale of such devices leads to novel balances in appropriate continuum theories when continuum theory is still valid. At the extreme limits of scale, modeling tools such as molecular dynamics become invaluable.

Micro- and Nano-Electromechanical Systems

Enter the word "nanotechnology" into the Google™ search engine and you will be inundated with more than 1.5 million hits. The acronym for micro-electromechanical systems, i.e., MEMS, returns slightly fewer at 857,000, while the word "nanoscience" returns a still respectable 134,000 sites.[1] This is just a crude measure of the popularity and importance of micro- and nanoscale science, but it makes clear the present overwhelming interest in these fields from both the scientific and lay communities.

The popularity of MEMS and NEMS technology is made more amazing by the fact that both fields are still relatively young. The roots of microsystem technology lie in technological developments accompanying World War II. In particular, wartime research in radar stimulated research in the synthesis of pure semi-conducting materials. These materials, especially silicon, became the platform on which MEMS technology was built.

Both MEMS researchers and nanotechnology proponents point to Richard Feynman's famous "There's plenty of room at the bottom" lecture as a seminal event in their respective fields. Showing remarkable prescience, in 1959 Feynman anticipated much of the next four decades of research in MEMS and NEMS:

[1]Google™ searches performed July 2004.

TABLE 4.1 Landmarks in the History of MEMS and NEMS[a]

1940s	Radar drives the development of pure semiconductors.
1959	Richard P. Feynman's famous "There's plenty of room at the bottom" lecture.
1960	Planar batch-fabrication process invented.
1964	H.C. Nathanson and team at Westinghouse produce the resonant gate transistor, the first batch-fabricated MEMS device.
1970	The microprocessor is invented, driving the demand for integrated circuits ever higher.
1979	The first micromachined accelerometer is developed at Stanford University.
1981	K. Eric Drexler's article, "Protein design as a pathway to molecular manufacturing," is published in the Proceedings of the National Academy of Sciences. This is arguably the first journal article on molecular nanotechnology to appear.
1982	The scanning tunneling microscope is invented.
1984	The polysilicon surface micromachining process is developed at the University of California, Berkeley. MEMS and integrated circuits can be fabricated together for the first time.
1985	The "Buckyball" is discovered.
1986	The atomic force microscope is invented.
1991	The carbon nanotube is discovered.
1996	Richard Smalley develops a technique for producing carbon nanotubes of uniform diameter.
2000s	The number of MEMS devices and applications continually increases. National attention is focused on funding nanotechnology research and education.

[a]Reprinted with permission from *Modeling MEMS and NEMS*, Pelesko and Bernstein, Chapman and Hall/CRC Press, Boca Raton, FL, 2002.

> It is a staggeringly small world that is below. In the year 2000, when they look back at this age, they will wonder why it was not until the year 1960 that anybody began to seriously move in this direction.

While Feynman's lecture inspired a few immediate developments, it was not until 5 years later that MEMS technology officially arrived. In 1964, H.C. Nathanson and his colleagues at Westinghouse produced the first batch fabricated MEMS device. Their resonant gate transistor exhibited all of the features of modern MEMS.

Especially notable is the key role played by *mathematical modeling* in the development of the resonant gate transistor. In fact, almost half of Nathanson's seminal paper concerns the development of a mathematical model. Today, the role of mathematical modeling in MEMS and NEMS is as important as ever. The high cost in both time and money needed to fabricate and test most MEMS and NEMS devices makes mathematical modeling an essential part of the design and optimization process. Further, an effective mathematical model provides the micro- or nanoresearcher with a new window into the small world below.

The Science of Scale

It is almost ridiculously obvious to state that the difference between macroscale and microscale engineering is one of size. Yet, this simple observation is crucial for understanding why and how micro- and nanoscale systems behave. It cannot be stated too forcefully: things change as length scales change. Consider taking a hot Thanksgiving turkey out of the oven. The aluminum foil covering the turkey cools from 400°F to room temperature in about a minute, while the turkey itself stays hot for hours. The difference is one of scale. The relevant length scale for the foil is its thickness, hence the ratio of the foil's volume to surface area is very small. Little thermal energy can be held, while lots of thermal energy can be convected away. In contrast, the relevant length scale for the turkey is much larger and its volume to surface area ratio much closer to one.

Scaling effects play a role in studying every aspect of MEMS and NEMS. In the microworld inertial effects are negligible compared to viscous effects, heat transfer is a fast process, and electrostatic forces dominate over almost every other type of force. The relative importance of various effects and how things change as system size changes can often be computed from simple scaling arguments. This is an important first step in the modeling process.

As an example of these types of arguments, let us examine how we would approach the study of a thermal-elastic actuator. A typical such system is sketched in Figure 4.8. In this design, pioneered by Y.C. Tai and his

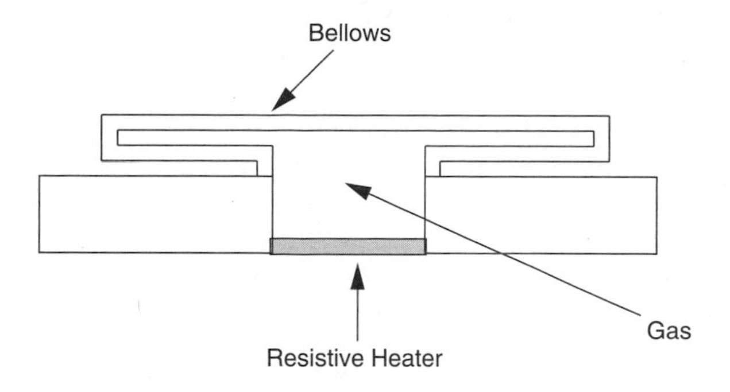

FIGURE 4.8 Sketch of micro-bellows actuator.

group at the California Institute of Technology, thermopneumatic forces are coupled to a "bellows-like" elastic structure in order to produce large deflections. A resistive heater in the base of the structure heats an enclosed volume of gas. Expansion of the gas causes the bellows to unfold and produces the desired displacement or force. A natural question is how quickly such a device could operate. The time limiting factor will be the cooling of system. That is, we expect the resistive heater to operate quickly compared to the time for the system to cool and the device to return to an undeflected state. A simple scaling argument to determine how long this cooling will take may be made as follows. Consider a sphere of radius a that has been heated uniformly to some temperature T_h. The time evolution of the temperature, T, of the sphere is governed by the *heat equation*:

$$\rho c_p \frac{\partial T}{\partial t} = k\nabla^2 T \tag{4.1}$$

where ρ is density, c_p specific heat, and k thermal conductivity. Since initially our system exhibits spherical symmetry, and since we will impose boundary conditions consistent with that fact, we can assume that T depends only on a radial variable, r', and time. With this assumption, the heat equation simplifies to

$$\rho c_p \frac{\partial T}{\partial t} = k\left(\frac{\partial^2 T}{\partial r^2} + \frac{2}{r}\frac{\partial T}{\partial r'}\right) \tag{4.2}$$

We write our initial condition explicitly as

$$T(r, 0) = T_h \tag{4.3}$$

and assume for simplicity that the sphere is immersed in a constant temperature bath of temperature T_b. Hence, we impose the boundary condition:

$$T(a, t) = T_b \tag{4.4}$$

This problem is easily solved using the method of separation of variables. From this solution we find that the center of the sphere cools to the fraction, f, of the initial temperature difference in time, t_c, given by

$$t_c = -\frac{4a^2 \log f}{9\pi^2 \kappa} \tag{4.5}$$

Here, $\kappa = k/(\rho c_p)$ and is called the thermal diffusivity. For illustrative purposes let us take $a = 1\ \mu$m, $f = 0.01$, and $\kappa = 0.02 \times 10^{-4}\ \mathrm{m^2/sec}$. The diffusivity is a typical value for silicon, a common construction material in MEMS. We find $t_c \approx 10^{-7}$ sec. Our sphere cools in a tenth of a microsecond. Assuming the sphere could be heated just as quickly, we find that our device can be operated at 5000 KHz.

This calculation represents the first step in the modeling process, i.e., performing a simple analysis in order to determine design feasibility. The estimate obtained of operating frequency is not meant to be definitive, but rather represents an order of magnitude calculation. If the order of magnitude of the estimates is in the desired range, more detailed models can now be constructed to guide the design process. Many more examples of simple scaling arguments may be found in Trimmer (1997) and Pelesko (2002).

Modeling Approaches

Once design feasibility has been ascertained, it is often desirable to create a more detailed and more realistic model of the system under consideration. A good model can guide design, help optimize the design, and explain phenomena observed during experimentation. There are no hard and fast rules concerning what modeling tools to use when studying MEMS and NEMS. Rather, the MEMS/NEMS researcher must be open to learning and employing a variety of tools as the situation warrants. There are, however, some tools that have proven of wide utility. We highlight some of these here.

Continuum Mechanics

The vast majority of mathematical models of MEMS and NEMS devices are based on the equations of *continuum mechanics*. The key test for the validity of continuum mechanics in the study of a particular MEMS/NEMS system is whether or not molecular details of the system may be ignored. Can the *continuum hypothesis* be assumed? If molecular details may be ignored then quantities such as temperature, pressure, and stress, can be treated as smoothly varying functions of spatial coordinates. If the continuum hypothesis is not valid, or quantum effects are important, an alternative approach is called for. Some alternative approaches are discussed below. Here, we review the principal equations of continuum mechanics. We note that the choice of boundary and initial conditions for these equations is highly dependent on the situation under consideration. Detailed discussions of boundary and initial conditions for the equations of continuum mechanics may be found in Segel (1987) and Lin (1988).

We have already encountered the *heat equation* which characterizes the thermal behavior of a body or a fluid:

$$\rho c_p \frac{\partial T}{\partial t} = k\nabla^2 T \tag{4.6}$$

This equation expresses conservation of energy. As written a homogeneous isotropic material is assumed. If the medium is inhomogeneous or anisotropic, the proper equation governing heat flow is

$$\rho c_p \frac{\partial T}{\partial t} = \nabla \cdot k\nabla T \tag{4.7}$$

Anisotropy may be modeled by treating k as a tensor. This allows the heat flux to vary as a function of direction within the material. The inhomogeneous nature of a material may be modeled by treating ρ, c_p, and k as functions of position.

The elastic behavior of a solid body is characterized in terms of *stress* and *strain*. The stress in a solid body is expressed in terms of the *stress tensor*, σ_{ij}. If you are unfamiliar with tensors, you can think of σ_{ij} as simply being a 3×3 matrix:

$$\begin{pmatrix} \sigma_{11} & \sigma_{12} & \sigma_{13} \\ \sigma_{21} & \sigma_{22} & \sigma_{23} \\ \sigma_{31} & \sigma_{32} & \sigma_{33} \end{pmatrix} \tag{4.8}$$

The *ij*th component of this matrix, σ_{ij}, denotes the force per unit area in the direction i exerted on a surface element with normal in the j direction. Balance of angular momentum within an elastic body requires that the stress tensor be symmetric, i.e.:

$$\sigma_{ij} = \sigma_{ji} \tag{4.9}$$

Or in matrix notation

$$\sigma_{ij} = \begin{pmatrix} \sigma_{11} & \sigma_{12} & \sigma_{13} \\ \sigma_{12} & \sigma_{22} & \sigma_{23} \\ \sigma_{13} & \sigma_{23} & \sigma_{33} \end{pmatrix} \tag{4.10}$$

so that we have only six independent components of the stress tensor. The strain in a solid body is also expressed in terms of a tensor, called the *strain tensor*, and is denoted ε_{ij}. For small displacements, the strain tensor is related to displacements of the elastic body by

$$\varepsilon_{ij} = \frac{1}{2}\left(\frac{\partial u_i}{\partial x_j} + \frac{\partial u_j}{\partial x_i}\right) \tag{4.11}$$

Here, u_i is the ith component of the displacement vector and the partial derivatives are taken with respect to the directions x_1, x_2, and x_3 in a Cartesian coordinate system. Note that Equation (4.11) is only valid for small displacements. This equation has been linearized by ignoring quadratic terms. In general, the strain tensor is

$$\varepsilon_{ij} = \frac{1}{2}\left(\frac{\partial u_i}{\partial x_j} + \frac{\partial u_j}{\partial x_i} + \frac{\partial u_k}{\partial x_i}\frac{\partial u_k}{\partial x_j}\right) \tag{4.12}$$

We have assumed the Einstein summation convention. This simply says that when you see a repeated index, it denotes summation over that index. Above, the repeated index of k indicates summation over k. The approximation of small displacements allows us to use Equation (4.11) in place of Equation (4.12). The basic equation of elasticity comes from applying conservation of momentum. That is, we apply Newton's second law to an appropriate control volume and obtain

$$\rho\frac{\partial^2 u_i}{\partial t^2} = \frac{\partial \sigma_{ij}}{\partial x_j} + f_i \tag{4.13}$$

where ρ is the density of the body and f_i is the body force per unit volume. For instance, in modeling an electrostatically actuated device, f_i would be computed from electrostatic forces while in a magnetic device f_i would be computed from magnetic forces. Note that Equation (4.13) is really a set of three equations, one for each of the components of the displacement vector.

To close the system we make a constitutive assumption. We assume a generalized Hooke's law:

$$\sigma_{ij} = 2\mu\varepsilon_{ij} + \lambda\varepsilon_{kk}\delta_{ij} \tag{4.14}$$

Equation (4.14) assumes that stress and strain are linearly related. Here, μ and λ are the *Lame constants* while δ_{ij} is called the *Kronecker delta*. In matrix terms, δ_{ij} is simply the 3×3 identity matrix. The Lame constants are related to the more familiar Young's modulus:

$$E = \frac{\mu(2\mu + 3\lambda)}{\lambda + \mu} \tag{4.15}$$

and Poisson ratio:

$$\nu = \frac{\lambda}{2(\lambda + \mu)} \tag{4.16}$$

Hence, Equation (4.14) may be rewritten as

$$E\varepsilon_{ij} = (1 + \nu)\sigma_{ij} - \nu\sigma_{kk}\delta_{ij} \tag{4.17}$$

Now, substituting Equation (4.14) into Equation (4.13), we obtain the Navier equations of elasticity:

$$\rho \frac{\partial^2 u_i}{\partial t^2} = \frac{\partial}{\partial x_j}(2\mu\varepsilon_{ij} + \lambda\varepsilon_{kk}\delta_{ij}) \tag{4.18}$$

Eliminating the strain tensor in favor of the displacement vector and using vector notation yields

$$\rho \frac{\partial^2 \mathbf{u}}{\partial t^2} = \mu\nabla^2\mathbf{u} + (\mu + \lambda)\nabla(\nabla \cdot \mathrm{u}) + f \tag{4.19}$$

Equation (4.19) is a set of equations called the Navier equations of linear elasticity.

When the elastic and thermal behaviors of a body are coupled, the equations of *linear thermoelasticity* are called for. In thermoelasticity, we incorporate a term in the heat equation that reflects the fact that elastic energy is converted into thermal energy. The modified heat equation is

$$\rho c_p \frac{\partial T}{\partial t} = \nabla \cdot k\nabla T - \alpha(3\lambda + 2\mu)T_0 \frac{\partial \varepsilon_{kk}}{\partial t} \tag{4.20}$$

Here, α is called the coefficient of thermal expansion and T_0 is a suitably defined reference temperature. The definition of the strain, ε_{ij}, remains unchanged from linear elasticity:

$$\varepsilon_{ij} = \frac{1}{2}\left(\frac{\partial u_i}{\partial x_j} + \frac{\partial u_j}{\partial x_i}\right) \tag{4.21}$$

as does the balance of linear momentum:

$$\rho \frac{\partial^2 u_i}{\partial t^2} = \frac{\partial \sigma_{ij}}{\partial x_j} + f_i \tag{4.22}$$

Also, as in linear elasticity, the stress tensor is symmetric $\sigma_{ij} = \sigma_{ji}$, reflecting the balance of angular momentum. The major modification to the linear elastic theory is to the constitutive law. A modified Hooke's law known as the Duhamel–Neumann relation is introduced. This modified Hooke's law contains a term expressing the fact that a rise in temperature creates a stress within a material:

$$\sigma_{ij} = 2\mu\varepsilon_{ij} + \lambda\delta_{ij}\varepsilon_{kk} - \delta_{ij}\alpha(3\lambda + 2\mu)(T - T_0) \tag{4.23}$$

Again, we have assumed the summation convention. Equation (4.20) to Equation (4.23) are known as the equations of linear thermoelasticity.

As with the Navier equations describing the motion of elastic bodies, the behavior of a fluid is characterized in terms of *stress* and *strain*. In fluids, however, in addition to conservation of momentum, we also have an equation derived from the principle of conservation of mass. If ρ denotes the density of fluid and u_i is a vector of fluid velocities, whose ith component is fluid velocity in direction i, then conservation of mass says

$$\frac{\partial \rho}{\partial t} + u_j \frac{\partial \rho}{\partial x_j} + \rho \frac{\partial u_i}{\partial x_i} = 0 \tag{4.24}$$

In contrast with elasticity, the reader should keep in mind that here we are working with *velocities* rather than *displacements*. This implies that it is convenient to define the strain rate tensor as opposed to the strain tensor. In particular, we define

$$\frac{\partial \varepsilon_{ij}}{\partial t} = \frac{1}{2}\left(\frac{\partial u_i}{\partial x_j} + \frac{\partial u_j}{\partial x_i}\right) \tag{4.25}$$

Stress in a fluid is expressed in terms of the stress tensor σ_{ij}, which, as with elasticity, may be thought of as the 3×3 matrix:

$$\begin{pmatrix} \sigma_{11} & \sigma_{12} & \sigma_{13} \\ \sigma_{21} & \sigma_{22} & \sigma_{23} \\ \sigma_{31} & \sigma_{32} & \sigma_{33} \end{pmatrix} \tag{4.26}$$

The ijth component of this matrix, σ_{ij} again, denotes the force per unit area in the direction i exerted on a surface element with normal in the j direction. The stress tensor is related to the rate of strain tensor through

$$\sigma_{ij} = -p\delta_{ij} + 2\mu\, \dot{\varepsilon}_{ij} + \lambda\, \dot{\varepsilon}_{kk}\, \delta_{ij} \tag{4.27}$$

Here, the dot denotes differentiation with respect to time, p is the pressure in the fluid, μ is the dynamic fluid viscosity, and λ is a second viscosity coefficient. Recall that repeated indices indicate summation and that δ_{ij} denotes the Kroneker delta or 3×3 identity matrix. The equation of conservation of momentum can now be written as

$$\rho \frac{\partial u_i}{\partial t} + \rho u_j \frac{\partial u_i}{\partial x_j} = \rho F_i + \frac{\partial \sigma_{ij}}{\partial x_j} \tag{4.28}$$

Using Equation (4.27) in Equation (4.28), we obtain

$$\rho \frac{\partial u_i}{\partial t} + \rho u_j \frac{\partial u_i}{\partial x_j} = \rho F_i - \frac{\partial p}{\partial x_i} + \frac{\partial}{\partial x_j}(2\mu\, \dot{\varepsilon}_{ij} + \lambda\, \dot{\varepsilon}_{kk}\, \delta_{ij}) \tag{4.29}$$

Equation (4.29) is usually called the Navier–Stokes equation of motion and Equation (4.24) and Equation (4.29) are called the Navier–Stokes equations. We may rewrite the Navier–Stokes equations in vector form:

$$\frac{\partial \rho}{\partial t} + \nabla \cdot (\rho \mathbf{u}) = 0 \tag{4.30}$$

$$\rho \frac{\partial \mathbf{u}}{\partial t} + \rho(\mathbf{u} \cdot \nabla)\mathbf{u} + \nabla p - \mu \nabla^2 \mathbf{u} - (\lambda + \mu)\nabla(\nabla \cdot \mathbf{u}) = \mathbf{f} \tag{4.31}$$

In Equation (4.31), we have eliminated the strain rate tensor in favor of the velocity vector and relabeled the body force vector as **f**.

Equation (4.30) and Equation (4.31), the Navier–Stokes equations for a viscous compressible fluid, are a system of four coupled nonlinear partial differential equations. Notice, however, that the system contains five unknown functions. The pressure, the density, and the three components of the velocity vector field are all unknown. To close this system one usually appends the equation of conservation of energy to the Navier–Stokes equations. This introduces one more equation and one more unknown function, the temperature T. The system is then completed by introducing an equation of state which relates ρ, p, and T. Various simplifications of the Navier–Stokes equations are possible. In particular, the so called Stokes equations are often of relevance in microfluidics.

Electromagnetic phenomena are described by Maxwell's equations. This system of four coupled partial differential equations describes the spatial and temporal evolution of the four vector fields, **E**, **D**, **B**, and **H**:

$$\nabla \cdot \mathbf{D} = \frac{\rho}{\varepsilon_0} \tag{4.32}$$

$$\nabla \times \mathbf{E} = -\frac{1}{c}\frac{\partial \mathbf{B}}{\partial t} \tag{4.33}$$

$$\nabla \cdot \mathbf{B} = 0 \tag{4.34}$$

$$\nabla \times \mathbf{H} = \frac{1}{c}\frac{\partial D}{\partial t} + \mathbf{J} \tag{4.35}$$

Here, ρ is the electrical charge density, **J** is the current density, and c is the speed of light in vacuum. To complete the description of the dynamics of charged particles in the presence of electromagnetic fields we must also supply the *Lorenz force law*:

$$\mathbf{F} = q(\mathbf{E} + \mathbf{v} \times \mathbf{B}) \tag{4.36}$$

where q is the electric charge of the particle and **v** its velocity. Note that the *conservation of charge*:

$$\frac{\partial \rho}{\partial t} + \nabla \cdot \mathbf{J} = 0 \tag{4.37}$$

is a consequence of Maxwell's equations.

The Maxwell equations are a system of 8 equations in the 12 components of **E**, **D**, **B**, and **H**. To close the system the *constitutive relations* of the materials involved are necessary. For *linear* materials these are usually written:

$$D_i = \varepsilon_{ij} E_j \tag{4.38}$$

$$B_i = \mu_{ij} H_j \tag{4.39}$$

The tensors ε_{ij} (the *permittivity tensor*) and μ_{ij} (the *magnetic permeability tensor*) are properties of materials which contain information about how they respond to the presence of external electric and magnetic fields. Note that this form does not apply to materials with permanent electric or magnetic moments (*ferroelectric* and *ferromagnetic* materials, respectively).

As an example, many materials respond to an electric field by generating a *dipole* moment. In addition, the dipole moment is independent of the direction of the applied field and its position in space. In this case, the material is said to be *homogeneous* and *isotropic* as well as linear and the permittivity tensor takes on the simple form $\varepsilon_{ij} = \varepsilon\delta_{ij}$; hence,

$$\mathbf{D} = \varepsilon \mathbf{E} \tag{4.40}$$

In this case, ε is the called the *dielectric constant* of the material. Note that while a large number of materials (called, naturally, *dielectrics*) fall into this category, most magnetic materials used in current technology are ferromagnetic as well as having a nonlinear response to external magnetic fields. *Paramagnetic* and *diamagnetic* materials, which do not have permanent magnetic moments and are linear in their response, are more the exception than the rule.

Mathematical models of MEMS and NEMS devices usually involve *coupled domains*. For example, a system may be thermoelectric and its study requires a model using both the heat equation and Maxwell's equations coupled through appropriate boundary and source terms. Perhaps the most prevalent coupled domains in MEMS systems are thermal–elastic systems such as thermoelastic actuators, electrostatic–elastic systems such as accelerometers or electrostatic actuators, and elastic–fluidic systems such as micropumps. Detailed examples of such models may be found in Pelesko (2002). One of the more interesting aspects of modeling MEMS and NEMS again is a consequence of scale. When a continuum based mathematical model has been constructed, the next step, as with all engineering theories, is to simplify the equations where possible. This involves determining the relative importance of various terms in the mathematical model. The small length scales involved in MEMS and NEMS often lead to novel balances of terms in continuum models. For example, inertial terms are often negligible whereas in the macro world they are usually dominant. This and other scale effects makes continuum modeling of MEMS and NEMS systems exciting and different than macro-engineering.

Other Tools

One of the key landmarks in the history of the development of MEMS and NEMS came in 1985 with the discovery by Curl, Kroto, and Smalley of C_{60}, the carbon "Buckeyball structure." The importance of this discovery was recognized almost immediately by the scientific community and, in 1996, the trio received the Nobel Prize for their work. The importance of the follow up discovery of carbon nanotubes promises to eclipse even the discovery of C_{60}. Nanotubes, often visualized as sheets of "chicken wire" rolled into a cylinder, exhibit fascinating thermal, elastic, and electrical properties. Technological developments based on nanotubes are proceeding apace.

When constructing a mathematical model of a device based on nanotube technology, molecular effects may become important. It is important to note the words "may become." This too is a question of scale. If, for example, one is interested in the bending of a nanotube serving as part of a nanotweezer system, the Navier equations of elasticity may be the basis for a perfectly valid model describing the elastic deflections of the tube. If, however, one is interested in the motion of a nanotube-based gear where individual atoms bound to the nanotube surface serve as gear teeth, a molecular scale model may be in order. In the latter case, *molecular dynamics* based simulation is often the only way to go.

In a typical molecular dynamics (MD) simulation, the location of each individual molecule is tracked. A potential, such as the Lenard–Jones potential, is used to model particle–particle interactions. Static configurations are then obtained by minimizing the energy of the system, while dynamic behaviors are simulated using classical mechanics for each particle and the appropriate potential to simulate particle–particle interactions. MD simulations are often computationally quite costly; however, rapid progress in nanoscale MD simulations is being made. The reader is referred to the listing below for further reading in this area.

Another area of micro- and nanotechnology showcasing rapidly developing mathematical modeling tools is the field of *self-assembly*. Our ability to fully exploit the potential of micro- and nano-electromechanical systems (MEMS and NEMS) technology is to a large extent dependent upon our capacity to efficiently fabricate and organize MEMS and NEMS *devices* and *systems*. Fabrication technologies used in MEMS are almost wholly derived from analogous technology used in the fabrication of integrated circuits. While this approach has been quite successful for MEMS, the feasibility of pushing this technology downward toward the nanoscale is doubtful. Rather, the few true NEMS devices fabricated have relied on costly, time-consuming, *ad hoc* methods, which do not easily scale to allow the production of batches of devices. Similarly, while many MEMS devices and several NEMS devices have been produced and even commercialized, the promise of MEMS and NEMS *systems* remains largely unfulfilled. The ideal of having thousands or tens of thousands of individual MEMS/NEMS devices working together as part of a system has yet to be widely realized.

To address these concerns, researchers in MEMS and NEMS have recently turned toward the study of self-assembly (SA) and self-organization (SO). Of course, the study of SA and SO did not originate with the MEMS and NEMS community, but rather has been an intense topic of research in many fields (Langton, 1995). It is worth noting, however, that the engineering perspective of the MEMS and NEMS community leads to a different take and different set of questions for studies of self-assembly and self-organization. Rather than attempting to describe the behavior of complex systems by assigning simple rules to individual agents, the MEMS and NEMS researcher seeks to construct a system with a desired complex behavior. The necessities of working on the micro- or nanoscale, make the individual-agent, simple-rules, emergent behavior approach particularly attractive. The mathematical tools used to model the self-assembly process are often very different than the tools used to model the behavior of an individual MEMS or NEMS device. A common approach borrows techniques from theoretical computer science. A set of rules, or a "grammar," defining how elements of the system can combine is constructed. Study of this grammar can then answer a myriad of questions about the self-assembling system. For example, what is the achievable complexity of a self-assembled system evolving according to a given rules set? Or, what is the statistical distribution of expected assemblies?

Of course, molecular dynamics and grammar based models are but two of the many new techniques being employed by MEMS and NEMS researchers. As the fields progress, and new challenges arise, undoubtedly those in the MEMS and NEMS field will draw on an ever widening range of mathematical tools.

Defining Terms

Constitutive relation: An equation relating several variables in a model based on continuum mechanics. The relation often captures material properties of the system.

Continuum hypothesis: The assumption that molecular details of a system may be ignored and variables such as pressure, temperature, and density treated as smooth functions of position.

Continuum mechanics: The partial differential equations expressing conservation of mass, momentum, and energy, and describing electromagnetic phenomena.

Coupled domain problem: The term used by the MEMS and NEMS community to describe a mathematical model involving more than one area of continuum theory. For example, a description of a MEMS resistive heater would involve both Maxwell's equations and the heat equation. These sets of equations would be coupled through boundary conditions and source terms.

Heat equation: The partial differential equation expressing conservation of energy and governing the flow of heat in a body.

Linear thermoelasticity: The linearized equations describing the coupling of elastic and thermal phenomena.

Mathematical modeling: The art of constructing a mathematical structure capturing the essence of a physical systems. In the modeling of MEMS and NEMS, continuum mechanics often forms the basis for such models.

Maxwell's equations: The partial differential equations describing electromagnetic phenomena.

MEMS: Acronym for microelectromechanical systems.

Molecular dynamics: An approach to the mathematical modeling of systems at the molecular level that involves simulating the motion of every molecule in the system under consideration.

Navier equations: The partial differential equations describing the elastic behavior of solid bodies.

Navier–Stokes equations: The partial differential equations describing the behavior of fluids.

NEMS: Acronym for nanoelectromechanical systems.

Self-assembly: A controllable, reversible process where components of a system order themselves without intervention by the experimenter.

References and Further Reading

New books on MEMS and NEMS are appearing almost as quickly as new MEMS and NEMS devices. Nevertheless, some of them are quite good. The text by Madou on fabrication is one of the best and contains numerous elementary mathematical models.

M.J. Madou, *Fundamentals of Microfabrication: The Science of Miniaturization*, 2nd ed., Boca Raton, FL: CRC Press, 2002.

The text by Pelesko and Bernstein focuses entirely on modeling and expands on many of the topics discussed here.

J.A. Pelesko and D. Bernstein, *Modeling MEMS and NEMS*, Boca Raton, FL: Chapman Hall/CRC Press, 2002.

The book by Maluf is a wonderful readable introduction to MEMS. It does not delve into modeling of MEMS or NEMS.

N. Maluf, *An Introduction to Microelectromechanical Systems Engineering*, Norwood, MA: Artech House, 1999.

Trimmer's collection of classic and seminal papers belongs on the shelf of anyone involved in MEMS and NEMS. The classic paper by Nathanson may be found in this collection. Trimmer's excellent article on scaling laws in MEMS also appears in this volume.

W. Trimmer Ed., *Micromechanics and MEMS: Classic and Seminal Papers to 1990*, Piscataway, NJ: Wiley-IEEE, 1997.

Two textbooks on MEMS worth owning are the texts by Elwenspoek and Senturia.

M. Elwenspoek and R. Wiegerink, *Mechanical Microsensors*, Berlin: Springer Verlag, 2001.

S.D. Senturia, *Microsystem Design*, Hingham, MA: Kluwer Academic, 2001.

A few papers that appear in the Trimmer collection but are worth highlighting are the articles by Nathanson and Feynman.

H.C. Nathanson, "The resonant gate transistor," *IEEE Trans. Elec. Dev.*, ED-14, 117–133, 1967.

R.P. Feynman, "here's plenty of room at the bottom," *J. Microelectromech. Sys.*, 1, 60–66, 1992.

An excellent book on heat transfer is the text by Carslaw and Jaeger.

H.S. Carlslaw and J.C. Jaeger, *Conduction of Heat in Solids*, Oxford: Oxford Science Publications, 1959.

An excellent introduction to continuum mechanics and related mathematical methods may be found in the series of books by Lin and Segel.

C.C. Lin and L.A. Segel, *Mathematics Applied to Deterministic Problems in the Natural Sciences*, Philadelphia, PA: SIAM, 1988.

L.A. Segel, *Mathematics Applied to Continuum Mechanics*, New York: Dover, 1987.

The text on thermoelasticity is now available in a Dover addition:

B.A. Boley and J.H. Weiner, *Theory of Thermal Stresses*, New York: Dover, 1988.

Jackson is considered the definitive work on electromagnetism.

J.D. Jackson, *Classical Electrodynamics*, 2nd ed., New York: Wiley, 1975.

Stratton is also a classic.

J.A. Stratton, *Electromagnetic Theory*, New York: McGraw-Hill, 1941.

There are many useful texts on fluid mechanics. The classics by Lamb and Batchelor are among the best.

H. Lamb, *Hydrodynamics*, Cambridge, MA: Cambridge University Press, 1993.

G.K. Batchelor, *An Introduction to Fluid Dynamics*, Cambridge, MA: Cambridge University Press, 1967.

Landau and Lifshitz is also a useful reference on fluid mechanics.

L.D. Landau and E.M. Lifshitz, *Fluid Mechanics*, Oxford: Butterworth Heinemann, 1959.

Several texts on microfluidics have been recently published.

G.E. Karniadakis and A. Beskok, *Microflows: Fundamentals and Simulations*, Berlin: Springer Verlag, 2001.

M. Koch, A. Evans, A. Brunnschweiler, and A. Brunnschweiler, *Microfluidic Technology and Applications*, Hertfordshire: Research Studies Press, 2000.
A nice introduction to modeling "emergent" behaviors may be found in the book by Langton.
C.G. Langton, *Artificial Life: An Overview*, Cambridge, MA: MIT Press, 1995.
Two entertaining popular treatments of nanotechnology are the books by Regis and Gross.
E. Regis, *Nano: The Emerging Science of Nanotechnology*, Boston, MA: Little, Brown and Company, 1995.
M. Gross, *Travels to the Nanoworld*, New York: Plenum Trade, 1995.

4.3 Micromechatronics

Victor Giurgiutiu and Sergey Edward Lyshevski

Micromechatronics is an area of great importance that has accomplished phenomenal growth over the past few years. Overall, these developments are based on far-reaching theoretical, applied, and experimental advances as well as the application of novel technologies to fabricate micromechatronics systems. These micromechatronics systems integrate motion devices, sensors, integrated circuits, and other components. The synergy of engineering, science, and technology is essential to design, fabricate, and implement micromechatronics systems. Recent trends in engineering and industrial demands have increased the emphasis on integrated synthesis, analysis, and design of micromechatronics systems. These synthesis, design, and optimization processes are evolutionary in nature, and revolutionary advances are sought. High-level physics-based synthesis is performed first in order to devise micromechatronics systems and their components by using a synthesis and classification concept. Then, comprehensive analysis, heterogeneous simulation, and design are performed applying the computer-aided design. Each level of the design hierarchy corresponds to a particular abstraction level and has a specified set of evolutionary learning activities, theories, and tools to be developed in order to support the design. The multidisciplinary synthesis and design require the application of a wide spectrum of paradigms, methods, computational environments, and fabrication technologies, which are reported in this section.

Introduction to Micromechatronics Systems

Micromechatronics systems integrate distinct components, and, in particular, actuators, sensors, and ICs. We focus our attention on high-performance micromechatronics systems. In their book, Giurgiutiu and Lyshevski (2004) covered the general issues in the design of micromechatronics systems (Figure 4.9). Important topics, focused themes, and issues will be outlined and discussed in this section. Micromechatronics systems are integrated high-performance electromechanical systems that include microscale motion devices that (1) convert physical stimuli to electrical or mechanical signals and vice versa, and (2) perform actuation and sensing. These motion devices are controlled by integrated circuits (ICs). Electromagnetic and electromechanical features of micromachines are basic of their operation, design, analysis, and fabrication. Correspondingly, ICs are designed taking into account possible system architectures. The step-by-step procedure in the design of micromechatronics systems is:

1. Define application and environmental requirements.
2. Specify performance specifications.
3. Devise (synthesize) actuators and sensors by researching operating principles, topologies, configurations, geometry, and electromagnetic, and electromechanical systems.
4. Perform electromagnetic, mechanical, and sizing-dimension estimates.
5. Define technologies, techniques, processes, and materials (permanent magnets, coils, insulators, etc.) to fabricate actuators and sensors.
6. Design ICs to control actuators and sensors.

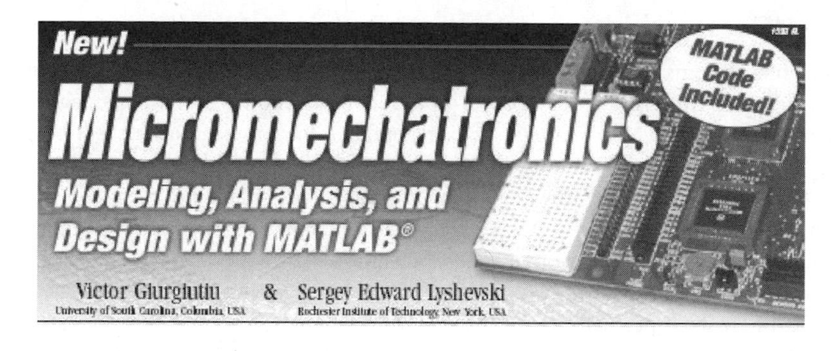

FIGURE 4.9 *Micromechatronics: Modeling, Analysis, and Design with MATLAB*, CRC Press, 2004.

7. Develop high-fidelity mathematical models with a minimum level of simplifications and assumptions to examine integrated electromagnetic, mechanical, vibroacoustic phenomena and effects.
8. Based upon data-intensive analysis and heterogeneous simulations, perform thorough electromagnetic, mechanical, thermodynamic, and vibroacoustic design with performance analysis and outcome prediction.
9. Modify and refine the design to optimize machine performance.
10. Design control laws to control micromechatronics systems and implement these controllers using ICs (this task itself can be broken down to many subtasks and problems related to control laws design, optimization, analysis, simulation, synthesis of ICs topologies, ICs fabrication, machine–ICs integration, interfacing, and communication).

Before being engaged in the fabrication, one must solve synthesis, design, analysis, and optimization problems. In fact, mechatronic systems' performance and its suitability/applicability directly depend upon synthesized topologies, configurations, and operating principles. The synthesis with modeling activities allows the designer to examine complex phenomena, and discover advanced functionality and new operating concepts. These guarantee synthesis of superior mechatronic systems with enhanced integrity, functionality, and operationability. Thus, through the synthesis, the designer devises machines that must be modeled, analyzed, simulated, and optimized. Finally, as shown in Figure 4.10, the devised and analyzed nano- and micromachines must be fabricated and tested.

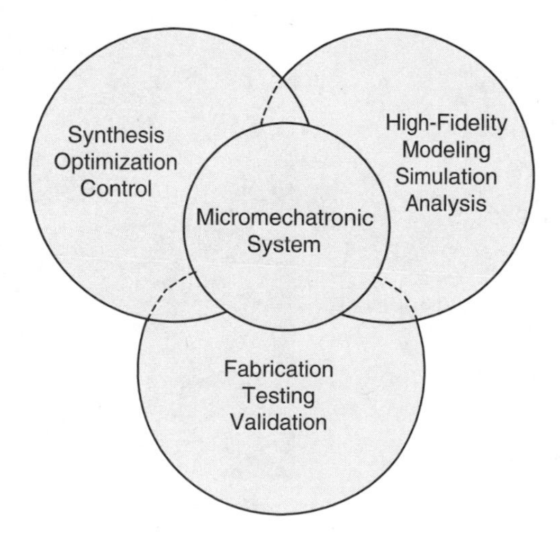

FIGURE 4.10 Synthesis design and fabrication of micromechatronics systems.

Synchronous Micromachines

In micromechatronics systems, rotational and translational micromachines (actuators and sensors), controlled by ICs, are widely used. Among various motion devices, synchronous permanent-magnet micromachines exhibit superior performance. The advantages of axial topology micromachines are feasibility, efficiency, and reliability. Simplicity of fabrication results because: (1) magnets are flat, (2) there are no strict shape requirements imposed on magnets, (3) rotor back ferromagnetic material is not required, and (4) it is easy to deposit planar wires on the flat stator. Utilizing the axial topology and endless electromagnetic system, we synthesize permanent-magnet synchronous micromachines (Lyshevski, 2001, 2004). The synthesized micromachine is shown in Figure 4.11.

Single- and two-phase axial permanent-magnet synchronous micromachines are illustrated in Figure 4.11. In particular, for two-phase micromachines, one supplies two phase voltages u_{as} and u_{bs}. While, for a single-phase micromachine, a phase voltage u_{as} or u_{bs} is applied. Assuming that the magnetic flux is constant through the magnetic plane (current loop), the torque on a planar current loop of any size and shape in the uniform magnetic field is given as

$$\mathbf{T} = i\mathbf{s} \times \mathbf{B} = \mathbf{m} \times \mathbf{B} \tag{4.41}$$

where i is the current in the loop (winding); $\mathbf{m}$ is the magnetic dipole moment (Am^2). The electromagnetic force is found as

$$\mathbf{F} = \oint_l i d\mathbf{l} \times \mathbf{B} \tag{4.42}$$

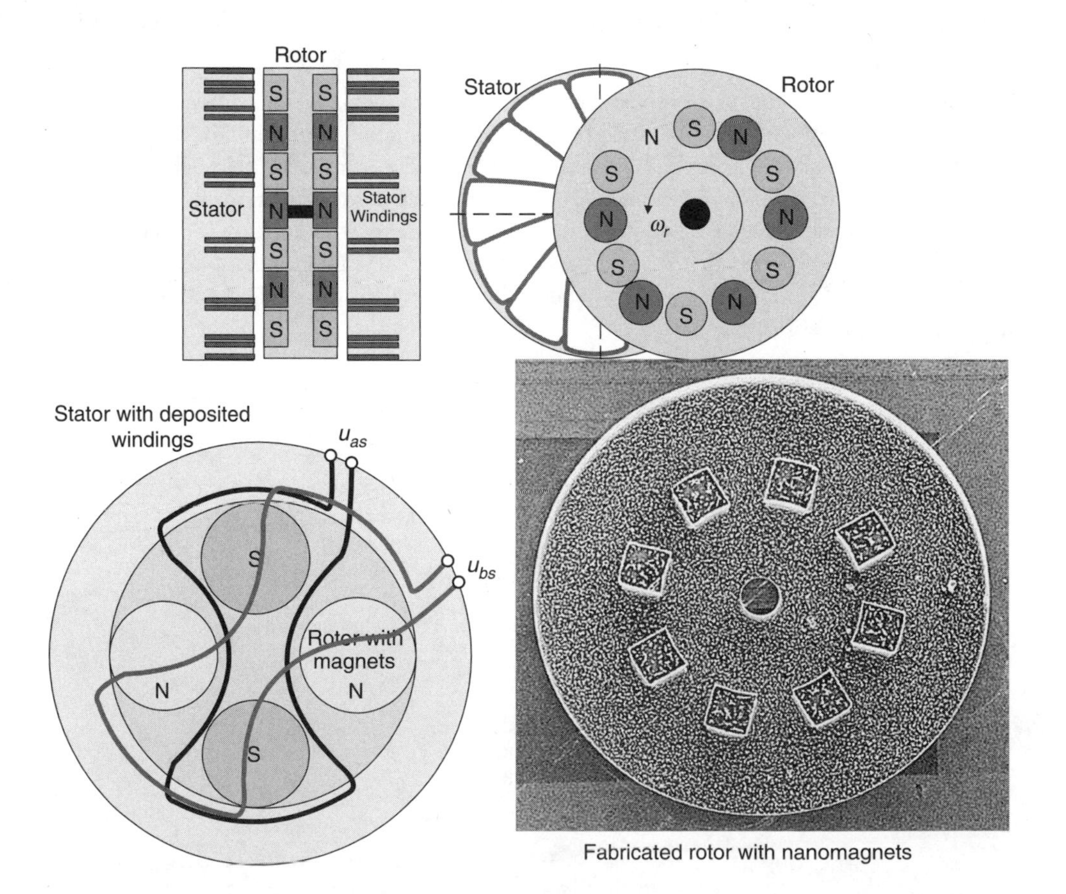

FIGURE 4.11 Axial permanent-magnet synchronous micromachine. (Lyshevski, 2001, 2004.)

The interaction of the current (in windings) and magnets will produce the rotating electromagnetic torque. Microscale synchronous transducers can be used as motors (actuators) and generators (sensors). Microgenerators (velocity and position sensors) convert mechanical energy into electrical energy, while micromotors–microactuators convert electrical energy into mechanical energy. A broad spectrum of synchronous microtransducers can be used in MEMS as actuators, e.g., electric microdrives, microservos, or microscale power systems.

Distinct electrostatic and electromagnetic micromachines can be designed and fabricated using the surface micromachining technology. However, all high-performance, high-power and torque density machines are electromagnetic, and these micromachines use permanent micromagnets. Therefore, the issues of fabrication and analysis of micromagnets are of great interest. Different soft and hard micromagnets can be fabricated using surface micromachining, e.g., Ni, Fe, Co, NiFe, and other magnets can be made. In general, four classes of high-performance magnets have been commonly used in electromechanical motion devices: neodymium iron boron ($Nd_2Fe_{14}B$), samarium cobalt (usually Sm_1Co_5 and Sm_2Co_{17}), ceramic (ferrite), and alnico (AlNiCo). The term *soft* is used to describe those magnets that have high saturation magnetization and a low coercivity (narrow BH curve). Another property of these micromagnets is their low magnetostriction. The soft micromagnets have been widely used in magnetic recording heads, and NiFe thin films with the desired properties have been fabricated. Hard magnets have wide BH curves (high coercivity) and, therefore, high-energy storage capacity. These nano- and micromagnets should be used in micromachines in order to attain high force, torque, and power densities. Unfortunately, limited progress has been made in the fabrication of hard micromagnets.

The energy density is given as the area enclosed by the BH curve, e.g., $w_m = \frac{1}{2}\mathrm{B} \cdot \mathrm{H}$. When micromagnets are used in micromachines, the demagnetization curve (second quadrant of the BH curve) is studied. A basic understanding of the phenomena and operating features of permanent magnets is extremely useful. Permanent magnets store, exchange, and convert energy. In particular, permanent magnets produce a stationary magnetic field without external energy sources.

We apply Kirchhoff's and Newton's laws to derive the equations of motion for axial topology permanent-magnet micro- and nanomotors. Using the axial permanent-magnet synchronous micromachine documented in Figure 4.11, we assume that this variation of the flux density is sinusoidal:

$$B(\theta_r) = B_{max}\sin^n\left(\frac{1}{2}N_m\theta_r\right), \quad n = 1, 3, 5, 7, \ldots, \tag{4.43}$$

where B_{max} is the maximum flux density in the airgap produced by the magnet as viewed from the winding (B_{max} depends on the magnets used, airgap length, temperature, etc.); N_m is the number of magnets; n is the integer that is a function of the magnet geometry and the waveform of the airgap B.

The electromagnetic torque developed by single-phase axial topology permanent-magnet synchronous micromotors is found using the expression for the co-energy $W_c(i_{as}, \theta_r)$ that is given as

$$W_c(i_{as}, \theta_r) = NA_{ag}B(\theta_r)i_{as} \tag{4.44}$$

where N is the number of turns and A_{ag} is the airgap surface area. Assuming that the airgap flux density obeys $B(\theta_r) = B_{max}\sin\left(\frac{1}{2}N_m\theta_r\right)$, we have $W_c(i_{as}, \theta_r) = NA_{ag}B_{max}\sin\left(\frac{1}{2}N_m\theta_r\right)i_{as}$, and the electromagnetic torque is

$$T_e = \frac{\partial W_c(i_{as}, \theta_r)}{\partial\theta_r} = \frac{\partial\left(NA_{ag}B_{max}\sin\left(\frac{1}{2}N_m\theta_r\right)i_{as}\right)}{\partial\theta_r} = \frac{1}{2}N_mNA_{ag}\,B_{max}\cos\left(\frac{1}{2}N_m\theta_r\right)i_{as} \tag{4.45}$$

As we feed the following current with the magnitude i_M to the micromotor winding $i_{as} = i_M\cos\left(\frac{1}{2}N_m\theta_r\right)$, the electromagnetic torque is

$$T_e = \frac{1}{2} N_m N A_{ag} B_{max} i_M \cos^2\left(\frac{1}{2} N_m \theta_r\right) \neq 0 \tag{4.46}$$

The mathematical model of the single-phase permanent-magnet micromotor is found by using Kirchhoff's and Newton's second laws:

$$u_{as} = r_s i_{as} + \frac{d\psi_{as}}{dt} \quad \text{(circuitry equation)} \tag{4.47}$$

$$T_e - B_m \omega_r - T_L = J \frac{d^2\theta_r}{dt^2} \quad \text{(torsional–mechanical equation)} \tag{4.48}$$

From the flux linkage equation $\psi_{as} = L_{as} i_{as} + N A_{ag} B(\theta_r)$, we have

$$\frac{d\psi_{as}}{dt} = L_{as}\frac{di_{as}}{dt} + N A_{ag}\frac{dB(\theta_r)}{dt} = L_{as}\frac{di_{as}}{dt} + \frac{1}{2} N_m N A_{ag} B_{max} \cos\left(\frac{1}{2} N_m \theta_r\right)\omega_r \tag{4.49}$$

Thus, a set of three first-order nonlinear differential equations results, which models a single-phase axial topology permanent-magnet synchronous micromotors. In particular:

$$\frac{di_{as}}{dt} = \frac{1}{L_{as}}\left(-r_s i_{as} - \frac{1}{2} N_m N A_{ag} B_{max} \cos\left(\frac{1}{2} N_m \theta_r\right)\omega_r + u_{as}\right) \tag{4.50}$$

$$\frac{d\omega_r}{dt} = \frac{1}{J}\left(\frac{1}{2} N_m N A_{ag} B_{max} \cos\left(\frac{1}{2} N_m \theta_r\right) i_{as} - B_m \omega_r - T_L\right) \tag{4.51}$$

$$\frac{d\theta_r}{dt} = \omega_r \tag{4.52}$$

Single-phase axial permanent-magnet synchronous micro- and nanomachines may have a torque ripple. To avoid this torque ripple, one must design two-phase machines. For two-phase machines, the co-energy and electromagnetic torque are given as

$$W_c(i_{as}, \theta_r) = N A_{ag} B_{max}\left(\sin\left(\frac{1}{2} N_m \theta_r\right) i_{as} - \cos\left(\frac{1}{2} N_m \theta_r\right) i_{bs}\right) \tag{4.53}$$

and the electromagnetic torque is

$$T_e = \frac{\partial W_c(i_{as}, \theta_r)}{\partial \theta_r} = \frac{1}{2} N_m N A_{ag} B_{max}\left(\cos\left(\frac{1}{2} N_m \theta_r\right) i_{as} + \sin\left(\frac{1}{2} N_m \theta_r\right) i_{bs}\right) \tag{4.54}$$

Thus, feeding the phase currents as

$$i_{as} = i_M \cos\left(\frac{1}{2} N_m \theta_r\right) \quad \text{and} \quad i_{bs} = i_M \sin\left(\frac{1}{2} N_m \theta_r\right) \tag{4.55}$$

we obtain

$$T_e = \frac{1}{2}N_m N A_{ag} B_{max} i_M \left(\cos^2\left(\frac{1}{2}N_m\theta_r\right) + \sin^2\left(\frac{1}{2}N_m\theta_r\right)\right) = \frac{1}{2}N_m N A_{ag} B_{max} i_M \quad (4.56)$$

The model developments and control issues are reported in Lyshevski (2001).

Fabrication Aspects

Micromachines can be fabricated through deposition of the conductors (coils and windings), ferromagnetic core, magnets, insulating layers, as well as other microstructures (movable and stationary members and their components including bearings). The subsequent order of the processes, sequential steps, and materials are different depending on the machines devised, designed, analyzed, and optimized. Several textbooks (Madou, 1997; Kovacs, 1998; Lyshevski, 2001, 2004; Giurgiutiu and Lyshevski, 2004) provide the reader with the basic fabrication features and processes involved in the micromachine fabrication. This section outlines the most viable aspects.

Complementary metal oxide semiconductor (CMOS), high-aspect-ratio (LIGA and LIGA-like), and surface micromachining technologies are key features for fabrication of nano- and micromachines and structures. The LIGA (Lithography–Galvanoforming–Molding, or, in German, *Lithografie–Galvanik–Abformung*) technology allows one to make three-dimensional microstructures with the aspect ratio (depth vs. lateral dimension is more than 100). The LIGA technology is based on x-ray lithography, which ensures short wavelength (from few to 10 Å) which leads to negligible diffraction effects and larger depth of focus compared with photolithography. The major processes in the machines' microfabrication are diffusion, deposition, patterning, lithography, etching, metallization, planarization, assembling, and packaging. Thin-film fabrication processes were developed and used for polysilicon, silicon dioxide, silicon nitride, and other different materials, e.g., metals, alloys, and composites. The basic steps are: lithography, deposition of thin films and materials (electroplating, chemical vapor deposition, plasma enhanced chemical vapor deposition, evaporation, sputtering, spraying, screen printing), removal of material (patterning) by wet or dry techniques, etching (plasma etching, reactive ion etching, laser etching, etc.), doping, bonding (fusion, anodic, and other), and planarization (Madou, 1997; Kovacs, 1998; Lyshevski, 2001, 2004).

To fabricate motion and radiating energy nano- and microscale structures and devices, different fabrication technologies are used (Madou, 1997; Kovacs, 1998; Lyshevski, 2001, 2004). New processes were developed and novel materials were applied to modify the CMOS, surface micromachining, and LIGA technologies. Currently, the state of the art in nanofabrication has progressed to nanocircuits and nanodevices (Lyshevski, 2004). Nano- and micromachines and their components (stator, rotor, bearing, coils, etc.) are defined photographically, and the high-resolution photolithography is applied to define two- (planar) and three-dimensional shapes (geometry). Deep ultraviolet lithography processes were developed to decrease the feature sizes of microstructures to 0.1 μm. Different exposure wavelengths λ (435, 365, 248, 200, 150, or 100 nm) are used. Using the Rayleigh model for image resolution, the expressions for image resolution i_R and the depth of focus d_F are given by

$$i_R = k_i \frac{\lambda}{N_A}, \quad d_F = k_d \frac{\lambda}{N_A^2} \quad (4.57)$$

where k_i and k_d are the lithographic process constants; λ is the exposure wavelength; N_A is the numerical aperture coefficient (for high-numerical aperture we have $N_A = 0.5$ to 0.6).

The g- and i-line IBM lithography processes (with wavelengths of 435 and 365 nm, respectively) allow one to attain 0.35-μm features. The deep ultraviolet light sources (mercury source or excimer lasers) with 248-nm wavelength enables the industry to achieve 0.25-μm resolution. The changes to short exposure wavelength possess challenges and present new highly desired possibilities. However, using CMOS technology,

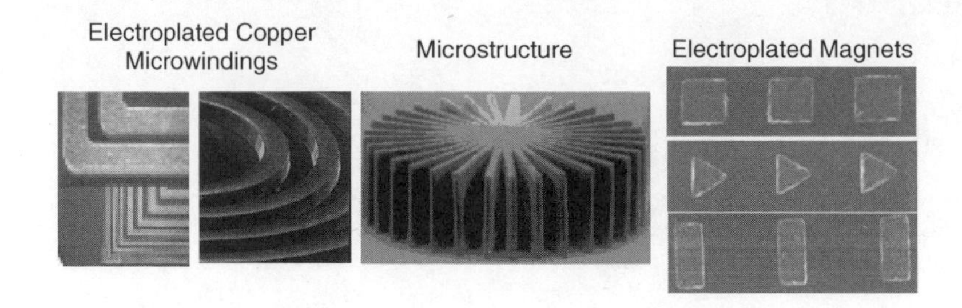

FIGURE 4.12 Deposited copper microwindings, microstructure, and permanent magnets.

50-nm features were achieved, and the application of x-ray lithography led to nanometer scale features (Madou, 1997; Kovacs, 1998; Lyshevski, 2001, 2004). Different lithography processes commonly applied are: photolithography, screen printing, electron-beam lithography, and x-ray lithography (high-aspect ratio technology).

Although machine topologies and configurations vary, magnetic and insulating materials, magnets, and windings are used in all motion devices. Figure 4.12 illustrates the electroplated 10-μm wide and thick with 10-μm spaced insulated copper microwindings (deposited on ferromagnetic cores), microstructures, and permanent magnets (electroplated NiFe alloy) as shown by Lyshevski (2001).

Electroactive and Magnetoactive Materials

Electroactive and magnetoactive materials are the building blocks of micromechatronics. The intrinsic active behavior of these materials, which change dimensions in response to electric and magnetic fields, make them ideal for actuation and sensing at the micro level.

Electroactive Materials

Electroactive materials can be divided into piezoelectric and electrostrictive. *Linear piezoelectric materials* obey the constitutive relations between the mechanical and electrical variables, which can be written in tensor notations as

$$S_{ij} = s^{E}_{ijkl} T_{kl} + d_{ijk} E_k + \delta_{ij} \alpha^{E}_{i} \theta \tag{4.58}$$

$$D_j = d_{jkl} T_{kl} + \varepsilon^{T}_{jk} E_k + \tilde{D}_j \theta \tag{4.59}$$

where S_{ij} is the mechanical strain, T_{kl} the mechanical stress, E_k the electrical field, and D_j the electrical displacement. The variable s^{E}_{ijkl} is the mechanical compliance of the material measured at zero electric field ($E = 0$), ε^{T}_{jk} is the dielectric permittivity measured at zero mechanical stress ($T = 0$), and d_{kij} is the piezoelectric coupling between the electrical and mechanical variables. The variable θ is the temperature, and α^{E}_{i} is the coefficient of thermal expansion under constant electric field. The coefficient $\tilde{D}_j$ is the electric displacement temperature coefficient. The stress and strain variables are second-order tensors, while the electric field and the electric displacement are first-order tensors. Since thermal effects only influence the diagonal terms, the respective coefficients, α_i and $\tilde{D}_j$, have single subscripts. The term δ_{ij} is the Kroneker delta ($\delta_{ij} = 1$ if $i = j$; zero otherwise). The physical explanation of the piezoelectric effect is represented schematically in Figure 4.13a.

Electromechanical coupling coefficient is the square root of the ratio between the mechanical energy stored and the electrical energy applied to a piezoelectric material, i.e.:

$$k = \sqrt{\frac{\text{mechanical energy stored}}{\text{electrical energy applied}}} \tag{4.60}$$

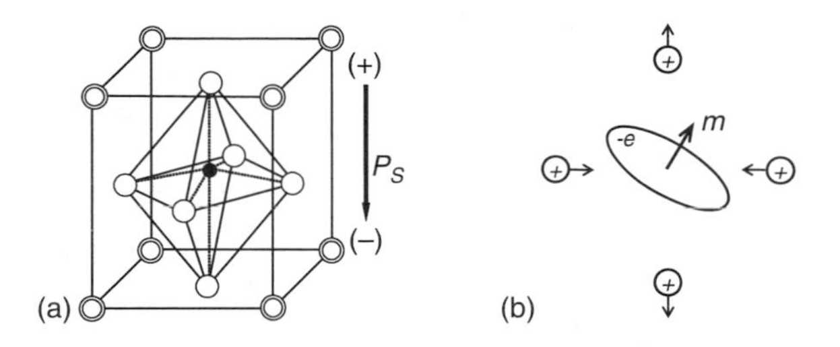

FIGURE 4.13 Physical explanation of induced-strain actuation: (a) piezoelectric response in a perovskite structure; (b) magetostrictive lattice deformation due to the rotation of the inner-shell charge-density oblate shape in a magnetic field.

For direct actuation, $k_{33} = d_{33}/\sqrt{s_{33}\varepsilon_{33}}$, where Voigt matrix notations are used. For transverse actuation, $k_{31} = d_{31}/\sqrt{s_{11}\varepsilon_{33}}$; for shear actuation, $k_{15} = d_{15}/\sqrt{s_{55}\varepsilon_{11}}$. For uniform inplane actuation, we obtain the planar coupling coefficient, $\kappa_p = \kappa_{13}\sqrt{2/(1-v)}$, where v is the Poisson ratio. The piezoelectric response in axial and shear directions is depicted in Figure 4.14.

In contrast with linear piezoelectricity, the *electrostrictive response* is quadratic in electric field. Hence, the direction of electrostriction does not change as the polarity of the electric field is reversed. The general constitutive equations incorporate both piezoelectric and electrostrictive terms:

$$S_{ij} = s^E_{klij} T_{kl} + d_{kij} E_k + M_{klij} E_k E_l \tag{4.61}$$

$$D_m = d_{mkl} T_{kl} + \varepsilon^T_{mn} E_n + 2M_{mnij} E_n T_{ij} \tag{4.62}$$

Note that the first two terms in each equation signify the linear piezoelectric behavior. The third term represents the nonlinear electrostrictive behavior. The coefficients M_{klij} are the electrostrictive coefficients.

Magnetoactive Materials

Most magnetoactive materials are based on the magnetostrictive effect. The *magnetostrictive constitutive equations* contain both linear and quadratic terms:

$$S_{ij} = s^E_{ijkl} T_{kl} + d_{kij} H_k + M_{klij} H_k H_l \tag{4.63}$$

$$B_m = d_{mkl} T_{kl} + \mu^T_{mk} H_k + 2M_{mnij} E_n T_{ij} \tag{4.64}$$

where, in addition to the already defined variables, H_k is the magnetic field intensity, B_j is the magnetic flux density, and μ^T_{jk} is the magnetic permeability under constant stress. The coefficients d_{kij} and M_{klij} are defined in terms of magnetic units. The magnetic field intensity in a rod surrounded by a coil with n turns per unit length depends on the coil current, I:

$$H = nI \tag{4.65}$$

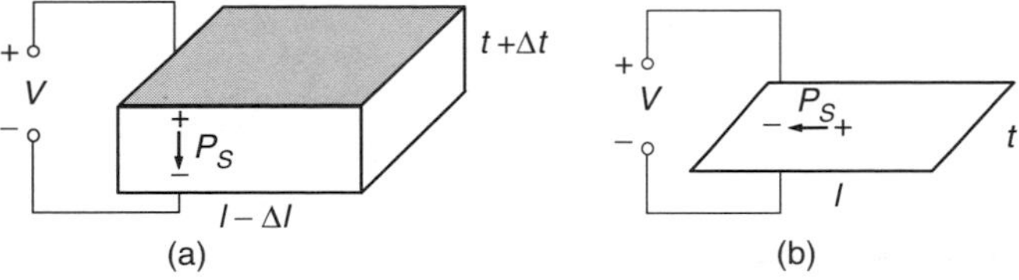

FIGURE 4.14 Induce-strain responses of piezoelectric materials: (a) axial strain; (b) shear strain.

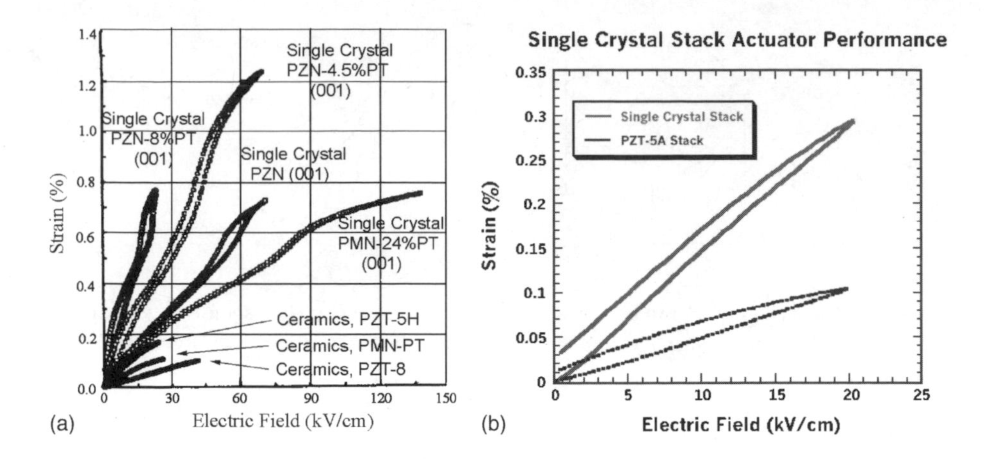

FIGURE 4.15 (a) Strain vs. electric field behavior of <001> oriented rhombohedral crystals of PZN–PT and PMN–PT compared to current piezoelectric ceramics (Park and Shrout, 1997); (b) single crystal stack actuator performance vs. conventional PZT-5A stack, as measured at TRS Ceramics, Inc. (http://www.trsceramics.com).

Magnetostrictive material response is quadratic in magnetic field, i.e., the magnetostrictive response does not change sign when the magnetic field is reversed. However, the nonlinear magnetostrictive behavior can be linearized about an operating point through the application of a bias magnetic field. In this case, *piezomagnetic* behavior, where response-reversal accompanies field reversal, can be obtained. In Voigt matrix notations, the equations of linear piezomagnetism are

$$S_i = s_{ij}^H T_j + d_{ki} H_k, \; i,j = 1,\ldots,6; \; k = 1,2,3 \tag{4.66}$$

$$B_m = d_{mj} T_j + \mu_{mk}^T H_k, j = 1,\ldots,6; \; k,m = 1,2,3 \tag{4.67}$$

where S_i is the mechanical strain, T_j is the mechanical stress, H_k is the magnetic field intensity, B_m is the magnetic flux density, and μ_{mk}^T is the magnetic permeability under constant stress. The coefficient s_{ij}^H is the mechanical compliance measured at zero magnetic field ($M = 0$). The coefficient μ_{mk}^T is the magnetic permeability measured at zero mechanical stress ($T = 0$). The coefficient d_{ki} is the *piezomagnetic constant*, which couples the magnetic and mechanical variables and expresses how much strain is obtained per unit applied magnetic field. A commercially available magnetoactive material with wide industrial applications is Terfenol-D ($Tb_{1-x}Dy_xFe_2$ where $x = 0.7$). Terfenol-D displays a large strain response of up to 0.2%. A full description of Terfenol-D properties is given in Table 4.9 of Giurgiutiu and Lyshevski (2004).

New active material developments include single-crystal piezoelectric ceramics, magnetic shape memory alloys, and others. The single crystal piezoelectric ceramics attain induced strain about an order of magnitude larger than conventional piezoelectric ceramics (Figure 4.15). Additional details of these and other active materials are given in Chapter 4 of Giurgiutiu and Lyshevski (2004).

Induced-Strain Actuators

Induced-strain actuators utilize active materials to produce force and displacement in response to applied electric or magnetic fields. Precise nano-positioning can be easily achieved with induced-strain actuators. The induced-strain actuators analysis differs from the analysis of conventional actuators because only a finite induced-strain displacement comes into play. The use of induced-strain actuators is preferred wherever a compact solid-state actuation solution is required.

Linearized Electromechanical Behavior of Induced-Strain Actuators

Induced-strain actuator vendor data usually contains the free-stroke, u_{ISA}, the corresponding maximum voltage, V, the internal stiffness, k_i, and the capacitance, C. Based on vendor data, one can calculate the apparent elastic compliance, s, electrical permittivity, ε, and piezoelectric strain coefficient, d, for full-stroke operation. For a piezoelectric stack:

$$s = \frac{A}{lk_i} \quad \text{(apparent zero − field elastic compliance)} \tag{4.68}$$

$$\varepsilon = \frac{C}{A}\frac{t^2}{l} \quad \text{(apparent zero − stress electrical permittivity)} \tag{4.69}$$

$$d = \frac{u_{ISA}}{V}\frac{t}{l} \quad \text{(apparent piezoelectric strain coefficient)} \tag{4.70}$$

where l, A, and k_i are the length, cross-sectional area, and internal stiffness, while t is the piezo layer thickness. The effective full-stroke electromechanical coupling coefficient of the piezoelectric stack actuator is obtained as

$$\kappa^2 = \frac{d^2}{s\varepsilon} = \frac{k_i u_{ISA}^2}{CV^2} \tag{4.71}$$

For magnetoactive actuators, a similar process is employed using current, I, and inductance, L, instead of voltage, V, and capacitance, C. As a result, the effective full-stroke electromechanical coupling coefficient of the magnetoactive actuator is obtained as

$$\kappa^2 = \frac{d^2}{s\mu} = \frac{k_i u_{ISA}^2}{LI^2} \tag{4.72}$$

The behavior of a typical piezoelectric induced-strain actuator under static and dynamic operation is given in Figure 4.16. Similar results for electrostrictive and magnetostrictive actuators can be found in Giurgiutiu and Lyshevski (2004) (Figure 4.19 and Figure 4.20).

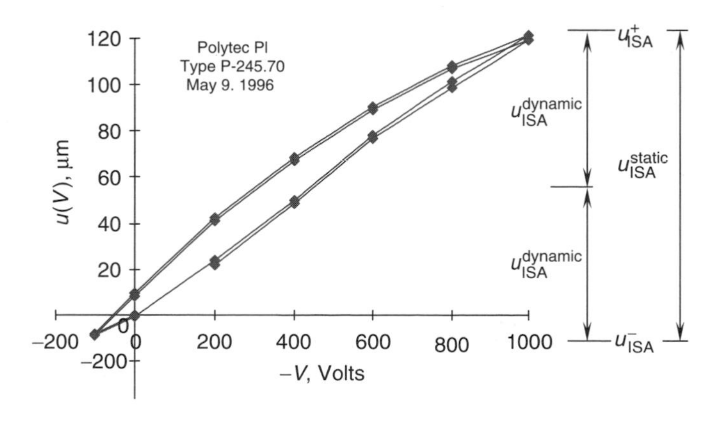

FIGURE 4.16 Induced-strain displacement vs. applied voltage for Polytec PI model P-245.70 piezoelectric (PZT) actuator.

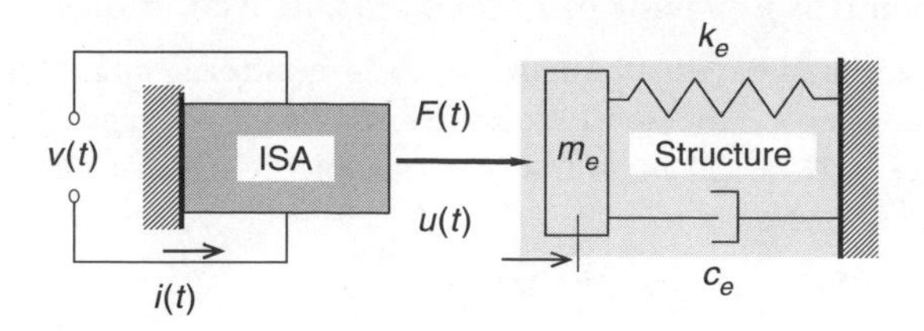

FIGURE 4.17 Interaction between an induced-strain actuator (ISA) and an elastic structure under dynamic conditions showing the frequency-dependent dynamic stiffness.

Power and Energy of Induced-Strain Actuators

The energy delivery of an induced-strain actuator depends on the relative relationship between the actuator internal stiffness, k_i, and the external stiffness, k_e, i.e., the stiffness of the desired application (Figure 4.17). Hence:

$$E_e = \frac{r}{(1+r)^2}\left(\frac{1}{2}k_i u_{ISA}^2\right) \tag{4.73}$$

where $r = k_e/k_i$ is the stiffness ratio. For dynamic operation, the stiffness ratio is frequency dependent and takes the form $r(\omega)$. The **matched stiffness** or **matched impedance** principle implies that maximum energy delivery is achieved when the internal and external stiffness values are equal (Figure 4.18). The maximum energy output that can be expected from a given induced-strain actuator is $E_e^{max} = \frac{1}{4}\left(\frac{1}{2}k_i u_{ISA}^2\right)$.

The electrical power and energy required for induced-strain actuation is calculated using induced-strain actuator admittance and impedance. For electroactive actuators:

$$Y_C(\omega) = i\omega C\left[1 - \kappa^2 \frac{\bar{r}(\omega)}{1+\bar{r}(\omega)}\right] = Y_C^R(\omega) + iY_C^I(\omega), \quad Z_C = Y_C^{-1} \tag{4.74}$$

For magnetoactive actuators:

$$Z_L(\omega) = i\omega L\left(1 - \kappa_L^2 \frac{\bar{r}(\omega)}{1+\bar{r}(\omega)}\right) \quad Y_L = Z_L^{-1} \tag{4.75}$$

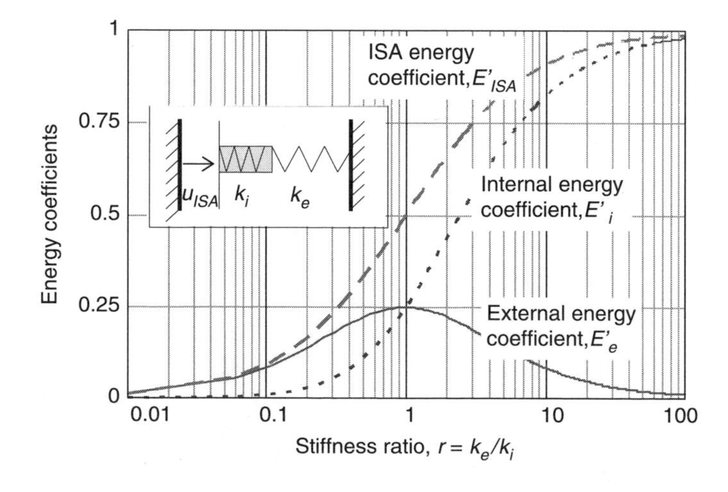

FIGURE 4.18 Variation of energy coefficients with stiffness ratio, r, under static operation.

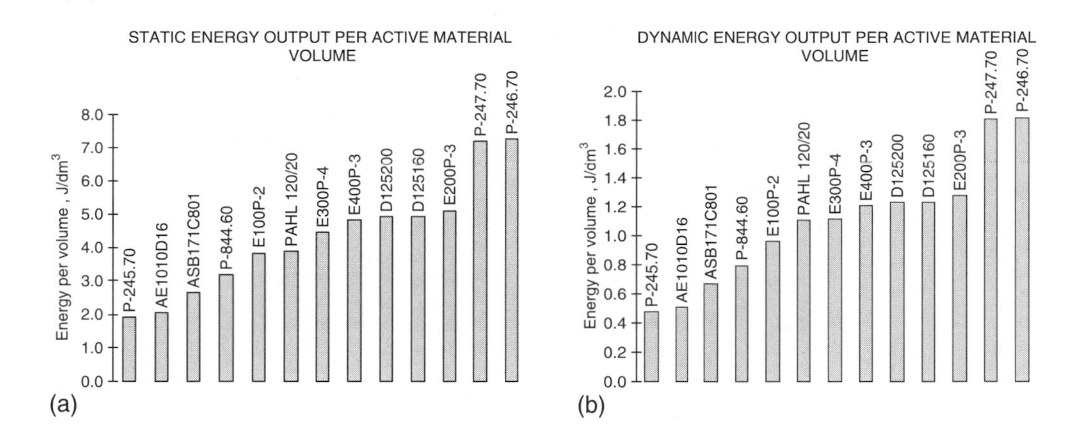

FIGURE 4.19 Energy density output per active material volume of commercially available induced-strain actuators: (a) static operation; (b) dynamic operation.

The energy density output calculated for a number of commercially available induced-strain actuators operating under static and dynamic conditions is presented Figure 4.19. Note that the dynamic energy density values are 1/4 of the static values, since the dynamic induced-strain stroke is half the static stroke. This specific aspect differentiates the analysis of induced-strain actuator from the analysis of conventional actuators. The complete analysis of induced-strain actuators power and energy, with a full complement of graphs and tables and extensive comparison data, is available in Sections 4.4 to 4.8 of Giurgiutiu and Lyshevski (2004).

Design with Induced-Strain Actuators

The design with induced-strain actuators must take into consideration their specific behavior. Induced-strain actuators can develop large forces but only a small finite stroke that must be judiciously used to achieve the design goals. By displacement-amplification (Figure 4.20), a tradeoff between stroke and force is obtained. Mitigation of the input/output requirements and induced-strain actuation capabilities is done during the design cycle.

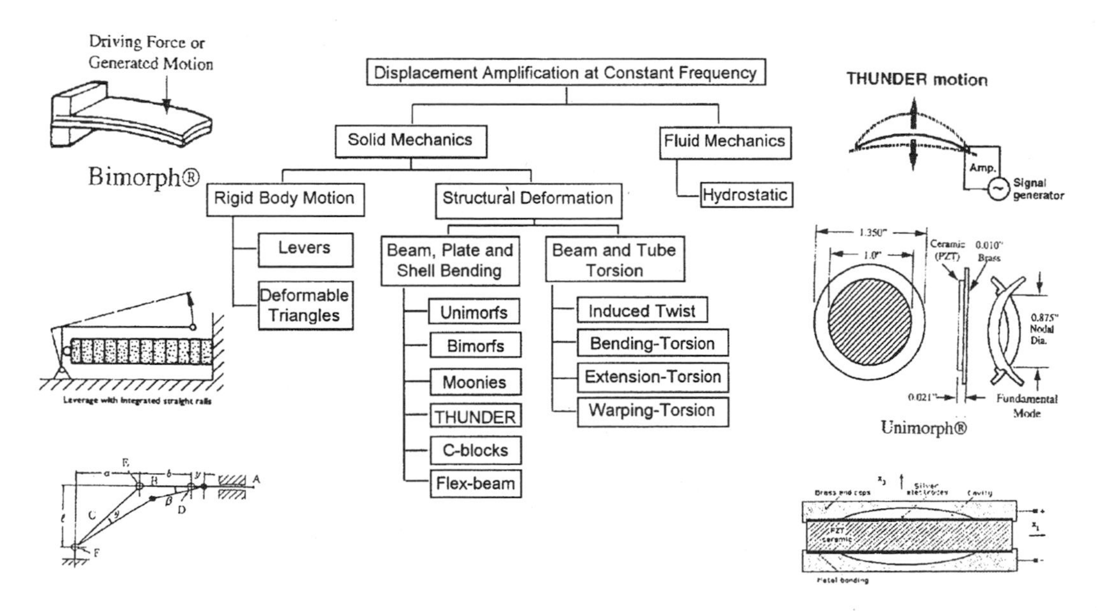

FIGURE 4.20 Family tree of displacement amplified induced-strain actuators.

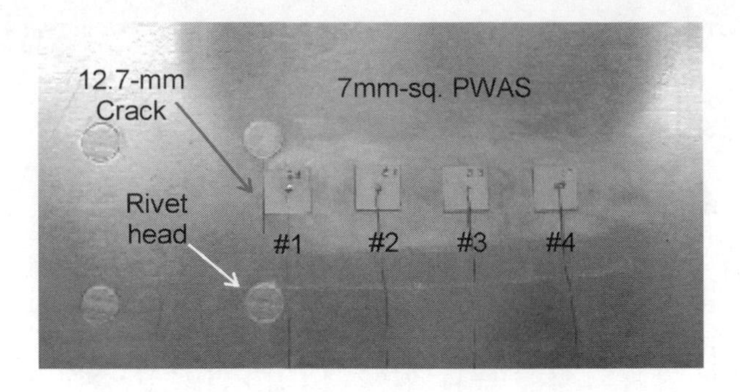

FIGURE 4.21 Piezoelectric wafer active sensors (PWAS) mounted on an aircraft panel.

Piezoelectric Wafer Active Sensors

Piezoelectric wafer active sensors (PWAS) are small and unobtrusive active-material devices that can act at both transmitters and receivers of elastic waves traveling in various materials (Figure 4.21). PWAS are the enabling technology for many micromechatronics applications, such as embedded sensing, vibration control, and structural health monitoring of cracks and defects.

PWAS Resonators

The analysis of PWAS resonators starts with the 1D analysis of rectangular PWAS and then extends to the 2D axisymmetric analysis of circular PWAS.

Rectangular PWAS Resonators

The 1D analysis of rectangular PWAS assumes that the ratio between length, width, and thickness is such that the respective vibrations can be considered uncoupled (Figure 4.22). Direct use of the constitutive Equation (4.58) yields the 1D wave equation:

$$\ddot{u}_1 = c^2 u_1'' \tag{4.76}$$

where $c^2 = 1/\rho s_{11}^E$ is the wave speed. For ac excitation, $E_3 = \hat{E}_3 e^{i\omega t}$, the solution is

$$\hat{u}_1(x) = \frac{d_{31}\hat{E}_3}{\gamma} \frac{\sin \gamma x}{\cos \frac{1}{2}\gamma l} \tag{4.77}$$

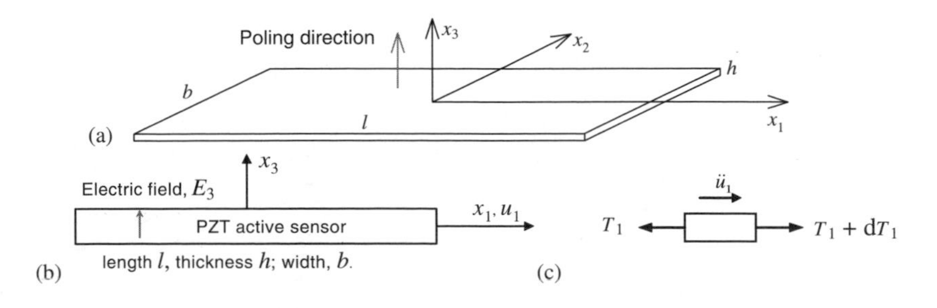

FIGURE 4.22 Schematic of a piezoelectric active sensor and infinitesimal axial element.

TABLE 4.2 Admittance and Impedance Poles for $k_{31} = 0.36$

Admittance poles, ϕ_Y (electromechanical resonances)		$3\frac{\pi}{2}$	$5\frac{\pi}{2}$	$7\frac{\pi}{2}$	$9\frac{\pi}{2}$	$11\frac{\pi}{2}$	...
Impedance poles, ϕ_Z (electromechanical resonances)	$1.0565\frac{\pi}{2}$	$3.021\frac{\pi}{2}$	$5.005\frac{\pi}{2}$	$\sim 7\frac{\pi}{2}$	$\sim 9\frac{\pi}{2}$	$\sim 11\frac{\pi}{2}$	...
Ratio ϕ_Z/ϕ_Y	1.0565	1.0066	1.0024	1.0012	1.0007	1.0005	...
Difference between ϕ_Z and ϕ_Y	5.6%	0.66%	0.24%	0.12%	0.07%	0.05%	

For electrical analysis, the solution substituted into the constitutive Equation (4.59) yields, after some manipulations:

$$\bar{Y} = i\omega \cdot \bar{C}\left[1 - \bar{k}_{31}^2\left(1 - \frac{1}{\bar{\varphi}\cot\bar{\varphi}}\right)\right], \quad \bar{Z} = \bar{Y}^{-1} \tag{4.78}$$

where $\bar{Y}$ and $\bar{Z}$ are the electric admittance and impedance, $\gamma = \omega/c$ γ is the wave number, $\phi = \frac{1}{2}\gamma l$, and $C = \varepsilon_{33}^T bl/h$ is the free capacitance. In addition, $\bar{k}_{13}^2 = d_{31}^2/(\bar{s}_{11}\bar{\varepsilon}_{33})$ is the complex coupling factor, $\bar{C} = (1 - \mathrm{i}\varepsilon)C$, $\bar{\varphi} = \varphi\sqrt{1 - \mathrm{i}\delta}$, $\bar{s}_{11} = s_{11}(1 - \mathrm{i}\eta)$, $\bar{\varepsilon}_{33} = \varepsilon_{33}(1 - \mathrm{i}\delta)$. The internal damping loss values η and δ vary with the piezoceramic formulation, but are usually small (η, δ, $> 5\%$). Of interest are the following resonance/antiresonance situations:

- **Electromechanical resonance**, when $Y \rightarrow \infty$, i.e., $Z = 0$
- **Electromechanical antiresonance**, when $Y=0$, i.e., $Z \rightarrow \infty$

Electromechanical resonances, i.e., admittance poles, exist for $\cos\phi = 0$, which gives the closed form solution $f_n^{\mathrm{EM}} = (2n - 1)c/2l$. Electromechanical resonances exist for $\frac{\tan\phi}{\phi} = -\frac{1 - k_{31}^2}{k_{31}^2}$. This is a transcendental equation that is solved numerically (Table 4.2). Practical measurements of the PWAS admittance and impedance are made with the impedance phase-gain analyzer (Figure 4.23).

Circular PWAS Resonators

The analysis of a circular PWAS resonator (Figure 4.24a) starts with the axisymmetric wave equation:

$$\frac{\mathrm{d}^2 u_\mathrm{r}}{\mathrm{d}r^2} + \frac{1}{r}\frac{\mathrm{d}u_\mathrm{r}}{\mathrm{d}r} - \frac{u_\mathrm{r}}{r^2} = -\frac{\omega^2}{c_\mathrm{p}^2}u_\mathrm{r} \tag{4.79}$$

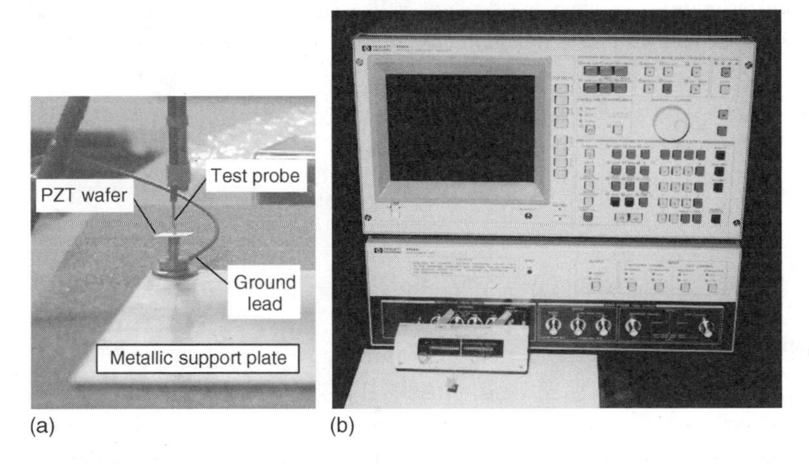

FIGURE 4.23 PWAS admittance and impedance measurement: (a) test jig ensuring unrestraint support, and (b) HP 4194A impedance phase-gain analyzer.

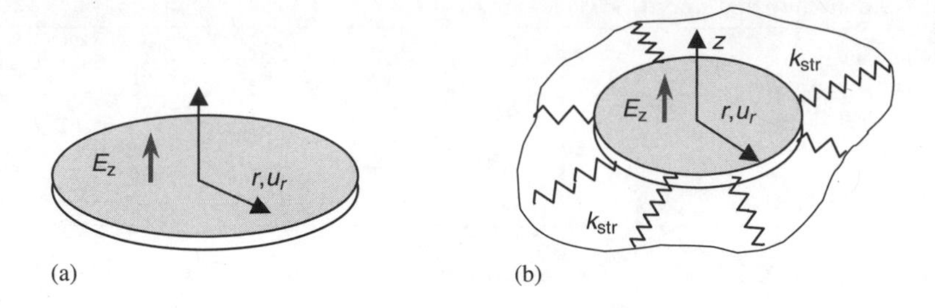

FIGURE 4.24 Analysis of circular PWAS: (a) free; (b) constrained by structural stiffness, $k_{str}(\omega)$.

where $c_p = \sqrt{1/\rho s_{11}^E(1-\nu^2)}$ is the wavespeed for radial vibrations. For ac excitation, $E_3 = \hat{E}_3 e^{i\omega t}$, the solution is expressed in terms of J_0 and J_1 Bessel functions as

$$u_r(r) = (d_{31}\hat{E}_3)a\frac{(1+\nu)J_1(\gamma r)}{(\gamma a)J_0(\gamma a) - (1-\nu)J_1(\gamma a)} \tag{4.80}$$

where a is the PWAS radius, ν is the Poisson ratio, and $\gamma = \omega/c_p$ is the wave number. The electromechanical admittance and impedance are given by

$$\bar{Y} = i\omega\bar{C}\left[(1-\bar{k}_p^2) - \bar{k}_p^2\frac{(1+\nu)J_1(\bar{\gamma}a)}{(\bar{\gamma}a)J_0(\bar{\gamma}a) - (1-\nu)J_1(\bar{\gamma}a)}\right], \quad \bar{Z} = \bar{Y}^{-1} \tag{4.81}$$

where $C = \varepsilon_{33}^T \pi a^2/h$. The bar above the quantities signifies that the complex values associated with internal damping are being used. The condition for mechanical resonance is

$$(\gamma a)J_0(\gamma a) - (1-\nu)J_1(\gamma a) = 0 \quad \text{(resonance)} \tag{4.82}$$

Numerical solution of Equation (4.82) for $\nu = 0.30$ yields

$$(\gamma a)_1 = 2.048652;\ (\gamma a)_2 = 5.389361;\ (\gamma a)_3 = 8.571860;\ (\gamma a)_4 = 11.731771\ldots \tag{4.83}$$

The corresponding resonance frequency is calculated as $f_n = (\gamma a)_n c/2\pi a$, where $n = 1, 2, 3, 4, \ldots$

The conditions for *electromechanical resonance and antiresonance* of a circular PWAS are:

$$zJ_0(z) - (1-\nu)J_1(z) = 0 \quad \text{(resonance)} \tag{4.84}$$

$$\frac{zJ_0(z)}{J_1(z)} = \frac{1-\nu-2k_p^2}{(1-k_p^2)} \quad \text{(antiresonance)} \tag{4.85}$$

These equations are transcendental and their solutions are found numerically.

PWAS Transmitters and Receivers of Elastic Waves

PWAS attached to structures act as good transmitters and receivers of elastic waves. In thin-wall structures, PWAS couple with symmetric and antisymmetric Lamb waves (Figure 4.25). In thicker structures, PWAS couple with Rayleigh waves. The first symmetric and antisymmetric Lamb wave modes, S_0 and A_0, approach the Rayleigh waves at very high frequency. At low frequency they can be approximated by the conventional axial and flexural waves (Figure 4.26).

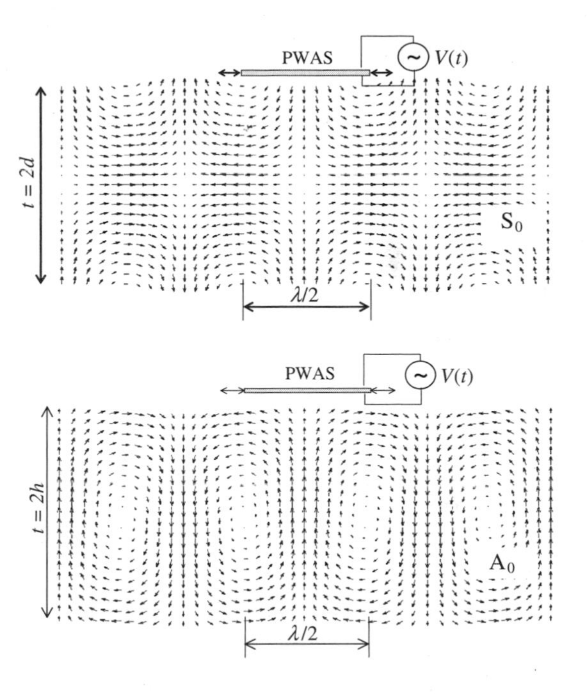

FIGURE 4.25 PWAS coupling with symmetric and antisymmetric Lamb waves, S_0 and A_0.

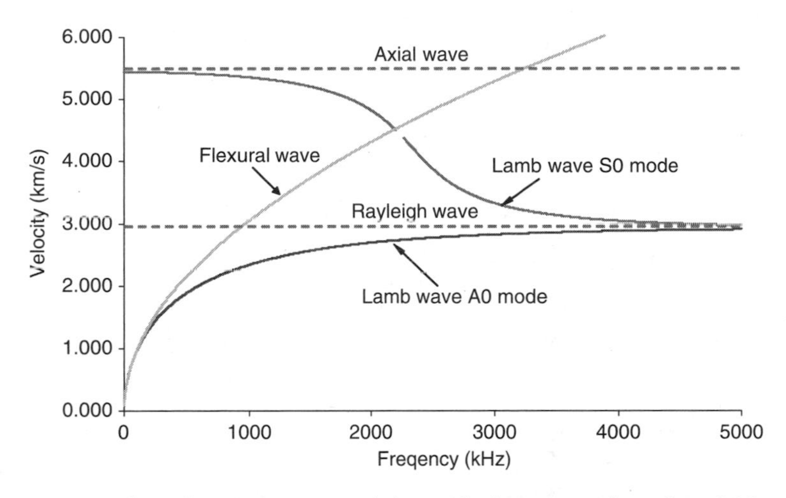

FIGURE 4.26 Frequency dependence of wave speed for axial, flexural, Lamb, and Rayleigh waves in 1-mm thick aluminum plate. The axial and flexural waves are the low-frequency asymptotes of the S_0 and A_0 Lamb wave modes. The Rayleigh wave is the high-frequency asymptote.

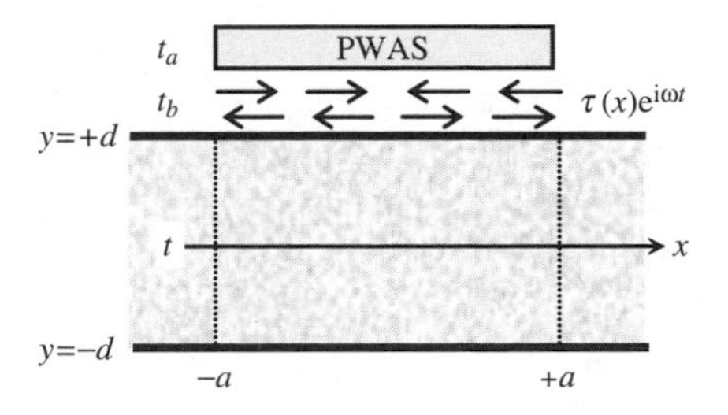

FIGURE 4.27 Interaction between the PWAS and the structure showing the bonding layer interfacial shear stress, $\tau(x)$.

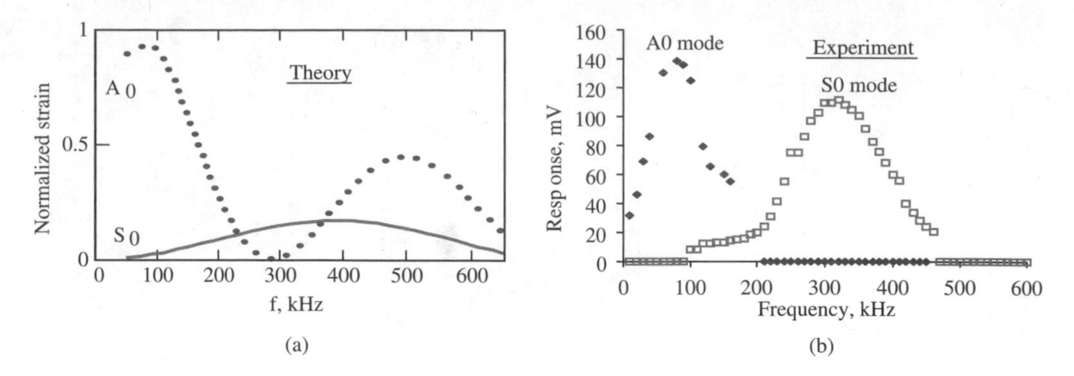

FIGURE 4.28 (a) Predicted Lamb wave strain amplitude from a 7-mm PWAS excitation in a 1.6-mm aluminum plate; (b) experimental verification of excitation sweet spot at 300 kHz.

The analysis of the interaction between the PWAS and the Lamb wave structure is performed assuming harmonic shear-stress boundary excitation applied to the upper surface of the plate (Figure 4.27), i.e.:

$$\tau_{\mathrm{a}}(x,h)=\begin{cases}\tau_0 \sinh(\Gamma x) & |x|<a \\ 0 & \text{otherwise}\end{cases} \tag{4.86}$$

Since the excitation is hasmonic, $\tau_{\mathrm{a}}(x)e^{-i\omega t}$, the solution is also assumed harmonic, in terms of the potentials ϕ and ψ satisfying the wave equations:

$$\frac{\partial^2\phi}{\partial x^2}+\frac{\partial^2\phi}{\partial y^2}+\frac{\omega^2}{c_{\mathrm{L}}^2}\phi=0, \qquad \frac{\partial^2\psi}{\partial x^2}+\frac{\partial^2\psi}{\partial y^2}+\frac{\omega^2}{c_{\mathrm{L}}^2}\psi=0 \tag{4.87}$$

where $c_{\mathrm{L}}^2=(\lambda+2\mu)/\rho$ and $c_{\mathrm{T}}^2=\mu/\rho$ are the longitudinal (pressure) and transverse (shear) wave speeds, λ and μ are Lame constants, and ρ is the mass density.

A salient result of this analysis, which is fully developed in Giurgiutiu and Lyshevski (2004), is that there are optimal conditions that permit the PWAS to preferentially excite one or another Lamb wave mode. For illustration, Figure 4.28a shows the predicted wave tuning into the A_0 Lamb wave mode at 100 kHz and into the S_0 Lamb wave mode at 300 kHz. The experimental validation of these predictions is shown in Figure 4.28(b). The equipment for the validation experiments is shown in Figure 4.29. For further details see Section 4.9 of Giurgiutiu and Lyshevski (2004).

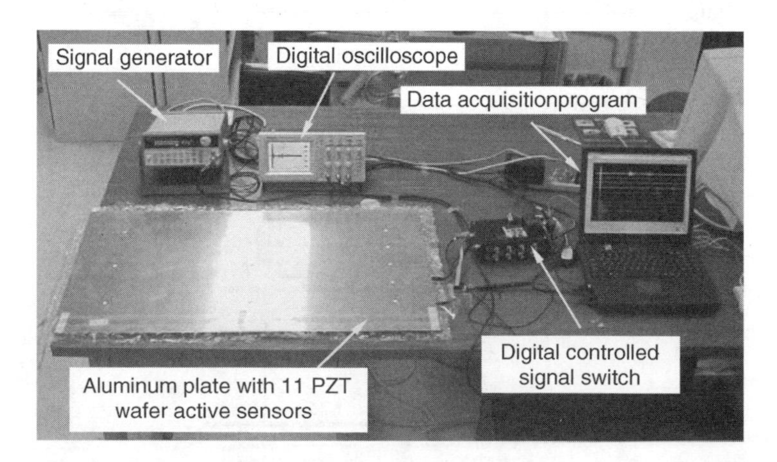

FIGURE 4.29 Experimental setup for wave propagation experiment with PWAS excitation and detection.

PWAS Phased Arrays

A remarkable result of PWAS Lamb wave tuning is the possibility of constructing the embedded ultrasonic structural radar (EUSR) utilizing the phased-array beamforming principles of the conventional electromagnetic radar and acoustic sonar (Figure 4.30). To understand the beam-forming principle, consider a linear array of M PWAS transducers as shown in Figure 4.31. If the PWAS are not fired simultaneously, but with some individual delays, δ_m, where $m = 0, 1, \ldots, M-1$, then the total signal received at a point P will be

$$s_{\mathrm{P}}(t) = \frac{1}{\sqrt{r}} \sum_{m=0}^{M-1} s_{\mathrm{T}}\left(t - \frac{r}{c} + \Delta_m(\phi) - \delta_m\right) \tag{4.88}$$

where $1/\sqrt{r}$ represents the decrease in the wave amplitude due to the omni-directional 2D radiation, and r/c is the delay due to the travel distance between the reference PWAS ($m = 0$) and the point P. Constructive interference between the received signals is achieved when $\delta_m = m\frac{d}{c}\cos(\phi_0)$, which yields

$$s_{\mathrm{P}}(t) = M \cdot \frac{1}{\sqrt{r}} s_{\mathrm{T}}\left(t - \frac{r}{c}\right) \tag{4.89}$$

At the target, the signal is backscattered with a backscatter coefficient, A. Hence, the signal received back at each PWAS will be $\frac{A \cdot M}{R} s_{\mathrm{T}}\left(t - \frac{2R}{c} + \Delta_m(\phi)\right)$. The receiver beamformer equation assembles the signals from

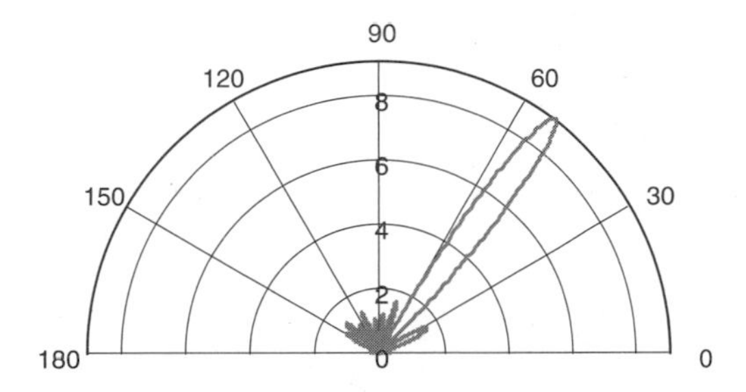

FIGURE 4.30 Beamforming pattern for a nine-sensor array (spacing $l = \lambda/2$) with 53° target azimuth.

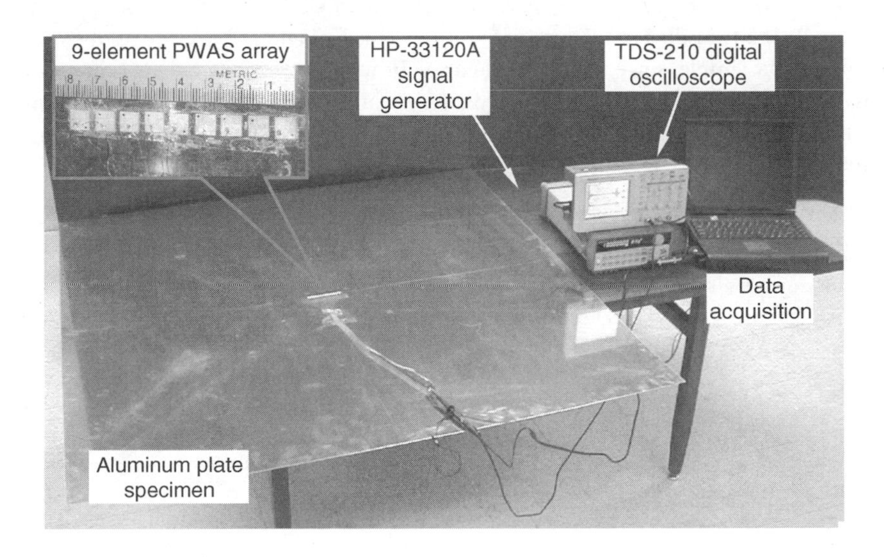

FIGURE 4.31 Experimental setup for the EUSR method showing the PWAS phased array.

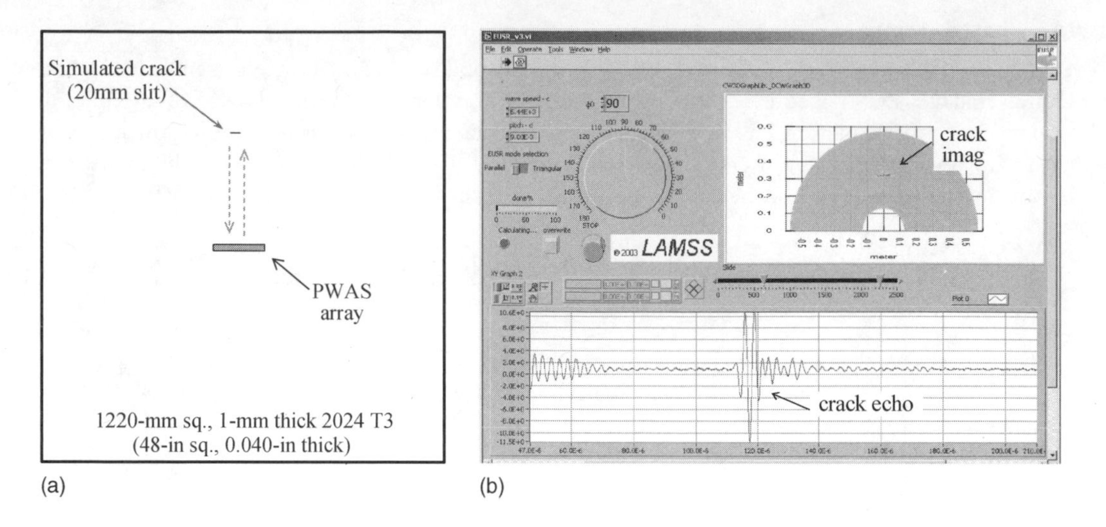

FIGURE 4.32 Crack detection in a plate: (a) schematic of crack location and size; (b) crack imaging and crack echo the EUSR algorithm window.

all the PWAS with the appropriate time delays, i.e.:

$$s_{\mathrm{R}}(t) = \frac{A \cdot M}{R} \sum_{m=0}^{M-1} s_{\mathrm{T}}\left(t - \frac{2R}{c} + \Delta_m(\phi) - \delta_m\right) \tag{4.90}$$

For $\delta_m = m\frac{d}{c}\cos(\phi_0)$, the receive signal will be again boosted M times. Hence:

$$s_{\mathrm{R}}(t) = \frac{A \cdot M^2}{R} \sum_{m=0}^{M-1} s_{\mathrm{T}}\left(t - \frac{2R}{c}\right) \tag{4.91}$$

The practical implementation of the EUSR principle in detecting small cracks in large metallic plates is illustrated in Figure 4.31 and Figure 4.32. Remarkable about the EUSR method is its simplicity, illustrated by two things: (a) the PWAS transducers are flush with the plate surface and hence quite unobtrusive; and (b) the signal acquisition is very simple, since all the phased array processing is done in virtual time using an array of elemental signals recorded in a round-robin fashion (Giurgiutiu and Lyshevski, 2004, Section 4.14). These aspects make this micromechatronics approach to phased-array technology much simpler than that of convention ultrasonics technology.

PWAS Modal Sensors and the Electromechanical Impedance Method

PWAS transducers can also act as *in-situ* modal sensors that can directly measure the high-frequency local impedance of the support structure. This remarkable property can be understood from the analysis of a constrained PWAS (Figure 4.33). The effect of the constraining stiffness is to modulate the electromechanical

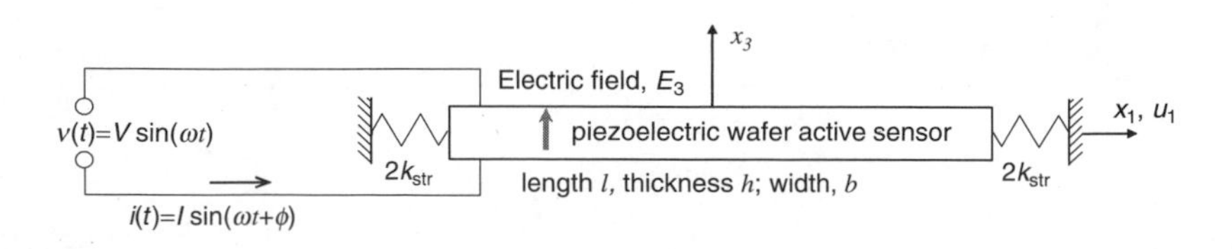

FIGURE 4.33 Schematic of a constraint piezoelectric wafer active sensor under harmonic ac excitation.

impedance with a term $\bar{r} = \bar{k}_{str}/\bar{k}_{PZT}$ that represents the dynamic stiffness ratio between the structural stiffness, k_{str}, and the PWAS stiffness, k_{PWAS}, i.e.:

$$\bar{Y} = i\omega \cdot \bar{C}\left[1 - \bar{\kappa}_{31}^2\left(1 - \frac{1}{\bar{\varphi}\cot\bar{\varphi} + \bar{r}}\right)\right], \quad \bar{Z} = \bar{Y}^{-1} \tag{4.92}$$

The structural stiffness $\bar{k}_{str}(\omega) = [k(\omega) - \omega^2 m(\omega)] - i\omega c(\omega)$ contains frequency dependent stiffness, mass, and damping coefficients. The PWAS stiffness is simply $k_{PWAS} = b_a t_a / s_{11}^E l_a$. A bar above the quantities signifies complex values resulting from the consideration of internal damping. The structural stiffness can be calculated in terms of axial and flexural vibration modes. For 1D vibrations, we have

$$k_{str}(\omega) = \frac{\hat{F}_{PZT}}{\hat{u}_{PZT}} = \rho A \left\{ \sum_{n_u} \frac{\left[U_{n_u}(x_a + l_a) - U_{n_u}(x_a)\right]^2}{\omega_{n_u}^2 + 2i\zeta_{n_u} - \omega^2} + \left(\frac{h}{2}\right)^2 \sum_{n_w} \frac{\left[W'_{n_w}(x_a + l_a) - W'_{n_w}(x_a)\right]^2}{\omega_{n_w}^2 + 2i\zeta_{n_w} - \omega^2} \right\}^{-1} \tag{4.93}$$

where n_u, ω_{n_u}, $U_{n_u}(x)$, and n_w, ω_{n_w}, $W_{n_w}(x)$ are the axial and flexural vibrations indices, frequencies, and mode shapes.

For a circular PWAS (Figure 4.24b), the constrained admittance is

$$Y(\omega) = \left\{ i\omega C(1 - k_p^2) \cdot \left[1 + \frac{k_p^2}{1 - k_p^2} \frac{(1 + \nu_a)J_1(\varphi_a)}{\varphi_a J_0(\varphi_a) - (1 - \nu_a)J_1(\varphi_a) - \frac{a}{r_a}\chi(\omega)(1 + \nu_a)J_1(\varphi_a)} \right] \right\} \tag{4.94}$$

For a circular plate, the structural stiffness can be calculated using the formula

$$k_{str}(\omega) = a^2 \rho \cdot \begin{bmatrix} \frac{2}{h}\sum_k \frac{\left[r_a R_k(r_a) - \int_0^a R_k(r) H(r_a - r) dr\right] R_k(r_a)}{(\omega_k^2 - 2i\varsigma_k \omega \omega_k + \omega^2)} \\ + \frac{h}{2}\sum_m \frac{\left[3Y_m(r_a) + r_a \cdot Y'_m(r_a)\right] \cdot Y'_m(r_a)}{(\omega_m^2 - 2i\varsigma_m \omega \omega_m + \omega^2)} \end{bmatrix}^{-1} \tag{4.95}$$

where $R_k(r)$, P_k and $Y_m(r)$, G_m are the modeshapes and the modal participation factors for axial and flexural vibrations of the circular plate. Experimental validation of the electromechanical impedance method is illustrated in Figure 4.34 for the case of 2D radial symmetric vibration of a circular plate. The structural resonances are reflected directly in the real part of the electromechanical impedance as measured at the PWAS terminals. A full treatment of the electromechanical impedance method and further experimental validation are given in Sections 4.15 to 4.17 of Giurgiutiu and Lyshevski (2004).

Microcontrollers Sensing, Actuation, and Process Control

Microcontroller-based devices and appliances can found in many areas of our everyday life. For example, the auto industry is putting tens of microcontrollers in a modern automobile, and plans to increase this number multifold as newer technologies are introduced. Figure 4.35a shows a generic computer architecture, while Figure 4.35b shows the architecture specific for microcontrollers. A **microcontroller** can be defined as a complete computer system on a chip, including CPU, memory, clock oscillator, and I/O devices. When some of these elements (such as the I/O or memory) are missing, the chip circuit would be called a **microprocessor**. The CPU in a personal computer is a microprocessor. Microcontrollers are commonly associated with embedded applications since they are placed directly inside a piece of machinery.

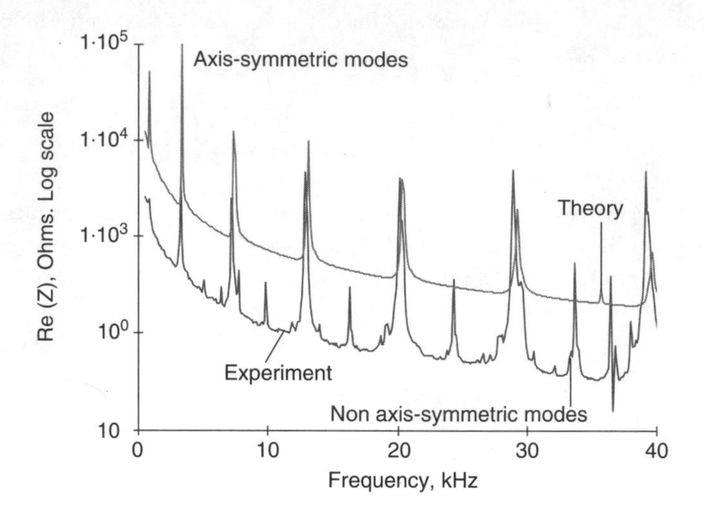

FIGURE 4.34 Experimental and calculated spectra for a circular plate specimen E/M impedance in the 0.5 to 40 kHz frequency range.

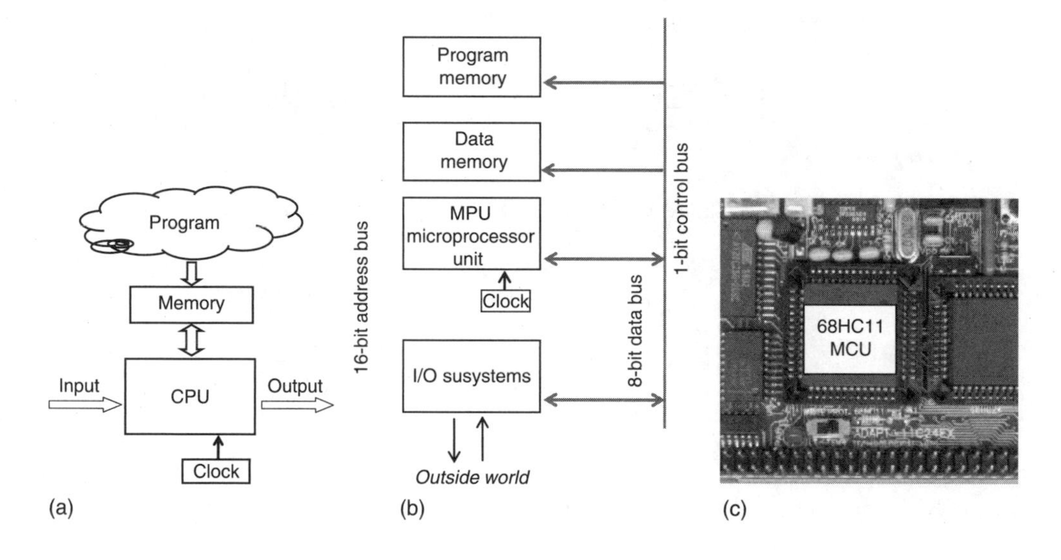

FIGURE 4.35 (a) Generic computer architecture; (b) microcontroller architecture; (c) 68HC11 microcontroller.

The MC68HC11 microcontroller family has an 8-bit architecture with advanced on-chip peripheral capabilities despite its small size (Figure 4.35c). The MC68HC11 has a nominal bus speed of 2 MHz, which is quite sufficient for many mechatronics applications that interface mechanical and electromechanical systems. A block diagram of the MC68HC11 microcontroller is shown in Figure 4.36. This diagram shows the major subsystems and the designation of the pins used by each subsystem: 6-bit free running timer (Port A); 8-bit parallel output (Port B); programmable bidirectional 8-bit parallel input/output port (Port C); two-pin asynchronous serial communications interface (SCI) and four-pin synchronous serial peripheral interface (SPI) as part of the six-pin Port D; four-channel 8-bit analog-to-digital (A/D) converter (Port E).

Two typical microcontroller applications are illustrated next. Figure 4.37 shows the use of the microcontroller for pulse width modulation (PWM) control of a dc motor. The experimental setup shown in Figure 4.37a includes the microcontroller mounted on an evaluation board (EVB), the driver circuit inside a transparent plastic case, the dc motor, and a multimeter. Figure 4.37b shows the experimental calibration

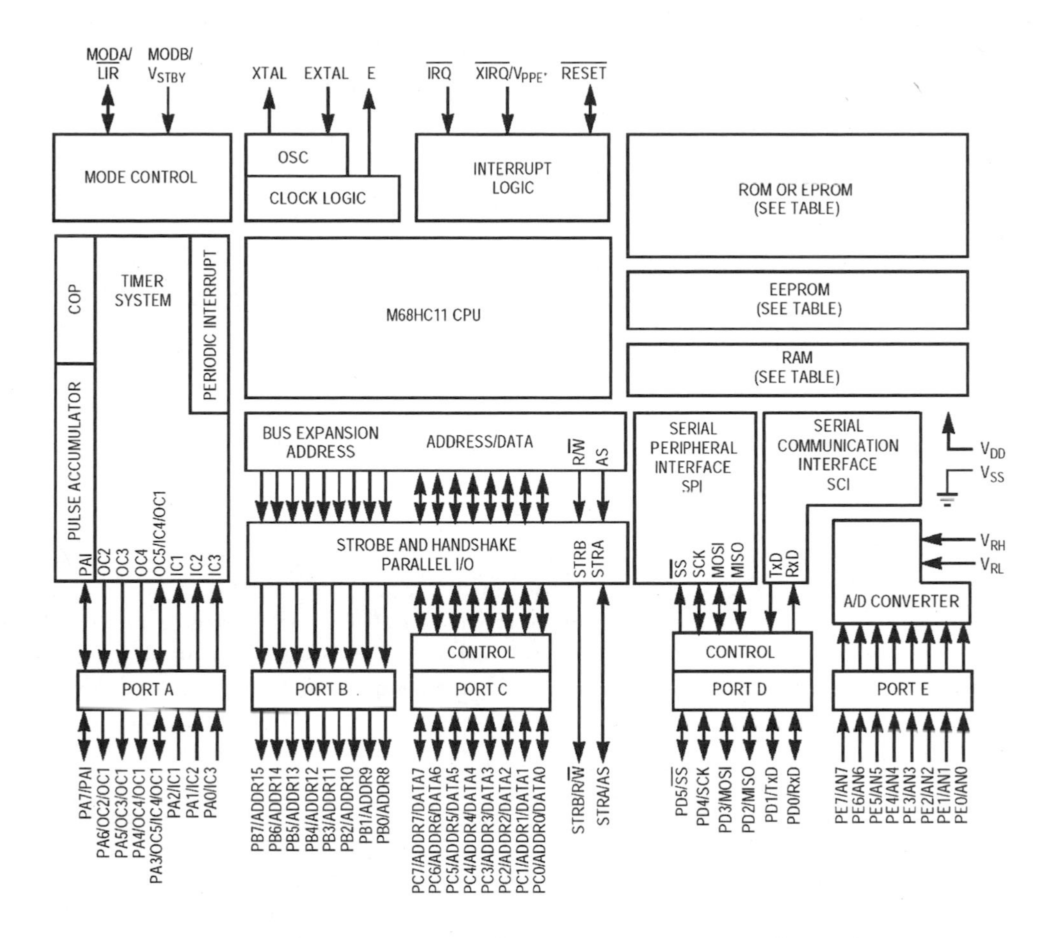

FIGURE 4.36 Block diagram of the MC68HC11 microcontroller family.

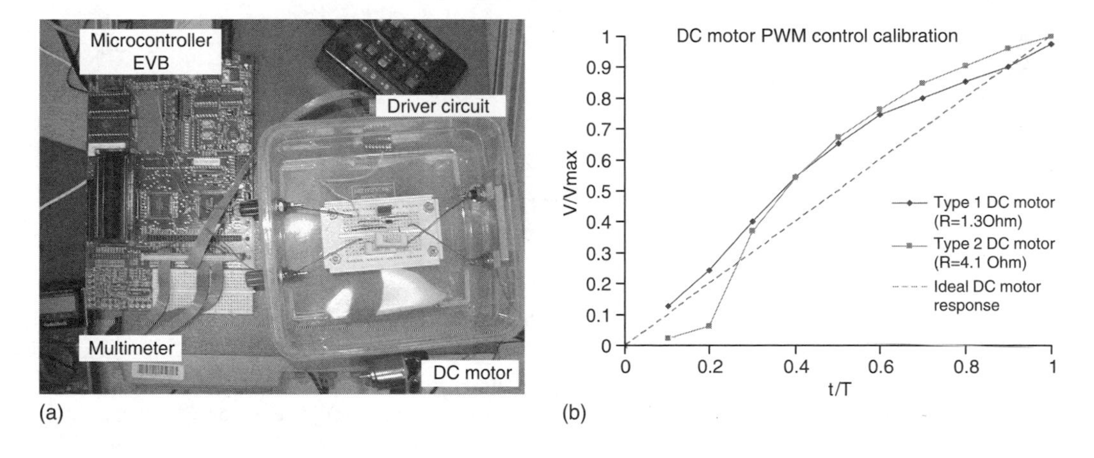

FIGURE 4.37 PWM control of a dc motor: (a) experimental setup; (b) experimental calibration curves.

curves raised for two dc motor types, and the ideally linear curve. It is apparent that motor nonlinearities differ from motor to motor.

The use of microcontrollers in process control is illustrated in Figure 4.38. In the case of open-loop control, the microcontroller is used to control the pump for a calibrated duration of time, based on the known pump

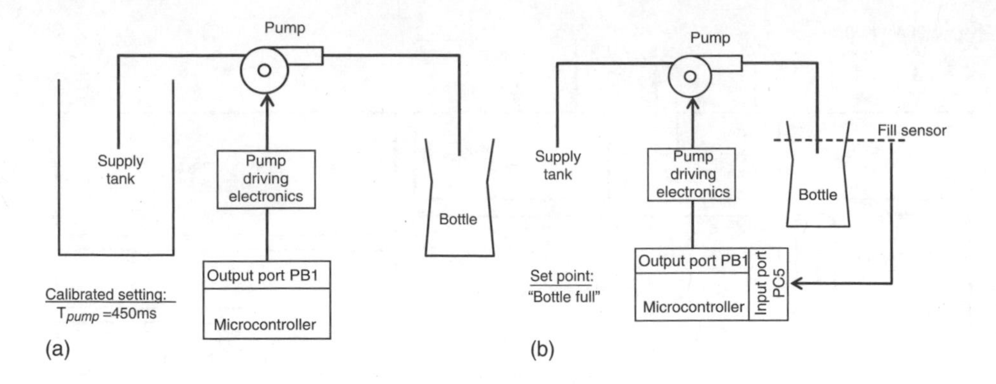

FIGURE 4.38 Schematic diagram of filling a bottle under microcontroller supervision: (a) open-loop control; (b) closed-loop control.

characteristics. However, should the pump characteristics or the fluid viscosity change, a new calibration would be required to achieve the desired fill level. This situation can be alleviated by the use of closed-loop control. In this case, a fill sensor is added to the system. The fill sensor signals to the microcontroller when the fill level has been reached and the microcontroller stops the pump. The closed-loop control, though initially more expensive to implement, it is more versatile and can save money over the plant life-cycle operation.

References

V. Giurgiutiu and S.E. Lyshevski, *Micromechatronics: Modeling, Analysis, and Design with MATLAB*, Boca Raton, FL: CRC Press, 2004.

G.T.A. Kovacs, *Micromachined Transducers Sourcebook*, Boston, MA: WCB McGraw-Hill, 1998.

S.E. Lyshevski, *MEMS and NEMS: Systems, Devices, and Structures*, Boca Raton, FL: CRC Press, 2001.

S.E. Lyshevski, *Nano- and Micro-Electromechanical Systems: Fundamental of Micro- and Nano-Engineering*, Boca Raton, FL: CRC Press, 2004.

M. Madou, *Fundamentals of Microfabrication*, Boca Raton, FL: CRC Press, 1997.

S.E. Park and T.R. Shrout, "Ultrahigh strain and piezoelectric behavior in relaxor ferroelectric single crystals," *J. Appl. Phys.*, vol. 82, no. 4, pp. 1804–1811, 1997.

4.4 Nanocomputers, Nano-Architectronics, and Nano-ICs*

Sergey Edward Lyshevski

This section discusses far-reaching developments in design, analysis, modeling, and synthesis of nano-computers using nanotechnology. In particular, nano-ICs can be applied to synthesize and design nano-computers utilizing two- and three-dimensional architectures. The nano-architectronics paradigm allows one to develop high-performance nano-ICs utilizing recently developed nanoelectronics components and devices, including nanoscale transistors, switches, capacitors, etc. Nanotechnology offers benchmarking opportunities to fabricate the components needed, and to date, different nanotechnologies are under development. Though molecular-, single-electron, carbon-, silicon-, GaAs-, and organic-based electronics have been developed to

*Parts of this section were published in: S.E. Lyshevski, Nanocomputer Architectronics and Nanotechnology, in *Handbook of Nanoscience, Engineering, and Technology*, W.A. Goddard, D.W. Brenner, S.E. Lyshevski, and G.J. Iafrate, Eds., CRC Press, Boca Raton, FL, 2003.

fabricate nanodevices, and promising pioneering results have been reported, it is difficult to accurately predict and envision the most promising high-yield affordable technologies and processes. Correspondingly, while covering some nanotechnologies to fabricate nanodevices and nano-ICs, this section focuses on the advanced concepts in fundamental and applied research in nanocomputers synthesis, design, and analysis. Mathematical models are developed using nanodevices and nano-ICs behavior description. The models proposed are straightforwardly applied to perform analysis, design, simulation, and optimization of nanocomputers. Novel methods in design of nanocomputers and their components are documented. Fundamental and applied results documented expand the horizon of nanocomputer theory and practice. It is illustrated that high-performance nanocomputers can be devised and designed using nano-ICs integrated within the *nanoarchitectronics* concept to synthesize two- and three-dimensional computer topologies with novel robust fault-tolerant organizations.

Introduction

Recently, meaningful applied and experimental results in nanoelectronic have been reported [1–15]. Though fundamental research has been performed in analysis of nanodevices, a limited number of feasible technologies has been developed to date to design applicable nanodevices operating at room temperature. However, the progress made in integrated carbon/silicon-based technology provides the confidence that nanoscale devices will be mass-produced in the nearest future. Unfortunately, no perfect nanodevices and large-scale nanodevice assemblies (matrices) can be fabricated. Correspondingly, novel adaptive and robust computing architectures, topologies, and organizations must be devised and developed. Our goal is to further expand and apply the fundamental theory of nanocomputers, develop the basic research toward sound nanocomputer theory and practice, as well as report the application of nanotechnology to fabricate nanocomputers and their components.

Several types of nanocomputers have been proposed. For the last one thousand years the synthesis and design of computers have been performed as a sequence of different paradigms and changes, e.g., from gears to relays, then to valves and to transistors, and more recently (in the 1980s) to integrated circuits [16]. Currently, IC technology progressed to the point that hundreds of millions of transistors are fabricated on a 1 cm^2 silicon chips. The transistors are downsized to hundreds of nanometers using 50- and 70-nm fabrication technologies. However, the silicon-based technology reaching the limit, and scaling laws cannot be applied due to the fundamental limitations and basic physics [17–26]. Nanotechnology allows one to fabricate nanoscale transistors that operate based on the quantum mechanics paradigms. Furthermore, computing can be performed utilizing quantum principles. Digital computers use bits (charged is 1 and not charged is 0). A register of 3 bits is represented by eight numbers, e.g., 000, 001, 010, 100, 011, 101, 110, and 111. In the quantum state (quantum computing), an atom (1 bit) can be in two places at once according to the laws of quantum physics. Therefore, two atoms (quantum bits or qubits) can represent eight numbers at any given time. For x number of qubits, 2^x numbers are stored. Parallel processing can take place on the 2^x input numbers, performing the same task that a classical computer would have to repeat 2^x times or use 2^x processors working in parallel. Therefore, a quantum computer offers an enormous gain in the use of computational resources in terms of time and memory. Unfortunately, limited progress has been made to date in practical application of this concept. Though conventional computers require exponentially more time and memory to match the power of a quantum computer, it is unlikely that quantum computers will become the reality in the near observable future. Correspondingly, experimental, applied, and fundamental research in nanocomputers has been performed to significantly increase the computational and processing speed, memory, and other performance characteristics utilizing novel nanodevices through application of nanotechnology (rather than solely rely on the quantum computing and possible quantum computers due to existing formidable challenges). Nanocomputers will allow one to compute and process information thousands of times faster than advanced computers.

Bioelectrochemical nanocomputers store and process information utilizing complex electrochemical interactions and changes. Bioelectrochemical nanobiocircuits that store, process, and compute exist in nature in enormous variety and complexity evolving through thousands of years of evolution. The development and prototyping of bioelectrochemical nanocomputer and three-dimensional circuits have progressed through engineering bioinformatic and biomimetic paradigms. Mechanical nanocomputers can be designed using tiny moving components (nanogears) to encode information. These nanocomputers can be considered as evolved Babbage computers (in 1822 Charles Babbage built a six-digit calculator that performed mathematical operations using gears). Complexity of mechanical nanocomputers is a major drawback, and this deficiency unlikely can be overcome.

First-, second-, third-, and fourth-generations of computers emerged, and tremendous progress has been achieved. The Intel® Pentium® 4 (3 GHz) processor was built using advanced Intel® NetBurst™ micro-architecture. This processor ensures high-performance processing, and is fabricated using 0.13-micron technology. The processor is integrated with high-performance memory systems, e.g., 8 KB L1 data cache, 12 K μops L1 Execution Trace Cache, 256 KB L2 Advanced Transfer Cache and 512 KB Advance Transfer Cache. Currently, 70 and 50 nm technologies are emerged and applied to fabricate high-yield high-performance ICs with billions of transistors on a single 1 cm^2 die. Further progress is needed, and novel developments are emerging. The fifth generation of computers will be built using emerging nano-ICs. This section studies the application of nanotechnology to design nanocomputers with nano-ICs. Synthesis, integration, and implementation of new affordable, high-yield nano-ICs are critical to meet Moore's first law. Figure 4.39 illustrates the first and second Moore laws (reported data and foreseen trends can be viewed as controversial and subject to adjustments; however, the major trends and tendencies are obvious, and most likely cannot be seriously argued and disputed) [10].

Nanotechnology and far-reaching fundamental progress eventually will lead to three-dimensional nano-ICs. This will result in synthesis and design of nanocomputers with novel computer architectures, topologies, and organizations. These nano-ICs and nanocomputers will guarantee superior level of overall performance. In particular, compared with the existing most advanced computers, in nanocomputers the execution time, switching frequency, bandwidth, and size will be decreased by the order of millions, while the memory capacity will be increased by the order of millions. However, significant challenges must be overcome particularly in synthesis and design of three-dimensional nanodevices, nanoelectronics, and nano-ICs. Many problems (novel nanocomputer architectures, advanced organizations, robust adaptive topologies, high-fidelity modeling, data-intensive analysis, heterogeneous simulations, optimization, reconfiguration, self-organization, robustness, utilization, and other) must be addressed, researched, and solved. Many of the above-mentioned problems have not been even addressed yet. Because of tremendous challenges, much effort must be focused to solve these problems. This section formulates and solves some long-standing fundamental and applied problems in synthesis, design, analysis, and optimization of nanocomputers utilizing nano-ICs. The fundamentals of nanocomputer *architectronics* are reported, and the basic organizations and topologies are examined progressing from the general system-level consideration to the nanocomputer subsystem/unit/device-level study.

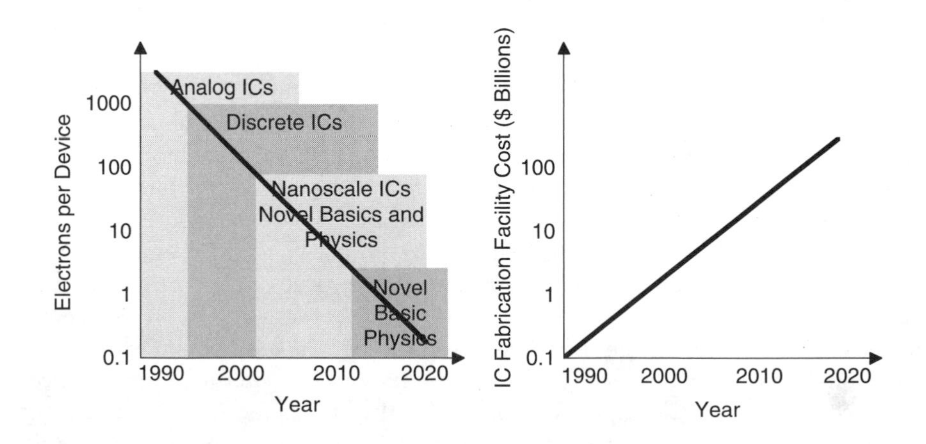

FIGURE 4.39 Moore's laws and nanotechnologies.

Nano-Electronics and Nanocomputer Fundamentals

In general, both reversible and irreversible nanocomputers can be designed. Nowadays, all existing computers are irreversible. The system is reversible if it is deterministic in the reverse and forward time directions. The reversibility implies that no physical state can be reached by more than one path (otherwise, reverse evolution would be nondeterministic). Current computers constantly irreversibly erase temporary results, and thus the entropy changes. The average instruction execution speed (in millions of instructions executed per second, I_{PS}) and cycles per instruction are related to the time required to execute instructions as given by $T_{inst} = 1/f_{clock}$. The clock frequency f_{clock} depends mainly on the ICs or nano-ICs used as well as upon the fabrication technologies (for example, the switching frequency 3 GHz was achieved in the existing Intel Pentium processors). The quantum mechanics implies an upper limit on the frequency at which the system can switch from one state to another. This limit is found as the difference between the total energy E of the system and ground state energy E_0. We have the following explicit inequality to find the maximum switching frequency $f_1 \leq \frac{4}{h}(E - E_0)$. Here, h is the Planck constant, and $h = 6.626 \times 10^{-34}$ J sec or J/Hz. An isolated nanodevice, consisting of a single electron at a potential of 1 V above its ground state, contains 1 eV of energy (1 eV $= 1.602 \times 10^{-19}$ J) and therefore cannot change its state faster than $f_1 \leq \frac{4}{h}(E - E_0) = \frac{4}{6.626 \times 10^{-34}} 1.602 \times 10^{-19} \approx 0.97 \times 10^{15}$ Hz. For example, the switching frequency can be achieved in the range up to 1×10^{15} Hz. We conclude that the switching frequency of nano-ICs can be significantly increased compared with currently used CMOS technology-based ICs.

In asymptotically reversible nanocomputers, the generated entropy is found as $S = b/t_t$, where b is the entropy coefficient that varies from 1×10^7 to 1×10^6 bits/GHz for ICs, and from 1 to 10 bits/GHz for quantum FETs; t_t is the length of time over which the operation is performed. Hence, the minimum entropy and processing (operation) rate for quantum nanodevices are $S = 1$ bit/operation and $r_e = 1 \times 10^{26}$ operation/sec cm^2, while CMOS technology allows one to fabricate devices with $S = 1 \times 10^6$ bits/operation and $r_e = 3.5 \times 10^{16}$ operation/sec cm^2.

The nanocomputer architecture integrates the functional, interconnected, and controlled hardware units and systems that perform propagation (flow), storage, execution, and processing of information (data). Nanocomputer accepts digital or analog input information, processes and manipulates it according to a list of internally stored machine instructions, stores the information, and produces the resulting output. The list of instructions is called a program, and internal storage is called memory.

In general, nanocomputer architecture can be synthesized utilizing the following major systems: (1) input–output, (2) memory, (3) arithmetic and logic, and (4) control units.

The input unit accepts information from electronic devices or other computers through the cards (electromechanical devices, such as keyboards, can be also interfaced). The information received can be stored in the memory, and then manipulated and processed by the arithmetic and logic unit (ALU). The results are output using the output unit. Information flow, propagation, manipulation, processing, and storage (memory) are coordinated by the control unit. The arithmetic and logic unit, integrated with the control unit, is called the processor or central processing unit (CPU). Input and output systems are called the input–output (I/O) unit. The memory unit integrates memory systems that stores programs and data. There are two main classes of memory, called *primary* (main) and *secondary* memory. The primary memory is implemented using nano-ICs that can consist of billions of nanoscale storage cells (each cell can store one bit of information). These cells are accessed in groups of fixed size called words. The main memory is organized such that the contents of one word can be stored or retrieved in one basic operation called a memory cycle. To provide consistent direct access to any word in the main memory in the shortest time, a distinct address number is associated with each word location. A word is accessed by specifying its address and issuing a control command that starts the storage or retrieval process. The number of bits in a word is called the word length. Word lengths vary, for example, from 16 to 64 bits. Personal computers and workstations usually have a few million words in the main memory, while nanocomputers can have hundreds of millions of words with the time required to access a word for reading or writing within the picosecond range. Although the main memory is essential, it tends to be expensive and volatile. Therefore, nano-ICs can be effectively used to implement the additional memory systems to store programs and data forming secondary memory.

Using the number of instructions executed (N), the number of cycles per instruction (C_{PI}), and the clock frequency (f_{clock}), the program execution time is found to be $T_{ex} = \frac{N \times C_{PI}}{f_{clock}}$. In general, the hardware defines the clock frequency f_{clock}, the software influences the number of instructions executed N, while the nanocomputer architecture defines the number of cycles per instruction C_{PI}.

One of the major performance characteristics is the time it takes to execute a program. Suppose N_{inst} is the number of the machine instructions needed to be executed. A program is written in high-level language, translated by compiler into machine language, and stored. An operating system software routine loads the machine language program into the main memory for execution. Assume that each machine language instruction requires N_{step} basic steps for execution. If basic steps are executed at the constant rate of R_T (steps/sec), then the time to execute the program is $T_{ex} = \frac{N_{inst} \times N_{step}}{R_T}$. The main goal is to minimize T_{ex}. Optimal memory and processor design allows one to achieve this goal. The access to operands in processor registers is significantly faster than access to the main memory. Suppose that instructions and data are loaded into the processor. Then they are stored in a small and fast cache memory (high-speed memory for temporary storage of copies of the sections of program and data from the main memory that are active during program execution) on the processor. Hence, instructions and data in cache are accessed repeatedly and correspondingly. The program execution will be much faster. The cache can hold small parts of the executing program. When the cache is full, its contents are replaced by new instructions and data as they are fetched from the main memory. A variety of cache replacement algorithms are used. The objective of these algorithms is to maximize the probability that the instructions and data needed for program execution can be found in the cache. This probability is known as the cache hit ratio. A high hit ratio means that a large percentage of the instructions and data are found in the cache, and the requirement to access the slower main memory is reduced. This leads to decreasing in the memory access basic step time components of N_{step}, and this results in a smaller T_{ex}. The application of different memory systems results in a memory hierarchy concept as will be studied later. The nanocomputer memory hierarchy is shown in Figure 4.40. As was emphasized, to attain efficiency and high performance, the main memory should not store all programs and data. Specifically, caches are used. Furthermore, virtual memory, which has the largest capacity but the slowest access time, is used. Segments of a program are transferred from the virtual memory to the main memory for execution. As other segments are needed, they may replace the segments existing in the main memory when the main memory is full. The sequential controlled movement of large program and data between the cache, main, and virtual memories, as programs execute, is managed by a combination of operating system software and control hardware. This is called the memory management.

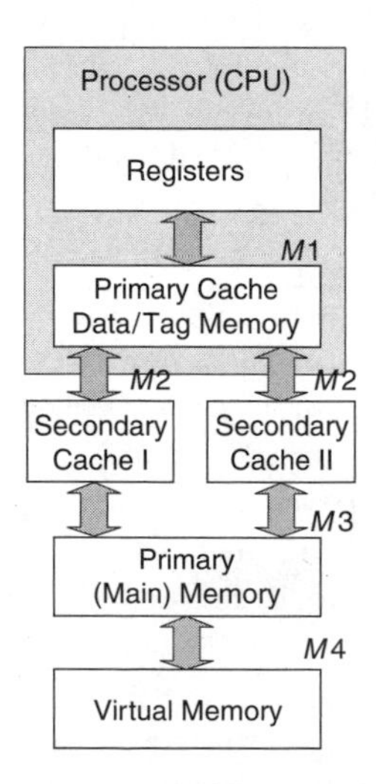

FIGURE 4.40 Processor and memory hierarchy in nanocomputer with cache (primary and secondary), primary (main) memory, and virtual memories.

Using the memory hierarchy illustrated in Figure 4.40, the CPU communicates directly only with M_1, and M_1 communicates with M_2, and so on. Therefore, for the CPU to assess the information, stored in the memory M_j, requires the sequence of j data transfer as given by

$$M_{j-1} := M_j, M_{j-2} := M_{j-1}, \ldots M_1 := M_2, \text{ CPU} := M_1$$

However, the memory bypass can be implemented and effectively used.

To perform computing, specific programs consisting of a set of machine instructions are stored in the main memory. Individual instructions are fetched from the memory into the processor for execution. Data used as operands are also stored in the memory. The connection between the main memory and the processor that guarantees the transfer of instructions and operands is called the bus. A bus consists of a set of address, data, and control lines. The bus permits transfer of program and data files from their long-term location (virtual memory) to the main memory. Communication with other computers is ensured by transferring the data through the bus. Normal execution of programs may be preempted if some IO device requires urgent control. To perform this, specific programs are executed, and the device sends an interrupt signal to the processor. The processor temporarily suspends the program that is being executed, and executes the special interrupt service routine instead. After providing the required interrupt service, the processor switches back to the interrupted program. During program loading and execution, the data should be transferred between the main memory and secondary memory. This is performed using the direct memory access.

Nanocomputers can be classified using different classification principles. For example, making use of the multiplicity of instruction and data streams, the following classification can be applied:

1. Single instruction stream/single data stream—conventional word-sequential architecture including pipelined nanocomputers with parallel arithmetic logic unit (ALU)
2. Single instruction stream/multiple data stream—multiple ALU architectures, e.g., parallel-array processor (ALU can be either bit-serial or bit-parallel)
3. Multiple instruction stream/single data stream
4. Multiple instruction stream/multiple data stream—the multiprocessor system with multiple control unit

The execution of most operations is performed by the ALU. In the ALU, the logic nanogates and nanoregisters used to perform the basic operations (addition, subtraction, multiplication, and division) of numeric operands, and the comparison, shifting, and alignment operations of general forms of numeric and nonnumeric data. The processors contain a number of high-speed registers, which are used for temporary storage of operands. A register, as a storage device for words, is a key sequential component, and registers are connected. Each register contains one word of data and its access time at least ten times faster than the main memory access time. A register-level system consists of a set of registers connected by combinational data-processing and data-processing nano-ICs. Each operation is implemented as given by the following statement:

$$\texttt{cond:}\ X := f(x_1, x_2, \ldots, x_{i-1}, x_i)$$

Thus, when the condition cond holds, compute the combinational function of f on x_1, x_2, ..., x_{i-1}, x_i and assign the resulting value to X. Here, cond is the control condition prefix which denotes the condition that must be satisfied; X, x_1, x_2, ..., x_{i-1}, x_i are the data words or the registers that store them; f is the function to be performed within a single clock cycle.

Suppose that two numbers located in the main memory should be multiplied, and the sum must be stored back into the memory. Using instructions, determined by the control unit, the operands are first fetched from the memory into the processor. They are then multiplied in the ALU, and the result is stored back in memory. Various nano-ICs can be used to execute data-processing instructions. The complexity of the ALU is determined by the arithmetic instruction implementation. For example, ALUs that perform fixed-point addition, subtraction, and word-based logic can be implemented as combinational nano-ICs. The floating-point arithmetic requires complex implementation and arithmetic coprocessors to perform complex numerical functions needed. The floating-point numerical value of a number X is (X_m, X_e), where X_m is the mantissa and X_e is the fixed-point number. Using the base b (usually, $b = 2$), we have $X = X_m \times b^{X_e}$. Therefore, the general basic operations are quite complex and some problems (biasing, overflow, underflow, etc.) must be resolved.

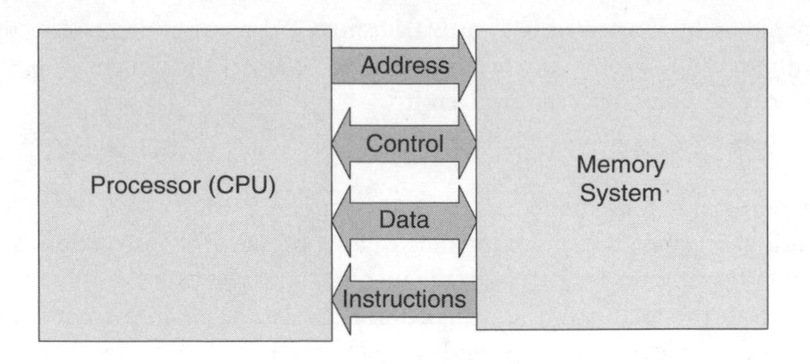

FIGURE 4.41 Memory–processor interface.

Memory–processor interface—A memory unit that integrates different memory systems stores the information (data). The processor accesses (reads or loads) the data from the memory systems, performs computations, and stores (writes) the data back to memory. The memory system is a collection of storage locations. Each storage location (memory word) has a numerical address. A collection of storage locations forms an address space. Figure 4.41 documents the data flow and its control, representing how a processor is connected to a memory system via address, control, and data interfaces. High-performance memory systems should be capable of serving multiple requests simultaneously, particularly for vector nanoprocessors.

When a processor attempts to load or read the data from the memory location, the request is issued and the processor stalls while the request returns. While nanocomputers can operate with overlapping memory requests, the data cannot be optimally manipulated if there are long memory delays. Therefore, a key performance parameter in the design of nanocomputer is the effective speed of its memory. The following limitations are imposed on any memory systems: the memory cannot be infinitely large, cannot contain an arbitrarily large amount of information, and cannot operate infinitely fast. Hence, the major characteristics are speed and capacity.

The memory system performance is characterized by the latency (τ_l) and bandwidth (B_w). The memory latency is the delay as the processor first requests a word from memory until that word arrives and is available for use by the processor. The bandwidth is the rate at which information can be transferred from the memory system. Taking note of the number of requests that the memory can service concurrently $N_{request}$, we have $B_w = \frac{N_{request}}{\tau_l}$. Using nano-ICs, it become feasible to design and build superior memory systems with desired capacity, low latency, and high bandwidth approaching the physical limits. Using nano-ICs, it will be possible to match the memory and processor performance characteristics.

Memory hierarchies provide decreased average latency and reduced bandwidth requirements, whereas parallel memories provide higher bandwidth. As was emphasized, nanocomputer architectures that utilize a small and fast memory located in front of a large but relatively slow memory, can tremendously enhance speed and memory capacity by making use of nano-ICs. This results in application of registers in the CPU, and most commonly accessed variables should be allocated at registers. A variety of techniques, employing either hardware, software, or a combination of hardware and software, are employed to ensure that most references to memory are fed by the faster memory. The locality principle is based on the fact that some memory locations are referenced more often than others. The implementation of spatial locality, due to the sequential access, provides one with the property that an access to a given memory location increases the probability that neighboring locations will soon be accessed. Making use of the frequency of program looping behavior, temporal locality ensures access to a given memory location, increasing the probability that the same location will be accessed again soon. It is evident that if a variable was not referenced for a while, it is unlikely that this variable will be needed soon.

As illustrated in Figure 4.40, the top of the memory hierarchy level consists of superior speed CPU registers. The next level in the hierarchy is a high-speed cache memory. The cache can be divided into multiple levels, and nanocomputers will likely have multiple caches that can be fabricated on the CPU nanochip. Below the cache memory is the slower but larger main memory, and then the large virtual memory, which is slower than the main memory. These levels can be designed and fabricated utilizing different nano-ICs. Three performance characteristics (access time, bandwidth, and capacity) and many factors (affordability, robustness, adaptability, reconfigurability, etc.) support the application of multiple levels of cache memory and the memory hierarchy concept. The time needed to access the primary cache should match with the clock frequency of the CPU, and the corresponding nano-ICs must be used. We place a smaller first-level (primary) cache above a larger second-level (secondary) cache. The primary cache is accessed quickly, and the secondary cache holds more data close to the CPU. The nanocomputer architecture, built using nanoelectronics integrated within nano-ICs assemblies, depends on the technologies available. For example, primary cache can be fabricated on the CPU chip, while the secondary caches can be an on- or out-of-chip solution.

Size, speed, latency, bandwidth, power consumption, robustness, affordability, and other performance characteristics are examined to guarantee the desired overall nanocomputer performance based upon the specifications imposed. The performance parameter, which can be used to quantitatively examine different memory systems, is the effective latency τ_{ef}. We have:

$$\tau_{ef} = \tau_{hit} R_{hit} + \tau_{miss}(1 - R_{hit}),$$

where τ_{hit} and τ_{miss} are the hit and miss latencies, R_{hit} is the hit ratio, and $R_{hit} < 1$.

If the needed word is found in a level of the hierarchy, it is called a hit. Correspondingly, if a request must be sent to the next lower level, the request is said to be a miss. The miss ratio is given as $R_{miss} = (1 - R_{hit})$. These R_{hit} and R_{miss} ratios are strongly influenced by the program being executed and influenced by the high-/low-level memory capacity ratio. The access efficiency E_{ef} of multiple-level memory ($i - 1$ and i) is found using the access time, and hit and miss ratios. In particular:

$$E_{ef} = \frac{1}{\dfrac{t_{\text{access time } i-1}}{t_{\text{access time } i}} R_{miss} + R_{hit}}$$

The hardware can dynamically allocate parts of the cache memory for addresses likely to be accessed soon. The cache contains only redundant copies of the address space. The cache memory can be associative or content-addressable. In an associative memory, the address of a memory location is stored along with its content. Rather than reading data directly from a memory location, the cache is given an address and responds by providing data that might or might not be the data requested. When a cache miss occurs, the memory access is then performed from main memory, and the cache is updated to include the new data. The cache should hold the most active portions of the memory, and the hardware dynamically selects portions of main memory to store in the cache. When the cache is full, some data must be transferred to the main memory or deleted. Therefore, a strategy for cache memory management is needed. Cache management strategies are based on the locality principle. In particular, spatial (selection of what is brought into the cache) and temporal (selection of what must be removed) localities are embedded. When a cache miss occurs, hardware copies a contiguous block of memory into the cache, which includes the word requested. This fixed-size memory block can be small (bit or word) or hundreds of bytes. Caches can require all fixed-size memory blocks to be aligned. When a fixed-size memory block is brought into the cache, it is likely that another fixed-size memory block must be removed. The selection of the removed fixed-size memory block is based on the effort to capture temporal locality. In general, this is difficult to achieve. Correspondingly, viable methods are used to predict future memory accesses. A least-recently-used concept can be the preferred choice for nanocomputers.

The cache can integrate the data memory and the tag memory. The address of each cache line contained in the data memory is stored in the tag memory (the state can also track which cache line is modified). Each line contained in the data memory is allocated by a corresponding entry in the tag memory to indicate the full address of the cache line. The requirement that the cache memory be associative (content-addressable) complicates the design because addressing data by content is more complex than by its address (all tags must be compared concurrently). The cache can be simplified by embedding a mapping of memory locations to cache cells. This mapping limits the number of possible cells in which a particular line may reside. Each memory location can be mapped to a single location in the cache through direct mapping. Although there is no choice of where the line resides and which line must be replaced, however, poor utilization results. In contrast, a two-way set-associative cache maps each memory location into either of two locations in the cache. Hence, this mapping can be viewed as two identical directly mapped caches. In fact, both caches must be searched at each memory access, and the appropriate data selected and multiplexed on a tag match hit and on a miss. Then, a choice must be made between two possible cache lines as to which is to be replaced. A single least-recently-used bit can be saved for each such pair of lines to remember which line has been accessed more recently. This bit must be toggled to the current state each time. To this end, an M-way associative cache maps each memory location into M memory locations in the cache. Therefore, this cache map can be constructed from M identical direct-mapped caches. The problem of maintaining the least-recently-used ordering of M cache lines is primarily due to the fact that there are $M!$ possible orderings. In fact, it takes at least $\log_2 M!$ bits to store the ordering. It can be envisioned that a two-, three-, or four-way associative cache will be implemented in nanocomputers.

Consider the write operation. If the main memory copy is updated with each write operation, then write-through or store-through technique is used. If the main memory copy is not updated with each write operation, write-back or copy-back or deferred writes algorithm is enforced. In general, the cache coherence or consistency problem must be examined due to the implementation of different bypass techniques.

Parallel Memories—Main memories can comprise a series of memory nanochips or nano-ICs on a single nanochip. These nano-ICs form a *nanobank*. Multiple memory nanobanks can be integrated together to form a parallel main memory system. Since each nanobank can service a request, a parallel main memory system with N_{mb} nanobanks can service N_{mb} requests simultaneously, increasing the bandwidth of the memory system by N_{mb} times the bandwidth of a single nanobank. The number of nanobanks is a power of 2, that is, $N_{mb} = 2^p$. An n-bit memory word address is broken into two parts: a p-bit nanobank number and an m-bit address of a word within a nanobank. The p bits used to select a nanobank number could be any p bits of the n-bit word address. Let us use the low-order p address bits to select the nanobank number, and the higher order $m = n - p$ bits of the word address is used to access a word in the selected nanobank.

Multiple memory nanobanks can be connected using *simple paralleling* and *complex paralleling*. Figure 4.42 shows the structure of a simple parallel memory system where m address bits are simultaneously supplied to all memory nanobanks. All nanobanks are connected to the same read/write control line. For a read operation, the nanobanks perform the read operation and deposit the data in the latches. Data can then be read from the latches one by one by setting the switch appropriately. The nanobanks can be accessed again to carry out another read or write operation. For a write operation, the latches are loaded one by one. When all latches have been written, their contents can be written into the memory nanobanks by supplying m bits of address. In a simple parallel memory, all nanobanks are cycled at the same time. Each nanobank starts and completes its

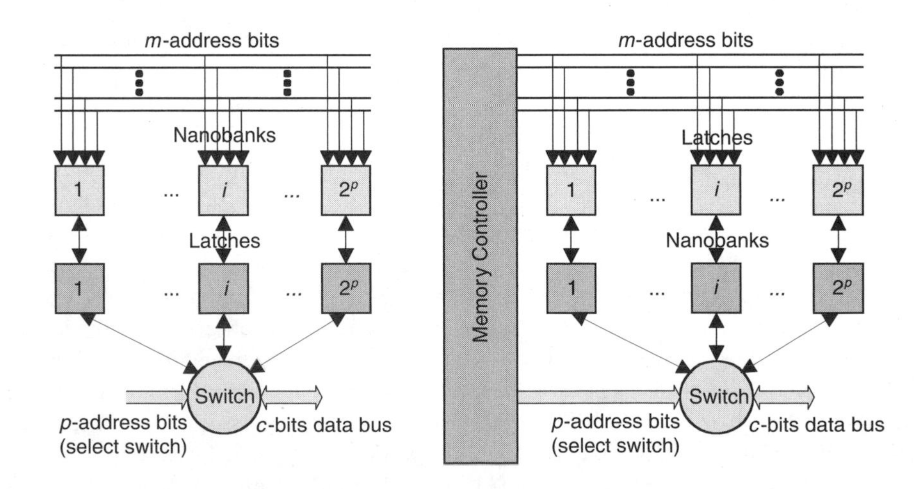

FIGURE 4.42 Simple and complex parallel main memory systems.

individual operations at the same time as every other nanobank, and a new memory cycle starts for all nanobanks once the previous cycle is complete.

A complex parallel memory system is documented in Figure 4.42. Each nanobank is set to operate on its own independent of the operation of the other nanobanks. For example, the ith nanobank performs a read operation on a particular memory address, while the $(i + 1)$th nanobank performs a write operation on a different and unrelated memory address. Complex paralleling is achieved using the address latch and a read/write command line for each nanobank. The *memory controller* handles the operation of the complex parallel memory. The processing unit submits the memory request to the memory controller, which determines which nanobank needs to be accessed. The controller then determines if the nanobank is busy by monitoring a busy line for each nanobank. The controller holds the request if the nanobank is busy, submitting it when the nanobank becomes available to accept the request. When the nanobank responds to a read request, the switch is set by the controller to accept the request from the nanobank and forward it to the processing unit. It can be foreseen that complex parallel main memory systems will be implemented in vector nanoprocessors. If consecutive elements of a vector are present in different memory nanobanks, then the memory system can sustain a bandwidth of one element per clock cycle. Memory systems in nanocomputers can have hundreds of nanobanks with multiple memory controllers that allow multiple independent memory requests at every clock cycle.

Pipelining—Pipelining is a technique to increase the processor throughput with limited hardware in order to implement complex datapath (data processing) units (multipliers, floating-point adders, etc.). In general, a pipeline processor integrates a sequence of i data-processing nano-ICs (nanostages) which cooperatively perform a single operation on a stream of data operands passing through them. Design of pipelining nano-ICs involves deriving multistage balanced sequential algorithms to perform the given function. Fast buffer registers are placed between the nanostages to ensure the transfer of data between nanostages without interfering with one another. These buffers should be clocked at the maximum rate that guarantees the reliable data transfer between nanostages.

As illustrated in Figure 4.43, the nanocomputers must be designed to guarantee the robust execution of overlapped instructions using pipelining. Four basic steps (fetch F_i–decode D_i–operate O_i–write W_i) with specific hardware units are needed to achieve these steps. As a result, the execution of instructions can be overlapped. When the execution of some instruction I_i depends on the results of a previous instruction I_{i-1} which is not yet completed, instruction I_i must be delayed. The pipeline is said to be stalled, waiting for the execution of instruction I_{i-1} to be completed. While it is not possible to eliminate such situations, it is important to minimize the probability of their occurrence. This is a key consideration in the design of the instruction set for nanocomputers and the design of the compilers that translate high-level language programs into machine language.

Multiprocessors—Multiple functional units can be applied to attain the nanocomputer operation when more than one instruction can be in the operating stage. The parallel execution capability, when added to the pipelining of the individual instructions, means that more than one instruction can be executed per basic step. Thus, the execution rate can be increased. This enhanced processor performance is called superscalar processing. The rate R_T of performing basic steps in the processor depends on the processor clock rate. This rate is on the order of

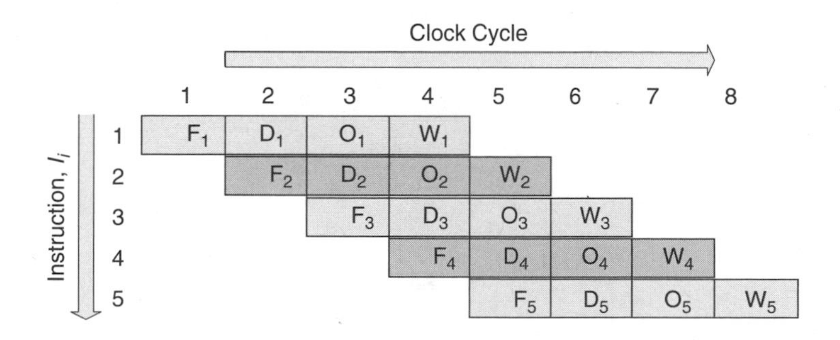

FIGURE 4.43 Pipelining of instruction execution.

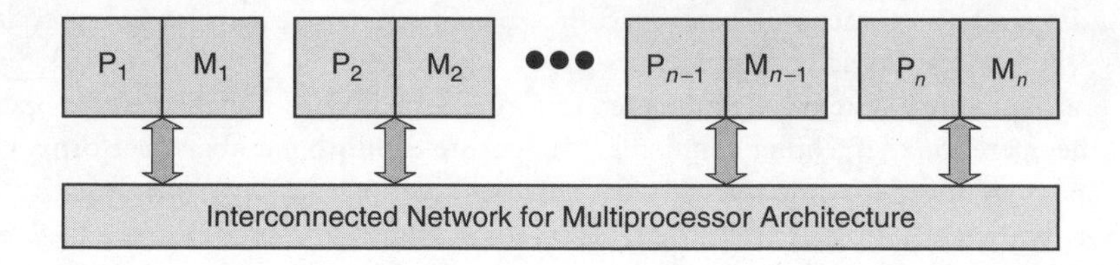

FIGURE 4.44 Multiprocessor architecture. The basic parallel organization for nanocomputers is represented in Figure 4.45.

billions steps per second in current high-performance nano-ICs. It was illustrated that physical limits prevent single processors from being speeded up indefinitely. Nanocomputers with multiprocessors will speed up the execution of large programs by executing subtasks in parallel. The main difficulty in achieving this is decomposition of a given task into its parallel subtasks and ordering these subtasks to the individual processors in such a way that communication among the subtasks will be performed efficiently and robustly. Figure 4.44 documents a block diagram of a multi-processor system with the interconnection network needed for data sharing among the processors P_i. Parallel paths are needed in this network in order to parallel activity to proceed in the processors as they access the global memory space represented by the multiple memory units M_i.

Nanocomputer Architectronics—The theory of computing, computer architecture, and networking is the study of efficient robust processing and communication, modeling, analysis, optimization, adaptive networks, architecture, and organization synthesis, as well as other problems of hardware and software design. These studies have emerged as a synergetic fundamental discipline (computer engineering and science), and many problems have not been solved yet. Correspondingly, a large array of questions remains unanswered. Nanocomputer *architectonics* is the theory of nanocomputers devised and designed using fundamental theory and applying nano-ICs. Our goal is to develop the nanocomputer achitectronics basics, e.g., fundamental methods in synthesis, design, analysis, modeling, computer-aided design, etc. Nanocomputer achitectronics, which is a computer science and engineering frontier, will allow one to solve a wide spectrum of fundamental and applied problems. Applying the nanocomputer achitectronics paradigm, this section spans the theory of nanocomputers and related areas, e.g., information processing, communication paradigms, computational complexity theory, combinatorial optimization, architecture synthesis, optimal organization, and their applications. Making of the nanocomputer achitectronics paradigms, one can address and study fundamental problems in nanocomputer architecture synthesis, design, and optimization applying three-dimensional organization, application of nano-ICs, multithreading, error recovery, massively parallel computing organization, shared memory parallelism, message passing parallelism, etc. The nanocomputer fundamentals, operation, and functionality can be devised through neuroscience. The key to understand learning, adaptation, control, architecture, hierarchy, organization, memory, intelligence, diagnostics, self-organization, computing, and other system-level

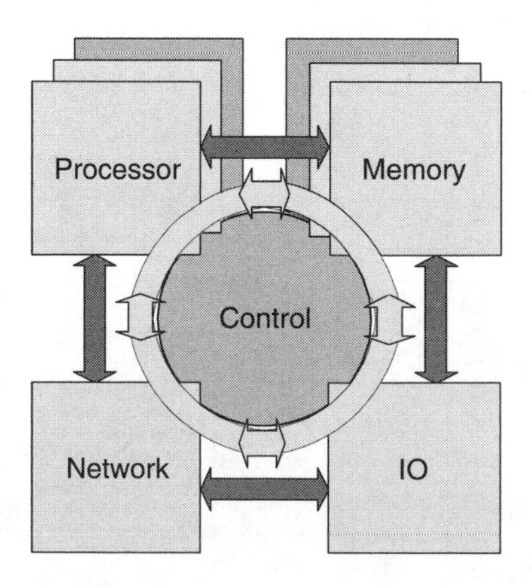

FIGURE 4.45 Parallel nanocomputer organization to maximize computer concurrency.

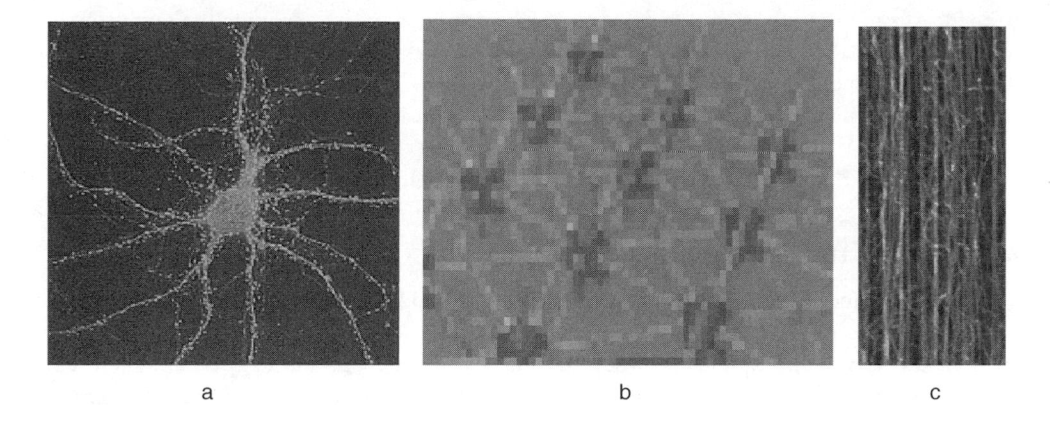

FIGURE 4.46 Vertebrate neuron (soma, axon with synaptic terminals, dendrites, and synapses), three-dimensional nano-ICs, aligned carbon nanotubes, and single C_{60} buckyballs on Si.

basics lies in the study of phenomena and effects in the central nervous system, its components (brain and spinal cord), and the fundamental building blocks, e.g., neurons. Neuronal cells have a large number of synapses. A typical nerve cell in the human brain has thousands of synapses, which establish communication and information processing. The communication and processing are not fixed, but constantly change and adapt. Neurons function in the hierarchically distributed robust adaptive network manner. During information transfer, some synapses on a cell are selectively triggered to release specific neurotransmitters, while other synapses remain passive. Neurons consist of a cell body with a nucleus (soma), axon (which transmits information from the soma), and dendrites (which transmit information to the soma) (see Figure 4.46). It becomes possible to implement three-dimensional nano-ICs structures using biomematic analogies as illustrated in Figure 4.46. For example, the complex inorganic dendrite-like trees can be implemented using the carbon nanotube-base technology (the Y-junction branching carbon nanotube networks ensure robust ballistic switching and amplification behavior desired in nano-ICs. Other nanodevices are emerged. For example, single isolated C_{60} molecules and multi-layered C_{60} can form nanodevices (superconducting transitions) (see Figure 4.46). Unfortunately, due to low temperature, the buckyball C_{60} solution in nanodevices is not feasible. However, the carbon-based technology is progressed to possible application in nano-ICs within three-dimensional architectures.

Two- and three-dimensional topology aggregation—There is a critical need to study the topology aggregation in the hierarchical distributed nanocomputer that will utilize two- and three-dimensional nano-ICs. One can examine how a hierarchical network with multiple paths and routing domain functions. Figure 4.47 shows the principle of topology aggregation of nanodevices in nano-ICs for nanocomputers. For example, the documented network consists of four routers (buffers) numbered 1, 2, 3, and 4, and interior (core) routers

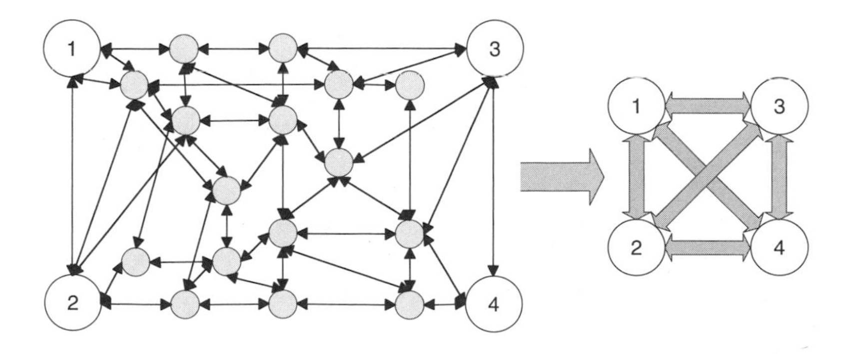

FIGURE 4.47 Network topology aggregation.

are illustrated. After the aggregation, a meshed network with four nodes represents the same topology. The difficulty in topology aggregation is to calculate the link metrics to attain the accuracy and to synthesize optimized network topologies. The aggregated link metrics can be computed using the methods used for multiplayer artificial networks. The bandwidth and delay are integrated to optimize the hierarchically distributed networks. We believe that the *distributed-memory* nanocomputers can be adaptively configured and reconfigured based upon *processing*, *communication*, and *control* (instruction) *parallelisms*.

Nanocomputer Architecture

System-level performance analysis is based on mathematical models used to examine nanocomputers and optimize their architectures, organization, topologies, and parameters, as well as to perform optimal hardware-software codesign. Computers process inputs, producing outputs accordingly. To examine the performance, one should develop and apply the mathematical model of a nanocomputer which comprises central processing, memory, input–output control, and other units. However, one cannot develop the mathematical model without explicitly specifying the nanocomputer architecture, identifying the optimal organization, and synthesizing the topologies. There are different levels of abstraction for nanocomputer architectures, organizations, models, etc.

Advanced nanocomputer architectures (beyond Von Neumann computer architecture) can be devised to guarantee superior processing and communication speed. Novel nanodevices that utilize new effects and phenomena to perform computing and communication are sought. For example, through quantum computing, the information can be stored in the phase of wavefunctions, and this concept leads to utilization of massive parallelism of these wavefunctions to achieve enormous processing speed.

The CPU executes sequences of instructions and operands, which are fetched by the program control unit (PCU), executed by the data processing unit (DPU), and then placed in memory. In particular, caches (high-speed memory where data is copied when it is retrieved from the random access memory improving the overall performance by reducing the average memory access time) are used. The instructions and data form instruction and data streams which flow to and from the processor. The CPU may have two or more processors and coprocessors with various execution units and multi-level instruction and data caches. These processors can share or have their own caches. The CPU datapath contains nano-ICs to perform arithmetic and logical operations on words such as fixed- or floating-point numbers. The CPU design involves trade-off analysis between the hardware, speed, and affordability. The CPU is usually partitioned on the control and datapath units, and the control unit selects and sequence the data-processing operations. The core interface unit is a switch that can be implemented as autonomous cache controllers operating concurrently and feeding the specified number (32, 64, or 128) of bytes of data per cycle. This core interface unit connects all controllers to the data or instruction caches of processors. Additionally, the core interface unit accepts and sequences information from the processors. A control unit is responsible for controlling data flow between controllers that regulate the *in* and *out* information flows. There is the interface to input/output devices. On-chip debug, error detection, sequencing logic, self-test, monitoring, and other units must be integrated to control a pipelined nanocomputer. The computer performance depends on the architecture and hardware components (which are discussed in this chapter). Figure 4.48 illustrates the possible nanocomputer organization.

In general, nanodevices ensure high density, superior bandwidth, high switching frequency, low power, etc. It is envisioned that in the near future nanocomputers will allow one to increase the computing speed by a factor of millions compared with the existing CMOS ICs computers. Three-dimensional, multiple-layered, high-density nano-IC assemblies, shown in Figure 4.49, are envisioned to be used. Unfortunately, the number of formidable fundamental, applied, experimental, and technological challenges arise, e.g., robust operation and characteristics of nano-ICs are significantly affected by the "second-order" effects (gate oxide and bandgap tunneling, energy quantization, electron transport, etc., and, furthermore, the operating principles for nanodevices can be based on the quantum effects), noise vulnerability, complexity, etc. It is well known that high-fidelity modeling, data-intensive analysis, heterogeneous simulation, and other fundamental issues even for a single nanodevice are not completely solved yet. In addition, the currently existing fabrication processes and technologies do not allow one to fabricate ideal nanodevices and nanostructures. In fact, even molecular

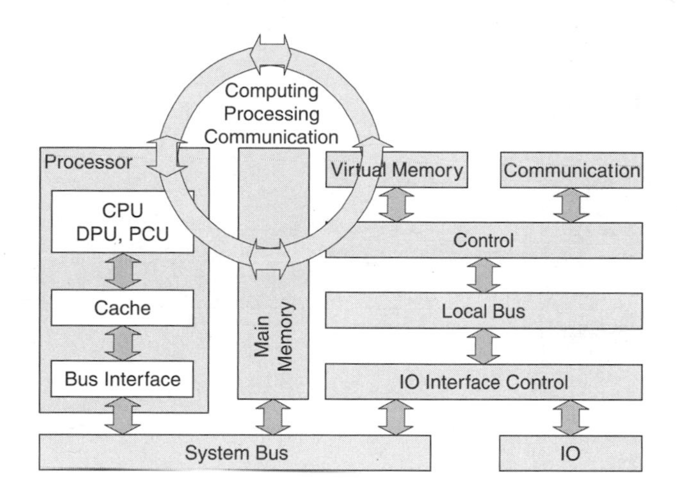

FIGURE 4.48 Nanocomputer organization.

wires are not perfect. Different fabrication technologies, processes, and materials have been developed to attain self-assembly and self-ordered features in fabrication of nanoscale devices [7–9] (see Figure 4.49). As an example, the self-assembled and aligned carbon nanotube array is illustrated in Figure 4.49.

One of the basic components of the current computers is CMOS transistors fabricated using different technologies and distinct device topologies. However, the CMOS technology and transistors fabricated by using even most advanced CMOS processes reach physical limits. Therefore, the current research developments have been concentrated on the alternative solutions, and leading companies (IBM, Intel, Hewlett-Packard, etc.), academia, and government laboratories develop novel nanotechnologies. We study computer hardware. Nanodevices (switches, logics, memories, etc.) can be implemented using the three-dimensional nanoelectronics arrays illustrated in Figure 4.49. It must be emphasized that the extremely high-frequency logic gates can be

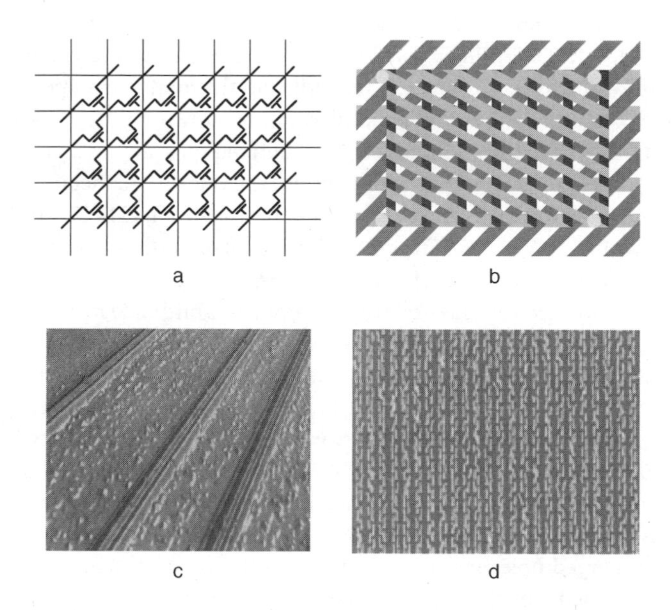

FIGURE 4.49 Three-dimensional multiple-layered high-density nanoIC assemblies (crossbar switching, logic, or memory arrays), 3 nm wide parallel (six-atom-wide) erbium disilicide ($ErSi_2$) nanowires (Hewlett-Packard), and carbon nanotube array.

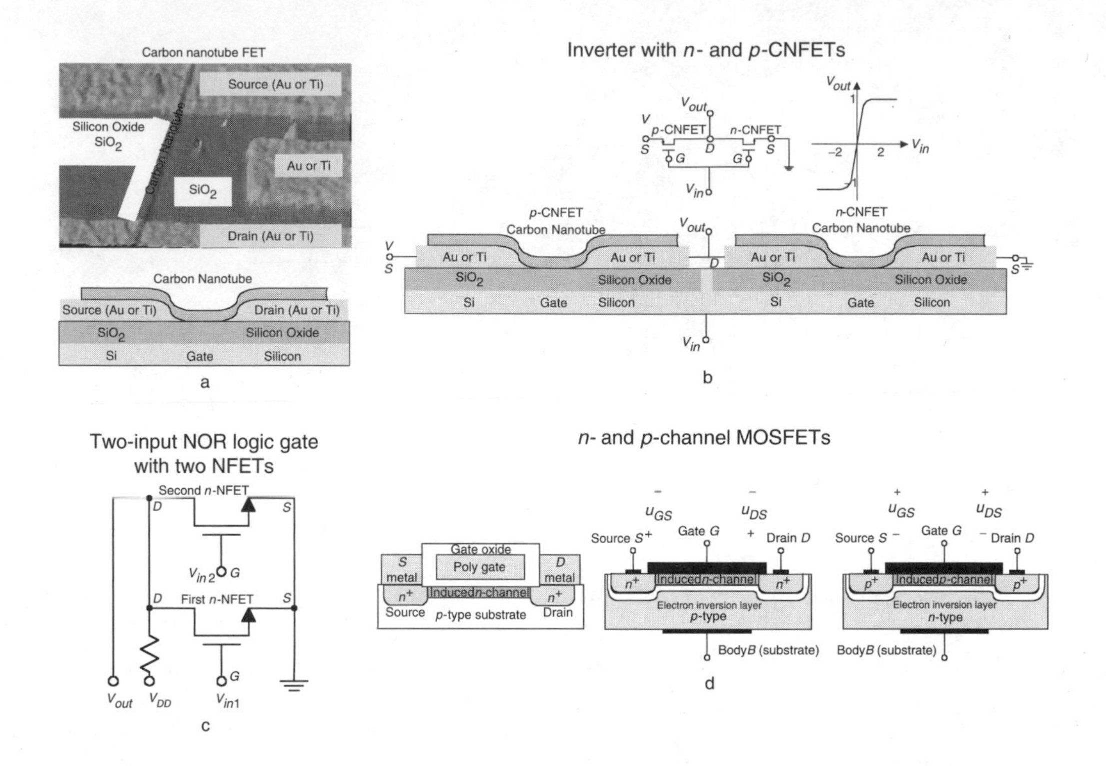

FIGURE 4.50 (a) Carbon nanotube FETs; (b) inverter with CNFETs; (c) NOR gate with NFETs; (d) n- and p-channel MOSFETs.

fabricated using carbon nanotubes, which are from 1 to 10 nm in diameter (100,000 times less than the diameter of human hair). *p*- and *n*-type carbon nanotube field-effect transistors (CNFETs) with single- and multi-wall carbon nanotubes as the channel were fabricated and tested [11]. The atomic force microscope image of a single-wall CNFET (50 nm total length) and CNFET are documented in Figure 4.50(a).

It should be emphasized that a two-dimensional carbon nanotube structure can be utilized to devise and build different transistors with distinct characteristics utilizing different phenomena [10,11]. For example, twisted carbon nanotubes can be used. Carbon nanotubes can be grown on the surface using chemical vapor deposition, deposited on the surface from solvent, etc. Photolithography can be used to attain the device-level structural and functional integration connecting source, drain, gate, etc. One concludes that different transistors topologies and configurations are available, and these results are reported in [11–13]. Taking note of this fact, we use nanoscale field-effect transistors (NFET) to synthesize and analyze the nano-ICs. The carbon nanotube inverter, formed using the series combination of p- and n-CNFETs, is illustrated in Figure 4.50.b. The gates and drains of two CNFETs are connected together to form the input and output. The voltage characteristics can be examined studying the various transistor bias regions. When the inverter input voltage V_{in} is either a logic 0 or a logic 1, the current in the circuit is zero because one of the CNFETs is cut off. When the input voltage varies in the region $V_{\text{threshold}} < V_{\text{in}} < V - |V_{\text{threshold}}|$, both CNFETs are conducting and a current exists in the inverter.

The current-control mechanism of the field-effect transistors is based on an electrostatic field established by the voltage applied to the control terminal. Figure 4.50(d) shows an *n*- and *p*-channel enhancement-type MOSFETs with four terminals (the gate, source, drain, and base [substrate] terminals are denoted as G, S, D, and B). Consider the *n*-channel enhancement-type MOSFETs. A positive voltage u_{GS}, applied to the gate, causes the free positively charged holes in the *n*-channel region. These holes are pushed downward into the *p*-base (substrate). The applied voltage u_{GS} attracts electrons from the source and drain regions into the channel region. The voltage is applied between the drain and source, and the current flows through the induced *n*-channel region. The gate and body form a parallel-plate capacitor with the oxide layer. The positive gate voltage u_{GS} causes the positive charge at the top plate, and the negative charge at the bottom is

TABLE 4.3 Two-input NOR Logic Circuit with Two NFETs

V_{in1}	V_{in2}	V_{out}
0	0	1
1	0	0
0	1	0
1	1	0

formed by the electrons in the induced *n*-channel region. Hence, the electric field is formed in the vertical direction. The current is controlled by the electric field applied perpendicularly to both the semiconductor substrate and to the direction of current (the voltage between two terminals controls the current through the third terminal). The basic principle of MOSFET operation is the metal-oxide-semiconductor capacitor, and high-conductivity polycrystalline silicon is deposited on the silicon oxide. As a positive voltage u_{DS} is applied, the drain current i_{D} flows in the induced *n*-channel region from source to drain, and the magnitude of i_{D} is proportional to the effective voltage $u_{GS} - u_{\text{GS1}}$. If u_{GS} is greater than the threshold value u_{GS1}, $u_{\text{GS}} > u_{\text{GS1}}$, the induced *n*-channel is enhanced. If one increases u_{DS}, the *n*-channel resistance is increased, and the drain current i_{D} saturates, and the saturation region occurs as one increases u_{DS}, to the u_{DSsat} value. The sufficient number of mobile electrons accumulated in the channel region to form a conducting channel if the u_{GS} is greater than the threshold voltage u_{GS}, which usually is 1 V, e.g., thousands of electrons are needed. It should be emphasized that in the saturation region, the MOSFET is operated as an amplifier, while in the triode region and in the cutoff region, the MOSFET can be used as a switch. A p-channel enhancement-type MOSFET is fabricated on an *n*-type substrate (body) with p^+ regions for the drain and source. Here, the voltages applied u_{GS} and u_{DS}, and the threshold voltage u_{GSt}, are negative.

We use and demonstrate the application of nanoscale field-effect transistors (NFETs) to design the logic nano-ICs. The NOR logic can be straightforwardly implemented when the first and second *n*-NFETs are connected in parallel; (see Figure 4.50(c)). Different flip-flops usually are formed by cross-coupling NOR logic gates. If two input voltages are zero, both *n*-NFETs are cut off, and the output voltage V_{out} is high. Specifically, $V_{\text{out}} = V_{\text{DD}}$, and if $V_{\text{DD}} = 1$ V, then $V_{\text{out}} = 1$ V. If $V_{\text{in1}} \neq 0$ (for example, $V_{\text{in1}} = 1$ V) and $V_{\text{in2}} = 0$, the first *n*-NFET turns on and the second *n*-NFET is still cut off. The first *n*-NFET is biased in the nonsaturation region, and V_{out} reaches the low value ($V_{\text{out}} = 0$). By changing the input voltages such as $V_{\text{in1}} = 0$ and $V_{\text{in2}} \neq 0$ ($V_{\text{in2}} = 1$ V), the first n-NFET becomes cut off, while the second n-NFET is biased in the nonsaturation region. Hence, V_{out} has the low value, $V_{\text{out}} = 0$. If $V_{\text{in1}} \neq 0$ and $V_{\text{in2}} \neq 0$ ($V_{\text{in1}} = 1$ V and $V_{\text{in2}} = 1$ V), both *n*-NFETs become biased in the nonsaturation region, and V_{out} is low ($V_{\text{out}} = 0$). Table 4.3 summarizes the result and explains how the NFET can be straightforwardly used in nanocomputer units.

The series–parallel combination of the NFETs is used to synthesize complex logic gates. As an example, the resulting carbon nanotube circuitry using n-NFETs to implement the Boolean output function $V_{\text{out}} = f\overline{(A \cdot B + C)}$ is illustrated in Figure 4.51. The n-NFETs executive OR logic gate $V_{\text{out}} = A \otimes B$ can be made; (see Figure 4.51). If $A = B =$ logic 1, the path exists from the output to ground trough NFET A and NFET B transistors, and the output goes low. If $A = B =$ logic 0 ($\bar{A} = \bar{B} =$ logic 1), the path exists from the output to ground trough NFET A1 and NFET B1 transistors, and the output goes low. For all other input logic signal

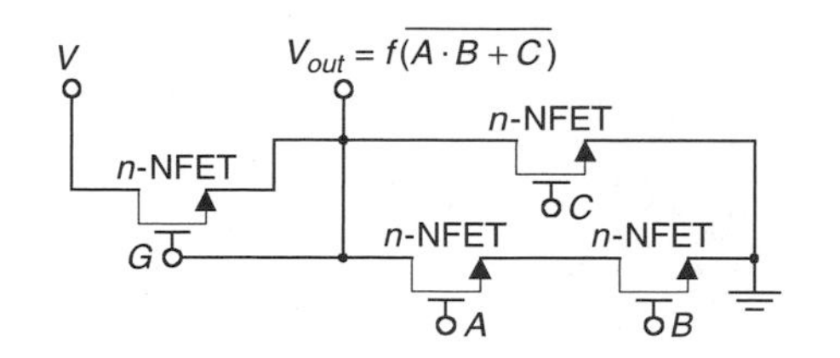

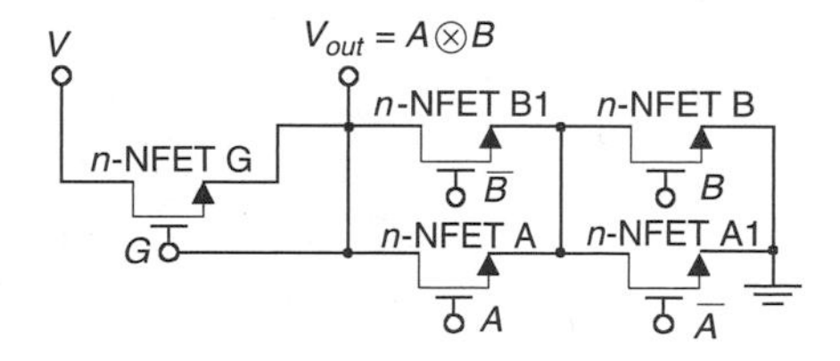

FIGURE 4.51 Static logic gates $V_{\text{out}} = f\overline{(A \cdot B + C)}$ and $V_{\text{out}} =$ A $\otimes$ *B* synthesized using *n*- and *p*-NFETs.

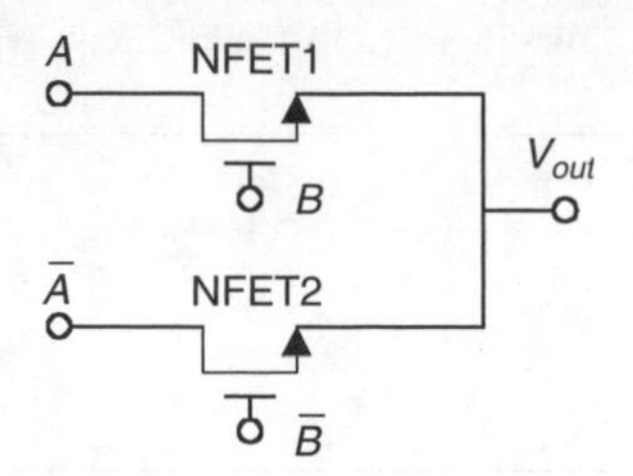

FIGURE 4.52 NanoICs pass network.

TABLE 4.4 Two-Input NOR Logic Circuit with Two NFETs

	Input Gate Control						
State	A	$\bar{A}$	B	$\bar{B}$	NFET1	NFET2	V_{out}
1	0	1	0	1	Off	On	1
2	1	0	0	1	Off	On	0
3	0	1	1	0	On	Off	0
4	1	0	1	0	On	Off	1
5	0	1	0	1	Off	On	1
6	1	0	0	1	Off	On	0
7	0	1	1	0	On	Off	0
8	1	0	1	0	On	Off	1

combinations, the output is isolated from ground, and, hence, the output goes high. Two logic gates $V_{out} = \overline{f(A \cdot B + C)}$ and $V_{out} = A \otimes B$ synthesized are the static nano-ICs (the output voltage is well defined and is never left floating). The static nano-ICs can be redesigned adding the clock.

The nano-IC pass networks can be easily implemented. Consider the nano-ICs with two n-NFETs documented in Figure 4.52. The nanoICs output V_{out} is determined by the conditions listed in Table 4.4. In states 1 and 2, the transmission gate of NFET2 is biased in its conduction state (NFET2 is on), while NFET1 is off. For state 1, $\bar{A}$ = logic 1 is transmitted to the output, and $V_{out} = 1$. For state 2, $\bar{A}$ = logic 0, and though A = logic 1, due to the fact that NFET1 is off, $V_{out} = 0$. In states 3 and 4, the transmission gate of NFET1 is biased, and NFET2 is off. For state 3, A = logic 0, we have $V_{out} = 0$ because NFET2 is off ($\bar{A}$ = logic 1). In contrast, in state 4, A = logic 1 is transmitted to the output, and $V_{out} = 1$. For other states the results are reported in Table 4.4. We conclude that the output V_{out} is a function of two variables, e.g., gate control and input (logic) signals.

The clocked nano-ICs are dynamic circuits that in general precharge the output node to a particular level when the clock is at a logic 0. The generalized clocked nano-ICs is illustrated in Figure 4.53, where F_N is the NFETs network that performs the particular logic function $F_N(X)$ of i variables, here $X = (x_1, x_2, \ldots, x_{i-1}, x_i)$.

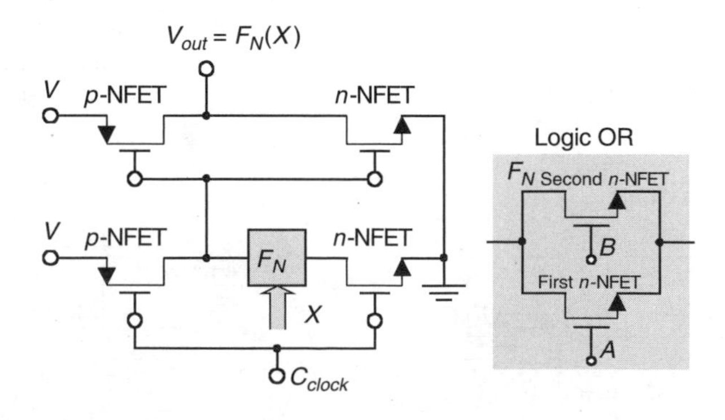

FIGURE 4.53 Dynamic generalized clocked nanoIC with logic function $F_N(X)$.

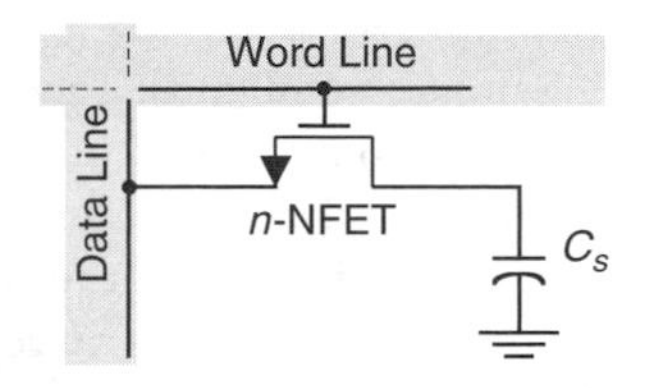

FIGURE 4.54 One n-NFET dynamic RAM with the storage capacitor.

The set of X inputs to the logic nano-ICs $F_N(X)$ is derived from the outputs of other static and dynamics nano-ICs. When $C_{\text{clock}} = \text{logic } 0$, the outputs of all inverters are a logic 0 during the precharged cycle, and during the precharged cycle all x variables of $X = (x_1, x_2, \ldots, x_{z-1}, x_z)$ are logic 0. During the precharge phase, all NFETs are cut off, and the transistor outputs are precharged to V. The transitions are possible only during the evaluation phase. The output of the nonoICs buffer change from 0 to 1. Specifically, the logic OR function is illustrated to demonstrate the generalized clocked nano-ICs in Figure 4.53.

Combination of logic gates is used to perform logic functions, addition, subtraction, multiplication, division, multiplexing, etc. To store the information, memory cell nano-ICs are used. A systematic arrangement of memory cells and peripheral nano-ICs (to address and write the data into the cells as well as to delete data stored in the cells) constitute the memory. The NFETs can be used to build superior static and dynamic random access memory (RAM is the read-write memory in which each individual cell can be addressed at any time), programmable and alterable read-only memory (ROM is commonly used to store instructions of a system operating systems). The static RAM (implemented using six NFETs) consists of a basic flip-flop nano-IC with two stable states (0 and 1), while dynamic RAM (implemented using one NFET and storage capacitor) stores one bit of information charging the capacitor. As an example, the dynamic RAM (DRAM) cell is documented in Figure 4.54. In particular, the binary information is stored as the charge on the storage capacitor C_s (logic 0 or 1). The DRAM cell is addressed by turning on the pass n-NFET via the world line signal S_{wl} and charge is transferred into and out of C_s on the data line (C_s is isolated from the rest of the nano-ICs when the n-NFET is off, but the leakage current through the n-NFET requires the cell refreshment to restore the original signal).

Dynamic shift registers are implemented using transmission gates and inverters, flip-flops are synthesized by cross-coupling NOR gates, while delay flip-flops are built using transmission gates and feedback inverters.

Though for many nano-ICs (we do not consider the optical, single-electron, and quantum nano-ICs) synthesis and design can be performed using the basic approaches, methods, and computer-aided design developed for conventional ICs (viable results exist for MOSFETs), the differences must be outlined. The major problems arise due to the fact that the developed technologies cannot guarantee the fabrication of high-yield perfect nano-ICs and different operating principles. In general, the secondary effects must be integrated (for example, even for NFETs, which are comparable to MOSFETs, the switching and leakage phenomena are different). Correspondingly, the simple scaling of ICs with MOSFETs to nano-ICs cannot be performed.

The direct self-assembly, nanopatterning, nano-imprinting, nano-aligning, nanopositioning, overlayering, margining, and annealing were shown to be quite promising. However, it is unlikely that near-future nanotechnologies will guarantee reasonable repeatable characteristics, high-quality, satisfactory geometry uniformity, suitable failure tolerance, and other important specifications and requirements imposed on nanodevices and nanostructures. Therefore, synthesis of robust defect-tolerant adaptive (reconfigurable) nanocomputer architectures (hardware) and software to accommodate failures, inconsistence, variations, nonuniformity, and defects is critical [10].

Hierarchical Finite-State Machines and Their Use in Hardware and Software Design

Simple register-level systems perform a single data-processing operation, e.g., summation $X{:=}x_1 + x_2$, subtraction $X{:}\,x_1 - x_2$, etc. To do, different complex data-processing operations, multifunctional register-level systems should be synthesized. These multifunctional register-level systems are partitioned as a data-processing unit (datapath) and a controlling unit (control unit). The control unit is responsible for collecting and controlling the data-processing operations (actions) of the datapath. To design the register-level systems, one studies a set of operations to be executed, and then designs nano-ICs using a set of register-level components that implement the desired functions satisfying the affordability and performance requirements. It is very difficult to impose meaningful mathematical structures on register-level behavior or structure using Boolean algebra and conventional gate-level design. Because of these difficulties, the heuristic synthesis is commonly accomplished as sequential steps listed below:

1. Define the desired behavior as a set of sequences of register-transfer operations (each operation can be implemented using the available components) comprising the algorithm to be executed.
2. Examine the algorithm to determine the types of components and their number to attain the required datapath. Design a complete block diagram for the datapath using the components chosen.
3. Examine the algorithm and datapath in order to derive the control signals with ultimate goal to synthesize the control unit for the found datapath that meet the algorithm's requirements.
4. Analyze and verify performing modeling and detail simulation (VHDL, Verilog, ModelSim, and other environments are commonly used).

Let us perform the synthesis of virtual control units that ensures extensibility, flexibility, adaptability, robustness, and reusability. The synthesis will be performed using the hierarchic graphs (HGs). A most important problem is to develop straightforward algorithms which ensure implementation (nonrecursive and recursive calls) and utilize hierarchical specifications. We will examine the behavior, perform logic synthesis, and implement reusable control units modeled as hierarchical finite-state machines with virtual states. The goal is to attain the top-down sequential well-defined decomposition in order to develop complex robust control algorithm step-by-step.

We consider datapath and control units. The datapath unit consists of memory and combinational units. A control unit performs a set of instructions by generating the appropriate sequence of micro instructions that depend on intermediate logic conditions or on intermediate states of the datapath unit. To describe the evolution of a control unit, behavioral models were developed [27,28]. We use the direct-connected HGs containing nodes. Each HG has an entry (*Begin*) and an output (*End*). Rectangular nodes contain micro instructions, macro instructions, or both.

A micro instruction U_i includes a subset of micro operations from the set $U = \{u_1, u_2, \ldots, u_{u-1}, u_u\}$. Micro operations $\{u_1, u_2, \ldots, u_{u-1}, u_u\}$ force the specific actions in the datapath (see Figure 4.55 and Figure 4.57). For example, one can specify that u_1 pushes the data in the local stack, u_2 pushes the data in the output stack, u_3 forms the address, u_4 calculates the address, u_5 pops the data from the local stack, u_6 stores the data from the local stack in the register, u_7 pops the data from the output stack to external output, etc.

A micro operation is the output causing an action in the datapath. Any macro instruction incorporates macro operations from the set $M = \{m_1, m_2, \ldots, m_{m-1}, m_m\}$. Each macro operation is described by another lower level HG. Assume that each macro instruction includes one macro operation. Each rhomboidal node contains one element from the set $L \cup G$. Here, $L = \{l_1, l_2, \ldots, l_{l-1}, l_l\}$ is the set of logic conditions, while $G = \{g_1, g_2, \ldots, g_{g-1}, g_g\}$ is the set of logic functions. Using logic conditions as inputs, logic functions are calculated examining predefined set of sequential steps that are described by a lower level HG. Directed lines connect the inputs and outputs of the nodes.

Consider a set $E = M \cup G$, $E = \{e_1, e_2, \ldots, e_{e-1}, e_e\}$. All elements $e_i \in E$ have HGs, and e_i has the corresponding HG Q_i which specifies either an algorithm for performing e_i (if $e_i \in M$) or an algorithm for calculating e_i (if $e_i \in G$). Assume that $M(Q_i)$ is the subset of macro operations and $G(Q_i)$ is the subset of logic functions that belong to the HG Q_i. If $M(Q_i) \cup G(Q_i) = \varnothing$, the well-known scheme results [10,27,28]. The application of HGs enables one to gradually and sequentially synthesize complex control algorithm concentrating the efforts at each stage on a specified level of abstraction because specific elements of the set E are used. Each component of the set E is simple and can be checked and debugged independently. Figure 4.55 reports HGs $Q_1, Q_2, \ldots, Q_i$ which describe the control algorithm.

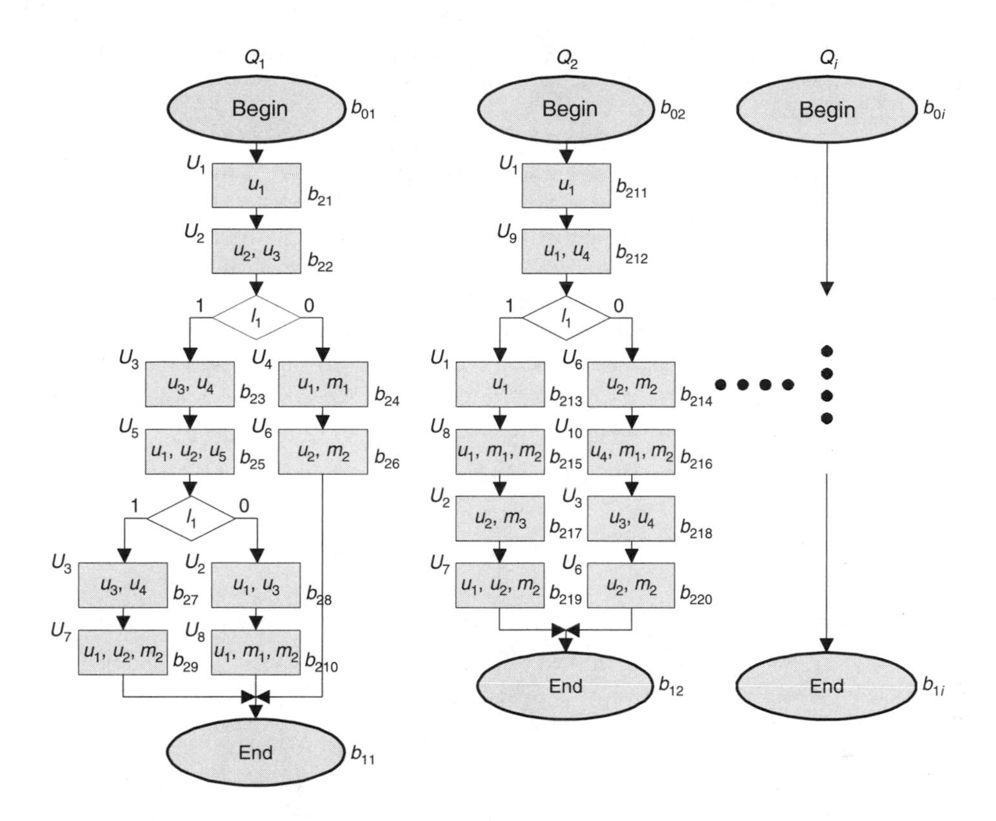

FIGURE 4.55 Control algorithm represented by HGs $Q_1, Q_2, \ldots, Q_i$.

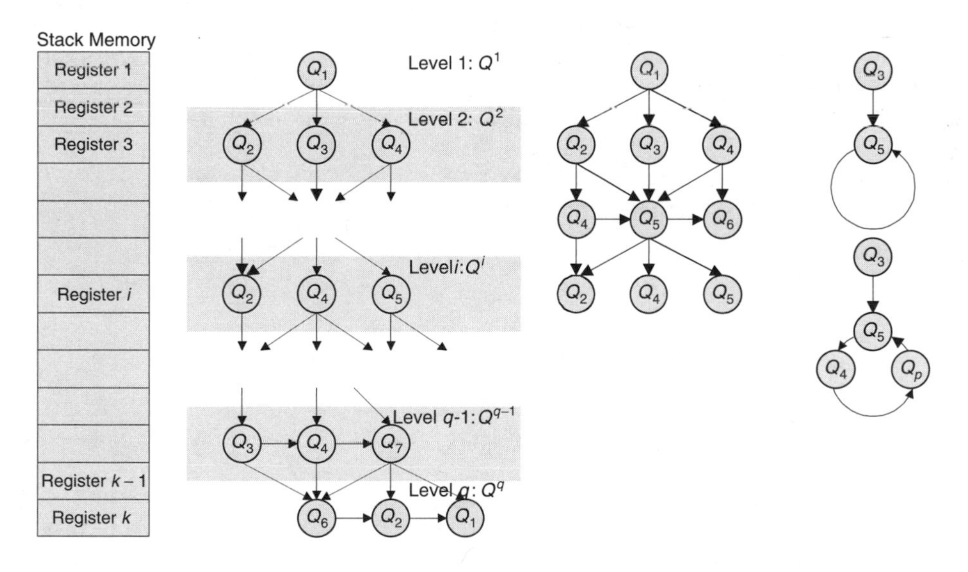

FIGURE 4.56 Stack memory with multilevel sequential HGs, with illustration of recursive call.

The execution of HGs is examined by studying complex operations $e_i = m_j \in M$ and $e_i = g_j \in G$. Each complex operation e_i that is described by a HG Q_i must be replaced with a new subsequence of operators that produces the result executing Q_i. In the illustrative example shown in Figure 4.56, Q_1 is the first HG at the first level Q^1, the second level Q^2 is formed by Q_2, Q_3, and Q_4, etc. We consider the following hierarchical sequence of HGs $Q_{1\,(\text{level }1)} \Rightarrow Q^2_{(\text{level }2)} \Rightarrow \cdots \Rightarrow Q^{q-1}_{(\text{level }q-1)} \Rightarrow Q^q_{(\text{level }q)}$. All $Q_{i\,(\text{level }i)}$ have the corresponding HGs. For example, Q^2 is a subset of the HGs that are used to describe elements from the set $M(Q_1) \cup G(Q_1) = \varnothing$, while Q^3 is a subset of the HGs that are used to map elements from the sets $\cup_{q\in Q^2} M(q)$ and $\cup_{q\in Q^2} G(q)$. In Figure 4.56, $Q^1 = \{Q_1\}$, $Q^2 = \{Q_2, Q_3, Q_4\}$, $Q^3 = \{Q_2, Q_4, Q_5\}$, etc.

Micro operations u^+ and u^- are used to increment and to decrement the stack pointer (SP). The problem of switching to various levels can be solved using a stack memory, see Figure 4.56. Consider an algorithm for $e_i \in M(Q_1) \cup G(Q_1) = \varnothing$. The SP is incremented by the micro operation u^+, and a new register of the stack memory is set as the current register. The previous register stores the state when it was interrupted. New Q_i becomes responsible for the control until terminated. After termination of Q_i, the micro operation u^- is generated to return to the interrupted state. As a result, control is passed to the state in which Q_f is called.

The synthesis problem can be formulated as: for a given control algorithm **A**, described by the set of HGs, construct the FSM that implements **A**.

In general, the synthesis includes the following steps:

- transforming the HGs to the state transition table
- state encoding
- combinational logic optimization
- final structure design

The first step is divided into substeps as: (1) marking the HGs with labels b (see Figure 4.56); (2) recording all transitions between the labels in the extended state transition table; and (3) convert the extended table to ordinary form.

The labels b_{01} and b_{11} are assigned to the nodes *Begin* and *End* of the Q_1. The label $b_{02}, \ldots, b_{0i}$ and $b_{12}, \ldots, b_{1i}$ are assigned to nodes *Begin* and *End* of $Q_2, \ldots, Q_i$, respectively. The labels $b_{21}, b_{22}, \ldots, b_{2j}$ are assigned to other nodes of HGs, inputs and outputs of nodes with logic conditions, etc. Repeating labels are not allowed. The labels are considered as the states. The extended state transition table is designed using the state evolutions due to inputs (logic conditions) and logic functions, which cause the transitions from $x(t)$ to $x(t+1)$. All evolutions of the state vector $x(t)$ are recorded, and the state $x_k(t)$ has the label k. It should be emphasized that the table can be converted from the extended to the ordinary form. To program the Code Converter, one records the transition from the state x_1 assigned to the *Begin* node of the HG Q_1, e.g., $x_{01} \Rightarrow x_{21}(Q_1)$. The transitions between different HGs are recorded as $x_{i,j} \Rightarrow x_{n,m}(Q_j)$. For all transitions, the data-transfer instructions are synthesized. The hardware implementation is illustrated in Figure 4.57.

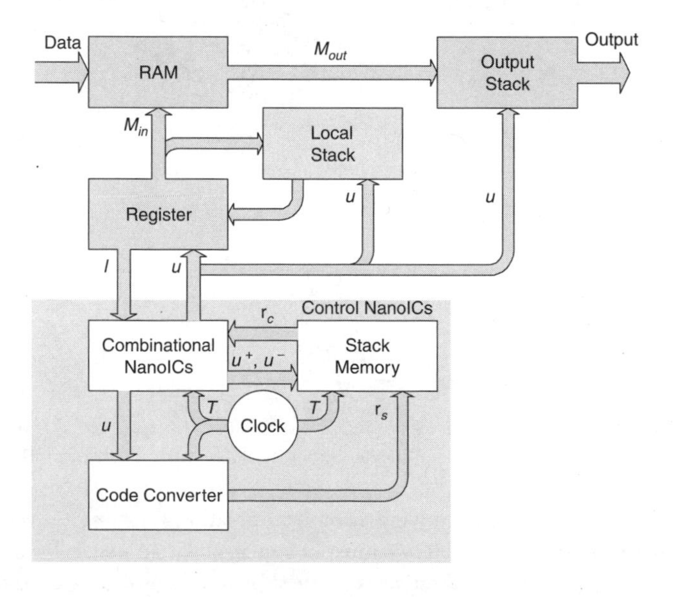

FIGURE 4.57 Hardware implementation.

Robust algorithms are synthesized and implemented using the HGs utilizing the hierarchical behavior specifications and top-down decomposition. The reported method guarantees exceptional adaptation and reusability features through reconfigurable hardware and reprogrammable software.

Reconfigurable Nanocomputers

To design nanocomputers, specific hardware and software solutions must be developed and implemented. For example, ICs are designed by making use of hardware description languages, e.g., very high speed integrated circuit hardware description language (VHDL) and Verilog. Making the parallel to the conventional ICs, the programmable gate arrays (PGAs) developed by Xilinx, Altera, Actel, and other companies, can serve as the meaningful inroad in design of reconfigurable nanocomputers. These PGAs lead one to the on-chip reconfigurable logic concept. The reconfigurable logic can be utilized as a functional unit in the datapath of the processor, having access to the processor register file and to on-chip memory ports. Another approach is to integrate the reconfigurable part of the processor as a coprocessor. For this solution, the reconfigurable logic operates concurrently with the processor. Optimal design and memory port assignments can guarantee the coprocessor reconfigurability and concurrency.

In general, the reconfigurable nanocomputer architecture synthesis emphasizes a high-level design, rapid prototyping, and reconfigurability in order to reduce time and cost improving performance and reliability. The goal is to device, design, and fabricate affordable high-performance high-yield nano-ICs arrays and application-specific nano-ICs (ASNICs). These ASNICs should be testable to detect the defects and faults. The design of ASNICs involves mapping application requirements into specifications implemented by nano-ICs. The specifications are represented at every level of abstraction including the system, behavior, structure, physical, and process domains. The designer should be able to differently utilize the existing nano-ICs to meet the application requirements. User-specified nano-ICs and ASNICs must be developed to attain affordability and superior performance.

The PGAs can be used to implement logic functions utilizing millions of gates. The design starts by interpreting the application requirements into architectural specifications. As the application requirements are examined, the designer translates the architectural specifications into behavior and structure domains. Behavior representation means the functionality required as well as the ordering of operations and completion of tasks in specified times. A structural description consists of a set of nanodevices and their interconnection. Behavior and structure can be specified and studied using hardware description languages. This nano-ICs hardware description language (NHDL) should manage efficiently very complex hierarchies which can include millions of logic gates. Furthermore, NHDLs should be translated into net-lists of library components using synthesis software. The NHDLs software, which is needed to describe hardware and must permit concurrent operations, should perform the following major functions:

- translate text to a Boolean mathematical representation
- optimize the representation based specified criteria (size, delays, optimality, reliability, testability, etc.)
- map the optimized mathematical representation to a technology-specific library of nanodevices

Reconfigurable nanocomputers should use reprogrammable logic units (e.g., PGAs) to implement a specialized instruction set and arithmetic units to optimize the performance. Ideally, reconfigurable nanocomputers can be reconfigured at real-time (runtime), enabling the existing hardware to be reused depending on its interaction with external units, data dependencies, algorithm requirements, faults, etc. The basic PGAs architecture is built using programmable logic blocks (PLBs) and programmable interconnect blocks (PIBs) (see Figure 4.58). The PLBs and PIBs will hold the current configuration setting until adaptation will be accomplished. The PGA is programmed by downloading the information in the file through a serial or parallel logic connection. The time required to configure a PGA is called the configuration time (PGAs could be configured in series or in parallel). Figure 4.58 illustrates the basic architectures from which most multiple PGAs architectures can be derived (pipelined architecture with the PGAs interfaced one to other is well fit for functions that have streaming data at specific intervals, while arrayed PGAs architecture is appropriate for

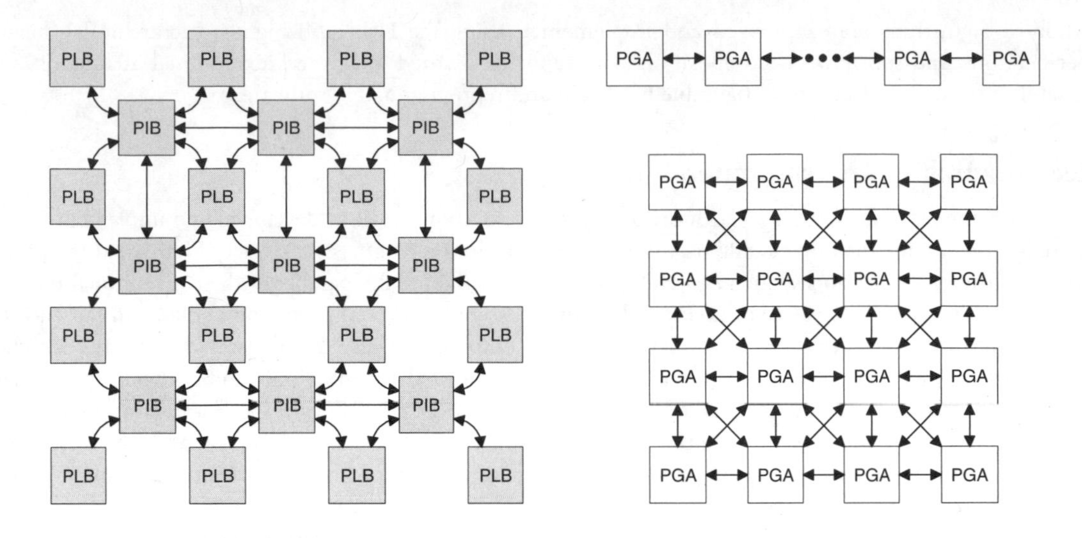

FIGURE 4.58 Programmable gate arrays and multiple PGA architectures.

functions that require a systolic array). A hierarchy of configurability is different for the different PGA architectures.

The goal is to design reconfigurable nanocomputer architectures with corresponding software to cope with less-than-perfect, entirely or partially defective and faulty nanoscale devices, structures, and connects (e.g., nano-ICs) encountered in arithmetic and logic, control, input-output, memory, and other units. To achieve our objectives, the redundant nano-ICs units can be used (the redundancy level is determined by the nanoscale ICs quality and software capabilities). Hardware and software evolutionary learning, adaptability and reconfigurability can be achieved through decision-making, diagnostics, health-monitoring, analysis, and optimization of software, as well as pipelining, rerouting, switching, matching, and controlling of hardware. We concentrate our research on how to devise–design–optimize–build–test–configurate nanocomputers. The overall objective can be achieved guaranteeing the evolution (behavior) matching between the ideal (C_I) and fabricated (C_F) nanocomputer, their units, systems, or components. The nanocompensator (C_{F1}) can be designed for the fabricated C_{F2} such that the response will match the evolution of the C_I, see Figure 4.59. The C_I gives the reference ideal evolving model, which analytically and/or experimentally maps the ideal (desired) input-output behavior, and the nanocompensator C_{F1} should modify the evolution of C_{F2} such that cf.

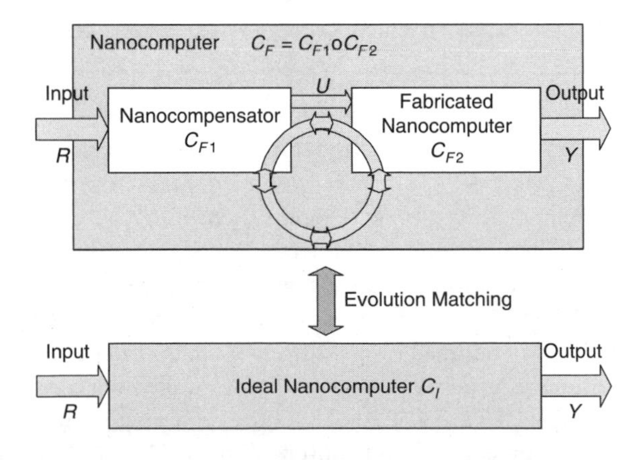

FIGURE 4.59 Nanocomputers and evolution matching.

described by $C_F = C_{F1} \circ C_{F2}$ (series architecture), matches the C_I behavior. Figure 4.59 illustrates the concept. The necessary and sufficient conditions for strong and weak evolution matching based on C_I and C_{F2} must be derived.

Mathematical Models for Nanocomputers

Sixtuple Nanocomputer Model

To address analysis, control, diagnostics, optimization, and design problems, the explicit mathematical models of nanocomputers must be developed and applied. There are different levels of abstraction in nanocomputer modeling, simulation, and analysis [10]. High-level models can accept streams of instruction descriptions and memory references, while the low-level (device-level) logic gates or memory modeling can be performed by making use of streams of input and output signals and nonlinear transient behavior of devices. The system- and subsystem-level modeling (medium-level) also can be formulated and performed. It is evident that one subsystem can contain millions of nanodevices. For example, computer systems can be modeled as queuing networks. Different mathematical modeling frameworks exist and have been developed for each level. In this section we concentrate on the high-, medium-, and low-level systems modeling of nanocomputer systems using the finite state machine concept.

The computer accepts the input information, processes it according to the stored instructions, and produces the output. There exist numerous computer models, e.g., Boolean models, polynomial models, information-based, etc. However, all mathematical models are the mathematical idealization based upon the abstractions, simplifications and hypotheses made. In fact, it is virtually impossible to develop and apply the complete mathematical model due to complexity and numerous obstacles.

It is possible to concurrently model nanocomputers by the sixtuple:

$$C = \{\mathbf{X}, \mathbf{E}, \mathbf{R}, \mathbf{Y}, \mathbf{F}, \mathbf{X}_0\}$$

where $\boldsymbol{X}$ is the finite set of states with initial and final states $\boldsymbol{x}_0 \in \boldsymbol{X}$ and $\boldsymbol{x}_f \subseteq \boldsymbol{X}$; $\boldsymbol{E}$ is the finite set of events (concatenation of events forms a string of events); $\boldsymbol{R}$ and $\boldsymbol{Y}$ are the finite sets of the input and output symbols (alphabets); $\boldsymbol{F}$ are the transition functions mapping from $\boldsymbol{X} \times \boldsymbol{E} \times \boldsymbol{R} \times \boldsymbol{Y}$ to $\boldsymbol{X}$ (denoted as $\boldsymbol{F_X}$), to $\boldsymbol{E}$ (denoted as $\boldsymbol{F_E}$) or to $\boldsymbol{Y}$ (denoted as $\boldsymbol{F_Y}$), $\boldsymbol{F} \subseteq \boldsymbol{X} \times \boldsymbol{E} \times \boldsymbol{R} \times \boldsymbol{Y}$ (we assume that $\boldsymbol{F} = \boldsymbol{F_X}$, e.g., the transition function defines a new state to each quadruple of states, events, references, and outputs, and $\boldsymbol{F}$ can be represented by a table listing the transitions or by a state diagram).

The nanocomputer evolution is due to inputs, events, state evolutions, and parameter variations (as explained at the end of this subsection), etc.

We formulate two useful definitions.

Definition 1. A vocabulary (or an alphabet) **A** is a finite nonempty set of symbols (elements). A world (or sentence) over **A** is a string of finite length of elements of **A**. The empty (null) string is the string which does not contain symbols. The set of all words over **A** is denoted as $\boldsymbol{A_w}$. A language over $\boldsymbol{A}$ is a subset of $\boldsymbol{A_w}$.

Definition 2. A finite-state machine with output $C_{FS} = \{\mathbf{X}, \mathbf{A_R}, \mathbf{A_Y}, \mathbf{F_R}, \mathbf{F_Y}, \mathbf{X_0}\}$ consists of a finite set of states $\boldsymbol{S}$, a finite input alphabet $\mathbf{A_R}$, a finite output alphabet $\mathbf{A_Y}$, a transition function $\boldsymbol{F_Y}$ that assigns a new state to each state and input pair, an output function $\boldsymbol{F_Y}$ that assigns an output to each state and input pair, and initial state $\boldsymbol{X_0}$.

Using the input-output map, the evolution of $\boldsymbol{C}$ can be expressed as

$$E_c \subseteq \mathrm{R} \times \mathrm{Y}$$

That is, if the computer in state $\boldsymbol{x} \in \boldsymbol{X}$ receives an input $\boldsymbol{r} \in \boldsymbol{R}$, it moves to the next state $f(\boldsymbol{x}, \boldsymbol{r})$ and produces the output $y(\boldsymbol{x}, \boldsymbol{r})$. Nanocomputers can be represented as the state tables that describe the state and output functions. In addition, the state transition diagram (direct graph whose vertices correspond to the states and edges correspond to the state transitions, and each edge is labeled with the input and output associated with the transition) is frequently used.

Nanocomputer Modeling with Parameters Set

Nanocomputers can be modeled using the parameters set ***P***. Designing reconfigurable fault-tolerant nanocomputer architectures, sets ***P*** and $\boldsymbol{P}_0$ should be integrated, and we have

$$\mathrm{C} = \{\mathbf{X}, \mathbf{E}, \mathbf{R}, \mathbf{Y}, \mathbf{P}, \mathbf{F}, \mathbf{X}_0, \mathbf{P}_0\}.$$

It is evident that nanocomputer evolution depends upon ***P*** and $\boldsymbol{P}_0$. The optimal performance can be achieved through adaptive synthesis, reconfiguration and diagnostics. For example, one can vary ***F*** and variable parameters $\boldsymbol{P}_v$ to attain the best possible performance.

Nanocomputer evolution, considering states, events, outputs, and parameters, can be expressed as

$$(x_0,e_0,y_0,p_0) \overset{\text{evolution 1}}{\Rightarrow} (x_1,e_1,y_1,p_1) \overset{\text{evolution 2}}{\Rightarrow} \cdots \overset{\text{evolution } j-1}{\Rightarrow} (x_{j-1},e_{j-1},y_{j-1},p_{j-1}) \overset{\text{evolution } j}{\Rightarrow} (x_j,e_j,y_j,p_j).$$

The input, states, outputs, events, and parameter sequences are aggregated within the model $\mathrm{C} = \{\mathbf{X}, \mathbf{E}, \mathbf{R}, \mathbf{Y}, \mathbf{P}, \mathbf{F}, \mathbf{X_0}, \mathbf{P_0}\}$. The concept reported allows us to find and apply the minimal, but complete functional description of nanocomputers. The minimal subset of state, event, output, and parameter evolutions (transitions) can be used. That is, the partial description $\mathrm{C}_{\text{partial}} \subset \mathrm{C}$ results, and every essential nanocomputer quadruple (x_i, e_i, y_i, p_i) can be mapped by $(x_i, e_i, y_i, p_i)_{\text{partial}}$. This significantly reduces the complexity modeling, simulation, analysis, and design problems.

Let the transition function ***F*** map from $\mathbf{X} \times \mathbf{E} \times \mathbf{R} \times \mathbf{Y} \times \mathbf{P}$ to ***X***, e.g., $\mathbf{F}: \mathbf{X} \times \mathbf{E} \times \mathbf{R} \times \mathbf{Y} \times \mathbf{P} \rightarrow \mathbf{X}$, $\mathbf{F} \subseteq \mathbf{X} \times \mathbf{E} \times \mathbf{R} \times \mathbf{Y} \times \mathbf{P}$. Thus, the transfer function ***F*** defines a next state $\boldsymbol{x}(t+1) \in \boldsymbol{X}$ based upon the current state $\boldsymbol{x}(t) \in \boldsymbol{X}$, event $e(t) \in \boldsymbol{E}$, reference $\boldsymbol{r}(t) \in \boldsymbol{R}$, output $\boldsymbol{y}(t) \in \boldsymbol{Y}$ and parameter $\boldsymbol{p}(t) \in \boldsymbol{P}$. Hence:

$$x(t+1) = F\big(x(t), e(t), r(t), y(t), p(t)\big) \text{ for } x_0(t) \in X_0 \text{ and } p_0(t) \in P_0.$$

The robust adaptive control algorithms must be developed. The control vector $\boldsymbol{u}(t) \in \boldsymbol{U}$ is integrated into the nanocomputer model. We have $\mathrm{C} = \{\mathbf{X}, \mathbf{E}, \mathbf{R}, \mathbf{Y}, \mathbf{P}, \mathbf{U}, \mathbf{F}, \mathbf{X}_0, \mathbf{P}_0\}$.

The nanocompensator synthesis procedure is reported in the following sections. This synthesis approach is directly applicable to design nanocomputers with two- and three-dimensional nano-ICs.

Nanocompensator Synthesis and Design Aspects

In this section we will design the nanocompensator. Two useful definitions that allow one to precisely formulate and solve the problem are formulated.

Definition 3. The strong evolutionary matching $C_F = C_{F1} \circ C_{F2} =_B C_I$ for given C_I and C_F is guaranteed if $E_{CF} = E_{CI}$. Here, $C_F =_B C_I$ means that the behaviors (evolution) of C_I and C_F are equivalent.~

Definition 4. The weak evolutionary matching $C_F = C_{F1} \circ C_{F2} \subseteq_B C_I$ for given C_I and C_F is guaranteed if $E_{C_F} \subseteq E_{CI}$. Here, $C_F \subseteq_B C_I$ means that the evolution of C_F is contained in the behavior C_I.~

The problem is to derive a nanocompensator $C_{F1} = \{X_{F1}, E_{F1}, R_{F1}, Y_{F1}, F_{F1}, X_{F10}\}$ such that for given $C_I = \{X_I, E_I, R_I, Y_I, F_I, X_{I0}\}$ and $C_{F2} = \{X_{F2}, E_{F2}, R_{F2}, Y_{F1}, F_{F2}, X_{F20}\}$ the following conditions:

$$C_F = C_{F1} \circ C_{F2} =_B C_I \text{ (strong behavior matching)}$$

or

$$C_F = C_{F1} \circ C_{F2} \subseteq_B C_I \text{ (weak behavior matching)}$$

are satisfied.

Here, we assume that the following conditions are satisfied:

- output sequences generated by C_I can be generated by C_{F2}
- the C_I inputs match the C_{F1} inputs

It must be emphasized that the output sequence means the state, event, output, and/or parameters vectors, e.g., the triple (x, e, y, p).

Lemma 1. If there exists the state-modeling representation $\gamma \subseteq X_1 \times X_F$ such that $C_I^{-1} \times {}_B^{\gamma} C_{F2}^{-1}$ (if $C_I^{-1} \times {}_B^{\gamma} C_{F2}^{-1}$, then $C_I \times {}_B^{\gamma} C_{F2}$), then the evolution matching problem is solvable. The nanocompensator C_{F1} solves the strong matching problem $C_F = C_{F1} \circ C_{F2} = {}_B C_I$ if there exist the state-modeling representations $\beta \subseteq X_1 \times X_{F2}$, $(X_{10}, X_{F20},) \in \beta$ and $\alpha \subseteq X_{F1} \times \beta$, $(X_{F10}, (X_{10}, X_{F20})) \in \alpha$ such that $C_{F1} = {}_B^{\alpha} C_1^{\beta}$ for $\beta \in \Gamma = \{\gamma | C_I^{-1} \times {}_B^{\gamma} C_{F2}^{-1}\}$. Furthermore, the strong matching problem is tractable if there exist C_I^{-1} and C_{F2}^{-1}.

The nanocomputer can be decomposed using algebraic decomposition theory, which is based on the closed partition lattice. For example, consider the fabricated nanocomputer C_{F2} represented as $C_{F2} = \{X_{F2}, E_{F2}, R_{F2}, Y_{F2}, X_{F20}\}$.

A partition on the state set for C_{F2} is a set $\{C_{F2\ 1}, C_{F2\ 2}, \ldots C_{F2\ i}, \ldots C_{F2\ k-1}, C_{F2\ k}\}$ of disjoint subsets of the state set X_{F2} whose union is X_{F2}, e.g., $\bigcup_{i=1}^{k} C_{F2i} = X_{F2}$ and $C_{F2i} \bigcap C_{F2j} = \varnothing$ for $i \neq j$. Hence, we can design and implement the nanocompensators (hardware) $C_{F1\ i}$ for given $C_{F2\ i}$.

References

1. J. Appenzeller, R. Martel, P. Solomon, K. Chan, P. Avouris, J. Knoch, J. Benedict, M. Tanner, S. Thomas, L.L. Wang, and J.A. Del Alamo, "A 10 nm MOSFET concept," *Microelectronic Engineering*, vol. 56, no. 1–2, pp. 213–219, 2001.
2. Y. Chen, D.A.A. Ohlberg, G. Medeiros-Ribeiro, Y.A. Chang, and R.S. Williams, "Self-assembled growth of epitaxial erbium disilicide nanowires on silicon (001)," *Appl. Phys. Lett.*, vol. 76, pp. 4004–4006, 2000.
3. V. Derycke, R. Martel. J. Appenzeller, and P. Avouris, "Carbon nanotube inter- and inramolecular logic gates," *Nano Lett.*, 2001.
4. J.C. Ellenbogen and J.C. Love, "Architectures for molecular electronic computers: Logic structures and an adder designed from molecular electronic diodes," *Proc. IEEE*, vol. 88, no. 3, pp. 386–426, 2000.
5. W.L. Henstrom, C.P. Liu, J.M. Gibson, T.I. Kamins, and R.S. Williams, "Dome-to-pyramid shape transition in Ge/Si islands due to strain relaxation by interdiffusion," *Appl. Phys. Lett.*, vol. 77, pp. 1623–1625, 2000.
6. S.C. Goldstein, "Electronic nanotechnology and reconfigurable computing," *Proc. Computer Society Workshop on VLSI*, pp. 10–15, 2001.
7. T.I. Kamins and D.P. Basile, "Interaction of self-assembled Ge islands and adjacent Si layers grown on unpatterned and patterned Si (001) substrates," *J. Electronic Materials*, vol. 29, pp. 570–575, 2000.
8. T.I. Kamins, R.S. Williams, Y. Chen, Y.L. Chang, and Y.A. Chang, "Chemical vapor deposition of Si nanowires nucleated by $TiSi_2$ islands on Si," *Appl. Phys. Lett.*, vol. 76, pp. 562–564, 2000.
9. T.I. Kamins, R.S. Williams, D.P. Basile, T. Hesjedal, and J.S. Harris, "Ti-catalyzed Si nanowires by chemical vapor deposition: Microscopy and growth mechanism," *J. Appl. Phys.*, vol. 89, pp. 1008–1016, 2001.
10. S.E. Lyshevski, Nanocomputer architectronics and nanotechnology, in *Handbook of Nano-science, Engineering, and Technology*, Eds W.A. Goddard, D.W. Brenner, S.E. Lyshevski, and G.J. Iafrate, Boca Raton, FL: CRC Press, pp. 6-1 to 6-38, 2003.
11. R. Martel, H.S.P. Wong, K. Chan, and P. Avouris, "Carbon nanotube field effect transistors for logic applications," *Proc. Electron Devices Meeting, IEDM Technical Digest*, pp. 7.5.1–7.5.4, 2001.
12. P.L. McEuen, J. Park, A. Bachtold, M. Woodside, M.S. Fuhrer, M. Bockrath, L. Shi, A. Majumdar, and P. Kim, "Nanotube nanoelectronics," *Proc. Device Research Conf.*, pp. 107–110, 2001.
13. R. Saito, G. Dresselhaus and M.S. Dresselhaus, *Physical Properties of Carbon Nanotubes*, London: Imperial College Press, 1999.
14. W.T. Tian, S. Datta, S. Hong, R. Reifenberger, J.I. Henderson, and C.P. Kubiak, "Conductance spectra of molecular wires," *Int. J. Chemical Physics*, vol. 109, no. 7, pp. 2874–2882, 1998.
15. K. Tsukagoshia, A. Kanda, N. Yoneya, E. Watanabe, Y. Ootukab, and Y. Aoyagi, "Nano-electronics in a multiwall carbon nanotube," *Proc. Microprocesses and Nanotechnology Conf.*, pp. 280–281, 2001.

16. E.K. Drexler, *Nanosystems: Molecular Machinery, Manufacturing, and Computations*, Wiley-Interscience, New York, 1992.
17. J. Carter, *Microprocessor Architecture and Microprogramming, a State Machine Approach*, Prentice-Hall, Englewood Cliffs, NJ, 1996.
18. V.C. Hamacher, Z.G. Vranesic, and S.G. Zaky, *Computer Organization*, McGraw-Hill, New York, 1996.
19. J.P. Hayes, *Computer Architecture and Organizations*, McGraw-Hill, Boston, MA, 1998.
20. J.L. Hennessy and D.A. Patterson, *Computer Architecture: A Quantitative Approach*, Morgan Kaufman, San Mateo, CA, 1990.
21. K. Hwang, *Computer Arithmetic*, Wiley, New York, 1978.
22. K. Likharev, "Riding the crest of a new wave in memory," *IEEE Circuits and Devices Magazine*, vol. 16, no. 4, pp. 16–21, 2000.
23. D.A. Patterson and J.L. Hennessey, *Computer Organization and Design—The Hardware/Software Interface*, Morgan Kaufman, San Mateo, CA, 1994.
24. L.H. Pollard, *Computer Design and Architecture*, Prentice-Hall, Englewood Cliffs, NJ, 1990.
25. A.S. Tanenbaum, *Structured Computer Organization*, Prentice-Hall, Englewood Cliffs, NJ, 1990.
26. R.F. Tinder, *Digital Engineering Design: A Modern Approach*, Prentice-Hall, Englewood Cliffs, NJ, 1991.
27. S. Baranov, *Logic Synthesis for Control Automata*. Kluwer, Norwell, MA, 1994.
28. V. Sklyarov, Synthesis of Finite State Machines Based on Matrix LSI. Science, Minsk, Belarus, 1984

4.5 Semiconductor Nano-Electronics and Nano-Optoelectronics

Nelson Tansu, Ronald Arif, and Zhian Jin

Introduction to Semiconductor Nanotechnology

This section presents the overview of semiconductor nanostructure devices, often also called semiconductor nanotechnology, which requires engineering of semiconductor structure with dimensions down to nanometer scale. The advancements in the field of semiconductor nanotechnology have significantly impacted various aspects of the physics and technologies of electronics and optoelectronics devices. New device concepts based on semiconductor nanotechnology have led to (1) novel devices which would not have been possible in the absence of nano-scale engineering of semiconductor structures, and (2) unique and significant improvement to device characteristics as a result of nanoscale device structures.

As the technology is rapidly moving toward the nanometer scale, classical physics fails to describe quantum phenomena observed in nanotechnology. Today, quantum physics has been the foundation of many applications in the fields of engineering, biology, and chemistry. Applications in the fields of engineering have included photonics, semiconductor lasers, semiconductor optoelectronic devices, resonant tunneling diodes, semiconductor transistors, quantum optics, and many other important novel applications that truly utilize quantum phenomena in their principles of operation.

In this section, three important aspects of semiconductor nanotechnology are discussed in subsections "Fundamental Physics of Semiconductor Nanotechnology," "Semiconductor Nanoelectronics – Resonant Tunneling Diode," "Semiconductor Nanoelectronics – Single Electron Transistor," and "Semiconductor Nano-optoelectronics." In "Fundamental Physics of Semiconductor Nanotechnology," the first topic is the fundamental physics of semiconductor nanotechnology, which examines the existence of quantum effects on nanoscale devices. The next three subsections cover the discussions of selected nanoscale devices on nano-electronics and nano-optoelectronics, respectively. Some selected nanoelectronics devices covered in "Semiconductor Nanoelectronics – Resonant Tunneling Diode" and "Semiconductor Nanoelectronics – Single Electron Transistors" are: (1) tunneling devices (resonant tunneling diode), and (2) single electron transistors. In "Semiconductor Nano-optoelectronics" several selected nano-optoelectronics topics covered include (1) fabrication and epitaxy methods, (2) novel nanostructure gain media for semiconductor lasers, including quantum wells and quantum dots, (3) novel telecom lasers for telecommunications, (4) Type-II quantum wells lasers, and (5) quantum intersubband lasers. Finally, there is a discussion of the future directions and a summary of some of the recent developments in the fields of semiconductor nanotechnology are discussed.

Fundamental Physics of Semiconductor Nanotechnology—Quantum Physics

Duality of Particle and Wave—Light as a Particle

At the end of the nineteenth century and the start of the twentieth century, scientists believed that they understood the most fundamental principles of nature. Classical mechanics, thermodynamics, and the theory of electromagnetism were the classical physics which scientists used to understand the behavior of nature. Atoms were solid building blocks of nature. People trusted Newtonian laws of motion to describe the motion of matter or particle. Maxwell's theory of electromagnetism was used to describe the behavior of radiation waves. Most of the problems of physics seemed to have been solved.

However, starting with Einstein's theory of relativity which replaced Newtonian mechanics, scientists gradually realized that their knowledge was far from complete. The inability of classical physics to explain various physical phenomena and experiments in the microscopic and sub-atomic scale also led to the need to replace classical physics. Of particular interest was the growing field of quantum mechanics, which completely altered the fundamental precepts of physics.

One of the most fundamental concepts in quantum mechanics is the dual behavior of matter as particle and wave. In many macroscopic engineering applications, classical physics is sufficient to explain many of the phenomena that we observe. As scientists and engineers are able to manipulate the size of semiconductor-based structures down to a critical dimension of several nanometers (often referred to as semiconductor nanotechnology or semiconductor nanostructure devices), quantum effects become increasingly important, and classical physics fails to explain these effects observed in quantum devices. Indeed, the understanding of applied quantum mechanics for engineers is a must for those working in the fields of semiconductor devices, photonics, nanoelectronics, and nano-optoelectronics.

Planck's explanation of the quantization of light energy, which accurately described the spectral energy density $u(v, T)$ for a blackbody radiation, led to the birth of quantum theory. In Planck's analysis, the light energy (E) with a frequency v is quantized by the relation $E = hv$, where h is called as Planck's constant. The spectral energy density derived based on Planck's Law can be expressed as

$$u(v,T) = \frac{8\pi \cdot h \cdot v^3}{c^3} \cdot \frac{1}{\exp\left(\frac{h \cdot v}{k_B \cdot T}\right) - 1} \tag{4.96}$$

By quantizing the light energy with frequency, the blackbody radiation spectral energy densities for various temperatures are found to be consistent with experimental results, as shown in Figure 4.60.

By extending Planck's idea of quantization of electromagnetic radiation, Einstein in 1905 proposed a theory to successfully explain the photoelectric effect phenomenon. The photoelectric effect itself was first observed in 1887, but classical physics failed to provide an accurate description which was supported by the experimental results. A schematic of the experiment is shown in Figure 4.61(a). In the photoelectric effect experiment, incident light is projected onto a metal surface, and the kinetic energy K of the ejected electrons from the metal surface is measured, as shown in Figure 4.61(b).

The experiment revealed several important discoveries for the photoelectric effect. If the frequency of incident light is smaller than v_0, no electron can be ejected from the surface of the metal (regardless of how high the incident light intensity is). If the frequency of incident light is higher than v_0, however, electrons will be ejected instantly, regardless of how low the incident light intensity is. For $v > v_0$, the number of ejected electrons is proportional to the light intensity. The kinetic energy K of the ejected electrons depends on the frequency/energy of the incident light, with its relation expressed by $K = hv - \phi_m$. Based on this idea, Einstein provided an explanation for the photoelectric effect by treating the light as particles with quantized energy packets of hv, in agreement with Planck's work. These quantized light particles are called quanta or photons.

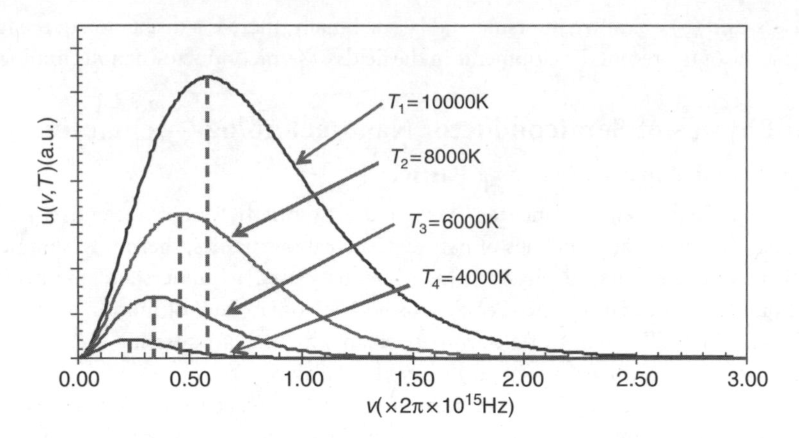

FIGURE 4.60 Spectral energy density of a blackbody object calculated using Planck's law, with its corresponding temperature and peak frequency.

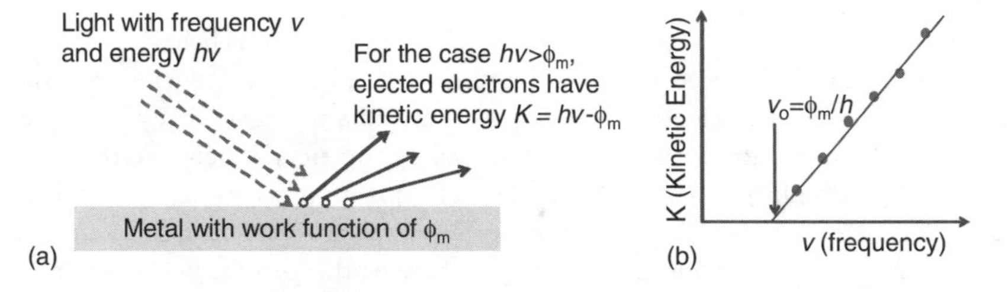

FIGURE 4.61 (a) Photoelectric effect experiment with incident light of energy hv and work function of ϕ_m. For the case of $hv > \phi_m$, electrons are ejected with kinetic energy of $K = hv - \phi_m$. (b) Typical relationship of kinetic energy K of electrons with the frequency v of the incident light. For the case of $v < v_0$, no electrons are ejected from the surface metal. For the case of $v > v_0$, electrons are ejected with certain kinetic energy $K = hv - \phi_m$.

In 1923, Arthur H. Compton conducted the experiment to demonstrate the particle characteristics of light radiation, by means of scattering x-rays off free electrons. In his experiment, Compton showed that light behaves as particles. The deflection of the x-rays scattered by free electrons gave strong confirmation that light (or the photon) behaves as a particle.

Duality of Particle and Wave—Electron as a Wave

The blackbody radiation, photoelectric effect, and Compton's scattering experiment provided the confirmation that light waves exhibit particle-like characteristics. In 1923, de Broglie suggested that not only does the light wave exhibit particle-like characteristics, but *all matter should also exhibit a particle-wave duality characteristic.* The particle-wave duality should be universal, which simply means that all matter exhibits both the particle and wave characteristics simultaneously. Obviously, this view is certainly very different from classical physics where particle and wave are mutually exclusive. In de Broglie's hypothesis, he speculated that this same relation holds for particles as well. In de Broglie's hypothesis, the relationship between wave and particle can be expressed as:

$$\lambda = \frac{h}{p} \quad \leftarrow \text{de Broglie's wavelength} \tag{4.97}$$

This relationship states that any matter with nonzero rest mass with momentum of p has de Broglie's wavelength λ associated with the matter.

To confirm de Broglie's hypothesis, which states that matter also exhibits wave behavior, Davisson and Germer of Bell Labs conducted an experiment that demonstrated the wave characteristics of electrons in 1927.

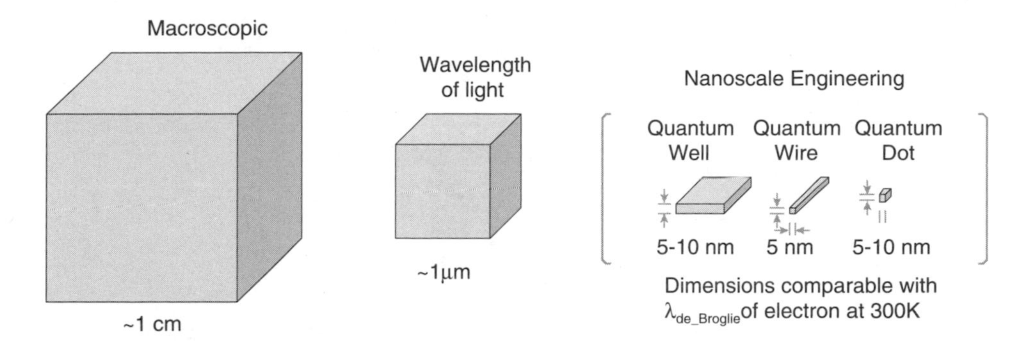

FIGURE 4.62 Comparison of dimension from macroscopic to nanoscale structures.

The experiment by Davisson and Germer demonstrated that electrons, which are considered only as particles in classical physics, can also cause interference patterns among themselves; obviously, interference phenomena demonstrate the existence of wave characteristics due to the phase information that wave carries.

Semiconductor Nanotechnology and Quantum Effects

The development of modern technology in semiconductor technology allows the engineering of nanoscale structure and devices. The nanoscale dimension of interest is typically in the range of de Broglie's wavelength ($\lambda_{\text{de\_Broglie}}$) for an electron at 300 K, which corresponds to dimensions smaller than ~50 nm.

Figure 4.62 provides a comparison of various dimensional scales used in this field of study. The dimension of interest for typical macroscopic matters is in the range of centimeters to meters. The dimension of interest for the light wavelength is of the order of 1 μm, leading to the typical dimension of optical waveguide in micron-size range. To achieve quantum confinement of electrons, one has to achieve dimensions in a range comparable to de Broglie's wavelength ($\lambda_{\text{de\_Broglie}}$) for an electron at 300 K. A typical quantum well structure consists of a sheet with thickness in the range of 5 to 10 nm, while a quantum wire structure provides 2D confinement of electrons with width and thickness in the range of 5 to 10 nm. All the dimensions of a quantum dot structure, however, are nanoscale, which leads to 3D confinement for an electron in the dot structure.

As shown in Figure 4.63 to Figure 4.68, many novel devices in modern technology require nanoscale engineering of matter, which requires in-depth understanding of quantum mechanics. The following are a few applications based on semiconductor nanotechnology: (1) semiconductor lasers, semiconductor optical amplifiers, semiconductor photodiodes, and semiconductor optical modulators that plays a major role in optical communication, (2) semiconductor transistors for integrated circuits in computer technology, (3) heterojunction bipolar transistor, resonant tunneling diode, and high electron mobility transistors that play important role in compound semiconductor electronics and wireless communication systems, (4) light-emitting diodes for high-efficiency and reliable visible solid-state lightings, (5) quantum intersubband devices

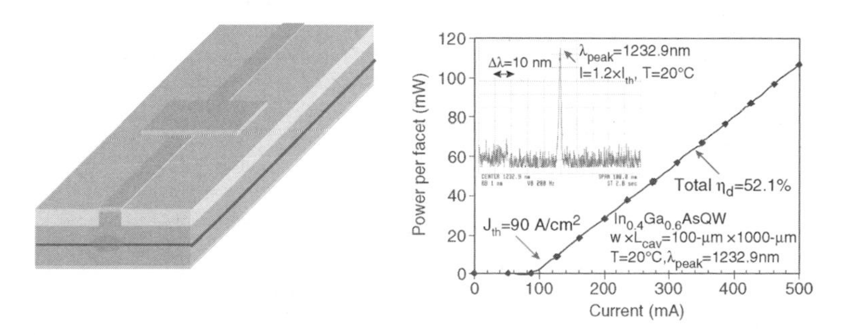

FIGURE 4.63 (a) Schematic of semiconductor edge-emitting ridge-guide lasers, and (b) the lasing characteristics of 60 Å, or about thickness of 20 atoms, InGaAs quantum-well laser grown on GaAs emitting at 1233-nm wavelength regime.

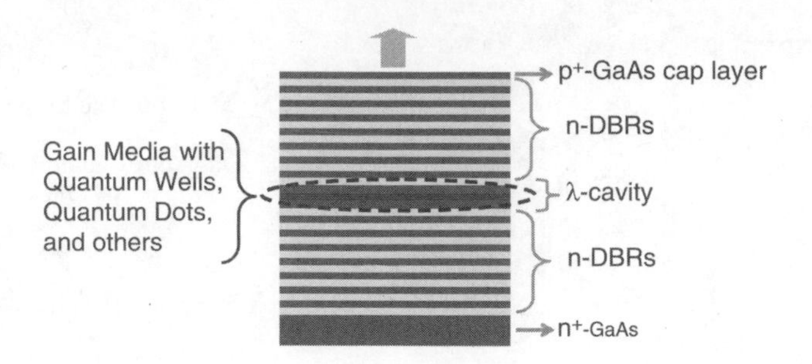

FIGURE 4.64 Schematic of vertical cavity surface emitting lasers (VCSELs) on GaAs substrate, utilizing gain media based on semiconductor nanostructure of quantum wells or quantum dots. Applications of VCSELs are mainly in the fields of optical communications.

for biochemical sensing and far-IR laser applications, (6) tunneling processes in semiconductor, (7) single electron transistors, (8) quantum computing and quantum information, and (9) many other important novel applications that use quantum phenomena in their operation principles. Several applications based on nanoscale engineering of semiconductor structure are shown in Figure 4.63 to Figure 4.68.

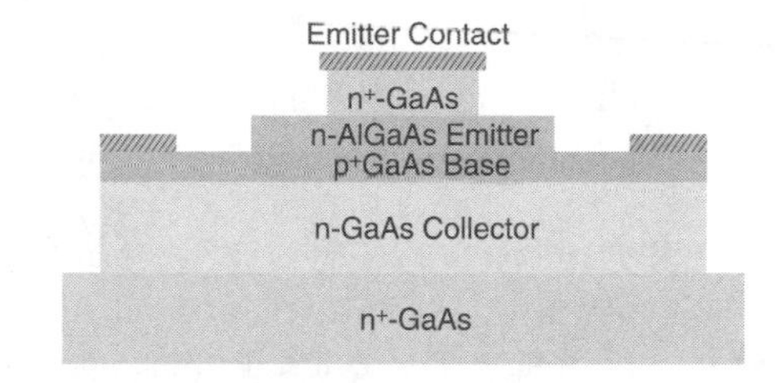

FIGURE 4.65 Schematic of heterojunction bipolar transistor, commonly utilized as a transmitter in wireless communication systems.

From the descriptions provided in Figure 4.63 to Figure 4.68, we observe how semiconductor nanostructure devices impact our lives in so many areas, such as high-speed electronics, current and future computers, optical communications, wireless communications, and biochemical sensors. Advancements in these areas have been made possible by semiconductor nanotechnology.

Semiconductor Nano-Electronics—Resonant Tunneling Diode

Nanoelectronics and Tunneling Phenomena

One of the operating principles for nanoelectronics devices is quantum tunneling phenomena. Tunneling elements in nanoelectronics are basically just two conducting materials separated by a very thin potential

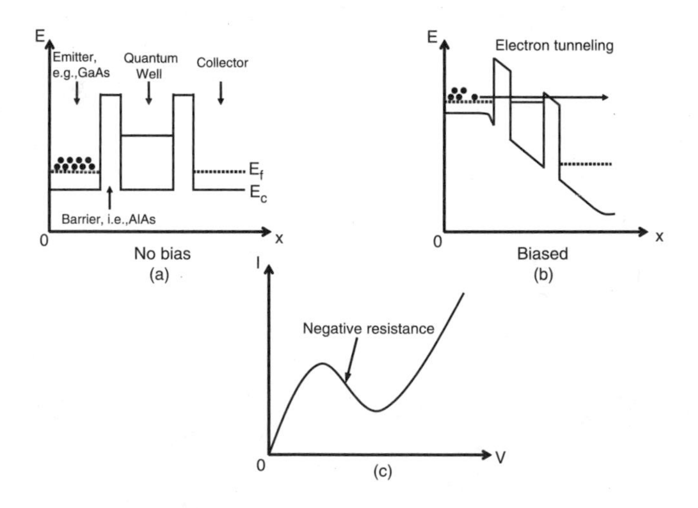

FIGURE 4.66 Schematic of resonant tunneling diode (RTD): (a) under thermal equilibrium, (b) under applied bias, and (c) its current–voltage characteristics.

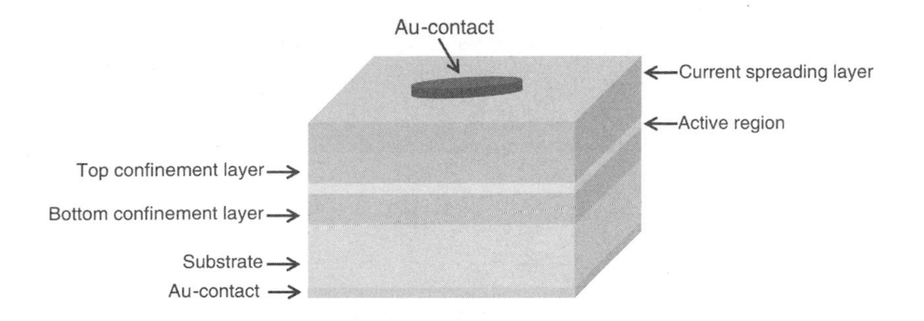

FIGURE 4.67 Schematic of light-emitting diodes (LEDs) for solid-state lighting.

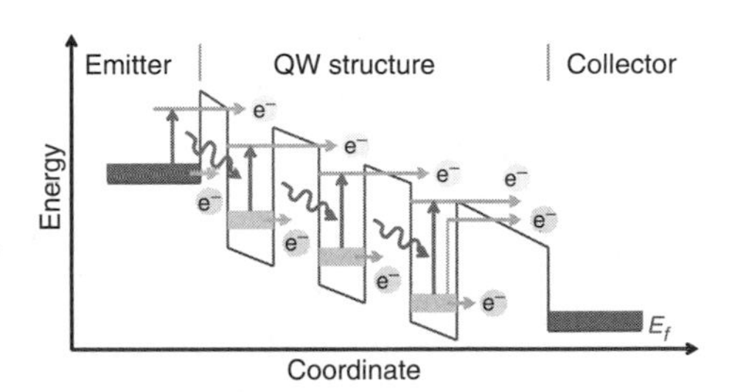

FIGURE 4.68 Schematic of quantum-well intersubband photodetector (QWIP) for far-IR imaging.

barrier; understanding of the tunneling element is of fundamental relevance for nanoelectronics, in particular for resonant tunneling diode (RTD) [1]. Compared to other nanoelectronics devices such as single electron transistor (SET), RTDs are the most mature. The engineering and realization of tunneling elements is achievable by advanced epitaxy technologies, such as molecular beam epitaxy (MBE) or metalorganic chemical vapor deposition (MOCVD). The term "tunneling" itself refers to particle (or matter) transport through a potential barrier where the total energy of the classical particle is lower than the energy barrier. In classical physics, this phenomenon is not possible. A review of quantum tunneling phenomena will be discussed below, followed by a discussion of various nanoelectronic devices.

Quantum Tunneling Phenomena

Tunneling phenomena is one of the true wave characteristics that does not exist in classical particle physics. The classical particle, with energy E smaller than potential barrier U_0, will not penetrate the barrier U_0 regardless of how thin the barrier is; this is due to the deterministic characteristic of the classical particle. Schematically, the phenomenon of the classical particle reflected by a thin potential barrier is shown in Figure 4.69.

Thus, all the incident classical particles will be reflected by the thin potential barrier. The incident particle with energy ($E < U_0$) has kinetic energy of K, in region I and each particle will move with velocity of v_1 as follows:

$$v_1 = \sqrt{\frac{2E}{m}}, \text{ with direction to the right } (+x) \tag{4.98}$$

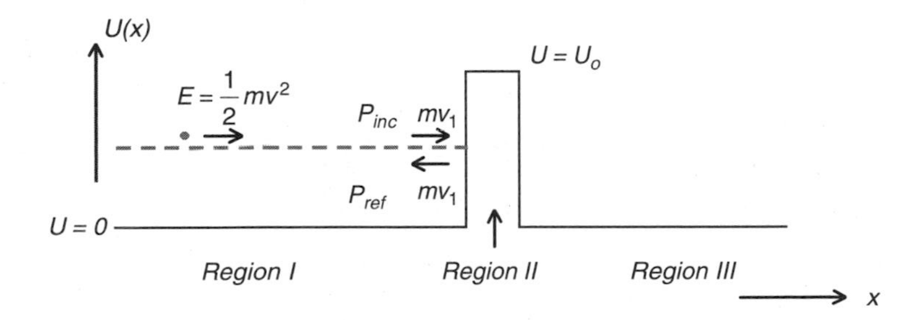

FIGURE 4.69 Schematic of classical picture for a particle with mass m and energy E ($E < U_0$), reflected by a thin potential barrier.

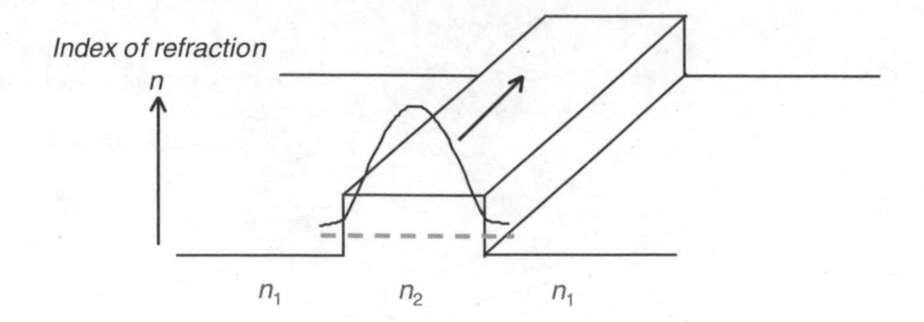

FIGURE 4.70 Light localization in the positive index waveguide. The light wave modes have quantized effective indices n_{eff}.

At the position where the potential barrier U_0 is introduced, the particles will be reflected by this potential barrier, U_0. The reflected particle will travel with velocity $-v_I$. The negative sign in the velocity indicates a direction of motion to the left. As all the particles were reflected back, no particles can be found in region II. As a result, no particle can also travel into region II.

Unlike the classical particle, tunneling phenomena are observed in classical waves. Obviously, one of the most common examples is light waves. A light wave can be guided by a positive index guide structure, using the well-known total internal reflection. Schematically, the guiding of light is shown in Figure 4.70.

The light localization phenomena described here are actually analogous to the localization of particle in a quantum well. Because of the wave nature of light, light has a nonzero field in its "forbidden" region (the region with index n_1). In the light forbidden region, the nonzero attenuation field of the light can be found.

The tunneling phenomena of light wave can be achieved by having light from one localized region (the so-called high index n_2 region) tunnel through a forbidden region (the so-called low index n_1 region) to another localized region (high index n_2 region again). This phenomenon is known as directional coupler in integrated optics. Schematically, the directional coupler is shown in Figure 4.71. At $z=0$, the light is localized inside guide 1, with only evanescent waves decaying in the n_1-region. If the evanescent wave of the light penetrates to guide 2, one can achieve complete transfer of light power from guide 1 to guide 2 at a distance $z = L$. This transfer of light wave energy through a "forbidden" region can be understood as a light wave tunnel through the forbidden region from guide 1 to guide 2.

In the quantum picture, the duality of matter as wave and particle results in the ability of matter to tunnel through a forbidden region by taking advantage of its wave characteristics. In the tunneling problem, obviously the energy E of the particle is smaller than the potential barrier $U(x)$ of the forbidden region ($E < U(x)$, for a forbidden region). As shown in Figure 4.72, the incident particle with energy E is scattered through a potential barrier $U(x)$. Fractions of the particle tunnel through, while the rest will be reflected back.

Note that classical particles are forbidden in region $E < U(x)$, which is region II in Figure 4.72. In contrast, there is the probability that the quantum particle will tunnel through the "classically forbidden" region ($E < U(x)$), as long as the potential barrier is "thin" enough.

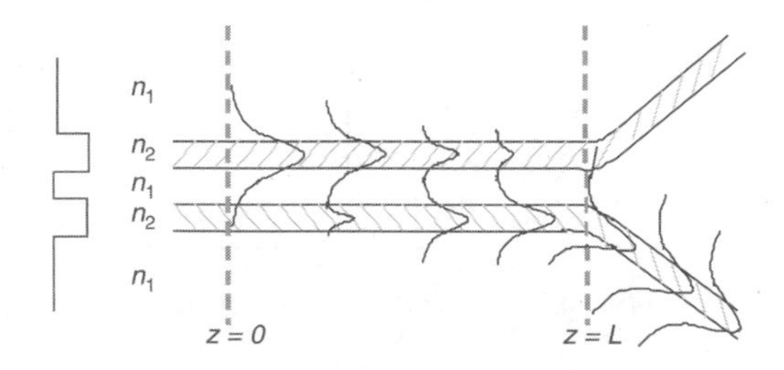

FIGURE 4.71 Schematic of directional coupler device, which demonstrates the tunneling phenomena of localized light from one waveguide to another waveguide through a "classically forbidden" region (region with index of n_1).

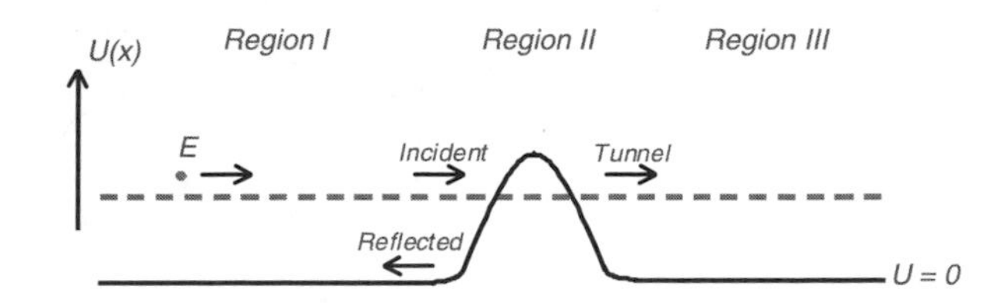

FIGURE 4.72 Schematic of reflection and tunneling phenomena of an incident quantum particle ($E < U_0$) scattered by a potential barrier $U(x)$.

Particle Tunneling through a Potential Barrier

Here, as in typical tunneling problems, the energy of the particle is smaller than the potential barrier. Let us take a look at Figure 4.73, which describes how a particle tunnels through a potential barrier.

The incident particle with mass m and energy E ($E < U_0$) travels from $x = -\infty$ to the right ($+x$) and is scattered by a potential barrier U_0 with thickness of L. Classically, all the particles would just be reflected back, but the quantum mechanical nature of the particles allow the nonzero fraction to be transmitted and the rest to be reflected back. To formulate this problem, one can solve the tunneling probability by solving the relation provided by Schrödinger's wave equation, resulting in tunneling probability as follows ($\hbar = h/2\pi$):

$$T = \frac{1}{1 + \frac{U_0^2}{4E \cdot (U_0 - E)} \cdot \sinh^2\left(\sqrt{\frac{2m}{\hbar^2}(U_0 - E)} \cdot L\right)} \tag{4.99}$$

One can observe from the expression above that there exists a nonzero transmission probability of the incident quantum particle into Region III despite the fact that $E < U_0$. Obviously, classically, no particle would be found in Region III for $E < U_0$.

Resonant Tunneling—Double Barrier Potential

In the case of particle tunneling through double or multiple potential barriers, the tunneling probability has strong resonance features associated with the quasi-bound states of the potential functions. The strong resonances found on the double or multiple barrier cases result in a "unity" tunneling rate ($E < U_0$) of the particle through the double or multiple barrier. The schematic of the double barriers potential for tunneling problems is shown in Figure 4.74 as follows.

In solving the problem related to double (or multiple) barriers, one can utilize the numerical or analytical formulation of the 1D Schrödinger wave equation. The tunneling coefficient T of particle tunneling through a double potential structure, as shown in Figure 4.74, can be expressed as:

$$T = |K|^2 \tag{4.100}$$

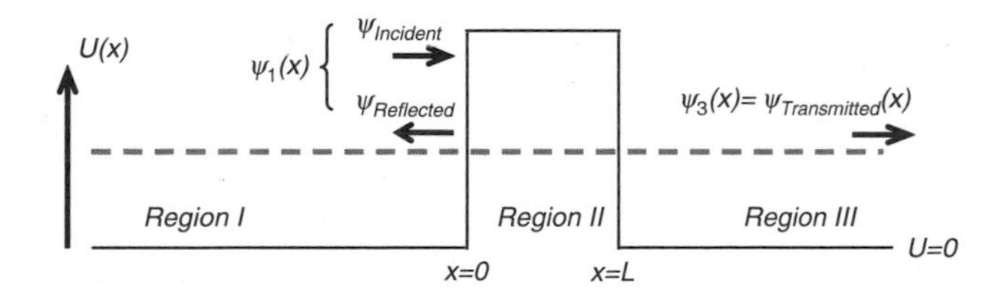

FIGURE 4.73 Tunneling and reflection phenomena of an incident quantum particle ($E < U_0$) scattered by a potential function $U(x)$ with rectangular barrier.

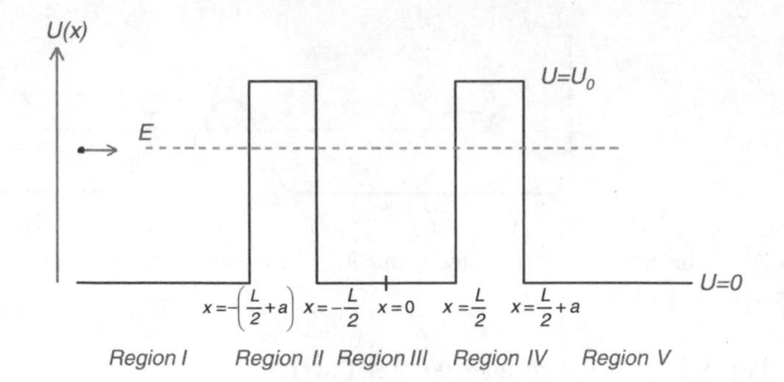

FIGURE 4.74 Schematic of double barrier potential function $U(x)$ for tunneling problems of an incident quantum particle with mass m and energy E.

with $1/K$ reads:

$$\frac{1}{K}=\frac{e^{i2k(\frac{L}{2}+a)}}{4\alpha^2\cdot k^2}\cdot\left\{\begin{matrix} e^{i2k\cdot L}\cdot(\alpha^2+k^2)^2\cdot\sinh^2(\alpha\cdot a)-(\alpha^4+k^4)\cdot\sinh^2(\alpha\cdot a) \\ +\alpha^2\cdot k^2\cdot[1+3\cosh(2\alpha\cdot a)]+i2\alpha\cdot k\cdot(\alpha^2-k^2)\cdot\sinh(2\alpha\cdot a)\end{matrix}\right\} \tag{4.101}$$

k and α can be expressed as:

$$k=\sqrt{\frac{2mE}{\hbar^2}} \tag{4.102}$$

$$\alpha=\sqrt{\frac{2m}{\hbar^2}(U_0-E)} \tag{4.103}$$

As an example, the transmission or tunneling coefficient T is plotted in Figure 4.75 for the case of $U_0=1.2$ eV, $L=6$ nm, and $a=1$ nm. From the example presented here, we observe the existence of three resonance states

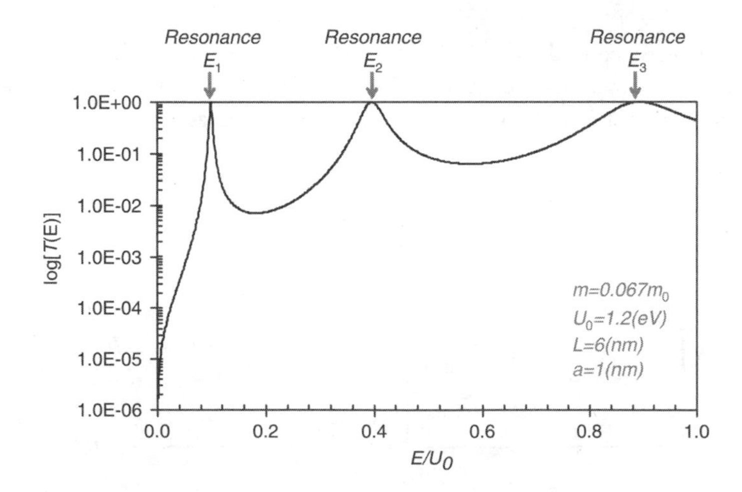

FIGURE 4.75 Tunneling coefficient as function of energy E for a particle with mass m, scattered by a double barrier potential. Notice the resonant features that occur at E_1, E_2, and E_3, which also correspond to the quasi-bound states.

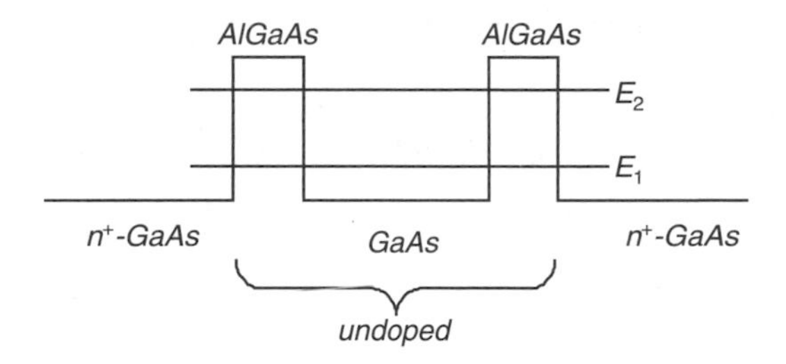

FIGURE 4.76 The conduction band of the GaAs-AlGaAs resonant tunneling diode. The double barrier potential is realized by the heterojunction of AlGaAs–GaAs layers.

at energy levels E_1, E_2, and E_3. The energy levels also correspond to the quasi-bound states of the middle-well-like region (*Region III*). As one extends the barrier thickness to infinity, the bound state energy levels in the well-like region (*Region III*) would be in the vicinity of E_1, E_2, and E_3. The tunneling processes through the "quasi-bound" states of the well region are what we call resonant tunneling.

Resonant Tunneling Diode—Application

The phenomenon of "resonant" tunneling through a double-barrier configuration is the concept behind the so-called resonant tunneling diode (RTD) devices [2,3]. RTD can be formed by epitaxially grown semiconductor layers of AlGaAs and GaAs. The GaAs layers provide the low potential region, as the AlGaAs layers serve as the barrier region. Schematically, the GaAs–AlGaAs RTD is shown in Figure 4.76 and Figure 4.77.

The cross-section of an RTD device is shown as follows. All the layers, except the n^+-GaAs substrate, can be grown either by metalorganic chemical vapor deposition or molecular beam epitaxy. By applying an electric field across RTD devices, one can achieve a negative resistance region.

To understand this principle of operation of RTD devices, one can observe the band lineup under various conditions as shown in Figure 4.78. In the absence of an electric field ($V = 0$), the electrons from region I cannot tunnel through the barriers, as the resonant level E_1 is far away from E_{f1}, thus the current is zero. At $V = V_{R1}$, we observe maximum resonant tunneling of current from region I to region V through the double barrier. The resonant tunneling through E_1 states allow current to flow from region I to region V. As we increase the voltage further above V_{R1}, we are moving away from the resonant condition, again resulting in low tunneling probability. This results in reduction of the current flowing in the RTD devices, which leads to the behavior of negative resistance (increasing voltage results in decreasing current, thus the differential resistance is negative). Note that the nonzero valley current at V_2 is typically due to the existence of thermionic emission. Applying a large bias voltage results in significant amount of thermionic current at $V >> V_2$.

The RTD, with its negative resistance region, is useful for low-power high-speed microwave digital devices. A similar concept of resonant tunneling also finds important applications in the injection of electrons in the

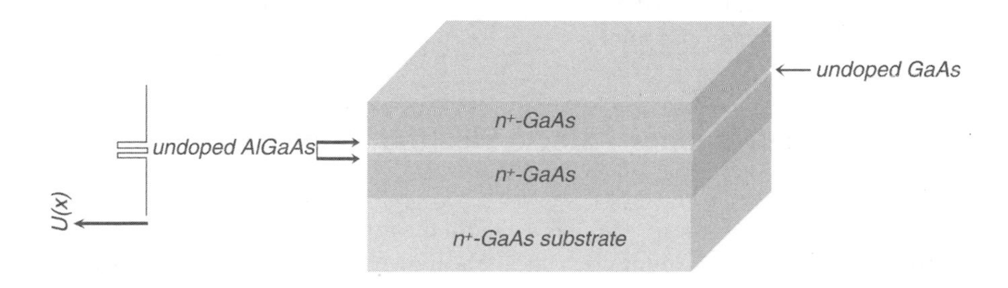

FIGURE 4.77 Cross-sectional schematic of resonant tunneling diode (RTD) with GaAs/AlGaAs structures. The RTD structure is grown on an n^+-GaAs substrate.

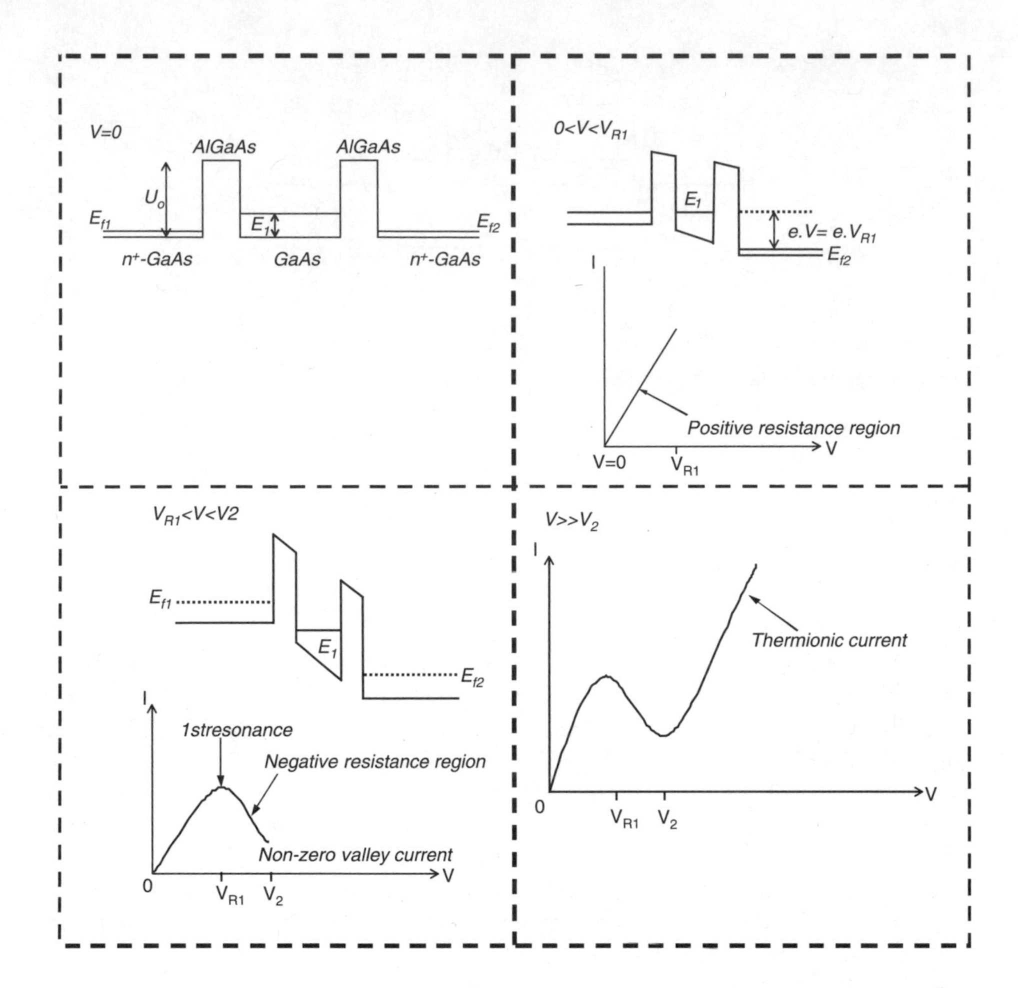

FIGURE 4.78 Schematic of band lineup for resonant tunneling diode (RTD) at various bias voltages, and their corresponding I–V characteristics.

quantum intersubband lasers. A different method to realize RTDs is by the use of three potential energy barriers and two quantum wells. In this case, typical I–V characteristics depend on the placement of the two quantum wells. Depending on the dimensions of the quantum wells, different configurations of energy levels are attainable. In brief, RTDs have very good switching properties with a downside of being a two-terminal device. In order to achieve isolation of gate input and output, a combination of electronic amplification and negative differential resistance is implemented. Monolithic integration of tunneling diodes with three terminal devices is a prerequisite for circuit manufacturing. These devices, basically a field effect transistor and bipolar transistor, offer the required input–output isolation and gain.

Semiconductor Nanoelectronics—Single Electron Transistors

Theoretical Basis

The operation of single electron transistor (SET) is based on the principle of electron tunneling and Coulomb blockade. Electron tunneling is a quantum mechanical phenomenon where, due to particle-wave duality, an electron can be made to tunnel through a sufficiently thin potential energy barrier as long as there are available states for the electron to exist on both sides of the barrier. This theory can be observed experimentally by using two metal electrodes separated by a thin section of dielectric layer, where electrons at the Fermi level can

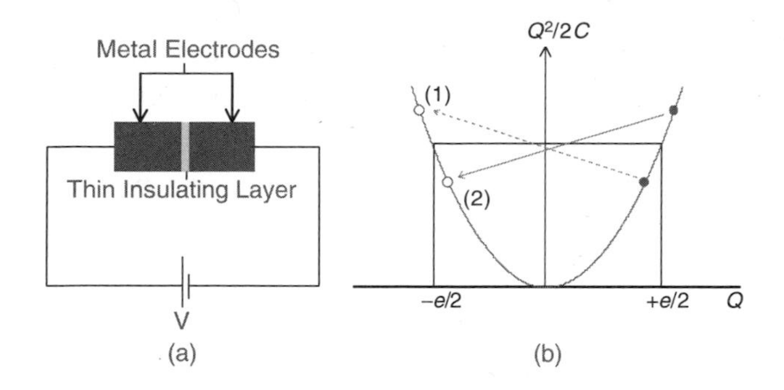

FIGURE 4.79 (a) A typical metal-thin insulator–metal junction under bias, and (b) total energy diagram of a capacitive junction.

tunnel through the insulator (in classical terms, this would not be possible since the energy of the electron is too low to overcome the potential barrier).

Coulomb blockade is a phenomenon of current flow inhibition, that until recently could only be observed at very low (cryogenic) temperature. Its principle can be described by Figure 4.79(a) and (b) [4].

When a potential difference is applied between the two metal electrodes, the ability (or inability) of current to flow across the junction follows an energetic requirement. Referring to Figure 4.79b, if the accumulated charge at the electrode–insulator interface is less than $e/2$, where e is electron charge, the total energy of the system will actually increase when a single electron transfer through tunneling process takes place, since energy is defined as $E = Q^2/2C$ (Q is total charge and C is the capacitance of the junction). This is not a favorable process (process 1 in Figure 4.79.b). Therefore, only when Q at the interface is greater than $e/2$ can charge transfer can take place (process 2 in Figure 4.79.b). This amount of charge corresponds to a potential difference of $V = e/2C$. An ideal I–V characteristics of such a junction at $T = 0$ K is shown in Figure 4.80.

At room temperature, such current flow blockade at low voltage is not readily observed. This is because thermal energy at room temperature is a few orders of magnitude higher than the Coulomb energy gap. However, a few modifications to the junction can still be made for cryogenic operation.

First, by using a double barrier sandwiching the electron pool in the middle, as shown in Figure 4.81. This method has been used to efficiently isolate the junction from the environmental (thermal) effect. The total capacitance (C_{total}) is then just the sum of two junction capacitances corresponding to the two junctions.

Second, the junction has to be made sufficiently resistive. Based on the Heisenberg uncertainty principle, $\Delta E \Delta t > \frac{1}{2}h$, we have to ensure that charging/discharging of the electron island does not happen too rapidly so that the quantum energy fluctuation is greater than $E = Q^2/2C$, or the Coulomb blockade will be destroyed.

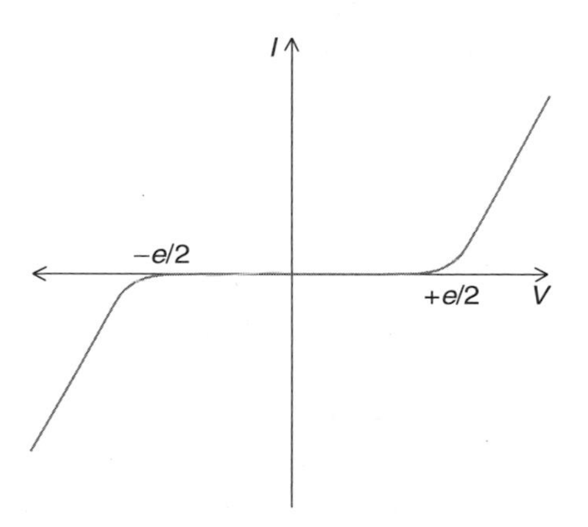

FIGURE 4.80 Ideal I–V characteristic of a capacitive junction with thin insulating layer between metal electrodes at 0 K.

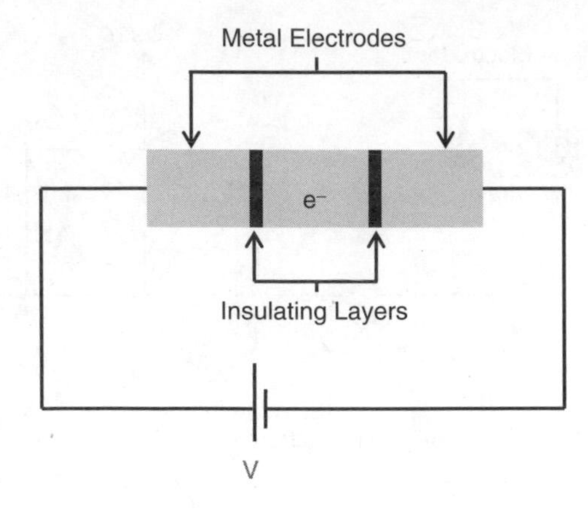

FIGURE 4.81 Double-barrier capacitive junction, with electron pool sandwiched by two insulating layers connected to metal electrode terminals.

Operation

From an application point of view, a single electron transistor is an ideal switching device. As an illustration, in a typical transistor, say MOSFET, in the "on" state, when the current flowing is 1 mA, then a charge of approximately 10^{-15} C will pass between the source and the drain terminal. This amount of charge corresponds to about 6000 electrons [4]. In other words, the information that we transfer using this 1 mA of current is carried over and thus depends on the properties of these 6000 electrons. In the off state, almost no current will flow.

For the case of SET, in the "on" state, only one electron can flow at a time across the island. Current flow is maintained by continuous, single, electron flow across the junction. This property makes SET suitable for the ultimate logic device, where "on" and "off" are represented by the presence and absence of only one electron at all times. One important requirement for the room-temperature switching operation of the SET is that we have to be able to tailor the total energy of the system. By applying a gate voltage (V_g) to the electron pool, the total energy (U) is now controllable by the gate voltage as follows [4]:

$$U(N, V_g) = \frac{(-N \cdot e + C_g \cdot V_g)^2}{2 \cdot C_{\text{total}}} \tag{4.104}$$

where N and C_g are the number of electrons and gate capacitance, respectively. One observes that the junction energy increases quadratically with applied gate voltage. This means, for a small applied voltage across the source and drain, no electron can hop onto the island and no current flow is observed (device is in "off" state). There exists a ΔV_g value, where $U(N,V_g) = U(N+1,V_g+\Delta V_g)$. When this happens, an additional electron can tunnel through the island, and the device is in the "on" state. Substituting this condition, it is trivial to show that $\Delta V_g = \frac{e}{C_g}$, as shown in Figure 4.82.

At this point, practical applications of SET at room temperature are still unrealizable. A considerable capacitance decrease (and thus total energy increase) corresponding to a reduction in size will have to be achieved.

Semiconductor Nano-Optoelectronics

Quantum-Effects Based Gain Media for Laser Applications

Semiconductor optoelectronics benefits significantly from the ability to realize nanometer-scale semiconductor structures, in particular those related to the engineering of its gain media for laser applications. To achieve lasing, semiconductor lasers require optical gain derived from bimolecular recombination and stimulated emission in the gain media. Several important device characteristics in designing semiconductor lasers are the threshold current density, external differential quantum efficiency, modulation speeds, and chirps for dynamic properties.

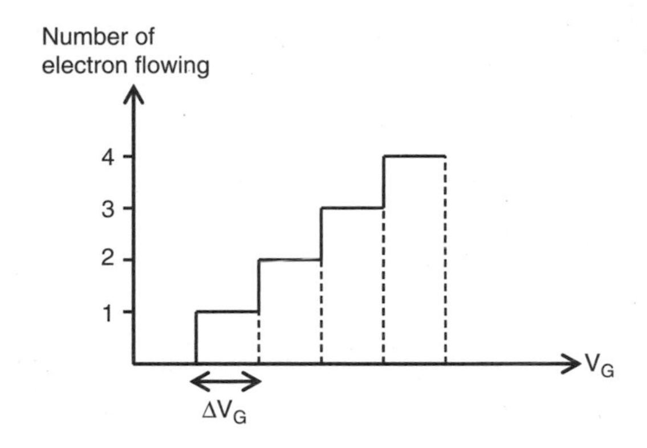

FIGURE 4.82 Number of electrons flowing across the junction increases in a staircase-like fashion with constant ΔV_G under small bias voltage.

A few of the many desirable features of semiconductor lasers include sharp emission, wavelength tunability, large modal gain, and low lasing threshold. It was first proposed in 1976 by Dingle and Henry [5] that quantum effects could be exploited to achieve those advantageous features. In 1982, Arakawa and Sasaki [6] also predicted the advantages of the quantum-confined gain media structures for laser applications, in particular for predicting the reduced temperature-sensitivity of lasers incorporating lower-dimensional gain media. The underlying idea is that quantum confinement of carriers in physical nanostructures leads to changes in the carrier density of states, which stems from a reduction of the carrier translational degree of freedom. However, the unavailability of appropriate technology at that time prevented practical realization of laser structures with 1D (quantum well), 2D (quantum wire) and 3D (quantum dot [QD]) carrier confinements.

As shown in Figure 4.83, the semiconductor gain media can be realized in the form of bulk, quantum wells, quantum wire, and quantum dots structures. Typical dimensions of the bulk structure ranges from 0.1 to 0.5 μm, which are many times the de Broglie wavelength of electrons. The carriers in semiconductors in bulk gain media are not confined, and thus free to move in all three directions.

In nanoscale gain media, at least one or more of the dimensions must be of the order of magnitude of the de Broglie wavelength of electrons, which range from 12 nm down to 2 to 3 nm, leading from weakly confined to strongly confined quantum structures. In the quantum well systems, the movement of electrons is confined in one direction (1D, i.e., in *z*-direction), resulting in step-like density of states as shown in the corresponding figure above. As we further confine the electron movement in 2D (i.e., quantum wire) and 3D (i.e., quantum dots), significant reduction in the density of states is observed as shown in Figure 4.83 above, resulting in an

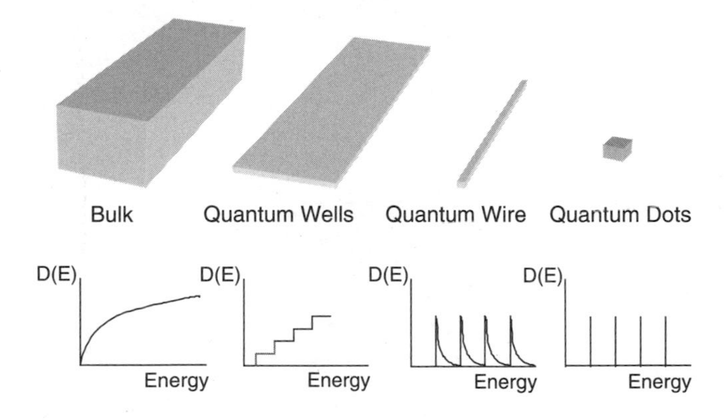

FIGURE 4.83 Schematic of gain media with structures of bulk, quantum wells, quantum wires, and quantum dots, with their corresponding density of states.

almost delta-function-like density function for the quantum dots. Engineering the dimensions of the nano-scale gain media also results in engineering of the transition energy of electrons and holes, allowing alteration of lasing wavelength on top of the bulk energy gap.

Implementation and Epitaxy of Gain Media into Devices

In semiconductor lasers, nano scale gain media (i.e., quantum wells, quantum dots, and others) can be incorporated into various devices to realize lasing in the horizontal (as shown in Figure 4.84) and vertical directions (as shown in Figure 4.85). In edge emitting lasers, the reflector of the lasers can be provided by the as-cleaved facets resulting in reflectance of approximately 30% with an in-plane resonator. For more sophisticated telecommunication lasers that require a single frequency, device structures employing distributed feedback lasers or distributed Bragg reflectors (DBRs) can be employed.

The principle of operation for vertical cavity surface emitting lasers (VCSELs) is different from that of edge-emitting lasers, in the sense that VCSELs emit the light out in the vertical direction. The cavity in VCSELs is formed by a λ-cavity sandwiched by the p-DBRs and n-DBRs. Typical DBR structures are formed by the GaAs–AlAs alternating quarter-wave stacked layers, forming a 1D photonic lattice with a range of the forbidden gap. The forbidden gap corresponds to the high reflectivity range for certain wavelengths, with typical stop band of approximately 50 to 100 nm. The center of the forbidden gap is typically aligned with the peak of the cavity resonance and the peak gain from the gain media.

The epitaxy of edge-emitting lasers and VCSELs devices with quantum-confined gain media can be realized by utilizing the molecular beam epitaxy (MBE) and metalorganic chemical vapor deposition (MOCVD). The MBE growth technique allows submonolayer deposition on a substrate, and it is based on a high-vacuum technique (10^{-11} Torr) with elemental crucibles serving as the growth sources. MOCVD is another epitaxy technique widely utilized in the compound semiconductor research and industry. Similar to MBE, MOCVD is also capable of realizing high-quality interfaces with precision in the monolayer range. MOCVD growth techniques do not require a high vacuum chamber; instead, typically, the reactor chamber is kept at low pressure (50 to 100 mbar).

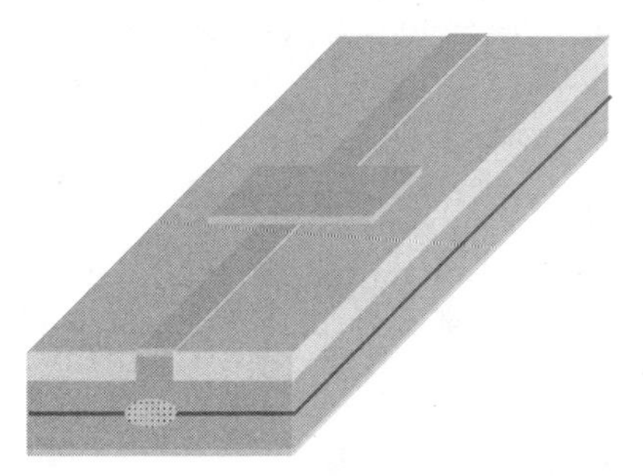

FIGURE 4.84 Schematic of ridge-guide edge emitting lasers.

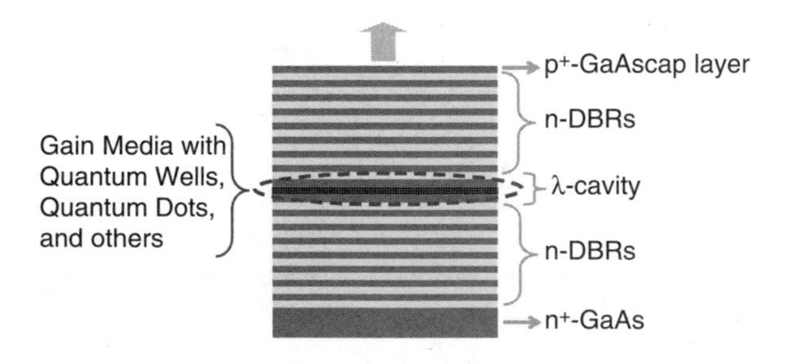

FIGURE 4.85 Schematic of vertical cavity surface emitting lasers (VCSELs).

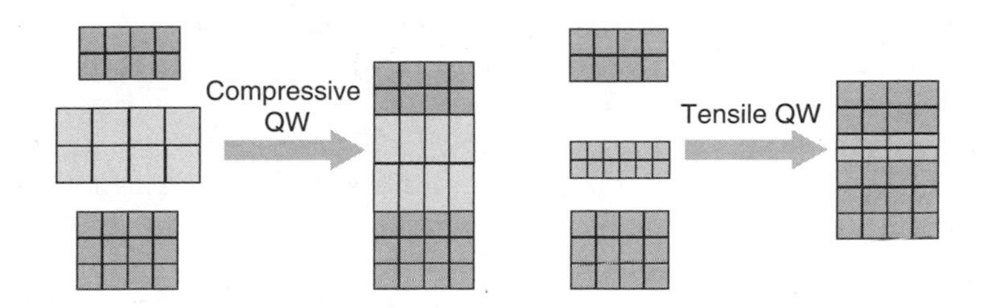

FIGURE 4.86 Schematic of compressive and tensile quantum wells.

Strained Quantum Well Lasers

It was first proposed by Yablonovitch and Kane [7,8], and independently by Adams [9], that the utilization of the strained quantum well structure should lead to improvements in lasing characteristics. The utilization of a strained quantum well structure allows the growth of material systems without lattice matching to the substrate, which achieves bandgap engineering for emission wavelength other than the bulk lattice matched materials. The strained quantum well also offers lower transparency current density as well as higher differential gain, which in turn results in lower threshold current density and higher speed diode lasers. The predicted theoretical advantages of the strain effect in quantum well lasers have been demonstrated experimentally for many different laser applications in telecommunications, mid-IR applications, red laser applications, and many other applications.

The compressive and tensile quantum well structures are shown in Figure 4.86. In the compressive quantum well structure, the lattice constant of the quantum well is larger than that of the substrate, while the lattice constant for tensile quantum well is smaller than that of substrate. These lattice mismatching of the strained quantum well materials with the lattice constant of the substrate results in biaxial strain in the layers. As the strain layer is made thicker, the biaxial strain in the layer leads to accumulation of strain energy. To ensure a high-quality strained quantum well, the layer should be grown under a pseudomorphic condition limited by a critical thickness (h_c). By growing the strained quantum well below a critical thickness, the accumulated surface strain energy is lower compared to the energy to form dislocations, which will in turn prevent the creation of defect during the epitaxy. Just as an example, the critical thickness of $In_xGa_{1-x}As$ QW ($x = 0.35$ to 0.4) grown on GaAs substrate is in the range of 60 to 80 Å.

The understanding of the improved performance of strained-layer QW lasers can be explained from the reduction of the density of states as shown in Figure 4.87. Lattice-matched QW active regions typically have degeneracy near the edge of the valence bands for the heavy holes and light holes. As biaxial strain is

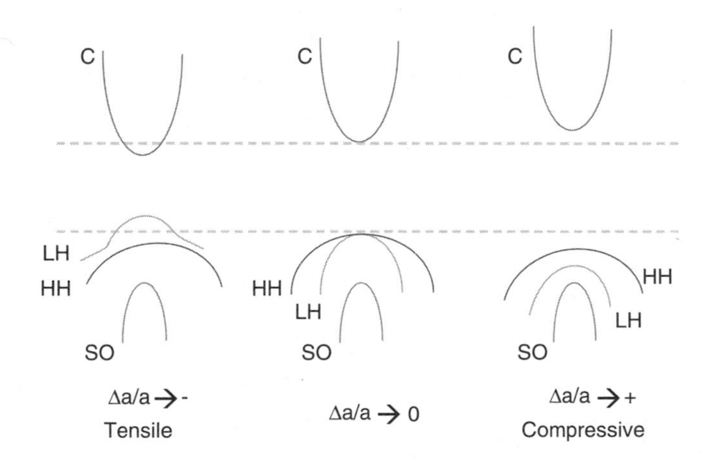

FIGURE 4.87 Effect of strain on the bulk band structure.

incorporated in the pseudomorphically grown QW active region, the degeneracy in the valence band edge is broken. For the compressively strained QW, typically the heavy holes (HH) band becomes the valence band maximum. This results in transverse-electric (TE)-like polarization for the optical gain of compressively strained quantum-well structure. In contrast to the case for a compressively strained QW, the light-hole (LH) band becomes the valence band maximum in a tensile strained QW. This leads to the transverse-magnetic (TM)-like polarization for the optical gain in the tensile strained QW.

The break in the degeneracy of the strained-layer QW active region leads to a reduced density of states. At the transparency condition, the separation of the quasi-Fermi level is identical to the separation of the conduction band minimum and the valence band maximum. The LH band is pushed further down from the HH band in the compressively strained QW structures, which leads to less filling of carriers in the LH band. The opposite case happens in the tensile strained QW, in which the HH is significantly less populated due to the lower band edge of the HH band in comparison to that of the LH band. Differential gain is also inversely proportional to the density of states, as a result of reduced state filling effect. The reduced density of states in a strained QW active region leads to a lower transparency carrier density and larger differential gain (dg/dn), which in turn will lead to reduced threshold carrier and current density.

Quantum Dots Lasers

Quantum dots (QD) gain media utilize a 3D carrier confinement in the dots. Some of the direct theoretical advantages of utilizing QDs in lasers include sharp band-to-band transitions that give an emission wavelength with narrow linewidth, high differential gain that leads to extremely low threshold current, and high characteristic temperature, T_0.

In the early development, quantum dots patterns were formed by patterning with electron beam lithography technique. By etching the patterns formed by lithography, one can realize the quantum dot structures. QD structures formed by lithography method are typically periodic, controllable, selective, and of high precision. Unfortunately, surface recombination and process-induced damages result in significant nonradiative recombination, thus leading to poor photonic devices.

In 1992, Tabuchi et al. proposed the use of Stransky–Krastanow (SK)-based self-assembled InAs islands on GaAs substrate as quantum dots [10], as shown in Figure 4.88. Thanks to advances in epitaxial growth technology, self-assembled growth of QDs is now the center of interest in the semiconductor material and device research field. Though the self-assembled QDs based on SK growth mode are inherently almost defect-free, the large inhomogeneous broadening of these QDs results in broad and low optical gain in comparison to that predicted theoretically. The large inhomogeneous broadening in the self-assembled QDs results from the random formation and large size distribution of the dots. Some of the common features of the self-assembled quantum dots gain media are controllable chirp (+, −, 0 chirp), extremely broad band gain (advantageous for optical amplifiers, but a disadvantage for lasers), low threshold current lasers, and potential for realizing high temperature insensitive lasers. Some common challenges of these self-assembled QDs are the difficulties in pushing the emission wavelength beyond 1300 nm on GaAs, large inhomogeneous broadening (from size distribution of QDs), and the challenges in achieving high maximum modulation speed for the SCH-QD. One of the methods of achieving high speed QD lasers is to utilize tunnel-injection QD structures, as proposed by Bhattacharya et al. [11].

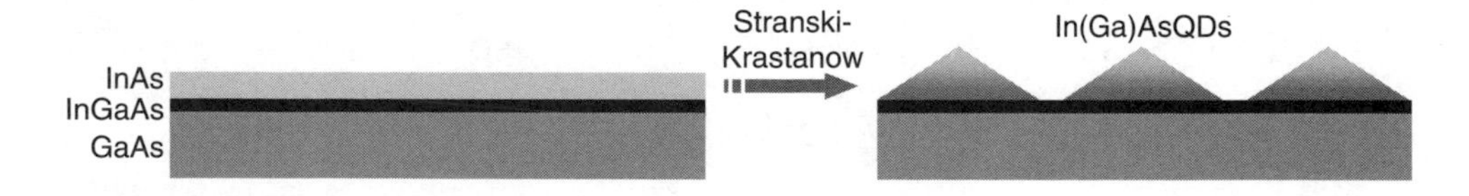

FIGURE 4.88 Schematic of Stranski–Krastanow epitaxy mode for self-assembled In(Ga)As QDs.

Novel Gain Media for Telecom Lasers: InGaAsN QWs and InAs QDs

One of the most important applications of semiconductor lasers is as the transmitter for optical fiber telecommunication. Because of the minimum dispersion and minimum attenuation in fiber, optical communication systems require semiconductor lasers at wavelength regimes of 1300 and 1550 nm, respectively. The ability to grow lattice-matched bulk and quantum-well InGaAsP material systems on InP substrates to achieve emission wavelengths of 1300 and 1550 nm led to significant research and development in the field of InP-based lasers for telecom applications, leading to the realization of some of the state-of-the-art telecom lasers. However, conventional InP-based long wavelength diode lasers, at $\lambda = 1300$ to 1550 nm, are unfortunately inherently highly temperature sensitive, due to strong Auger recombination, large carrier leakage from the gain media, intervalence band absorption, and a strongly temperature-dependent material gain parameter. These poor temperature characteristics of InGaAsP–InP lasers lead to the need for additional electronics to maintain thermal stability, which in turn lead to a significant increase in packaging cost.

The demand for higher bandwidth and longer transmission distance requires low-cost, single-mode, 1300 to 1550 nm transmitter sources, without any temperature controller. Transmitters based on 1300-nm edge emitters or VCSELs operating at a modulation bandwidth of 10 Gb/sec, for the metro application using single mode fiber, should allow data transmission up to a distance of 20 to 30 km. In order to realize low-cost (uncooled), 1300 to 1550 nm-based optical communications systems, high-performance (i.e., temperature insensitive) diode lasers (either in-plane or VCSELs) are needed that operate up to 85°C. Another major factor motivating the development of 1300 to 1550 nm GaAs-based diode lasers is the ease in forming high-quality GaAs/AlAs distributed Bragg reflectors (DBRs) on GaAs substrates. The ability to fabricate high-quality AlGaAs-based DBRs has allowed the GaAs-based VCSELs to have performance comparable to GaAs-based in-plane diode lasers.

Several approaches to realize novel nano-scale gain media have been explored for emission wavelengths of 1300 to 1550 nm on GaAs substrate, utilizing semiconductor nanostructure of InGaAsN (dilute nitride), InAs, GaAsSb, and others. The lists of novel approaches on GaAs and InP (i.e., InGaAlAs quantum wells) here are not meant to be exhaustive; rather, the discussion here will be limited to only *selected* approaches that utilize InGaAsN quantum wells and InAs quantum dot lasers.

An attractive approach for achieving long-wavelength laser emission on GaAs substrates is the use of highly strained InGaAsN QWs. The reduction in the bandgap of the InGaAsN materials (as shown in Figure 4.89),

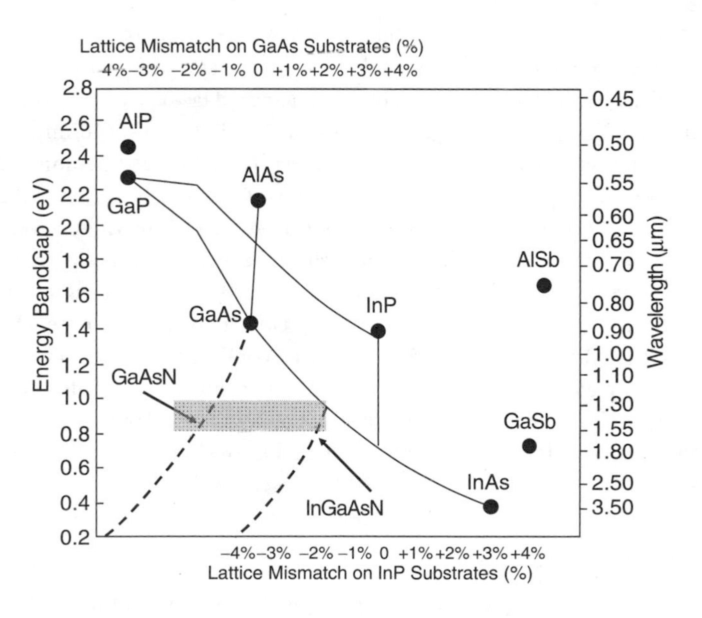

FIGURE 4.89 Schematic of energy bandgap for GaAsN and InGaAsN material systems with their corresponding strain and bulk emission wavelengths.

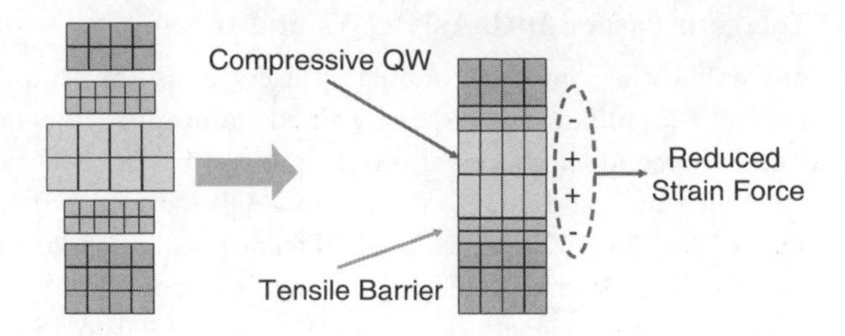

FIGURE 4.90 Schematic of strain-compensated InGaAsN QW with GaAsP tensile barriers.

pioneered by M. Kondow et al. [12], due to the existence of the N, is also followed by reduction in the compressive strain of the material due to the smaller native lattice constant of the InGaN compound. The early development of InGaAsN QW lasers employed nearly-lattice-matched low-In content and high–N content InGaAsN QW active regions [12,13]. Because of the smaller native lattice constant of the InGaN compound, the incorporation of N into the compressively strained InGaAs material system can result in a nearly-lattice-matched InGaAsN QW.

Some of the best lasing characteristics for InGaAsN devices have been realized by MBE [14–19] and MOCVD techniques [20–27] with threshold current densities in the range of 200 to 210 A/cm^2 for emission wavelength at around 1280 to 1320 nm. One of the most promising approaches is by utilizing the compressively strained InGaAsN QW surrounded by tensile barriers of GaAsP, for strain compensation purpose as shown in Figure 4.90. Prior analysis [22] indicates that heavy hole leakage and temperature sensitivity of material gains for dilute-nitride lasers are the contributing factors in limiting its high-temperature performance. By suppressing the heavy hole leakage phenomenon in InGaAsN QW (utilizing higher bandgap GaAsP barriers to surround the QW), significant reduction in threshold current density and increase in the external differential efficiency of the InGaAsN QW lasers are achieved. As a result of reduced heavy hole escape rate, InGaAsN lasers with higher bandgap barriers also showed reduction in the temperature sensitivities of both the threshold current density and slope efficiencies. Utilizing the larger bandgap barrier design of $GaAs_{0.67}P_{0.33}$, threshold current density of only 400 A/cm^2 were measured for InGaAsN QW lasers at a heat sink temperature of 100°C [20,22].

Some of the recent MOCVD structures with InGaAsN QWs and GaAsN barriers have demonstrated low threshold current densities for $\lambda = 1378$ nm, and InGaAsN lasers with a carefully chosen QW growth condition, barrier material and annealing temperature have achieved lasing to $\lambda = 1410$ nm. Threshold current densities were 563 and 1930 A/cm^2 for the lasers emitting at $\lambda = 1378$ and 1410 nm, respectively [20,28].

Low-threshold current density MBE-grown InAs QD lasers have also been demonstrated by several groups [11,29–32] at emission wavelengths around 1.3 μm. In contrast to that of MBE, low threshold current density MOCVD-grown In(Ga)As QD lasers have only been demonstrated up to emission wavelengths around 1150 to 1180 nm [33,34]. TU Berlin reported MOCVD-grown three-stacked $In_{0.5}Ga_{0.5}As$ QD as-cleaved lasers with threshold current density of approximately 100 A/cm^2 ($L_{cav} = 1000$ μm) emitting at 1150 nm [33]. Utilizing strain-relieving layers of $In_{0.12}Ga_{0.88}As$, the group at the University of Tokyo reported threshold current density of 147 A/cm^2 for HR/HR-coated MOCVD-grown InAs QD laser devices emitting at 1180 nm [34].

As of 2004, the best-reported InAs QD laser (by MBE) at 1.46 μm was reported by TU Berlin, with high-threshold current density of 2.3 kA/cm^2 [35]. The existence of very large strain and large quantum-size-effects in InAs QD grown on GaAs have led to significant challenges in pushing its emission wavelength to 1550 nm for laser devices.

Type-II Quantum Well Lasers

Type-I quantum well structures confine both electrons and holes in the same spatial layer, similar to the quantum well structures discussed above. The type-II "W" structure was originally proposed by Meyer and coworkers [36], and this idea has been successfully implemented in mid-IR diode lasers on GaSb substrates.

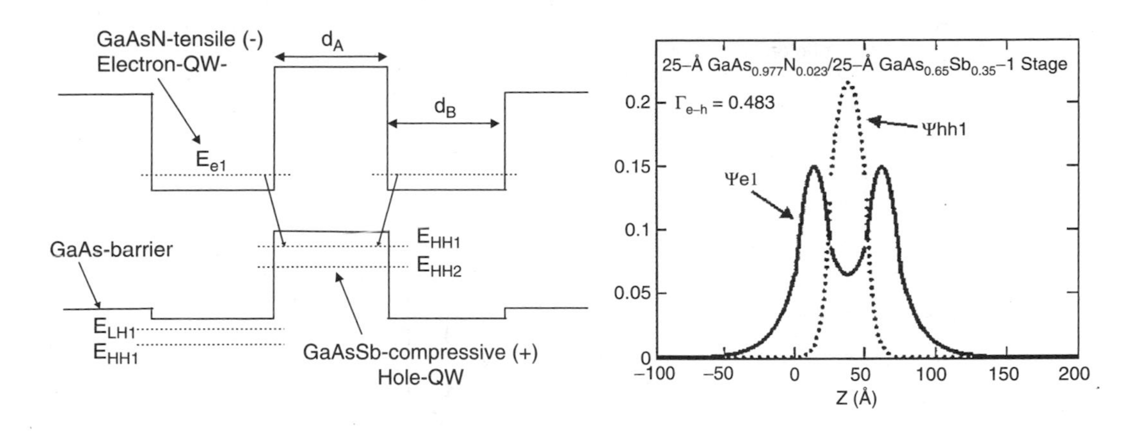

FIGURE 4.91 Type-II QW of GaAsN–GaAsSb, with their respective electron and hole wavefunctions.

In contrast to the type-I quantum well structure, electrons and holes are confined in different spatial layers for the case of type-II quantum well structures [37], as shown in Figure 4.91 for the GaAsN–GaAsSb structure. Figure 4.91 shows an example in which the electrons and holes are confined in the GaAsN and GaAsSb quantum wells, respectively [37]. Typical materials chosen for electron quantum well in this type-II configuration are materials with large electron confinement energy, similar to that of the GaAsN layer. In contrast to that, the GaAsSb is chosen for confining the holes, due to the large valence band confinement energy. One of the unique characteristics of this type-II quantum well structure is that the electron and hole transition energy is determined by the band discontinuity of the semiconductor layers, rather than their fundamental bulk band gaps.

In the example discussed here [37], the electron wells consist of GaAsN layers and the hole-wells consist of GaAsSb layers. The arrangement of this design is made possible due to the large disparity of the band lineup of the GaAsN and GaAsSb compounds with that of GaAs. The weak type-II band lineup near the valence band of the GaAsN/GaAs, results in a large conduction band offset (ΔE_c). The GaAsSb/GaAs system has a large type-II band lineup in the conduction band, which results in the large valence band offset (ΔE_v). This particular structure allows one to achieve emission wavelength at 1550 nm on GaAs substrate, which is the wavelength of interest for long-haul optical communication systems. One of the additional advantages of this structure is the potential for reduced Auger recombination in type-II structures [38], which is a highly temperature sensitive process. Suppression of Auger recombination in laser applications leads to reduced threshold and less temperature sensitive lasers. The drawback of this type-II quantum well structure is related to the reduced electron-hole wavefunctions overlap as shown in Figure 4.91, which is due to the fact that the electrons and holes are confined in different spatial layers. Though low electron-hole wavefunctions overlap will impact the optical gain of this quantum well structure, careful bandgap engineering of the active media can allow optimization of the gain achievable from this structure.

Quantum Intersubband Lasers

The possibility of using unipolar intersubband transition as a means of light amplification was first proposed by Kazarinov and Suris in 1971 [39]. However, due to significant theoretical and technical difficulties, the next 20 years saw little progress in utilizing the concept to build a practical laser device. Finally in 1994, Faist and Capasso et al. from AT&T Bell Labs, first demonstrated the first quantum cascade intersubband laser emitting at 4.3 μm [40].

Compared to the larger, more common family of interband laser, quantum cascade intersubband lasers are theoretically intriguing and technologically important at the same time. To begin with, they are intriguing because light amplification, or gain, is provided by carrier relaxation from higher to lower discrete energy levels in a quantum-confined physical structure, commonly referred to as a well. This means that emission

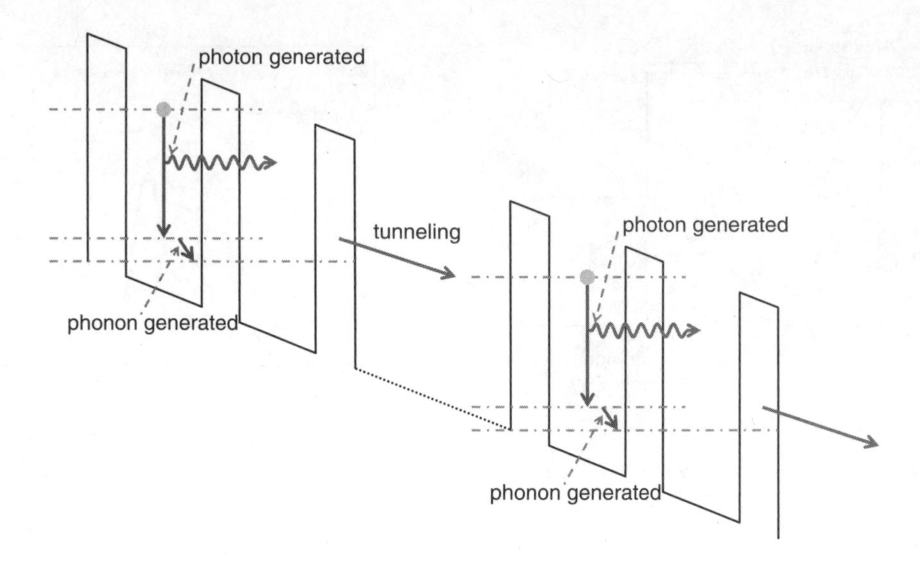

FIGURE 4.92 Energy band lineup schematic of quantum cascade intersubband laser under bias.

wavelength is no longer restricted to the energy gap of materials. Wavelength tailoring can now be done simply by changing the dimension of the quantum well. The relaxed carriers then quantum mechanically "tunnel" through potential energy barriers (by the application of potential difference) and cascade down the energy ladder while providing light amplification. Please refer to Figure 4.92 for clarity.

Quantum cascade intersubband lasers are also technologically important since they cover wavelengths in the mid- to far-IR range, which were previously unattainable by interband lasers. Mid- to far-IR spectra are important because they contain fundamental absorption lines of most molecules. This property allows compact mid-IR sources to find applications in highly sensitive trace gas analysis such as pollution monitoring and biomedical sensing [41].

Future: Quantum Effects and Semiconductor Nanotechnology

The capabilities of nanoscale engineering of semiconductor materials has allowed the realization of various electronics and optoelectronics devices utilizing quantum effects as its operating principles. The overview presented in this chapter only covers selected choices of semiconductor nano-electronics and nano-optoelectronics devices.

For semiconductor nano-electronics devices, resonant tunneling diodes and single electron transistors were discussed. The utilization of 2D electron gas for the high electron mobility transistors has also led to the realization of record high speed electronics devices. The pursuit of semiconductor nano-electronics based on emerging GaN-based compound semiconductor material systems has not matured to the extent of GaAs and InP material systems. The development of resonant tunneling diodes on GaN-based material systems is important not only for electronics application, but also as an injector for optoelectronics utilizing quantum intersubband processes. Improvement in the GaN-based material epitaxy should improve the performance of GaN-based RTDs and high electron mobility transistors (HEMTs).

The section on semiconductor nano-optoelectronics only discussed selected topics on quantum wells and quantum dots laser devices. The understanding of the semiconductor optical amplifier (SOA) based on quantum dots is still lacking, and the QD-SOA should provide a mechanism to achieve higher-speed amplifiers in comparison to that achievable by bulk or QW gain media. The development of the dilute-nitride semiconductor nanostructure is also very interesting, as it provides a mechanism to achieve 1550-nm (or beyond) emission wavelength on a GaAs substrate. The utilization of dilute-nitride type-II quantum well gain media should also provide a potential mechanism to achieve mid-IR lasers from InP substrates [42].

The development of the quantum intersubband devices based on GaN material systems is still lagging behind that of the GaAs/InP material systems, mainly due to the difficulty in reducing the defect density in the GaN material systems. As the material quality of GaN-based epitaxy is improved, the device physics and performance of the GaN-based intersubband devices should be feasible for laser and switching applications. Though self-assembled InAs QD lasers have demonstrated excellent lasing characteristics, the development of InN QD lasers is still immature and requires further investigation.

References

1. K. Goser, P. Glosekotter, and J. Dienstuhl, *Nanoelectronics and Nanosystems: from Transistors to Molecular and Quantum Devices*, Germany: Springer, 2004.
2. L. Esaki, *Phys. Rev.*, 109, 603, 1958.
3. L. Esaki, *IEEE Trans. Electron. Dev.*, ED-23, 644, 1976.
4. Keith Barnham and Dimitri Vvedenski, Eds., *Low-Dimensional Semiconductor Structures: Fundamentals and Device Applications*, United Kingdom: Cambridge University Press, 2001.
5. R. Dingle, W. Wiegmann, and C.H. Henry, *Phys. Rev. Lett.*, vol. 33, p. 827, 1974.
6. Y. Arakawa and H. Sasaki, *Appl. Phys. Lett.*, 40, 939, 1982.
7. E. Yablonovitch and E.O. Kane, *IEEE J. Lightwave Technol.*, LT-4, 504, 1986.
8. E. Yablonovitch and E.O. Kane, *IEEE J. Lightwave Technol.*, LT-4, 961, 1986.
9. A.R. Adams, *Electron. Lett.*, 22, 249, 1986.
10. M. Tabuchi et al., *Science and Technology of Mesoscopic Structures*, 1992, pp. 379–384.
11. S. Ghosh, S. Pradhan, and P. Bhattacharya, *Appl. Phys. Lett.*, 81, 3055, 2002.
12. M. Kondow, T. Kitatani, S. Nakatsuka, M.C. Larson, K. Nakahara, Y. Yazawa, M. Okai, and K. Uomi, *IEEE J. Select. Topic Quant. Electron.*, 3, 719–730, 1997.
13. J.S. Harris, Jr., *IEEE J. Select. Topics Quant. Electron.*, vol. 6, no. 6, pp. 1145–1160, 2000.
14. D.A. Livshits, A.Yu. Egorov, and H. Riechert, *Electron. Lett.*, vol. 36, no. 16, pp. 1381–1382, 2000.
15. J. Wei, F. Xia, C. Li, and S.R. Forrest, *IEEE Photon. Technol. Lett.*, 14, 597, 2002.
16. K.D. Choquette, J.F. Klem, A.J. Fischer, O. Blum, A.A. Allerman, I.J. Fritz, S.R. Kurtz, W.G. Breiland, R. Sieg, K.M. Geib, J.W. Scott, and R.L. Naone, *Electron. Lett.*, vol. 36, no. 16, pp. 1388–1390, 2000.
17. W. Ha, V. Gambin, M. Wistey, S. Bank, S. Kim, J.S. Harris, Jr., *IEEE Photon. Technol. Lett.*, vol. 14 no. 5, 2002.
18. C.S. Peng, T. Jouhti, P. Laukkanen, E.-M. Pavelescu, J. Konttinen, W. Li, and M. Pessa, *IEEE Photon. Technol. Lett.*, vol. 14, no. 3, pp. 275–277, 2002.
19. W. Li, T. Jouhti, C.S. Peng, J. Konttinen, P. Laukkanen, E.-M. Pavelescu, and M. Pessa, *Appl. Phys. Lett.*, vol. 79, no. 21, pp. 3386–3388, 2001.
20. N. Tansu, J.Y. Yeh, and L.J. Mawst, *IOP J. Phys.: Condens. Matter Phys.*, 16, 2004 (August).
21. N. Tansu, N.J. Kirsch, and L.J. Mawst, *Appl. Phys. Lett.*, vol. 81, no. 14, pp. 2523–2525, 2002.
22. N. Tansu, J.Y. Yeh, and L.J. Mawst, *Appl. Phys. Lett.*, vol. 83, no.11, pp. 2112–2114, 2003.
23. N. Tansu, J.Y. Yeh, and L.J. Mawst, *Appl. Phys. Lett.*, vol. 83, no. 13, pp. 2512–2514, 2003.
24. S. Sato, *Jpn. J. Appl. Phys.*, 39, 3403–3405, 2000 (June).
25. F. Hohnsdorf, J. Koch, S. Leu, W. Stolz, B. Borchert, and M. Druminski, *Electron. Lett.*, vol. 35, no. 7, pp. 571–572, 1999.
26. M. Kawaguchi, T. Miyamoto, E. Gouardes, D. Schlenker, T. Kondo, F. Koyama, and K. Iga, *Jpn. J. Appl. Phys.*, 40, L744-L746, 2001 (July).
27. T. Takeuchi, Y.-L. Chang, M. Leary, A. Tandon, H.-C. Luan, D.P. Bour, S.W. Corzine, R. Twist, and M.R. Tan, *IEEE LEOS 2001 Post-Deadline Session*, San Diego, CA, 2001 (November).
28. J.Y. Yeh, N. Tansu, and L.J. Mawst, *IEE Electron. Lett.* 40, 739 2004.
29. O.B. Shchekin and D.G. Deppe, *Appl. Phys. Lett.*, vol. 80, no. 18, pp. 3277–3279, 2002.
30. A.R. Kovsh, N.A. Maleev, A.E. Zhukov, S.S. Mikhrin, A.R. Vasil'ev, Yu.M. Shemyakov, M.V. Maximov, D.A. Livshits, V. Ustinov, Zh.I. Alferov, N.N. Ledentsov, and D. Bimberg, *Electron. Lett.*, vol. 38, no. 19, pp. 1104–1106, 2002.

31. V. Tokranov, M. Yakimov, A. Katsnelson, M. Lamberti, and S. Oktyabrsky, *Appl. Phys. Lett.*, vol. 83, no. 5, pp. 833–835, 2003.
32. G.T. Liu, A. Stintz, H. Li, K.J. Malloy and L.F. Lester, *Electron. Lett.*, vol. 35, no. 14, pp. 1163–1165, 1999.
33. R.L. Sellin, I. Kaiander, D. Ouyang, T. Kettler, U.W. Pohl, D. Bimberg, N.D. Zakharov, and P. Werner, *Appl. Phys. Lett.*, vol. 82, no. 6, pp. 841–843, 2003.
34. J. Tatebayashi, N. Hatori, H. Kakuma, H. Ebe, H. Sudo, A. Kuramata, Y. Nakata, M. Sugawara, and Y. Arakawa, *Electron. Lett.*, vol. 39, no. 15, pp. 1130–1131, 2003.
35. N.N. Ledentsov, A.R. Kovsh, A.E. Zhukov, N.A. Maleev, S.S. Mikhrin, A.P. Vasil'ev, E.S. Semenova, M.V. Maximov, Yu.M. Shernyakov, N.V. Kryzhanovskaya, V.M. Ustinov, and D. Bimberg, *Electron. Lett.*, vol. 39, no. 15, pp. 1126–1128, 2003.
36. J.R. Meyer, C.A. Hoffman, F.J. Bartoli, and L.R. Ram-Mohan, *Appl. Phys. Lett.*, 67, 757, 1995.
37. N. Tansu and L.J. Mawst, *IEEE J. Quantum Electron.*, vol. 39, no. 10, pp. 1205–1210, 2003.
38. J.R. Meyer, C.L. Felix, W.W. Bewley, I. Vurgaftman, E.H. Aifer, L.J. Olafsen, J.R. Lindle, C.A. Hoffman, M.J. Yang, B.R. Bennett, B.V. Shanabrook, H. Lee, C.H. Lin, S.S. Pei, and R.H. Miles, *Appl. Phys. Lett.*, vol. 73, no. 20, pp. 2857–2859, 1998.
39. R.F. Kazarinov and R.A Suris, *Fiz. Tekh. Poluprovodn.*, 5, 797, 1971.
40. J. Faist, F. Capasso, D.L. Sivco, C. Sirtori, A.L. Hutchinson, and A.Y. Cho, *Science*, 264, 553, 1994.
41. Hong K. Choi, Ed., *Long Wavelength Infrared Semiconductor Lasers*, New Jersey: Wiley, 2004.
42. I. Vurgaftman, J.R. Meyer, N. Tansu, and L.J. Mawst, *J. Appl. Phys.*, vol. 96, no. 8, pp. 4653–4655, 2004.

5

Instruments and Measurements

5.1 Electrical Equipment in Hazardous Areas 5-1
Fundamentals of Explosion Protection • Hazardous Areas Classification • Classification Methods • Division Classification • Marking • Zone Classification • Marking • Enclosure Types and Requirements • Protection Methodologies • Making Field Devices Intrinsically Safe • Ignition Curves • Certification and Approval • IS Ground Rules

5.2 Portable Instruments and Systems 5-27
Introduction • Features of Portable Instruments • Sensors for Portable Instruments • Communication and Networking of Portable Instruments • Applications of Portable Instruments • Conclusions

5.3 G (LabVIEW™) Software Engineering 5-36
Data Types • Polymorphism • Units • Data Coercion • Error Handling • Shortcuts • GOOP • Code Distribution • Application Building (Creating Executables) • Open Source G: Distributed Development

Sam S. Khalilieh
Tyco Infrastructure Services

Halit Eren
Curtin University of Technology

Christopher G. Relf
National Instruments Certified LabVIEW Developer

5.1 Electrical Equipment in Hazardous Areas

Sam S. Khalilieh

The safety and economic impact of unintentional ignition of explosive mixtures is something that should never be underestimated when processing, storing, generating or transporting combustible liquids, gases or dusts. Where hazardous atmospheres can exist, electricity should be a primary concern of every engineer and system designer. Hazardous atmospheres can exist not only in the more common surroundings of industrial, chemical, and environmental facilities, but also in many less obvious environs where dust is present, where gas can accumulate, and where combustible gas-forming reactions occur. To minimize risks in such areas, it is necessary to design specific hazard-reducing electrical systems. Most electrical equipment is built to specific standards aimed to reduce the incidence of fires and human casualties. The majority of such incidents can be attributed to poor or defective installations, improper use of approved equipment, deteriorated equipment, and accidental applications. In combination with an explosive atmosphere, these factors can result in extremely dangerous conditions. Designing an electrical system for a hazardous location requires careful planning, research, engineering, and ingenuity in using proper protection techniques to develop better applications and classifications that reduce hazards.

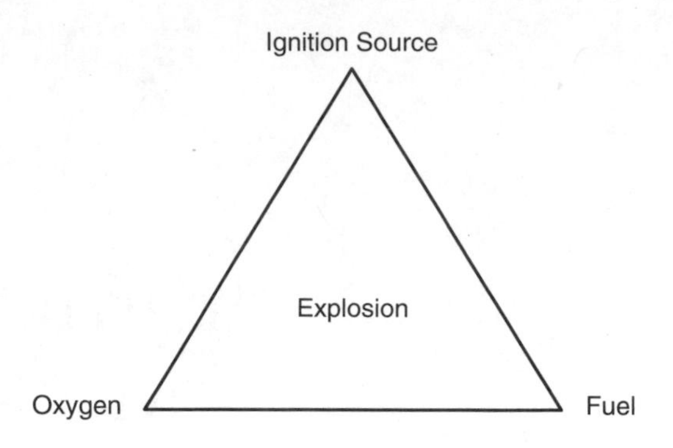

FIGURE 5.1 Explosion triangle.

Fundamentals of Explosion Protection

Safety of personnel and equipment present in hazardous areas should never be taken for granted. In 1913, a massive methane gas explosion in a coal mine in Glamorganshire, South Wales claimed the lives of 439 mine workers. After months of research and studies, a group of experts and scientists concluded that the explosion was caused by a small amount of electrical energy stored in the circuit. This small amount of energy, combined with the presence of an explosive gas and air mixture and the absence of proper protection, proved to be fatal for the mine workers.

To understand the dangers associated with electrical equipment in hazardous areas, one must first understand the basics. Chemically speaking, oxidation, combustion, and explosions are all exothermic reactions where heat is given off at different reaction speeds. For these reactions to occur, three components must be present simultaneously in certain concentrations (Figure 5.1). These components are: (1) fuel (liquid, gas, or solids); (2) sufficient amount of oxygen (air); and (3) ignition source (electrical or thermal). After ignition, an exothermic reaction in the explosive atmospheres will concurrently and simultaneously propagate at a total pressure and temperature ranging from 11.6 PSI to almost 16 PSI and -20°C to 60°C, respectively.

Some of the obvious ignition sources that can be potentially hazardous include: (1) hot surfaces (motor windings, heat trace cable, light fixtures); (2) electric sparks and arcs (when circuits are opened and closed, short circuits); and (3) mechanic sparks (friction, grinding). Some less obvious but just as dangerous ignition sources include: (1) electrostatic discharge ESD (separation process in which at least one chargeable substance is present); (2) lightning; and (3) radiation, compression, and shock waves.

Explosions are usually violent and perilous, and all the protection techniques pale in comparison to one method — avoidance. It is by far the cheapest, safest, and most preferable technique in dealing with explosions. Some of the "avoidance techniques" that follow can be employed alone or in combinations:

1. Air movement/ventilation — This concept focuses on preventing the formation or accumulation of explosive gases in a confined area. Ventilation usually requires the introduction of mechanical equipment specifically designed to inject air into a specific area at higher volumes than natural ventilation. In typical areas above ground level and without artificial air, the air will be removed and replaced at one air change per hour (1 ACPH). If such a technique is chosen, a good designer will take into account the implications of equipment failure.
2. Concentration — This concept focuses on keeping the explosive mixture concentration outside its flammable limits (see flammable limits below), and therefore preventing the buildup of explosive atmospheres.
3. Avoid flammable or ignitable material — This concept is self explanatory. Wherever possible, avoid the use of flammable material or substitute with one that is incapable of producing or forming an explosive mixture.

4. Adjusting the flash point (see definition below) — Raising the flash point temperature of the flammable substance usually does the trick. For a water soluble mixture, this can be easily achieved by adding water.
5. Oxygen starvation — This concept focuses on limiting the oxygen to less than 10% of volume. This is usually accomplished by introducing a high volume of what is commonly known as inert gases, such as nitrogen, to the mixture causing the ratio of inert gas to explosive mixture to exceed 25 to 1. At such a ratio, the buildup of explosive concentration is virtually impossible regardless the volume of air (oxygen) added.

When dealing with electrical equipment in hazardous locations, it is important to understand the following terms as they are use frequently when it comes to hazardous areas

1. Flash Point (FP) — The minimum temperature at normal air pressure at which a combustible or flammable material releases sufficient vapors ignitible by an energy source. FP provides an indication of how easily a chemical may burn. The lower the FP, the greater the hazard. Depending on the flash point, flammable liquids are divided into four classes of hazard: (1) AI ($FP < 21°C$), (2) AII ($21 < FP < 55°C$), (3) AIII ($55°C < FP < 100°C$), and (4) B ($FP < 21°C$ at 15°C dissolving in water).
2. Flammable Liquids — Are generally volatile and give off vapors with vapor density over 1.0, and therefore collect at low points. They also have a flash point below 100°F (37.8°C) with a vapor pressure below 40 PSI.
3. Combustible Liquids — Have most of the characteristics of flammable liquids, except that their flash point is above 100°F (37.8°C).
4. Ignition Temperature — The minimum temperature under normal operating pressure at which a dangerous mixture ignites independently of the heating or heated element.
5. Flammable Limits (FL) — The upper flammable limit (UFL), also known as the upper explosive limit (UEL), or the maximum concentration ratio of vapor to air mixture above which the propagation of flame does not occur when exposed to an ignition source. Here, the mixture is said to be "too rich" to burn. The lower flammable limit (LFL), also know as lower explosive limit (LEL), is the minimum concentration ratio of vapor to air mixture below which the propagation of flame does not occur when exposed to an ignition source. Also, here, the mixture is said to be "too lean" to explode. Significant attention must be given to LEL, since it provides the minimum quantity of gas necessary to create a hazardous mixture. Generally, the flammable limits are indicated in percent by volume, which is abbreviated % vol. Note that the explosion of a mixture in the middle the of UEL and LEL is much more violent than if the mixture were closer to either limit.
6. Maximum Surface Temperature — The maximum temperature generated by a piece of electrical equipment under normal or fault conditions. This temperature must be below the minimum ignition temperature of the potentially explosive surrounding atmosphere. Equipment used in hazardous locations must be clearly marked to indicate class, group, and maximum surface temperature or range referenced to 40°C (104°F) ambient temperature. Table 5.1 shows that an apparatus with a specific "T" class can be used in the presence of all gases having an ignition temperature higher than the "T" temperature class of the device. For added safety, it is recommended that the maximum surface temperature be not more than 80% of the minimum ignition temperature of the surrounding gas. The reader is cautioned not to confuse maximum working (operating) temperature with maximum surface temperature, which is measured under worst-case conditions of the electrical apparatus. An electrical apparatus designed to operate with a maximum ambient temperature of 70°C — even in the worst conditions of the expected temperature range — must not have a temperature rise greater than a safety margin of 10°C to be classified as T6 or 5°C for classes T3, T4, and T5 (Table 5.1).
7. Vapor Density — The weight of a volume of pure vapor gas compared to the weight of an equal volume of dry air under the same normal atmospheric pressure and temperature. It is calculated as the ratio of molecular weight of the gas to the average molecular weight of air (28.96). Methane gas (CH_4) with molecular weight of 16 and vapor density of 0.6 tends to rise, while Acetone (C_3H_6O) with molecular weight of 58 and vapor density of 2 tends to settle closer to ground levels. A vapor density of 0.75 is typically considered the limit between lighter and heavier gases.

TABLE 5.1 Maximum Surface Temperature under All Operating Conditions

Maximum Temperature		
°C	°F	Identification Number
450	842	T1
300	572	T2
280	536	T2A
260	500	T2B
230	446	T2C
215	419	T2D
200	392	T3
180	356	T3A
165	329	T3B
160	320	T3C
135	275	T4
120	248	T4A
100	212	T5
85	185	T6

Note: Surface temperature of electric apparatus during operation must not exceed limitations of the hazard present. Reprinted with permission from NEPA 70-1996, the *National Electrical Code*®, Copyright© 1995, National Free Protection Association, Quincy, MA. This reprinted Protection Association, on the referenced subject which is represented only by the standard in its entirety.

8. Air Current and Ventilation — Air movement/current can be both helpful and disastrous. A strong air movement/current can help dilute the gas concentration and consequently reduce, if not eliminate the hazard. A soft air movement/current can easily extend the perimeter of the hazardous area into an adjacent safe area.
9. Vapor Dispersion — Where solid boundaries (walls, enclosures, panels, etc.) do not exist, vapor dispersion will depend predominately on gas vapor density and velocity. Lighter vapors tend to disperse vertically and outward, while heavier vapors tend to settle downward and out.
10. Fuels — Fuels of all forms — solid, liquid, and gas — are chemical substances that may be burned in oxygen to generate heat, and are made up predominately of carbon and hydrogen and occasionally sulfur. The ingredients of a combustion process are called reactants, while the outputs are called products.

Hazardous Areas Classification

In the United States, the National Electrical Code (NEC) defines a hazardous area as "an area where a potential hazard may exist under normal or abnormal conditions because of the presence of flammable, combustible, or ignitible materials." This general description is divided into different classes, divisions, and groups to properly assess the extent of the hazard and to design and specify safe operating electrical systems.

The need for classification is important not only for safety, but for economic reasons as well. Proper application, good engineering, and experience can reduce the extent of the most volatile areas (Class I, Division 1) within reasonably safe distances of potential leaks and ignition sources. Under Class I, Division 1, equipment and installation costs can become an economic burden because the equipment is considerably more expensive and must pass stringent tests to ensure proper and safe operation under normal or abnormal conditions. The National Fire Protection Association (NFPA 497 A & B) and the American Petroleum Institutes "Recommended Practice for Classification of Locations for Electrical Installations at Petroleum Facilities" (ANSI/API RP 500) are excellent resources for defining hazardous area boundaries.

Classification of a hazardous area within a facility is usually determined by highly-qualified personnel, including chemical engineers, process engineers, and safety officers. Their primary objective is to determine where a potentially hazardous atmosphere exists, under what conditions it exists, and how long it exists. Careful study and design of electrical installations, especially in hazardous areas, are crucial for the safe operation of electrical equipment and prevention of an accidental ignition of flammable materials. The NEC, which has been adopted by many states, agencies, and companies as the basis for inspections, describes the requirements and procedures for electrical installations in hazardous areas. Articles 500–505 contain the requirements of electrical equipment and wiring for all voltages in locations where fire or explosion hazards may exist due to flammable gases or vapors, flammable liquids, combustible dust, or ignitible fibers or flyings.

In order to make a safe, cost-effective, and sound assessment of area classification, we first must ask some rudimentary questions. Perhaps the most critical aspect of area classification is the ability of qualified personnel to ask the right questions while simultaneously visualizing and possibly modeling or simulating different abnormal conditions and leaking scenarios under different circumstances (pressure, temperature, etc.). These questions are by no means the only questions to ask, but rather a sample of the systematic process needed when assessing hazardous areas.

1. What is the process?
2. What type of material and what are the properties of the raw materials, finished products, and byproducts?
3. What is the potential or likelihood that hazardous conditions are present at each potential leak source?
4. What are the volumes, pressures, and temperatures throughout the process?
5. What type of ventilation is available and what is its purpose?
6. What is the impact/enormity of a potential explosion?

Classification Methods

There are currently two recognized classification methodologies: the traditional method — the NEC Division Classification and the International Electrotechnical Commission (IEC) — Zone Classification. The IEC methodology, which was added to the NEC (Article 505) in 1996, has been contentious for many reasons including economic reasons, market monopoly, politics, and safety concerns. For the Zone Classification, the NEC addresses only Class I (gases and vapors) areas and therefore, it [NEC] cannot be applied to Class II (Combustible Dusts) or III (Fibers) areas. The NEC handbook clearly states that these two classification methodologies are not to be intertwined or partially used. One method or the other should be chosen when a facility is classified. Figure 5.2 graphically reflects the relation between division and zone areas.

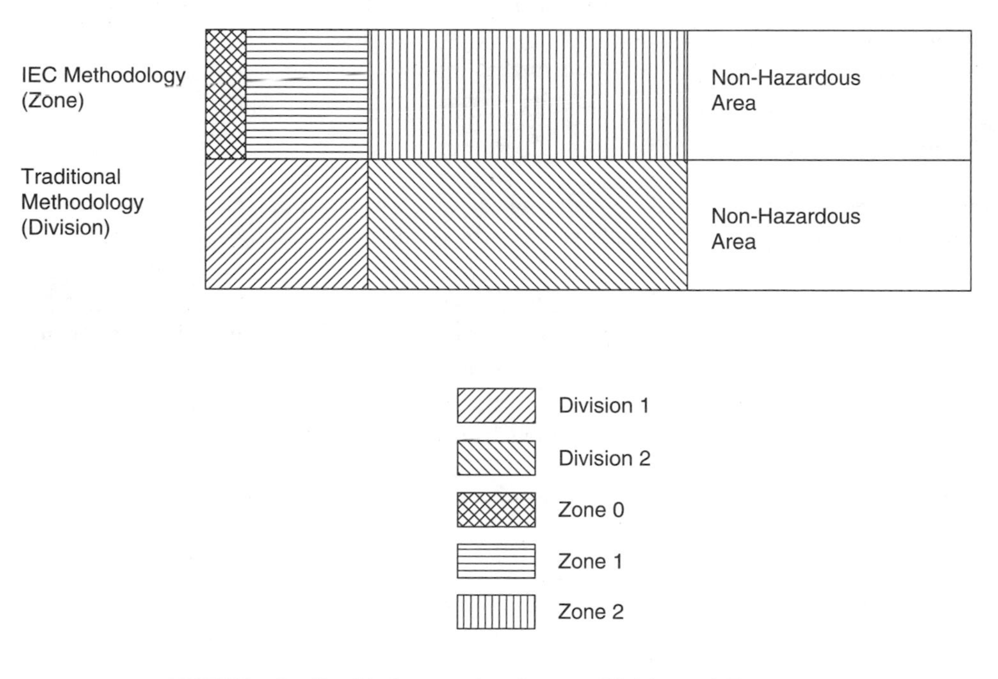

FIGURE 5.2 Graphical comparison between Division and Zone areas.

TABLE 5.2 Area Classification Based on NEC

Division 1—Hazard Is Present under Normal Operating Conditions	
Class I	Gases and Vapor
Group A	e.g., Acetylene
Group B	e.g., Hydrogen
Group C	e.g., ethylene
Group D	e.g., methane
Class II	Combustible dusts
Group E	Metal dust
Group F	Coal dust
Group G	Grain dust
Class III	Fibers
Division 2—Hazard Is Present only under Abnormal Operating Conditions	

Division Classification

In North America, hazardous areas are separated by classes, divisions, and groups. Article 500 of the NEC and Table 5.2 describe hazardous locations by Class, Division, and Group. The Class defines the physical form of combustible material mixed with oxygen molecules. The Division defines the probability of an explosive fuel to air mixture being present. The Group indicates the type of vapor or dust present. The NEC gives the following definitions:[1]

Class I, Division 1 Locations

1. Where ignitible concentrations of flammable gases or vapors can exist under normal operating conditions; may exist frequently because of repair or maintenance operations or because of leakage; and where breakdown or faulty operation of equipment or processes might release ignitible concentrations of flammable gases or vapors, and cause simultaneous failure of electric equipment.

Class I, Division 2 Locations

1. Where volatile flammable liquids or flammable gases are handled, processed, or used but where the liquids, vapors, or gases will normally be confined within closed containers or closed systems from which they can escape only in case of accidental rupture or breakdown of such containers or systems, or in case of abnormal operation of equipment;
2. Where ignitible concentrations of gases or vapors are normally prevented by positive mechanical ventilation, and where they might become hazardous through failure or abnormal operation of the ventilating equipment;
3. Adjacent to Class I, Division 1 locations, and where ignitible concentrations of gases or vapors might occasionally be communicated; unless such communication is prevented by positive-pressure ventilation from a source of clean air, and effective safeguards against ventilation failure are provided.

[1]Reprinted with permission from NFPA 70–2005, National Electrical Code®, Copyright© 2004, National Fire Protection Association. This reprinted material is not the complete and official position of the NFPA, on the referenced subject which is represented only by the standard in its entirety. National Electrical Code® and NEC® are registered trademarks of the National Fire Protection Association, Inc., Quincy, MA 02169.

Class II, Division 1 Locations

1. Where combustible dust is in the air under normal operation conditions in quantities sufficient to produce explosive or ignitible mixtures;
2. Where mechanical failure or abnormal operation of machinery or equipment might cause such explosive or ignitible mixtures to be produced, and also might provide a source of ignition through simultaneous failure of electric equipment, operation of protective devices, or from other causes;
3. Where combustible dusts of an electrically conductive nature may be present in hazardous quantities.

Class II, Division 2 Locations

Where combustible dust normally is not in the air in quantities sufficient to produce explosive or ignitible mixtures, and dust accumulations normally are insufficient to interfere with the safe dissipation of heat from electrical equipment, or may be ignitible by abnormal operation or failure of electrical equipment.

Class III, Division 1 Locations

Where easily ignitible fibers or materials producing combustible flyings are handled, manufactured, or used.

Class III, Division 2 Locations

Where easily ignitible fibers are stored or handled. Quantities and properties of hazardous materials are the basis upon which the NEC classifies hazardous locations. Each hazardous location must be evaluated carefully to determine the appropriate classification to facilitate the design process and to help specify the correct equipment.

Marking

All equipment used in hazardous area must be clearly marked to reflect class, group and operating temperature referenced to 40°C (104°F) or temperature class (e.g. Class I, Division 1, Group D, T6). Sometime, Division (or Div.) is not shown on the equipment nameplate, such equipment not marked to indicate division or marked "Division 1" or "Div.1" can be used in both Division 1&2 locations. However, equipment marked "Division 2" or "Div 2" can only be used in Division 2. locations. If temperature class is used it shall indicate the "T Code" referenced in Table 5.1. Some equipment is provided with thermally protected (TP) sensors, designed specifically to limit the temperature to that marked one on the equipment. Without such TPs, operating these equipment in an ambient temperature higher than 40°C (104°F), will increase the operating temperature of the equipment. Equipment marked for use in Class I and II, shall be marked with the maximum safe operating temperature, based on simultaneous exposure to the combination of Class I and Class II conditions.

Zone Classification

In Europe and countries (outside of North America), classification of hazardous areas is accomplished-differently. BS EN 60079–10 is the standard for determining the classification of hazardous areas, giving guidance in determining the area classification and recommendations for detailing the zones on drawings. The standard also gives details about the protective measures that need to be applied to reduce the risk of explosions. In the United States, Article 505 of the NEC describes hazardous locations by Class, Zone, and Group. The Class defines the physical form of combustible material mixed with oxygen molecules. The Zone classification defines the probability of an explosive fuel to air mixture being present. The Group indicates the type of vapor or dust present. Table 5.3a defines area classification under the IEC methodology and compares it to the Division methodology. The zone classification is defined by the IEC. Hazardous locations are classified depending on the properties of the flammable vapors, liquids, or gases that may be present and the likelihood that a flammable or combustible concentration is present. From Table 5.3a we can see that Division 2 is equivalent to Zone 2, while Division 1 is split between Zone 1 and Zone 0. It is worth noting that equipment approved for the Divisional area may and can be used in the equivalent Zone area. Because of the idiosyncrasies such as supervision of work, dual classifications and area reclassification associated with

TABLE 5.3 Division vs. Zone Comparison Based on the National Electrical Code (Traditional Method vs. IEC)

Table 3a—Area Classification Comparison

Traditional Method	IEC Method
Division 1: Where ignitable concentrations of flammable gases, vapors or liquids can exist all of the time or some of the time under normal operating conditions	*Zone 0:* Where ignitable concentrations of flammable gases, vapors or liquids can exist all of the time or for long periods of time under normal operating conditions
	Zone 1: Where ignitable concentrations of flammable gases, vapors or liquids can exist some of the time under normal operating conditions
Division 2: Where ignitable concentrations of flammable gases, vapors or liquids are not likely to exist under normal operating conditions.	*Zone 2:* Where ignitable concentrations of flammable gases, vapors or liquids are not likely to exist under normal operating conditions.

Table 3b—Protection Method Comparison

Traditional Method	IEC Method
Division 1:	*Zone 0:*
Explosion proof	Intrinsically safe "n" (2 fast)
Intrinsically safe (2 fast)	Class I, Div. 1 Intrinsically safe (2 fast)
Purged pressurized (Type X or Y)	
	Zone 1:
	Encapsulation, "m"
	Flameproof, "o"
	Increased safety, 'e'
	Intrinsically safe, "b" (1 fast)
	Oil immersion, "o"
	Powder filling, "q"
	Purged pressurized, "p"
	Any Class I, Zone 0 method
	Any Class I, Div. 1 method
Division 2:	*Zone 2:*
Hermetically sealed	Hermetically sealed, "nC"
Nonincentive	Nonincentive "nC"
Non-sparking	Non-sparking, "nA"
Oil immersion	Restricted breathing, "nR"
Purge pressurized (Type Z)	Sealed device, "nC"
Sealed device	Any Class I, Zone 0 or 1 method
Any Class I Div. 1 method	Any Class I, Div. 1 or 2 method

Table 3c—Temperature Code Comparison

Traditional Method		IEC Method
T1	450°C/842°F	T1
T2	300°C/572°F	T2
T2A	250°C/536°F	–
T2B	260°C/500°F	–
T2C	230°C/446°F	–
T2D	215°C/419°F	–
T3	200°C/392°F	T3
T3A	180°C/356°F	–
T3B	165°C/329°F	–
T3C	160°C/320°F	–

TABLE 5.3 (Continued)

Traditional Method		IEC Method
T4	135°C/275°F	T4
T4A	120°C/248°F	–
T5	100°C/212°F	T5
T6	85°C/185°F	T6

Table 3d—Gas Group Comparison

Traditional Method	IEC Method
A (acetylene)	IIC (acetylene & hydrogen)
B (hydrogen)	IIC (acetylene & hydrogen)
C (ethylene)	IIB (ethylene)
D (propane)	IIA (propane)

Table 3e—Marking Comparison

Traditional Method	IEC Method
Divisions 1 or 2	Zones 0, 1 or 2
Gas Groups A, B, C or D	Gas Groups IIA, B, or IIC
Temperature Codes T1-T6	Temperature Codes T1-T6

Zone Classification, it is usually used in new construction or areas requiring major process and upgrades. Zone classification is divided into six categories:

Zone 0 Locations

Where ignitable concentrations of flammable gases, vapors or liquids can exist all of the time or for long periods of time under normal operating conditions.

Zone 1 Locations

Where ignitable concentrations of flammable gases, vapors or liquids can exist some of the time under normal operating conditions

Zone 2 Locations

Where ignitable concentrations of flammable gases, vapors or liquids are not likely to exist under normal operating conditions.

Zone 20 Locations

Where an explosive atmosphere in the form of a cloud of combustible dust in air is present continuously, or for long periods or frequently.

Zone 21 Locations

Where an explosive atmosphere in the form of a cloud of combustible dust in air is likely to occur in normal operation occasionally.

Zone 22 Locations

Where an explosive atmosphere in the form of a cloud of combustible dust in air is not likely to occur in normal operation but, if it does occur, will persist for a short period only.

Marking

As with division marking, all equipment used in hazardous area must be marked to reflect five points that must be clearly shown in order on the equipment nameplate:

1. Class I, Zone 1: Indicates area classification
2. AEx: Indicates equipment built to US standards (EEx for Europe)
3. ia: Indicates protection methodologies
4. IIB: Indicates gas group
5. T4 : Indicates temperature classification

Enclosure Types and Requirements

When it comes to choosing the right enclosure to house electrical equipment, this task must not be taken lightly. Choosing the proper type of enclosure for electrical equipment is important for two reasons:

1. Personnel protection against accidental contact with enclosed electrical equipment.
2. Protection of internal equipment against outside harm.

Enclosures are designated by a type number indicating the degree of protection and the condition for which they are suitable. In some applications, enclosures have a dual purpose and therefore, are designated by a two-part type number shown with the smaller number first (e.g., 7/9). The following enclosure types, with their enclosed equipment, have been evaluated in accordance with Underwriters Laboratories, Inc. UL 698, "Industrial Control Equipment for Use in Hazardous Locations," and are marked to show the class and group letter designations.

Type 7 Enclosures

Type 7 enclosures are non-ventilated, intended for indoor applications, and classified for Class I, Group A, B, C, and D as defined in Table 5.2. The letters A-D sometimes appear as a suffix to the designation Type 7 to give the complete designation. According to UL 698, Type 7 enclosures must be designed to withstand an internal explosion pressure of specific gases and to prevent such an explosion from igniting a hazardous mixture outside the enclosure (Explosion Test). In addition, Type 7 enclosures fabricated from sheet steel are designed to withstand two times the internal explosion pressure for 1 minute without permanent deformation and three times the explosion pressure without rupture. If constructed of cast iron, the enclosure must be capable of withstanding four times the explosion pressure without rupture or deformation. This test may be waived if calculations show a safety factor of five to one for cast metal or four to one for fabricated steel. The enclosed heat generating devices are specifically designed to prevent external surfaces from reaching temperatures capable of igniting explosive vapor-air mixtures outside the enclosure (Temperature Test).

Type 8 Enclosures

Type 8 enclosures are non-ventilated, intended for indoor applications, and intended for Class I, Group A, B, C, and D as outlined in Table 5.2. The letters A-D appear as a suffix to the designation Type 8 to give the complete designation. According to UL 698, the oil-immersed equipment must be able to operate at rated voltage and most severe current conditions in the presence of flammable gas-air mixtures without igniting these mixtures.

Type 9 Enclosures

Type 9 enclosures are non-ventilated, intended for indoor applications, and classified for Class II, Group E, F, and G as outlined in Table 5.2. The letters E, F, or G appear as a suffix to the designation Type 9 to give the complete designation. According to UL 698, the enclosure with its enclosed equipment is evaluated in accordance with UL 698 in effect at the time of manufacture. This evaluation includes a review of dimensional requirements for shaft opening and joints, gaskets material, and temperature rise under a blanket of dust. The device is operated at full rated load until equilibrium temperatures are reached, and then allowed to cool to ambient temperature over a period of at least 30 hours while continuously subjected to circulating dust of specified properties. No dust shall enter the enclosure (Dust Penetration Test). Furthermore, Type 9 enclosures must also pass the "Temperature Test with Dust Blanket," which is similar to the temperature rise test except the circulating dust is not aimed directly at the device during testing. The dust in contact with the enclosure shall not ignite or discolor from heat, and the exterior surface temperature based on 40°C (104°F) shall not exceed specific temperatures under normal or abnormal conditions. Where gasketed enclosures are used, gaskets shall be of a noncombustible, non-deteriorating, vermin-proof material and shall be mechanically attached. Type 9 ventilated enclosures are the same as non-ventilated enclosures, except that ventilation is provided by forced air from a source outside the hazardous area to produce positive pressure within the enclosure. The enclosure must also meet temperature design tests.

Type 10 Enclosures

Type 10 enclosures are non-ventilated and designed to meet the requirements of the U.S. Bureau of Mines which relate to atmospheres containing mixtures of methane and air, with or without coal dust present.

It is important to note that enclosures for hazardous applications are designed for specific applications and must be installed and maintained as recommended by the enclosure manufacturer. Any misapplication or alteration to the enclosure may jeopardize its integrity and may eventually cause catastrophic failure of the system. All enclosures should be solidly grounded and properly labeled with a warning sign reminding the operator of the importance of de-energizing the incoming power to the enclosure prior to its servicing.

Protection Methodologies

Choosing a protection technique that suits each application can appear complicated because safety, reliability, cost, and maintenance factors all must be considered. Over the years, a few hazardous area safety protection methodologies have been used. Although methodologies differ in application and principles of operation, they all have one common goal: to eliminate one or more components necessary for combustion. There are different methods used in hazardous area protection environment protection. A good hazardous area assessor recognizes that no one method alone is sufficient or suitable for all installations because of specifications and regulatory issues. The final design is usually a combination of different methodologies designed to meet the hazardous area specific needs. The protection methodologies can be separated into two categories:

Most widely used and popular methods include:

1. Intrinsic Safety
2. Explosion-Proof
3. Dust Ignition-Proof
4. Purging and Pressurization

Less popular methods include:

1. Powder (Sand) Filled
2. Oil Immersed
3. Non Sparking
4. Encapsulation
5. Increased Safety
6. Combustible Gas Detection System

Intrinsic Safety "i"

Simply stated, intrinsic safety (IS) is all about preventing explosions. Intrinsic safety is based on the principle of limiting the thermal and electrical energy levels in the hazardous area to levels that cannot cause an ignition of a specific hazardous mixture in its most ignitable concentration. Under normal or abnormal operating conditions (fault conditions are expected and are the essence of design for IS systems), the energy levels and power generated are never sufficient to cause explosion by igniting a specific hazardous mixture present. IS can only be used on instruments, control and sensing circuits where the voltage is typically 24VDC and less than 100mA. Intrinsic safety pertains to the minimum ignition temperature and the minimum ignition electrical energy required causing a specific group to ignite. The energy level provided by an IS circuit is low ($\approx$ 1 W) and is used only to power up instruments with a low energy demand. An IS circuit incorporates an Intrinsically Safe Apparatus (field device), and Associated Apparatus, and interconnecting wiring system. Designing intrinsically safe systems begins with studying the field device. This will help determine the type of

Associated Apparatus that can be used so the circuit functions properly under normal operating conditions, but is still safe under fault conditions. Field devices can be simple, such as resistance temperature devices (RTDs), thermocouples, mechanical switches, proximity switches, and light emitting diodes (LEDs), or they can be non-simple, such as transmitters, solenoid valves, and relays. A field device is considered and recognized as a "simple device" if its energy storing or generating values do not exceed 1.2 V, 0.1 A, 25 mW (or 20 μJ) in an intrinsically safe system under normal or abnormal conditions.

The "simple device" may be connected to an intrinsically safe circuit without further certification or approval. However, the fact that these devices do not have the ability to store or generate high levels of energy does not mean they can be installed in a hazardous area without modification. They must always be used with an Associated Apparatus to limit the amount of energy in the hazardous area, since a fault outside the hazardous area can cause sufficient high levels of energy to leak into the hazardous area. A non-simple device (e.g., relay, and transmitter) is capable of generating and storing energy levels exceeding the aforementioned values. Such devices require evaluation and approval under the Entity concept (described later) to be used in conjunction with an intrinsically safe circuit. Under the Entity concept, these devices have the following entity parameters: V_{max} (maximum voltage allowed), I_{max}(maximum current allowed), C_i (internal capacitance) and L_i (internal inductance). Under fault conditions, voltage and current must be kept below the V_{max} and I_{max} of the apparatus to prevent any excess heat or spark, which can be disastrous in hazardous areas. C_i and L_i indicate the ability of a device to store energy in the form of internal capacitance and internal inductance, and their value must be less than C_a and L_a of the Associated Apparatus (Table 5.4).

An Associated Apparatus (Figure 5.3), also known as a safety barrier, is an energy-limiting device needed to protect a field device located in a hazardous area from receiving excessive voltage or current. An Associated Apparatus is normally installed in a dust and moisture-free enclosure (NEMA 4) located in a non-hazardous

TABLE 5.4 Comparison of Entity Values of a Field Device and a Safety Barrier

Field Device (Intrinsically Safe Apparatus)		Safety Barrier (Associated Barrier)
V_{max}	$\geqslant$	V_{oc}
I_{max}	$\geqslant$	I_{sc}
C_i	$\leqslant$	C_a (maximum allowed capacitance)
L_i	$\leqslant$	L_a (maximum allowed inductance)

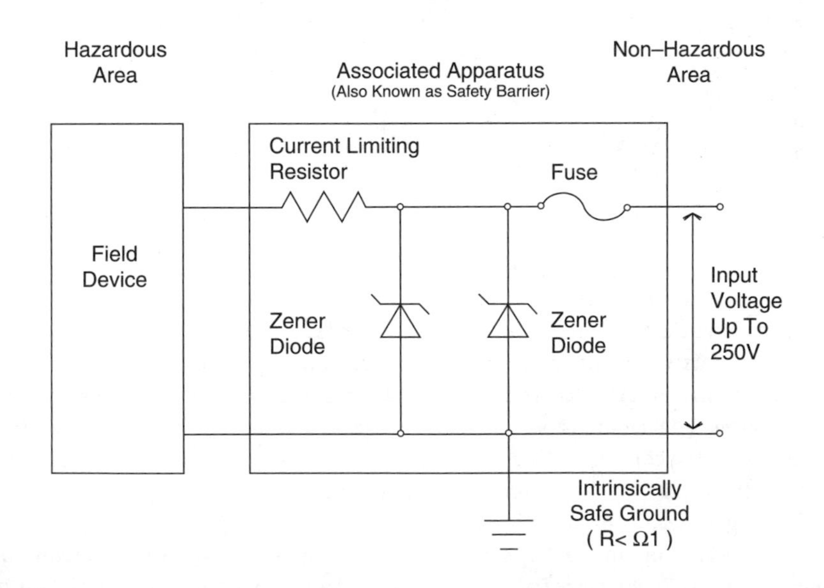

FIGURE 5.3 Major components of barrier circuit.

area, as close as possible to the hazardous area to minimize the capacitance effect of the cable. If installed in a hazardous area, the Associated Apparatus must be installed in an explosion-proof enclosure (e.g., NEMA 7D).

Figure 5.1 shows the three major components of a Zener-type safety barrier (note that there are other types of barriers such as isolation and repeater types). The components are:

1. The current limiting resistor, which limits the current to a specific value known as short circuit current (I_{sc}).
2. The fuse, which acts as an interrupter or protective device in case of a diode failure (fuse will blow if diode conducts).
3. The Zener diode, which limits the voltage to a specific value known as open circuit voltage (V_{oc}). Zener diodes are unique in their ability to conduct current under reverse bias conditions. When voltage is applied to the Zener diode in the reverse direction, a small amount of current known as leakage current is passed through. This current remains small until the bias voltage exceeds the Zener breakdown voltage. Exceeding the breakdown voltage causes the inherently high resistance of the Zener diode to drop to a very low value, thus allowing the current to abruptly increase. This sudden current increase forces the Zener diode to become a conductor, thereby diverting the excess voltage to ground. If the current continues to flow above and beyond the fuse rating, the fuse will open and the circuit will be completely interrupted. Most safety barriers incorporate at least two diodes in parallel to provide maximum protection in case one diode fails (redundant safety).

In 1988, ANSI/UL 913 allowed the use of intrinsic safety barriers with replaceable fuses as follows: "if it is accessible for replacement, and the fuse on a fuse protected shunt diode barrier shall not be replaceable by one of higher rating." The fuses are housed in tamper-proof assemblies to prevent confusion or misapplication. The diodes have specific power ratings that must not be exceeded. The Zener diodes and fuses are governed by a very specific set of parameters that allow the fuse to operate at one-third the power rating of the Zener diode and to avoid irreversible damage to the Zener diode. The power rating for the Zener diode can be determined as follows:

$$Z_w = 1.5 \times V_{oc} \times 2 \times I_f$$

where

Z_w = minimum power rating of the Zener diode
V_{oc} = maximum Zener diode open-circuit voltage
I_f = fuse current rating

Selecting the best barrier for the application depends on the field device and requires analysis to ensure proper operation of the intrinsically safe circuit under normal or abnormal conditions. Three of the more important characteristics requiring examination are: (1) internal resistance, (2) rated voltage, and (3) circuit polarity. Regardless of the selected barrier, each has an internal resistance (R_i) which limits the short circuit current under fault conditions. As current passes through R_i, it creates a voltage drop across the barrier that must be accounted for ($V = IR$). The rated voltage of the safety barrier must be equal to or reasonably greater than the supply voltage. The word *reasonably* is significant because excessive supply voltage can cause the diode to conduct, rushing high current through the fuse and blowing it. The use of a regulated power supply can significantly reduce problems associated with excessive supply voltage. To complete an analysis, the circuit polarity must be established. AC barriers can be connected with either positive or negative power supply, while DC barriers can be rated to either positive or negative.

Making Field Devices Intrinsically Safe

Resistance temperature devices (RTDs) and thermocouples can be made intrinsically safe by using isolated temperature converters (ITCs) that convert a low DC signal from the field device into a proportional 4–20 mA signal. These ITCs require no ground connection for the safe and proper operation of the IS circuit. Because of their ability to store energy, transmitters are considered non-simple devices and must be approved as intrinsically safe. If they are third-party approved, their entity parameter must be carefully considered.

Transmitters (4–20 mA) convert physical measurements in hazardous areas, such as pressure and flow, into electrical signals that can be transmitted to a controller in a safe area. Depending upon the conditions, 4–20 mA signals can be made intrinsically safe by using a repeater barrier, which duplicates the output signal to match the input signal. Repeaters can be grounded or ungrounded. Ungrounded repeater barriers are known as "transformer-isolated barriers," since the incoming voltage or signal is completely isolated from the outgoing voltage or signal via a transformer. Digital inputs, such as mechanical and proximity switches, which are simple devices, can be made intrinsically safe by using a switch amplifier. A switch amplifier is simply a relay or an optocoupler (a high-speed relay that uses optical isolation between the input and the output) that transfers a discrete signal (e.g., on/off) from the hazardous area to a safe area. Grounded safety barriers are passive devices designed specifically to prevent excessive energy in a non-hazardous area from reaching a hazardous area. These barriers can be used with most field devices. In order for such barriers to function properly, we must emphasize the need for a solid, low impedance ($<1\Omega$) connection to ground to prevent ground loops and induced voltages, which can hinder operation of the system.

Ignition Curves

All electrical circuits possess certain electrical characteristics that can be classified under three categories: resistance, inductance, and capacitance. To some extent, all circuits possess these three characteristics.

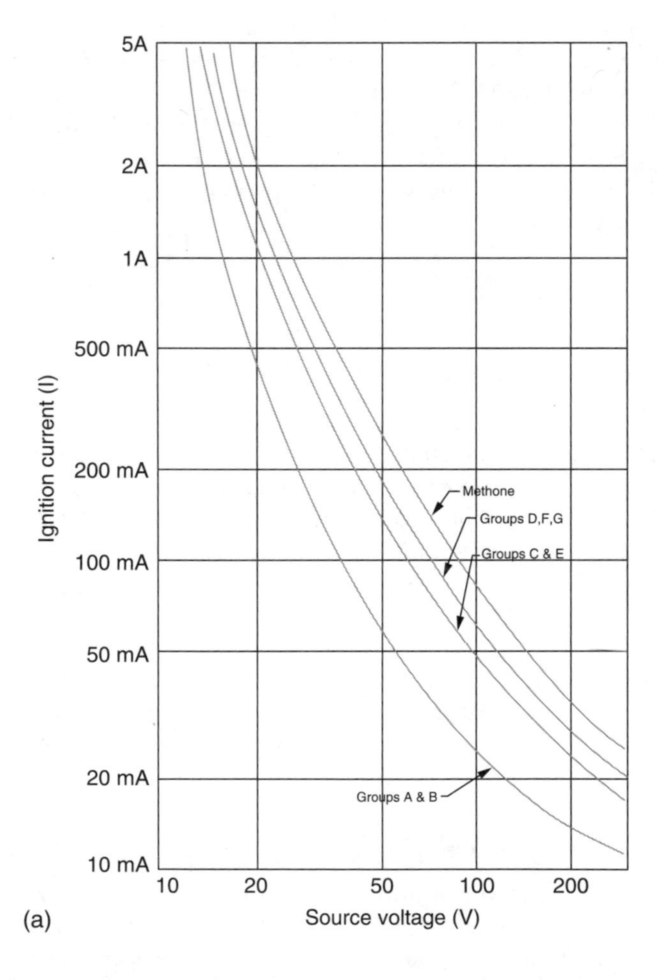

FIGURE 5.4 (a) Resistance circuit ignition curves for all circuit metals; (b) inductance circuit ignition curves at 24 V for all circuit metals; (c) capacitance circuit ignition curves for groups A and B for all circuit metals.

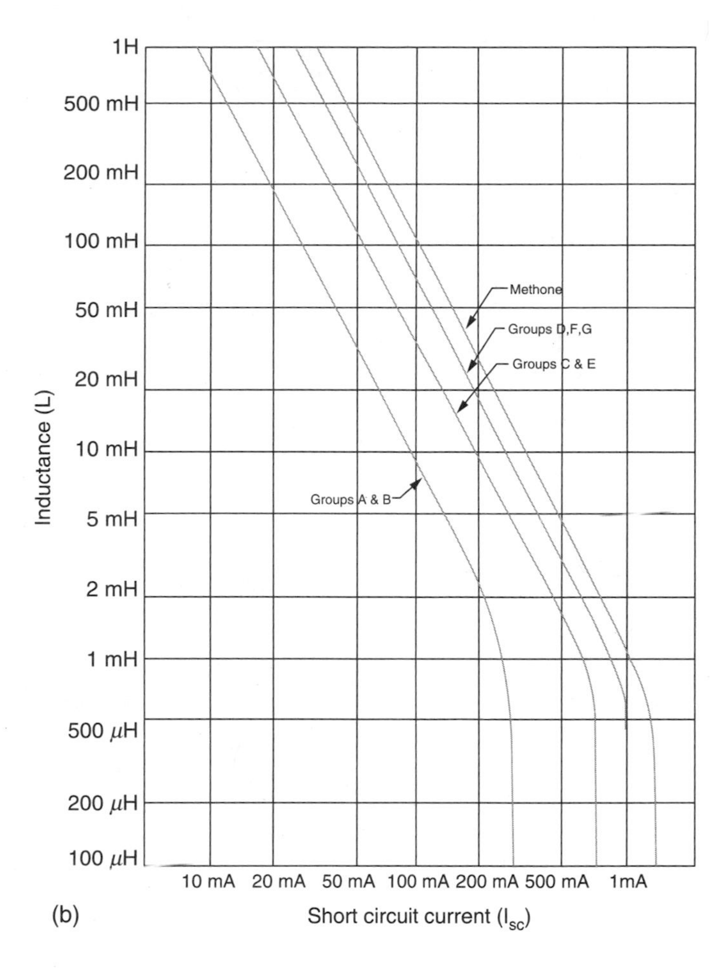

FIGURE 5.4 (Continued)

However, some of these characteristics may be so small that their effects are negligible compared with that of the others; hence the terms resistive, inductive, and capacitive circuit. Since the concept of Intrinsic Safety is based on the principle that a large electric current can cause an explosion in a hazardous area and the lack of it cannot, we must identify the ranges of currents that are safe and those that are dangerous.

What is a dangerous amount of electrical energy? The answer lies in the ignition curves. Ignition curves are published in most intrinsic safety standards, such as ANSI/UL 913. Three of the most referenced curves are shown in Figure 5.4. The curves show the amount of energy required to ignite various hazardous atmospheric mixtures in their most easily ignitible concentration. The most easily ignitible concentration is determined by calculating the percentage of volume-to-air between the upper and lower explosive limits of a specific hazardous atmospheric mixture. In the three referenced curves, the energy levels (voltage and current) below the group curve are not sufficient to cause an ignition of the referenced group.

Since specific ignition temperature is directly related to the amount of voltage and current consumed, both V_{oc} and I_{sc} of the safety barrier must be less than V_{max} and I_{max}. When designing an intrinsically safe system, the cable resistance R (Ω/m), the inductance L (μH/m), and the capacitance C (pF/m), which are inherently distributed over the length of the cable, must be considered. The capacitance and inductance can be readily obtained from the cable manufacturer's literature. If these parameters are not available, certain default values can be used based on NFPA 493/78 (A-4–2). They are C_c=200 pF/m (60 pF/FT), L_c=0.66 μH/m, and (0.2 μH/FT). To determine the maximum wiring distance required to ensure proper operation, the capacitance

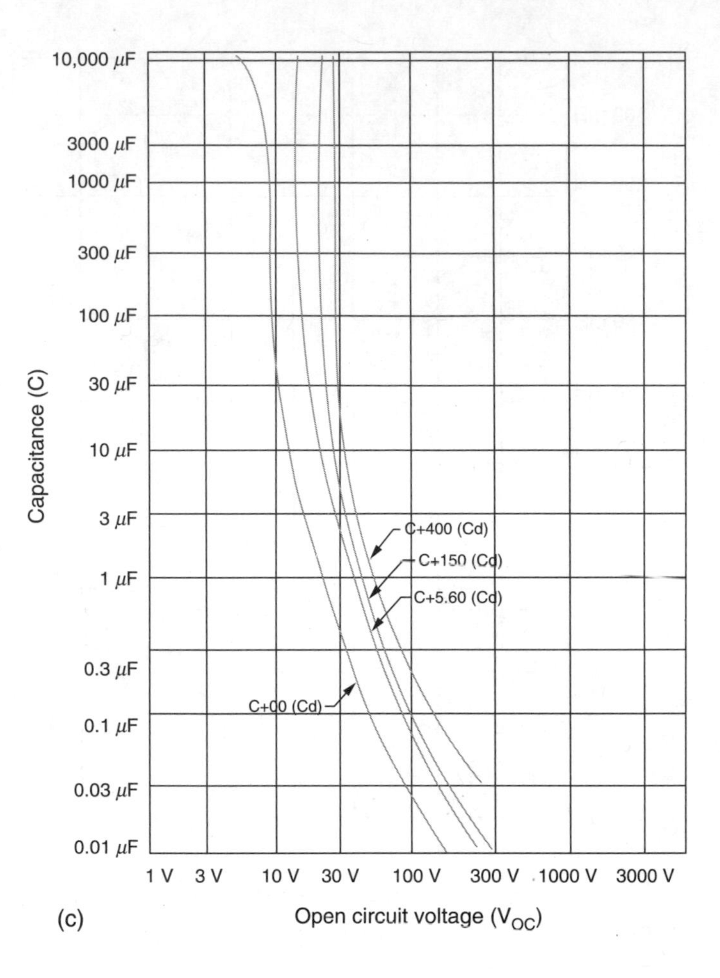

FIGURE 5.4 (Continued)

and inductance must be calculated. One common approach uses "lumped parameters," in which the voltage and current of both the Intrinsically Safe Apparatus and the Associated Intrinsically Safe Apparatus are compared and matched according to Equation (5.1) and Equation (5.2). Any deviation from either Equation (5.1) or Equation (5.2) can compromise the integrity of the system and introduce hazardous conditions. The reactive parts of the system must also be considered and verified to demonstrate that C_a and L_a values of the Associated Apparatus are not be exceeded by the field device and the field wiring values as shown in Equation (5.3) and Equation (5.4). This method, although simple and effective, tends to exaggerate the wiring capacitance and inductance effect, which can be limiting in some applications. Another method takes advantage of the relation between the cable resistance and inductance. This method can be used if the L/R ratio of the Associated Apparatus is higher than the calculated L/R ratio of the cable. Under these conditions, the lesser D_a (maximum allowed distance) value can be ignored and the cable length can be extended to the higher D_a value. This method is more flexible where cable length is an issue. Figure 5.5 and the following example illustrate these methods.

Lumped parameters method:

$$V_{oc} \leqslant V_{max} \tag{5.1}$$

$$I_{sc} \leqslant \mathrm{I}_{max} \tag{5.2}$$

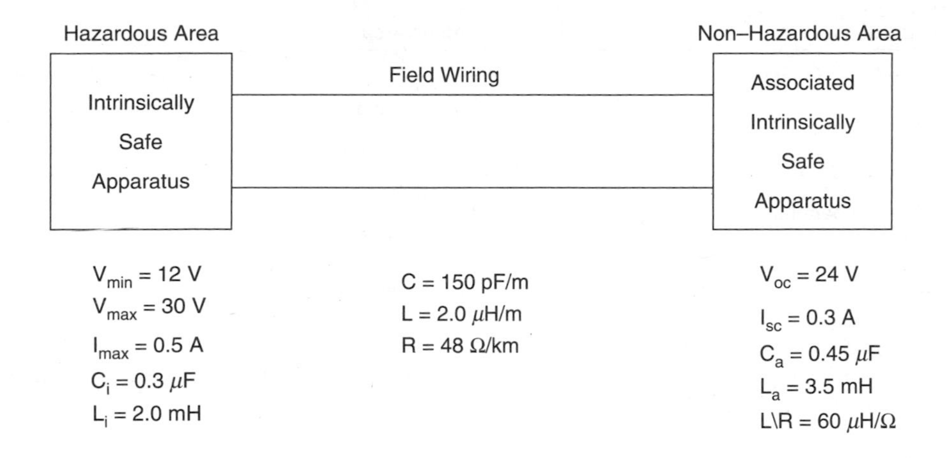

FIGURE 5.5 Analysis of an intrinsically safe system.

$$C_c \leqslant C_a - C_i \quad 0.45\mu\text{F} - 0.30\mu\text{F} = 0.15\mu\text{F} \tag{5.3}$$

$$L_c \leqslant L_a - L_i \quad 3.5\,\text{mH} - 2.0\,\text{mH} = 1.5\,\text{mH} \tag{5.4}$$

The maximum length of the field wiring, referred to its capacitance and inductance, is the lesser value of D_a.

$$D_a = 0.15\,\mu\text{F}/150\,\text{pF/m} = 1,000\,\text{m}$$

$$D_a = 1.5\,\text{mH}/2.0\,\mu\text{H/m} = 750\,\text{m (maximum distance of field wiring)}$$

L/R ratio method:

Since the cable *L/R* ratio of 41.6 μH/Ω (2 μH/m / 48 Ω/km) is less than the given Associated Apparatus *L/R* ratio, the inductive effect can be ignored and the maximum distance can be increased to 1,000 m.

Certification and Approval

Although approval and certification processes help to provide safety, careful planning, designing, and engineering are still necessary. Intrinsic safety standards, procedures, and tests are recognized worldwide. Testing authorities include Underwriters Laboratories Inc. (UL) and Factory Mutual Research Corp. (FM) in the United States, Canadian Standards Association (CSA) in Canada, and Physikalisch-Technische Bundesanstalt (PTB) in Europe. Intrinsically safe products are suitable for all Classes, Divisions, and Groups outlined in Table 5.2. It is imperative that the Intrinsically Safe product must be rated and classified for each specific application (zone/class, division and group). Since air is made up of 79% nitrogen and 21% oxygen, IS approvals are based on 21% oxygen concentration. A typical UL label identifies that the device is suitable for intrinsic safe application in specific Zone/Class, Division and Group. A 21% oxygen concentration is common within the industry and the approving agencies that test and certify instruments as intrinsically safe for normal oxygen concentration. Oxygen concentration can vary; depending on the situation certain conditions can exist well over 21% causing what is commonly called an "enriched environment" and can consequently increase the risk of flammability.

In the United States, FM adopted two methods for testing and approving equipment to be used in hazardous areas:

1. Loop (System) Approval — Where an Intrinsically Safe Apparatus is evaluated in combination with a specific Associated Apparatus and is approved to be installed in this manner. Any changes to the circuit require re-evaluation and certification (Figure 5.6).

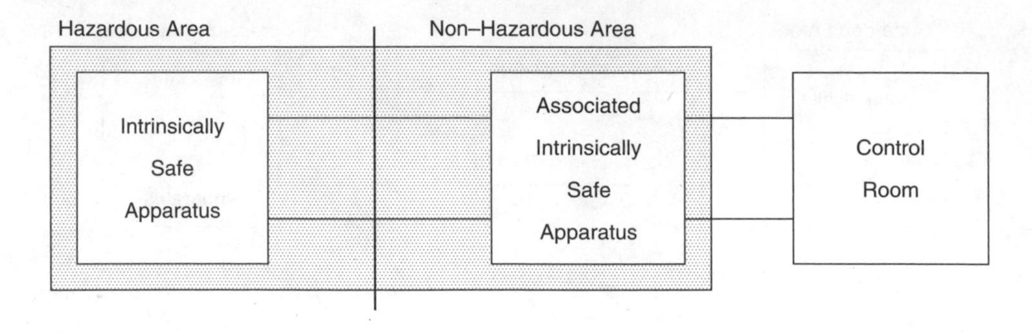

FIGURE 5.6 Loop approval. Intrinsically safe apparatus and associated apparatus are evaluated together. Shaded area indicates evaluated for loop approval.

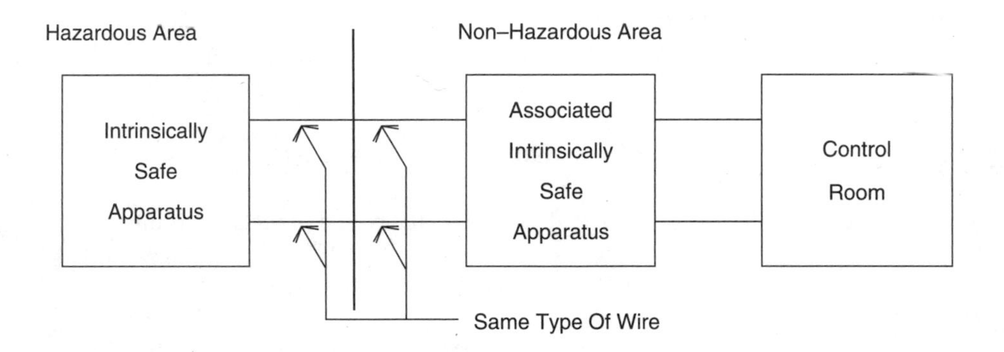

FIGURE 5.7 Entity approval. Intrinsically safe apparatus and associated apparatus are evaluated separately.

2. Entity Approval — Where an Intrinsically Safe Apparatus and the Associated Apparatus are separately evaluated and given their own electrical entity parameters (Figure 5.7). The correct application matches the entity parameters shown in Table 5.3. When examining the safety of a circuit, it is crucial to compare the entity values of an Intrinsically Safe Apparatus with an Associated Apparatus.

Most safety barriers are entity approved for all hazardous locations. Since most field devices have the ability to store energy, they must have loop approval or entity approval for the proper construction and operation of an intrinsically safe system.

Intrinsic safety engineers often advocate the use of intrinsically safe equipment for the following reasons:

1. Safety. No explosion can occur in an intrinsically safe system under any operating condition. Intrinsically safe equipment operates on lower power levels and prevents shocks, excess thermal energy, and arcing. In different systems and under various scenarios, shocks, thermal energy, and arcing may cause a hazard.
2. Reliability. The components and assemblies of intrinsically safe circuits are tested for reliability before they are labeled and certified. Most intrinsically safe equipment is designed with special circuitry to provide surge suppression and to prevent spikes and transients.
3. Ease of handling and installation. Intrinsically safe systems tend to be small and do not require expensive, bulky accessories such as enclosures, seals, and rigid metallic conduits which increase the initial investment.
4. Economy. In some geographical locations, facilities containing hazardous conditions must carry special liability insurance. With the proper installation of intrinsically safe circuits and equipment,

the probability of an explosion is 10^{-18} [8], or nearly nonexistent. As a result, insurance rates tend to be lower.

5. Maintenance. Equipment may be calibrated and maintained without disconnecting power, thereby resulting in less downtime.

The wiring of intrinsically safe systems is similar to any other application, but to ensure a proper operating system, certain guidelines regarding identification and separation must be strictly followed. All intrinsically safe components including terminal blocks, conductors, and intrinsically safe apparatus must be explicitly marked and labeled. The conventional color used to identify intrinsically safe equipment is blue. In an open wiring installation, intrinsically safe conductors must be physically separated from non-intrinsically safe conductors by at least 50 mm (2 in.) so an induced voltage does not defeat the purpose of intrinsic safety. Where intrinsically safe conductors occupy a raceway, the raceway should be labeled, "Intrinsically Safe Circuits." Intrinsically safe conductors should not be placed with non-intrinsically safe conductors. Where a cable tray is used, a grounded sheet metal partition may be used as an acceptable means of separation. Where intrinsically safe and non-intrinsically safe conductors occupy the same enclosure, a 50 mm (2 in.) separation must be maintained. In addition, a grounded metal partition shall be in place to prevent contact of any conductors that may come loose. Insulation deterioration of intrinsically safe conductors of different circuits occupying the same raceway or enclosure can be detrimental to the operation of the system. Intrinsically safe conductors must have an insulation grade capable of withstanding an AC test voltage of 550 V root-mean-square (rms) or twice the operating voltage of the intrinsically safe circuit. Non-intrinsically safe conductors in the same enclosure with intrinsically safe conductors must have an insulation grade capable of withstanding an AC test voltage of $2U+1{,}000$ V, with a minimum of 1,500 V rms, where U is the sum of rms values of the voltages of the intrinsically safe conductors. A commonly used and highly recommended practice utilizes separate compartments for intrinsically safe and non-intrinsically safe conductors. In addition to physical separation of IS conductors and non-IS conductors, sealing of conduits and raceways housing IS conductors is essential to prevent the passage of gases, vapors, and dusts from hazardous to non-hazardous areas. According to the NEC, Seal-Offs are not required to be explosion-proof. Where an Associated Apparatus is installed in an explosion-proof enclosure in a hazardous area, Seal-Offs must be explosion-proof. Although it is not required by Code, it is a good engineering practice to install explosion-proof Seal-Offs on conduits housing IS conductors, as shown in Figure 5.8.

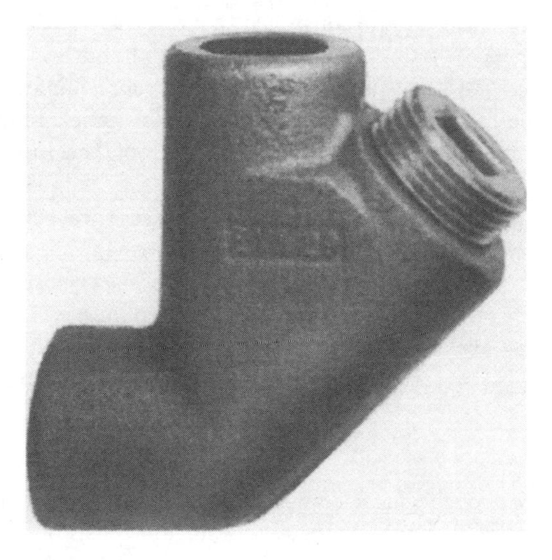

FIGURE 5.8 Explosion-proof seal-off fitting. (Photography copyright of Cooper Crouse-Hinds.)

IS Ground Rules

Grounding of IS systems is one of the most important design features. A properly grounded system will help ensure the proper performance of the IS system, while a poorly designed IS ground system can potentially create more hazard by creating noise on the circuit or altering the signals. Examples of grounding systems are shown in Figure 5.9. The first step in IS ground design is to understand and identify the type of barrier used. There are two types of barriers:

1. Grounded barriers: usually small, less expensive and require a separate ground connection.
2. Isolated barriers: usually bulky, more expensive and do not require a ground connection.

A properly designed IS ground system includes:

1. Low resistance path to earth (less than 1 ohm)
2. Properly sized grounding wire (minimum of 12 AWG)
3. Solid, secure, permanent, and most importantly, visible ground connection
4. A separate and isolated ground wire to avoid different ground potentials
5. One ground connection to earth
6. Redundant ground wire (although not required, it is a good engineering practice)

Explosion-Proof "d"

Explosion-proof design is a mechanical concept that relies heavily on the mechanical construction of an enclosure and the narrow tolerances between its joints, threads, and flanges to safely contain, cool, and vent any internal explosion that may occur. By definition, explosion-proof enclosures must prevent the ignition of explosive gases or vapors that may surround it (Type 7 and Type 10 enclosures only). In hazardous areas, Class I, Divisions 1 and 2, arcing devices, such as switches, contactors, and motor starters must be enclosed in an explosion-proof enclosure specifically rated for that area. Contrary to popular belief, explosion-proof enclosures are not and should not be vapor-tight. Succinctly stated, an explosion inside an enclosure must be prevented from starting a larger explosion outside the enclosure. Unlike intrinsic safety, explosion-proof enclosures address the maximum internal pressure (see NEMA Type 7 enclosures). Figure 5.10 illustrates the rugged construction of a standard explosion-proof panelboard.

In addition to its durability and strength, explosion-proof enclosures must also be "flame-tight." The joints or flanges must be held within narrow tolerances to allow cooling of hot gases resulting from internal explosions. In this way, if any gases are released into the outside hazardous atmosphere, they are cool enough not to cause ignition outside the enclosure and consequently, create a hazard outside the enclosure. Explosion-proof enclosures tend to be bulky (making them easy to identify) and heavy, requiring conduit seals and careful handling. Unlike intrinsically safe equipment, explosion-proof equipment operates on normal power levels, which are necessary due to the high power requirements of some circuits and equipment. With the proper equipment, installation, and maintenance, explosion-proof enclosures can safely and effectively distribute high levels of voltage and power into hazardous areas.

Where ignitible amounts of dust are present, enclosures housing electrical equipment must be dust-ignition-proof. These enclosures must exclude combustible dusts from entering, while preventing arcs, sparks, or heat generated internally from igniting dust surrounding the exterior of the enclosure. These enclosures must also efficiently dissipate the heat generated internally, since many types of dust will ignite at relatively low temperatures. Unlike Class I, Division 1 explosion-proof enclosures (Type 7), Class II, Division 1 dust-ignition-proof enclosures (Type 9) are designed to prevent an explosion. Subsequently, dust-ignition-proof enclosures need not be as strong or have walls as thick as explosion-proof enclosures, since there will be no internal explosion.

Dust-Ignition Proof

By far, dust explosions are one of the most complex and least understood hazards and thus, the most dangerous. Dust is a solid material no larger than 500 μ (1 micron equals one millionth of a meter) in cross section. The smaller the dust particles, the more explosive they are. Dust alone is not explosive; therefore, it must be disturbed so that every particle is surrounded by oxygen (air) in order to create a hazardous

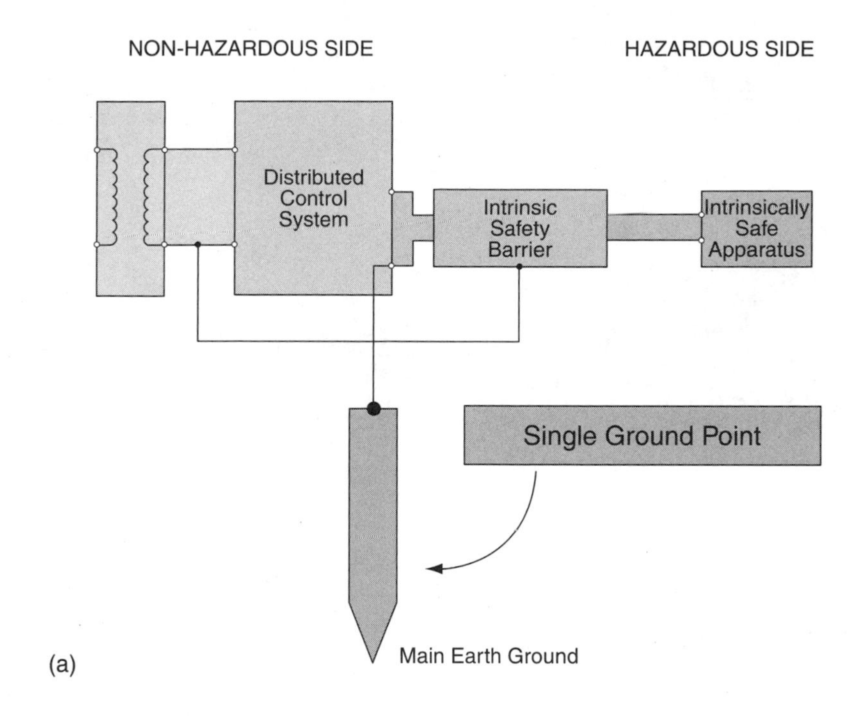

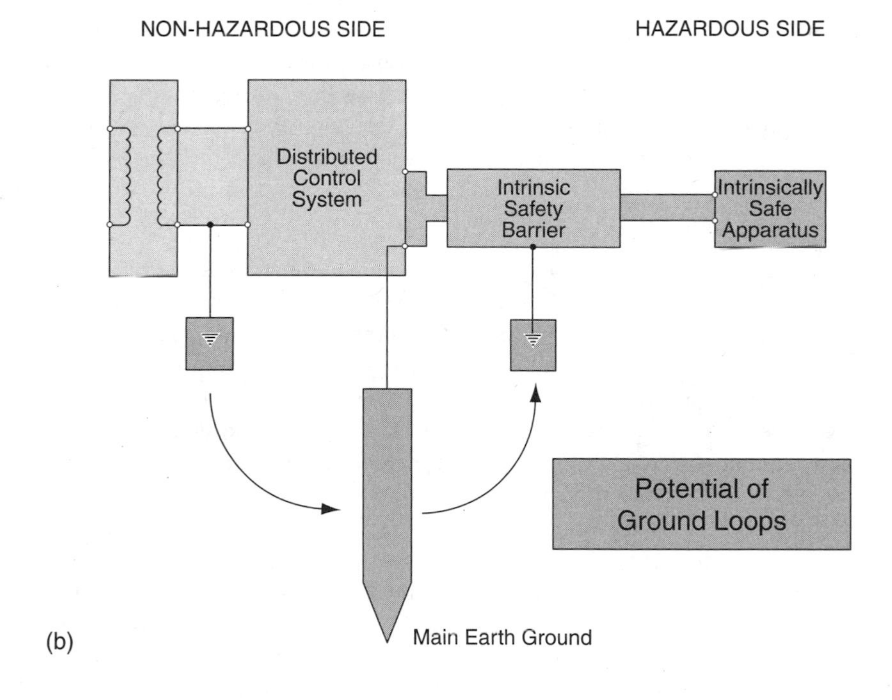

FIGURE 5.9 (a) Example of a properly grounded I.S. System (photography copyright of Cooper Crouse-Hinds); (b) example of a poorly grounded I.S. System (photography copyright of Cooper Crouse-Hinds).

condition. A dust-ignition-proof component prevents dust entering from outside. Arcs, sparks, and heat generated inside of the enclosure will not be allowed to ignite the exterior surroundings near the component. Dust explosion requires five ingredients: (1) ignitable dust; (2) confinement (with enough concentration); (3) suspension (disturbed dust); (4) oxygen; and (5) source of ignition.

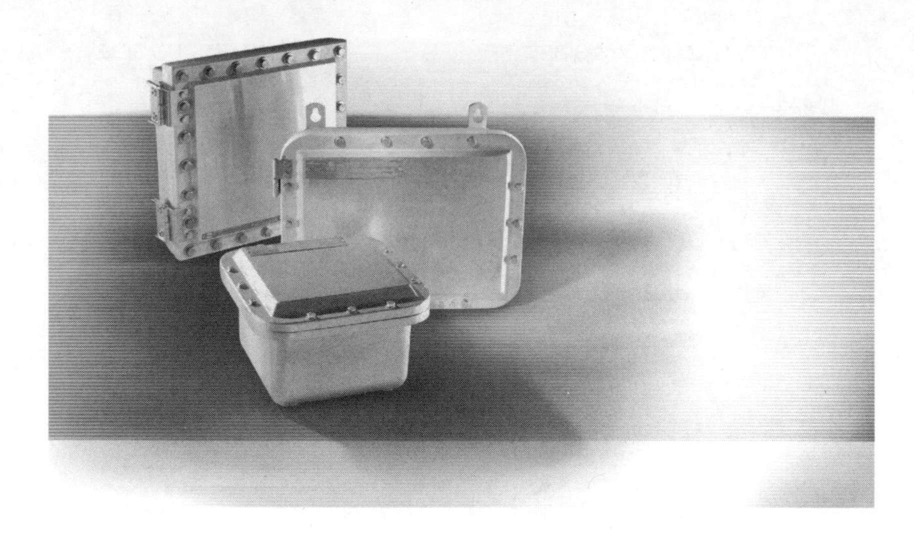

FIGURE 5.10 Explosion-proof junction box. (Photography copyright of Cooper Crouse-Hinds.)

Purging and Pressurization "p"

This methodology allows the safe operation of electrical equipment where hazardous conditions exist and where no other methodology is applicable because of the imperative high-energy demands and actual physical dimensions. This is true for large-sized motors and switchgear units where they are not commercially available for Class I, Group A and B. In addition, this methodology is used when control panels that house the instruments and electrical equipment must be located in hazardous areas. Purging and pressurization (P&P) is a protection method that relies on clean air or non-explosive gas (e.g., nitrogen) to be continuously supplied to the enclosure at sufficient flow and volume to keep the equipment adequately cooled and to provide adequate internal pressure to prevent the influx of combustible atmospheres into the enclosure. Although the enclosures are not explosion-proof, they must be relatively vapor-tight and must have adequate strength to perform safely and satisfactorily. A typical P&P system consists of:

1. Clean Air (or non-explosive gas) Supply: Careful study and analysis is of crucial importance to this process because the air supplied must be reasonably free of contaminants. Finding a safe location for an air intake requires skill and ingenuity. Consulting with an HVAC specialist is recommended. Other factors such as vapor density, location, wind pattern, and surrounding environment should also be considered. Where compressors and blowers are used to supply compressed air, caution must be exercised when selecting the proper compressor or blower size and location in order to meet air flow requirements without compromising the main objective of safety and reliability.
2. Purging: A pressurized enclosure that has been out of service for some time tends to collect a combustible mixture. Before energizing, clean or non explosive gas and positive pressure must provide a sufficient initial clean air volume to minimize the concentration of any combustible mixture that may be present. For typical applications, a flow of five times the internal volume of the enclosure is usually sufficient to minimize the concentration of combustible mixture that may exist. For unusual applications, the flow volume must be carefully calculated to ensure the success of the purging process.
3. Pressurization "p": This process uses the concept of pressure differential between the outside and the inside of the enclosure to keep flammable materials from entering. This is accomplished by maintaining a higher pressure on the inside of the enclosure. For safe operation, the protected enclosure must be constantly maintained at a positive pressure of at least 25 Pa [2] (0.1 in. water) above the surrounding atmosphere during the operation of the protected equipment.

If the purging phase is stalled or interrupted due to insufficient time or drop in flow or simply because the enclosure fails to maintain a positive internal pressure, the enclosure/equipment must be de-energized and an alarm indication is initiated for Zone 1and Zone 2 respectively. If either purging or pressurization fail to complete its cycle, the purging cycle starts be restarted and the two passed must be fully completed before power is applied. The P&P process is normally controlled by a Purge Control Unit (PCU) which is required to measure flow (air volume- purging) and pressure (internal/external), and time. Just like any other piece of equipment to be used in hazardous areas, the operation of the PCU must also be assessed under abnormal operating conditions such as fault conditions, relay failure, etc., since improper operation of the PCU can have enormous safety impact. As a minimum, the enclosure that encapsulates the apparatus must conform to IP 40 protection (protection against solid foreign bodies ≥1 mm in diameter). The enclosure must have sufficient mechanical integrity to withstand impacts, overpressures while at the same time allow for ease of flow of air. The enclosure must prevent the communication of flames, sparks to the explosive surrounding outside the enclosure. One way to do that is by installing a spark arrestor on the air outlets, or by venting the air to a non-hazardous area free of explosive mixtures. There are two types of pressurization, namely:

1. Static Pressurization (SP): Also known as constant flow. Air supplied and pressurized continuously from a non-hazardous area to avoid the influx of flammable gases/vapor inside the protected enclosure. After a pre-set time, power is applied to the enclosure.
2. Dynamic Pressurization (DP): Also known as leakage compensation. A process that depends on maintaining pressure in a protected enclosure or area. Normally after purging the protective gas is passed continuously through the enclosure at a pressure just above that of the specified minimum to maintain positive pressure.
3. Signals and Alarms: When positive pressure is lost, warnings and alarms are essential. Three types of pressurization and alarms can be used, depending on the nature of the enclosure's controls and the degree of hazard outside. In addition, door interlocks are required to prevent opening of the protected enclosure while the circuit is energized.

According to NFPA 496, there are three types of pressurization. They are:

Type X — reduces the classification within the protected enclosure from Division 1 to non-classified. This usually involves a source of ignition housed in a tight enclosure located in a potentially hazardous atmosphere. Type X requires a disconnecting means (flow or pressure switch) to completely and automatically de-energize power to the protected enclosure immediately upon failure of the protective gas supply (loss of either pressure or flow). The disconnecting means must be explosion-proof or intrinsically safe, as it is usually located in the hazardous area.
Type Y — reduces the classification within the protected enclosure from Division 1 to Division 2. The protected enclosure houses equipment rated for Division 2 and does not provide a source of ignition. Therefore, no immediate hazard is created. Type Y requires a visual or audible alarm in case of system failure. Caution: Safeguards must be established to ensure that any malfunction in the system does not raise the external surface temperature of the enclosure to over 80% of the ignition temperature of the combustible mixture present.
Type Z — reduces the classification within the protected enclosure from Division 2 to non-classified. Type Z requires a visual or audible alarm to be activated if failure to maintain positive pressure or flow within the protected enclosure has been detected.

More information regarding the Ex-p requirements can be found in IEC60079–2

Powder Filled "q"

The filling medium used for this application can include quartz sand (the origin of the "q"), glass beads, or powder. This method of protection is used primarily for small electrical components that have no moving parts (e.g., capacitor). The methodology uses a sealed enclosure (normally with a vent) containing any of the filling mediums to cover the enclosed electrical components capable of producing a spark. This ensures that under normal use no arc can be created that is able to ignite the explosive mixture inside the enclosure and the surrounding hazardous area. The enclosure construction requirements are specific and can be one of two types: 1) pressure test of 0.5 bar over-pressure for one minute and, if not protected by another enclosure, a minimum Ingress Protection of IP 54, the same requirement for Ex-e enclosures; 2) if the component is protected by another enclosure, no specific requirements for the type of IP protection is required. It is absolutely essential that the enclosure filled with the "q" medium. The maximum distance from live parts of electrical components to earth fitted inside the metal enclosure or metal screen can vary from 10 to 50 mm, depending on the voltage applied. If the enclosure is permanently factory sealed and the voltage does not exceed 500 volts, the minimum distance between live parts or live parts to earth can be reduced by 5 mm. If there are "flying leads" from the apparatus, they must be connected to Ex-e certified terminals. Ex "q" is used in Europe for heavy equipment and is not used in instrumentation applications. More information regarding the Ex "q" requirements can be found in IEC60079–5.

Oil Immersion "o"

The Oil Immersion concept has been predominantly reserved for heavy-duty, high voltage switchgear. As the name implies (oil immersion) the electrical parts are immersed in mineral (nonflammable or explosive) oil, which will prevent any exposure of the arcing or sparking to an explosive atmosphere that may be present above the surface of the oil. Furthermore the oil is designed and used to quench arcs and limit the temperature rise on electrical parts. To ensure compliance with the oil immersion protection requirements, two issues must be addressed: 1) All parts capable of producing arcs or sparks must be immersed in the oil no less than 25 mm in depth; and 2) An acceptable and reliable method to check the oil level must be provided. Depending on the type of mineral oil used, caution must be exercised, as some mineral oils are capable of producing explosive gases (e.g., acetylene and hydrogen) gas when arcing occurs and consequently create a hazardous condition that this methodology was intended to reduce. More information regarding the Ex-o requirements can be found in IEC60079–6.

Non Sparking (Nonincendive) "n"

This methodology is straight forward type of protection. Type "n" apparatus is standard equipment which, under normal operation will not produce arcs, sparks, or generate surface temperatures high enough to cause ignition and a fault capable of causing ignition is not likely to occur. Examples of normally arcing equipment are relays, circuit breakers, adjustable resistors, switches, and motor brushes.

Nonincendive circuit

A circuit in which any arc or thermal effect produced under intended operating conditions of the equipment is not capable, under the test conditions specified, of igniting the specified flammable gas- or vapor- air mixture.

Nonincendive component:

A component having contacts for making or breaking an incendive circuit and the contacting mechanism shall be constructed so that the component is incapable of igniting the specified flammable gas- or vapor-air mixture. The housing of a nonincendive component is not intended contain an explosion or to exclude the flammable atmosphere..

This methodology does not have power level restrictions and is primarily used in Zone 2 hazardous areas. More information regarding the Ex-n requirements can be found in IEC60079–15.

Encapsulation "m"

Encapsulation is finding increased usage for printed circuit boards that are assembled in small rail mounted housings similar to terminals. The Encapsulation concept is a type of protection in which sparking or heating parts are enclosed in a compound in such a way that the explosive atmosphere cannot be ignited under operating or installation conditions. The encapsulating compound is thermosetting, thermoplastic, epoxy, resin (cold curing), or elastomeric material with or without fillers and/or additives, in their solid state. The temperature range must satisfy the requirements of an appropriate standard for this type of protection. (Thermal stability at maximum operating temperature.) The following must be considered:

1. I_{sc} of a component during abnormal conditions (fault).
2. Controlled and limited temperature rise of the wiring and components.

3. Resistors, capacitors, diodes etc., must operate at no more than 66% of their rated voltage.
4. Air pockets and gaps must be avoided.

More information regarding the encapsulating compound for this type of protection can be found in IEC60079–18

Increased Safety "e"

As the name may imply, the increased safety concept relies on added measures and precautions to be taken to prevent the source of ignition (spark, heat, etc.,) from accruing either internally or externally to the apparatus under normal operating conditions. Therefore, devices such as switches and contactors are not allowed to be used since arching and sparking is part of the operation of the device under normal cooperating conditions. Increased Safety is most suited for non-sparking devices such as transformers and terminal boxes and is primarily used in Zone 1 area. The enclosures housing devices that incorporate the Increased Safety methodology must confirm to certain guidelines. The apparatus has an ingress protection (IP) rating, which is similar to NEMA enclosure ratings such as NEMA 4. As a minimum the following must be met:

1. IP 54 (dust and water splash) for enclosures containing live parts
2. IP 44 (solid foreign bodies $\geqslant$1 mm in diameter and water splash)
3. Thermal tolerance
4. Resistance to chemicals (solvents)
5. Mechanical integrity/strength

Where terminals are used inside these enclosures, they must also confirm to certain guidelines such as:

1. Means to prevent the conductors from coming loose
2. Sufficient contact pressure
3. Temperature limitations
4. Maximum voltage rating
5. Terminals de-rating for both current and the conductors

Hermetically Sealed

The equipment is protected against the external atmosphere to prevent the entry of hazardous gases or vapors. The seal is made by fusion, such as soldering, brazing, welding, or the fusion of glass to metal. A typical sealed device that is constructed so that it cannot be opened, has no external operating mechanisms, and is sealed to restrict entry of an external atmosphere without relying on gaskets. The device may contain arcing parts or internal hot surfaces. Figure 5.11 shows a valve positioner with hermetically sealed feed switches. For additional information refer to UL1604

Combustible Gas Detection System

Depending on the industrial facility, hundreds of industrial gases are usually present and used in different manufacturing processing. Examples of some of these gases include Acetylene C_2H_2 - is a group A gas (2.8% LFL and 31.0 UFL) that is lighter than air (0.9 vapor density), odorless, and colorless in its pure state. It can be a health hazard since it is considered a simple asphyxiant. Acetylene can decompose spontaneously if pressure exceeds 15 PSIG. Acetylene is the simplest member of unsaturated hydrocarbons known as alkynes or acetylenes. Because of its LFL and wide flammability range, it is considered one of the most easily ignitible gases.

Another commonly used gas in commercial applications and the oldest refrigerant known and still used today is Ammonia — NH_3 — a group D gas (15% LFL and 28% UFL). Ammonia is lighter than air (0.6 vapor density), colorless, with a sharp odor, reactive, and corrosive. Anything more than a sniff and ammonia can be fatal. Ammonia is a toxic product that is highly irritating to the mucous membranes and eyes. Contact with the skin causes severe burns. Normally ammonia is shipped as a liquified gas (LG) under its own vapor pressure of 114 PSIG. Its most extensive use is in soil fertilization. This application is used in the form of salts, nitrates, and urea. Ammonia has many important uses including bulk chemicals, plastic, and explosive

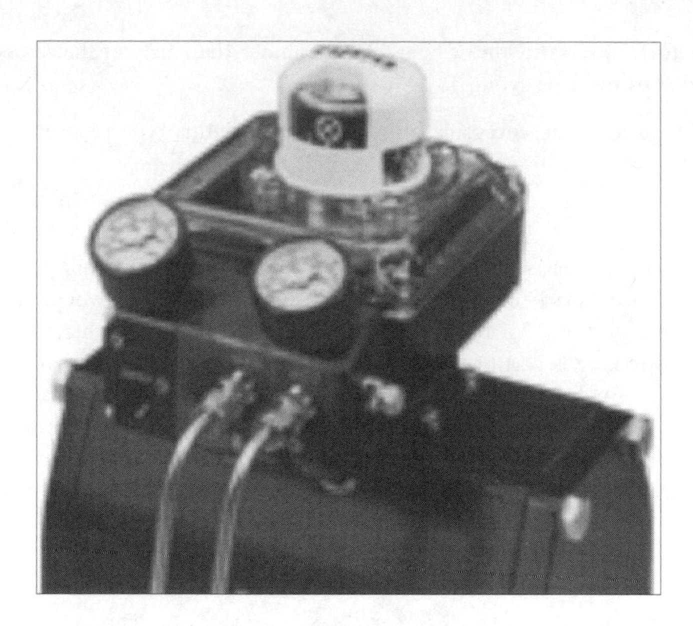

FIGURE 5.11 Analog Positioner (EaziCal®) with hermetically sealed feed switches. (Photography Copyright of Tyco Valves.) EaziCal is a registered trademark of Tyco International.

compounds. Because of its limited flammability range and high LFL, small ammonia leaks generally do not create a flammable mixture in air.

Combustible Gas Detection Systems (CGDS) can be used as a means of protection in industrial areas that meet certain strict requirements. Some of these requirements include restricted public access and dedicated qualified personnel to service such systems. To ensure code compliance and proper operation, CGDS must be tested and listed for the specific gas or vapor present in the area. The equipment must adhere to a strict maintenance program and calibration procedure. CGDS can be separated into two categories: (1) Passive Systems[14] — the most common type is electrocatalytic type, which is a single point detector. The principle of operation is rudimentary yet very reliable. Oxidized combustible gases produce heat, which generates temperature that is converted using a Wheatstone Bridge to a signal which is usually tied to a distributed control system (DCS) capable of activating alarms and possibly shutting down systems, and (2) Infrared Detectors [14] — operate on the principal of absorption of infrared radiation at specific wavelengths as it passes through a volume of gas. For these detectors to function properly, the light source and the light detector must work together to measure the light intensity at two specific wavelengths: active and reference. As the gas passes between the light source and the detector, the amount of light in the active wavelength hitting the detector is reduced while the amount of light in the reference wavelength stays unchanged. The difference between the two wavelengths is calculated and the result is the gas concentration that generates a signal to activate certain alarms or to initiate fire prevention response.

Equipment Use and Hierarchy

Equipment tested and used for the most stringent conditions can always be used in less stringent conditions of the same gas or vapor. Equipment can also be listed and labeled for a specific gas, vapor, or any specific combination. The lower the number, the more stringent the conditions. Zone 0 equipment can be used in Zone 1 and 2, and Zone 1 equipment can be used in Zone 2. But although the previous statements are true, one must always exercise caution when evaluating the use of electrical equipment in hazardous areas given the conditions present, such as type of gases, temperature, and possible ignition sources. Area classification is always specific for the hazard and conditions.

Recognizing and understanding the potential danger associated with the use of electricity in hazardous areas is a crucial part of selecting the best protection. Techniques for most applications, where the need for different energy demands is required, will likely involve a combination of various methodologies and specialized technologies. Properly performed analysis and investigation may appear to be time-consuming and expensive, but for those who are willing to adhere to the established guidelines and solid engineering practices, the process will help ensure the highest level of compliance while yielding tremendous savings and preventing property damage and injuries.

Defining Terms

Inductance: The ability of an electrical apparatus to store an electrical charge (energy). An inductor will release this energy when the circuit is opened (broken).

Oxidation: The process where negatively charged ions (anions) lose electrons at the anode during electrochemical process. For anions to become neutral, they must lose electrons.

RTD: A device that measures temperature based on change of resistance.

Ground: A conducting connection, whether intentional or accidental, between an electrical circuit or equipment and the earth or to some conducting body that serves in place of the earth.

Zener diode: A nonlinear solid state device that does not conduct current in reverse bias mode until a critical voltage is reached. It is then able to conduct current in reverse bias without damage to the diode. Zener diodes have almost constant voltage characteristics in the reverse-bias region (usual operation).

Normal Operation: Refers to the equipment and installation operation within their design parameters.

References

1. NFPA 70 (ANCI C1 - 2004), *National Electrical Code 2004,* Quincy.
2. National Fire Protection Association (NFPA), Articles 493, 496, 497, Quincy.
3. American Petroleum Institute 500 (RP 500), 1st ed., Washington, DC, June 1991. *Recommended Practice For Classification of Location For Electrical Installation at Petroleum Facilities.*
4. Elcon Instruments, Inc., *Introduction To Intrinsic Safety,* 3rd print, Norcross, 1990.
5. Underwriters Laboratories, Inc., Pub. UL 913, 4th ed., Northbrook, 1988, *Standard for Intrinsically Safe Apparatus & Associated Apparatus For Use In Class I, II, III, Division 1 Hazardous Locations.*
6. Underwriters Laboratories, Inc., Pub. UL 508, *Industrial Control Equipment.*
7. Babiarz, P., Cooper Industries, Crouse-Hinds, *InTech Engineer's Notebook,* Syracuse, 1994.
8. R. Stahl, Inc., RST 49, *Comprehensive Applications and Data Catalog,* Woburn, 1992.
9. Oudar, J., *Intrinsic Safety,* Journal of the Southern California Meter Association, October, 1981.
10. Alexander, W., *Intrinsically Safe Systems,* InTech, April 1996.
11. Tyco Thermal Controls, H56895, August 2003
12. Sean Clarke, Epsilon Technical Services Limited
13. Copper Crouse-Hinds 2004 EX Digest
14. General Monitors, Fundamentals of Combustible Gas Detection

5.2 Portable Instruments and Systems

Halit Eren

Introduction

Measurement, a process of gathering information from the physical world, is carried out by using measuring instruments. Instruments are man-made devices that are designed to maintain prescribed relationships between the parameters being sensed and the physical variable under investigation. Modern measuring instruments can be categorized in a number of ways based on operational principles, application areas, and physical characteristics of the instruments. Physical characteristics differentiate measuring instruments into two broad groups:

- Portable instruments with self-powering capabilities
- Non-portable or fixed instruments that require external power

Further, portable instruments can be divided into three main groups:

- *Portable and hand-held instruments* that are built for specific applications
- *Intelligent-sensors* in a single chip that function as a complete instrument
- *Portable data systems* that contain portable or fixed devices and are capable of communicating with other digital systems

All three forms of portable instruments are used in a variety of applications, including: science and engineering, laboratories, medicine, environmental monitoring systems, chemical processes, biology, oil and gas industry, aerospace, manufacturing, military, navigation, personal security, and hobby devices. In recent years, many devices conventionally known as bench-top instruments are being replaced by their portable counterparts thanks to improvements in supporting technologies. As the electronic components for all instruments get smaller in the form of microelectronics, and the software support becomes widely available, the physical dimensions of conventional instruments become smaller day by day. As a result, the trend of miniaturization of larger and bulkier instruments opens up many new avenues for development and applications of portable instruments.

In previous years, due to the unique nature of instrumentation hardware, customized software support was necessary from instrument to instrument. Nevertheless, today's portable instruments are largely software-driven and can be programmed by commonly available software tools. Therefore, many standards such as the IEEE-1451 can now be implemented in portable devices; hence the front-end and back-end analog and digital hardware of portable instruments can now be standardized to address large classes of similar applications.

In this section, a general concept for portable instruments will be introduced and recent progress in this area will be discussed. Further information can be found in the publications listed in the Reference section.

Features of Portable Instruments

Portable instruments have special features that are decided and shaped in the early stages of design and construction. Compared to non-portables, portable instruments are centered on the trade-offs between instrument cost, performance, small size, less weight, low power consumption, user-friendly interface options, ruggedness, and ability to operate in a diverse range of environments. Due to their portability, these devices must be able to withstand accidental or deliberate abuses such as drops and knocks, be able to operate under harsh conditions in extreme heat and cold, even in rain and water. Often they may be handled by untrained users. Consequently, portable instruments require finely tuned features that balance performance against power consumption, weight against ruggedness, and simple user interface needs against convenience of operations, at the same time maintaining reasonable cost.

Portable instruments have the following general features that differentiate them from nonportables:

- Available power is limited.
- Voltage level to supply the electronic components will generally be low, usually less than 12 V.
- Under normal operating conditions, power supply voltage levels may vary considerably due to diminishing stored power. Even if the portable instruments are kept on shelves without being used the power of batteries may diminish due to leakage.
- Conditions of use and environments in which portable instruments operate may vary often. The possibility of portable instruments being subjected to severe variations in temperature moisture, and intense electromagnetic noise increases.
- Likelihood of the portable instruments being operated by unskilled and untrained users is greater.
- The human-machine interface of electronic portable instruments may be very different from that of nonportable counterparts.
- Weight and size may be dominant factors.

Important features of portable instruments are discussed in the following subsections.

Power Requirements of Portable Instruments

Power available in portable instruments is limited. Therefore, the restriction of power consumption is perhaps the most significant problem in their design and application. As a rule, better performance demands more power, while the desire to keep instruments small and light in weight precludes the use of larger battery packs. Additionally, the desire to operate longer without the need for battery recharge or replacement puts further pressure on power consumption. Nevertheless, recent advances in battery technology, although less significant than the impact of the new generation of semiconductor devices, have led to the development of many different types of light and compact portable instruments with somewhat enhanced features.

Both primary and rechargeable batteries can be used for the supply of power, although primary batteries maintain an edge in energy and weight in relation to volume. Solar and wind power are viable alternatives to batteries, particularly in remote applications for long-term monitoring and measuring purposes. As many of today's portable instruments are digital, they might be equipped with control features that slow down operations or turn off nonessential parts to save power. For example, if operator intervention is not detected for a set period of time, the instrument may slow down the measurement rate and eventually puts itself to "sleep," expecting to be woken upon request. In some cases, this approach can result in a reduction of power consumption by a factor of five to ten. Another simple way to save battery power is to allow operation from an external power source, usually a small wall transformer, whenever an ac power source is available.

Digital Portable Instruments

Today's portable instruments are predominantly digital due to the advantages that this technology offers. The use of low-voltage digital components, and the easy availability of microsensors and intelligent sensors have eased the design complexities of portable instruments and increased the application areas. A general scheme of an intelligent sensor-based instrument is illustrated in Figure 5.12. In this particular example, the instrument is under microprocessor control. The memory may contain the full details of the instrument's characteristics for troubleshooting, calibration, gain adjustment, power saving, and diagnostic purposes.

Currently, there is a full range of commercially available low-power and low-voltage digital signal processors, memories, converters, and other supporting components. These components have varying degrees of performance, power consumption, physical size, and software support. Similarly, recent developments in analog signal processing components contribute to the improvement of portable instruments in operational bandwidths, sensitivity, and accuracy of measurements. In addition, faster and more sensitive analog-to-digital (A/D) and digital-to-analog (D/A) converters are available with reasonably low cost. The introduction of novel converter architectures that incorporate internal digital antialiasing filters and sigma-delta ($\Sigma\Delta$) converters allow designers to shrink analogue hardware to small sizes, thereby extending benefits of the digital approach in their design and construction. Digital technology has also resulted in the development of user-friendly instruments and high-volume production, thus lowering costs further.

It is important to emphasize that a recent and essential improvement in portable instruments took place largely due to wide application of low-voltage and low-power electronics. Since the beginning of the 1990s, there has been much concentration on the development of devices and circuits capable of operating at low supply voltages and with reduced power consumption. In this respect, complementary metal-oxide semiconductor (CMOS) integrated circuits find wide applications in portable devices. More and more companies offer low-power, low-voltage analog and digital devices suitable for portables. A typical example is the XE88LC03 microcontroller

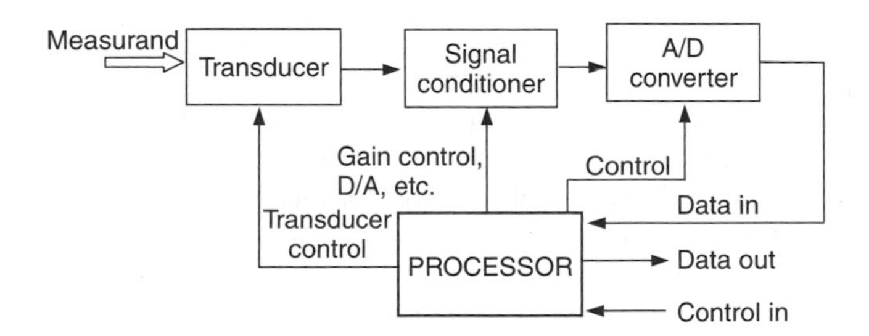

FIGURE 5.12 Block diagram of a typical intelligent sensor-based portable instrument.

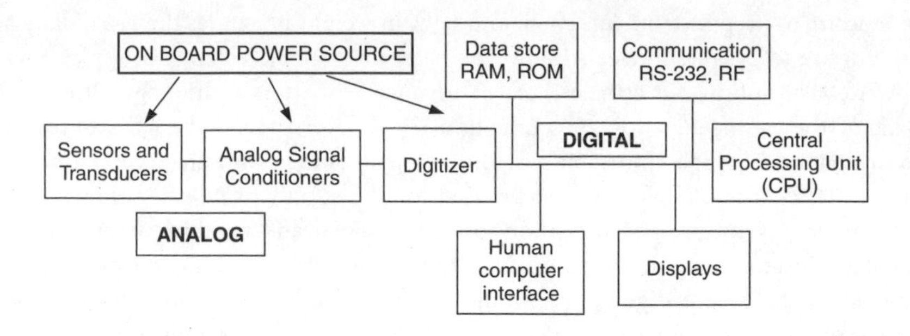

FIGURE 5.13 Block diagram of a digital portable instrument.

manufactured by IXMICS. Such components are designed to have high efficiency at 2.4-V supplies. Some low-power microcontrollers can draw currents less than 300 μA at 1 MIPS operation.

Figure 5.13 illustrates the block diagram of a typical digital portable instrument. Such instruments can implement very complex and sophisticated measurement techniques, store the results, display them graphically, and also operate automatically or remotely by using advanced communication techniques. They can communicate with other devices at high speeds and therefore can easily be integrated in complex measurement systems.

Sensors for Portable Instruments

Sensors and transducers are the primary and most basic elements of all instruments. Recent advances made in embedded controllers, microelectronics, and micromachining achieved cost breakthroughs that allowed a leap forward in the manufacture and use of sensors suitable for portable instruments. Micromachining technology, combined with semiconductor processing provides microsensing of mechanical, optical, magnetic, chemical, and biological data. Batch-processing techniques are suitable for making it possible to efficiently produce high-volume, low-cost sensors for portable instruments.

Semiconductor sensors provide easier-to-interface, lower cost, and more reliable inputs to follow-up circuits. In this respect, particularly, CMOS technology allows integration of many sensors in a single chip. Most microsensors and semiconductor sensors interface with a master controller unit (MCU) without requiring any analog-to-digital conversion or additional external components. This can be achieved either by inherent digital output sensors or by the integration of on-chip processing electronics within the sensing unit. Examples of single chip use include ion detectors, moisture sensors, electrostatic discharge sensors, strain gauges, and corrosion detectors. In broad terms, advanced semiconductor sensors can be classified as:

- Micro electromechanical systems (MEMS)
- Capacitive and piezo-effect sensors
- Optical sensors
- Biological sensors
- Gas and pollution sensors
- Radiation sensors, etc.

In many applications, more than one sensor is required to provide sufficient information about a process. In this respect, there is considerable effort to integrate many sensors on the same silicon wafer together with signal conditioning circuits and other computational components to make sensing arrays. These sensing arrays can include a number of sensors for different measurements such as pressure, flow, temperature, and vibration. The multiple sensors are used to increase the range and provide redundancy. A good example of sensor arrays is in chemical applications where different chemicals can be measured by the same instrument by using a range of different sensors often based on different principles. For instance, multi-element devices are developed by using different thin film detectors as in the case of a four-element gas analyzer.

Nowadays many portable instruments use intelligent sensors. Intelligent sensors contain the primary sensor, analog and digital signal processors, and input/output circuits in a single chip. Intelligent sensors are appearing in the marketplace as pressure sensors and accelerometers, biosensors, chemical sensors, optical sensors, and magnetic sensors. Some of these sensors are manufactured with neural networks and other intelligence techniques on the chip. There are many variations of these devices, such as neural processors, intelligent vision systems, and intelligent parallel processors.

Sensor Standards

As rapid developments in hardware and software occur, some new standards are emerging, thus making a revolutionary contribution to electronic portable instruments. Although not specifically addressing portable instruments, the IEEE-1451 is one example of such standards that define interfaces, network-based data acquisition and control of smart sensors and transducers. The IEEE-1451 standard aims to make it easy to create solutions using existing networking technologies, standardized connections, and common software architectures. The standards allow application software, field networks, and transducer decisions to be made independently. It offers flexibility to choose the products and vendors that are most appropriate for a particular application. As the new sensors are developed and these standards are coupled with wireless communication technology, we would expect good growth in the application possibilities and variety of portable instruments.

There are positive signs that many companies are producing devices in compliance with IEEE-1451. For example, National Instruments is actively promoting and introducing Plug and Play Sensors complying with IEEE-1451.4. There are many other intelligent sensors available in the marketplace complying with these standards such as some accelerometers and pressure transducers.

Communication and Networking of Portable Instruments

Today almost all portable instruments have some form of communication capabilities that enhances their usability, hence enriching their range of applications. We can list two levels of communications; the first one being the internal communication at the sensor and component level, the second being the instrument communication that takes place with external devices. The external communication is realized either by wires or wireless methods by using infrared, RF, or microwave techniques.

Many modern portable instruments contain at least an RS-232 port for communication and networking purposes. Once equipped with an RS-232 port, all portable instruments can be made to operate in wireless mode. Many companies are offering radio frequency RS-232 systems for remote data transmission. The transmission speed can be set to certain baud rates such as: 1200, 2400, 4800, 9600, 19,200, and 38,400 bits per second or higher. It is also possible to see some commercial portable instruments equipped with other communication ports such as the USB, EIA-485, and IEEE-488.

A dosimeter is a typical example of a portable instrument equipped with wireless communication capabilities. In some dosimeters, the information exchange between an electronic reader and the dosimeter is provided through an infrared (IR) device operating through an RS-232 port. When the dosimeter is placed on the reader window, the IR emitter forms signals in accordance with an exchange protocol. By using suitable software, the operator can register the dosimeter, enter user's personal information, create a database for the registered dosimeter, and transmit the accumulated dose data from memory to a PC for storage in the database. Once the information is on the computer, historical information in the database can be viewed and the dose levels over a period of time can be assessed. Another example is a portable multiple-sensor toxic gas detector that is equipped with a wireless modem that allows the unit to communicate and transmit readings and other information on a real-time basis to a remotely located base station. The real-time data transmission from the sensors can be realized by the use of a base-station computer located at a distance of a few kilometers away from the sensor.

In industrial applications, several standards for digital data transmission are available that are suitable for integrating portable instruments into the system. These standards are commonly known as *fieldbuses.*

Among many others, some of these standards are widely accepted and used in portable instrument applications, such as the WordFIP, Profibus, and Foundation Fieldbus. The fieldbuses are supported by hardware and software that allows increases in the data rates suitable for high-speed protocols.

Wireless Portable Instruments and Networks

Many modern portable instruments are equipped with wireless communication features. Wireless instruments are devices that can measure or monitor physical variables and communicate the information with other devices without the need for wired connections. A typical construction of wireless instruments is illustrated in Figure 5.14. Although not applicable to all, wireless portable instruments tend to have many additional features such as self-diagnostics, self-calibration, and artificial intelligence.

Wireless portable instruments and instrumentation systems enjoy a wide variety of software support at various levels. These levels can be summarized to be at the chip, instrument, communication, and network levels. Some of the supporting software is explained below:

- If commercial microprocessors are selected in the instrument design, standard languages, algorithms, and library tools can be used.
- At the system programming level, low-level languages such as assembly and machine language standing alone, or backed up with C++, are used.
- High level programming can be conducted by using Forth, C, C++, VB, HTML/ASP, SQL, and Visual Basic.
- Embedded systems tools such as Extreme Programming (XP), PICBasic, Embedded C or Verilog. eMbedded Visual C++, eMbedded, and Visual Basic find extensive applications.
- Structured programming tools such as the LabView and MATLAB are used in some design and implementations.
- The use of software for communication protocols such as Bluetooth are used in combination with JAVA, e.g. Java APIs for Bluetooth wireless technology (JABWT) are common.

There are various wireless communication techniques suitable for portable instruments, as illustrated in Figure 5.15. These methods can be summed up as: electromagnetic methods, such as the RF and the microwave; optical methods, such as infrared and laser; sonic methods, such as ultrasonic; and electrical or magnetic field methods.

In wireless applications, communication by means of radio frequencies (RF) is well established. RF communication can be realized by standardized or nonstandard methods. The choice of these methods for a particular portable instrument depends on its application requirements and complexity. For example, some RF techniques have high levels of power consumption.

Wireless Networks

Wireless portable instruments enjoy a wide variety of network options. Apart from well-established networks, there are many new and different types that are either being researched and/or offered by vendors. At the moment, common LAN/WAN networks appear to be applicable for wireless portable instruments. Many existing communication protocols such as Bluetooth, Wi-Fi, IEEE-1451X are commonly used. Wireless portable instruments can be networked in two configurations:

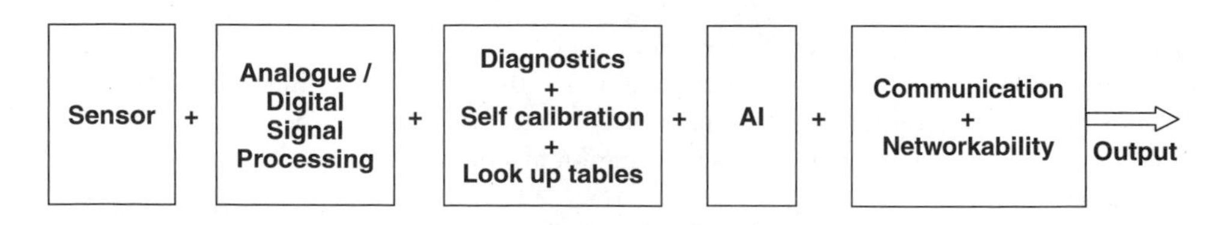

FIGURE 5.14 Wireless-instrument architecture.

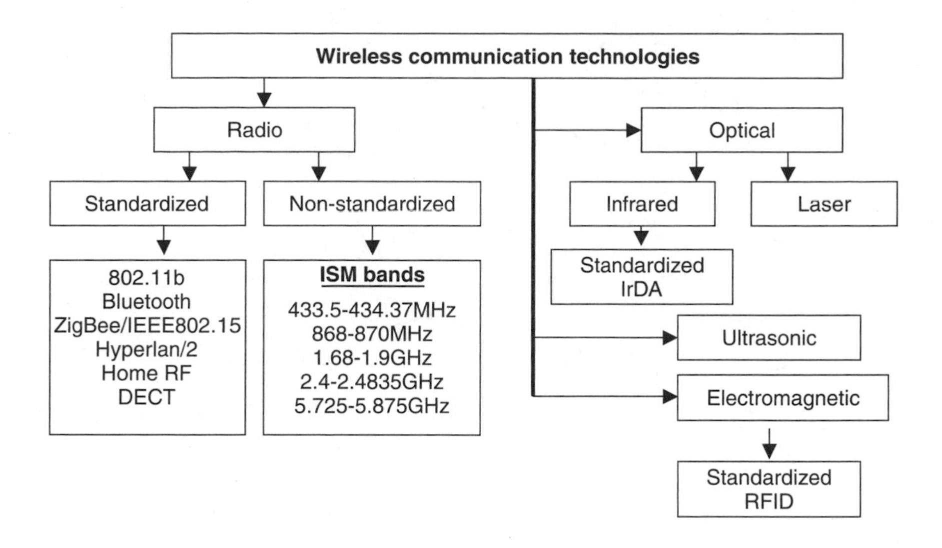

FIGURE 5.15 Wireless communication methods for portable instruments.

1. *Self-organized*, such as wireless integrated sensor networks (WINS) and smart wireless autonomous microsystems (SWAMs), and scatternet
2. *Structured*, such as wireless sensor networks (WSN)

The networks for wireless portable instruments can be thought of in three layers, as shown in Figure 5.16. These layers are essentially at the physical level of the ISO seven-layer reference model. By the use of routers and gateways, networks can be realized by *sensor-sensor*, *sensor-computer*, and *human-system* communications.

A typical example of a wireless instrument system is the scatternet network as illustrated in Figure 5.17. This method is used in military and environmental monitoring applications where mobility is the primary concern. In this system, self-organization takes place as each device communicates with its nearest neighbor, forming clusters. Clusters form chains by those belonging to two or more groups, thus passing information from one cluster to the next. The protocols support handover capabilities from one device to the next to realize mobility.

Applications of Portable Instruments

Portable instruments are becoming available in diverse ranges and capabilities with improved or added features. They are manufactured to be small enough to fit in wristwatches, as altimeters and pulse measuring devices for personal use, and large enough to be mobile geological surveying and mineral prospecting

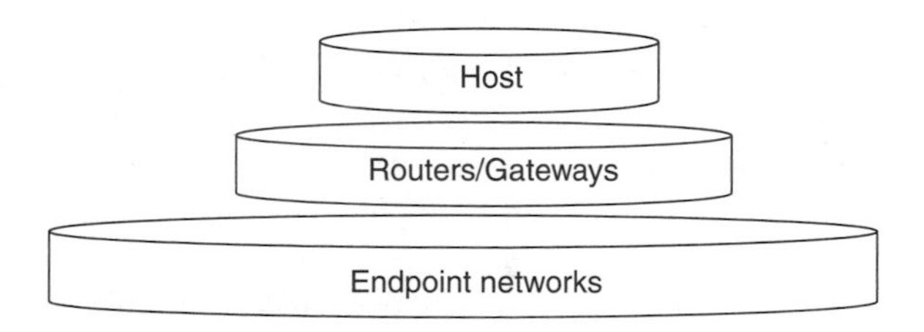

FIGURE 5.16 Wireless instrument network layers.

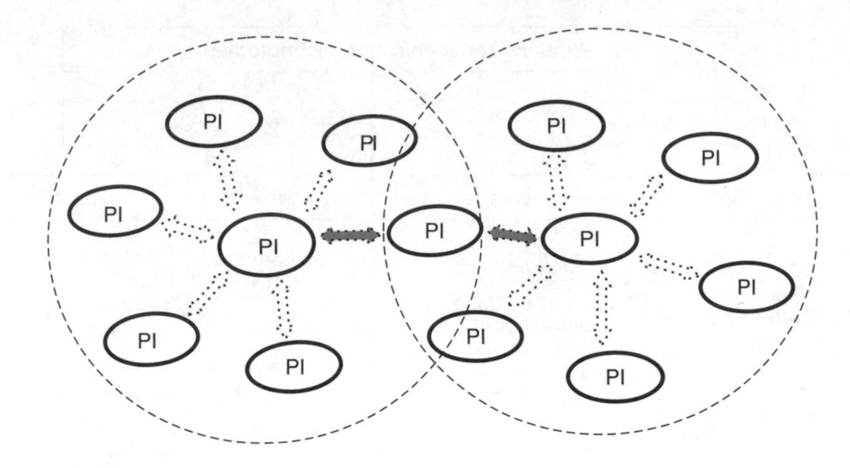

FIGURE 5.17 A typical scatternet-based network.

instruments and instrumentation in environmental applications. It is not possible to cover all ranges of portable instruments in this section, but they can be grouped in nine different major classes. These are:

1. Laboratory instruments and oscilloscopes
2. Environmental instruments
3. Chemical instruments
4. Biomedical instruments
5. Mechanical, sound, and vibration instruments
6. Radiation instruments
7. GPS and telemetry-based instruments
8. Computer-based and intelligent instruments
9. Domestic, personal, hobby and leisure portable instruments

Laboratory instruments are among the first and most commonly available portable instruments. They were used in the measurement of currents, voltage, and resistances, such as the well-known analog AVOmeters. Today, there are many different types of instruments suitable for laboratory applications, ranging from simple multimeters to measure currents and voltages, to highly advanced digital storage oscilloscopes.

There are many different types of portable instruments used in environmental applications, ranging from water quality measurements to soil and atmospheric pollution analyzers. For example, in water analysis, they are used for measuring water quality to determine biological and chemical pollution levels.

Portable instruments are used as chemical analyzers in diverse applications: for safety reasons in industry; monitoring of the performance of combustion engines; environmental safety; pharmaceutical testing; geological and scientific explorations; in emergency situations, where accurate information is required to determine the chemical make-up of air, liquids or solids; or in the day-to-day operations of manufacturing and processing plants.

Portable biomedical instruments are extensively used in clinical applications and home healthcare. They are frequently used as patient monitors, pacemakers, defibrillators, and also for ambulatory electrocardiographic (ECG) and blood pressure recording. Most of the patient monitors are now computer-based instruments that contain many elements of basic digital electronics. The portable patient monitors vary in size from compact to palm-sized instruments. Depending on the their sophistication, portable patient monitors may measure many vital parameters, such as heart rate, respiration rate, arterial blood oxygen saturation, and non-invasive blood pressure measurement. Some of these measurements are performed continuously and others intermittently. Most patient monitors include alarms and more sophisticated units may also include some diagnostic functions, such as arrhythmia detection.

In mechanical measurements, portable instruments are used for acceleration and velocity measurements; mass, volume, density, and weight measurements; power and torque measurements; force, stress, and strain measurements; displacement measurements; rotation and distance measurements; and pressure measurements.

Portable radiation measuring devices are used in medical and pharmaceutical instruments, nuclear weapons research and manufacturing, genetic engineering, nuclear reactor plants, accelerators, biomedical and materials research, space radiation studies, food processing, and environmental monitoring. They need to be reliable and consistent for administrative, legal, technical, medical, educational, and psychological reasons.

GPS-based portable instruments are used in many applications for personal use such as hiking, hunting, camping, boating, flying, and driving; and in industrial applications for fleet-tracking and geological surveying. They find extensive military applications from aircraft and missiles to individual soldiers. Consequently, there are many competitors in the marketplace offering a diverse range of products. These products vary from simple handheld receivers to mountable systems backed up with accessories to perform specific tasks such as ship and aircraft navigation.

There are a number of different types of computer-based electronic portable instruments. Laptop and palm computers are used as portable instruments. Computers are also used as base stations receiving information from portable instruments and intelligent sensors via wireless communications and telemetry. In the third type of these instruments, the instrument itself is so powerful that it contains a computer as part of its normal operation.

Personal hobby and leisure instruments constitute a large section of portable instruments with many vendors competing in the marketplace. Because of the market size, diverse instruments are offered in many ranges from simple disposable types to highly sophisticated and robust instruments. In some of these instruments, power efficiency is of paramount importance as in the case of biomedical applications; while in others, power efficiency is not considered at all as in the case of more disposable types of instruments.

Conclusions

Portable instruments are going through a revolutionary phase, rapidly replacing conventional benchtop instruments. The progress in portable instruments can largely be attributed to recent advances in microsensor technology. In recent years, due to easy and cost-effective availability of RF hardware and software, portable instruments find freedom to communicate wirelessly with other devices. This capability offers many advantages over conventional instruments finding many novel and complex applications. Open standards like Bluetooth, IEEE 802.XX and IEEE-1451.5 are becoming key supporting elements for the proliferation of electronic portable instruments.

Semiconductor-based, intelligent sensors and instruments are paving the way for wide applications of wireless portable instrument networks. There are many products and complete systems appearing in the marketplace offered by diverse interest vendors.

References

1. T. Brooks, “Wireless technology for industrial sensor and control networks,” SIcon/01, in *Proc. First ISA/IEEE, Sensors for Industry Conference*, pp. 73–77, 2001.
2. M. Dunbar, “Plug-and-play sensors in wireless networks”, *IEEE Instru. Meas. Mag.* vol. 4, no. 1, pp. 19–23, 2001.
3. S.A. Dyer, Ed., *Survey of Instrumentation and Measurement*, New York: Wiley, 2001.
4. R. Frank, *Understanding Smart Sensors*, Norwood, MA: Artech House, 1996.
5. H. Eren, *Electronic Portable Instruments-Design and Applications*, Boca Raton, FL: CRC Press, 2004.
6. J. Fraden, *AIP Handbook of Modern Sensors-Physics, Design and Application*, New York: American Institute of Physics, 1993.
7. A. Girson, “Handheld devices, wireless communications, and smart sensors: what it all means for field service,” *Sensors*, vol. 19, no. 1, 14; see also pp. 16–20, 2002.
8. P.J. Lee, Ed., *Engineering Superconductivity*, New York: Wiley, 2001.
9. J.G. Webster, Ed., *Wiley Encyclopedia of Electrical and Electronic Engineering*, New York: Wiley, 1999.

5.3 G (LabVIEW™) Software Engineering

Christopher G. Relf

The LabVIEW (Laboratory Virtual Instrument Engineering Workbench) development system has certainly matured beyond its original role of simple laboratory bench experiment automation and data collection—it has become a full-featured programming language (known as G) in its own right. Although National Instruments (the creators of LabVIEW) continues to push its rapid prototyping and code development virtues, an increasing number of G software developers are relying on advanced programming techniques, far beyond those initially apparent.

The documentation that ships with a standard LabVIEW installation is sufficient to assist the development of simple applications by users not initially familiar with LabVIEW, and the various online documents provided by National Instruments and third-party vendors extend that learning experience. This chapter attempts to describe some of the features, methods, and more obscure tidbits of programming expertise that are of use to the advanced G software engineer.

Data Types

Like most modern programming languages, G code uses various data types. These data types allow for efficient data storage, transmission, manipulation, and processing of information. Simple data types include the integer, floating point, strings, paths, arrays, clusters, and reference numbers (*refnums*). The method G uses to store data depends on its type, and it is important to understand the way data will reside in memory. Savvy use of data types decreases the overall memory footprint of an application, minimizes data coercion errors, and improves system performance.

Figure 5.18 lists representations of the standard numerical data types available to G. Others exist, including the extended-precision float, although its representation is platform dependent, as shown in Figure 5.19. (The representation of an extended-precision float is identical to a double-precision float when using HP-UX.)

Unlike numerical values, strings are represented by dimension-defined arrays (Figure 5.20). Each array consists of a 4-byte integer that contains the number of characters required to represent the string, and

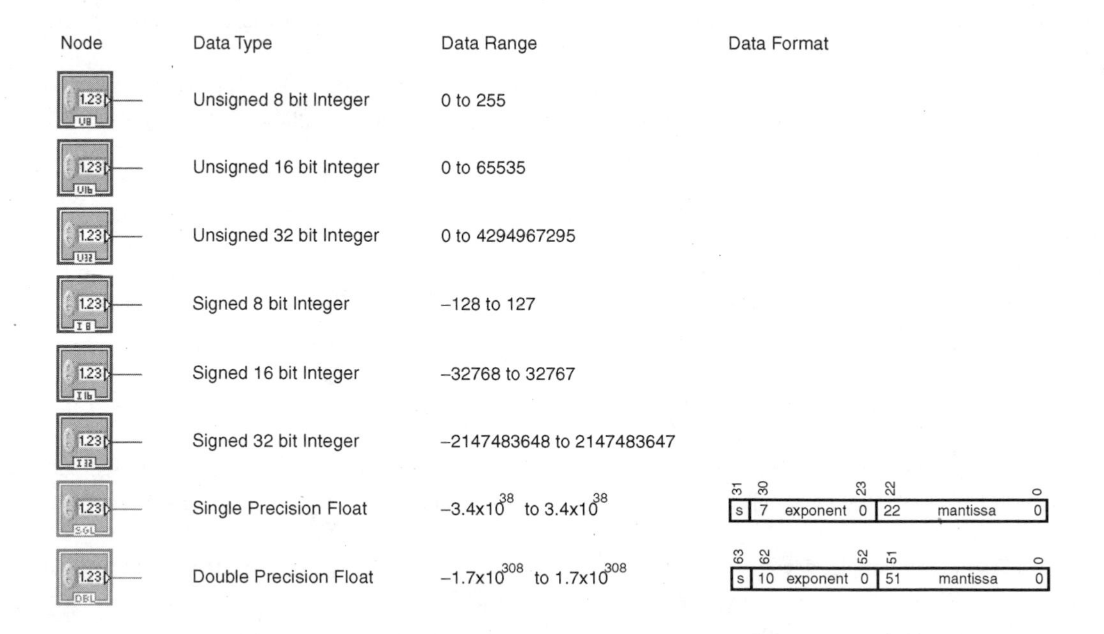

FIGURE 5.18 Numerical data types.

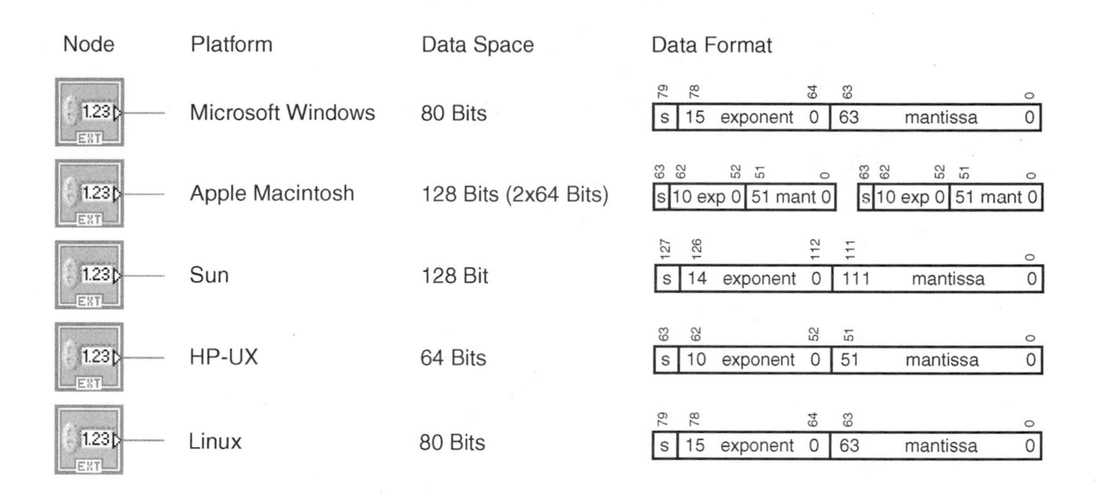

FIGURE 5.19 Extended precision data type.

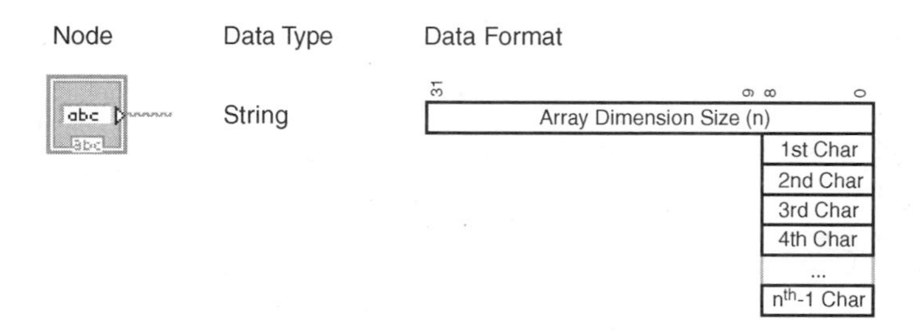

FIGURE 5.20 String data type.

subsequent byte integers that represent each character. Therefore, as the highest number that will fit into a 4-byte word is 4,294,967,296, the longest string that can be continuously represented has 4,294,967,296 characters.

Paths are also stored as arrays, although the format is different from strings. The first element of a path array data format describes the *path type*, which is determined as shown in Table 5.5.

The second element of the path array data format defines the *number of path components*. For example, the following path

```
\\PC_NAME\DATA\TEMP.DAT
```

contains three components: the PC name, then a folder, and a file. Each of the components is then described in the array as a double-element pair—the first element is a byte that represents the character length of the

TABLE 5.5 Path Type Descriptions

Path Type	Description	Microsoft Windows Examples
0	Absolute	C:\DATA\TEMP.DAT
1	Relative	\DATA\TEMP.DAT
2	Undefined	
3	Universal naming convention	\\PC_NAME\DATA\ TEMP.DAT
$4 \rightarrow \infty$	Undefined	

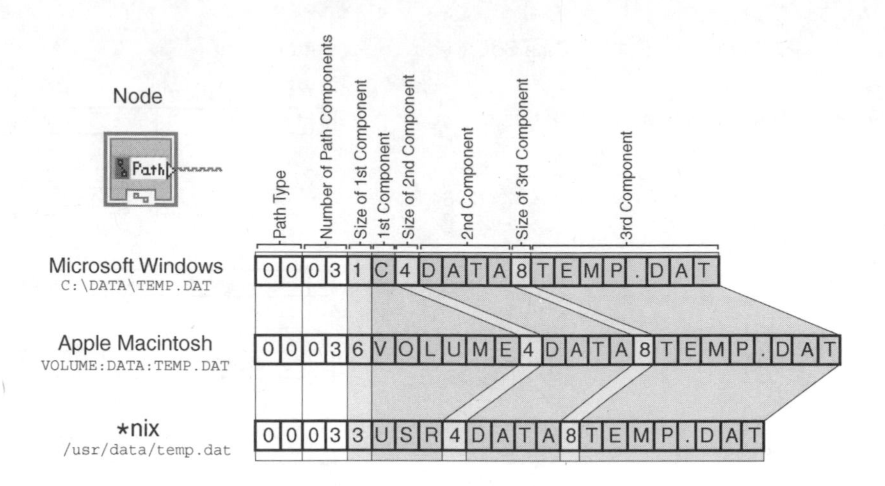

FIGURE 5.21 Path data type representations.

component, and the second element is the component. As might be expected, path representations are platform dependent, as shown in Figure 5.21.

Polymorphism

Considered a generally underrated technique, polymorphic virtual instruments (VIs) are simply a collection of related VIs that can perform functions on differing data types. For example, a VI that loads a waveform from a file could return the result as an array of values or the waveform data type (Figure 5.22).

While it is valid to create two separate VIs to perform these functions, it often makes more sense combining them into one polymorphic library (Figure 5.23). When a polymorphic VI is dropped onto a wiring diagram, the user can select the data "type" to use, and the appropriate VI is loaded (as shown in Figure 5.24).

It is considered good form to include a polymorphic VI and its daughter VIs in one LabVIEW library, as a polymorphic VI alone contains no code, only references to its daughters. Using this method assists in

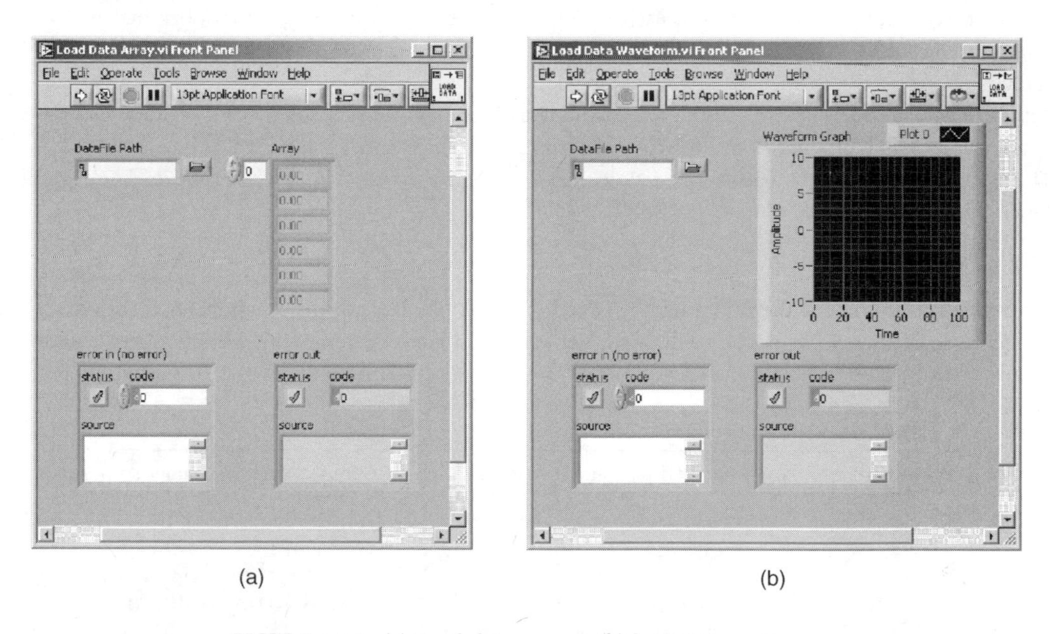

FIGURE 5.22 (a) Load data array, 5; (b) load data waveform.

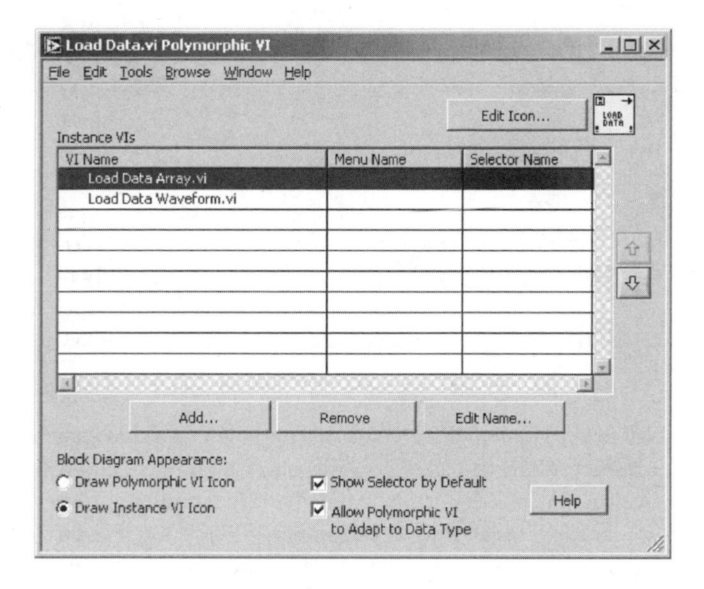

FIGURE 5.23 Creating a polymorphic VI.

code distribution, and minimizes the incidence of broken polymorphic VIs unable to find their daughters. Using polymorphic VIs can increase the size of an application, as all of its daughters, irrespective of whether they are used in the application, are saved in the application.

Polymorphism is already used in several vi.lib VIs, including many of those found in the data acquisition function subpalette.

Units

Associating units to raw data adds an additional level of numerical checking when evaluating expressions and formulas. Incorporating units also adds the ability to display data to the user in dynamically controlled units, without the need for code to perform conversions.

A data node's unit association can be found by right-clicking on the node, and selecting Visible Items → Units (as shown in Figure 5.25). Once the unit label is displayed, the user can enter a unit type (a comprehensive list can be found in the LabVIEW online help), such as g for "grams." Now that a unit is

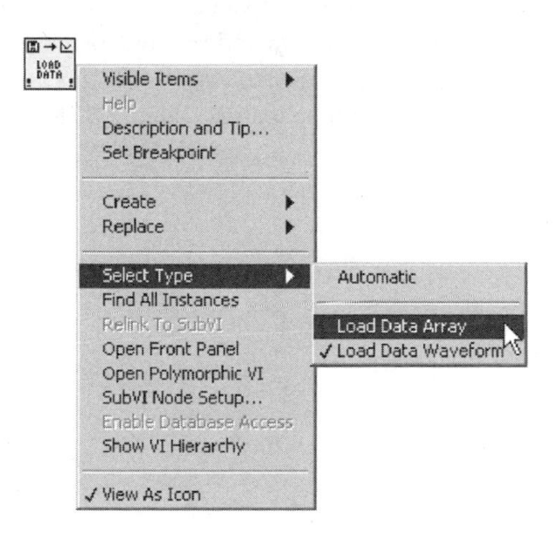

FIGURE 5.24 Select polymorphic type.

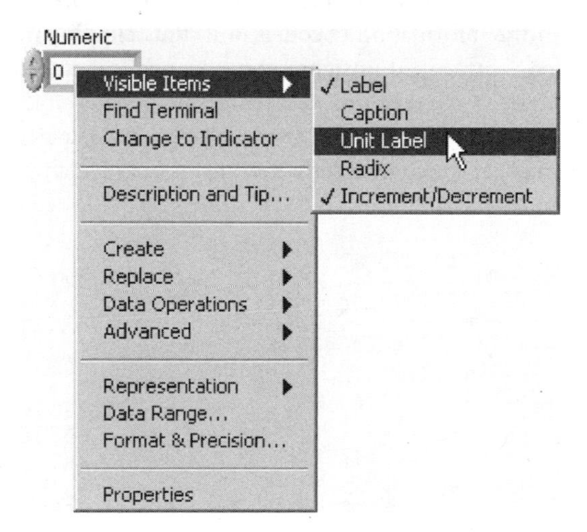

FIGURE 5.25 Selecting unit label.

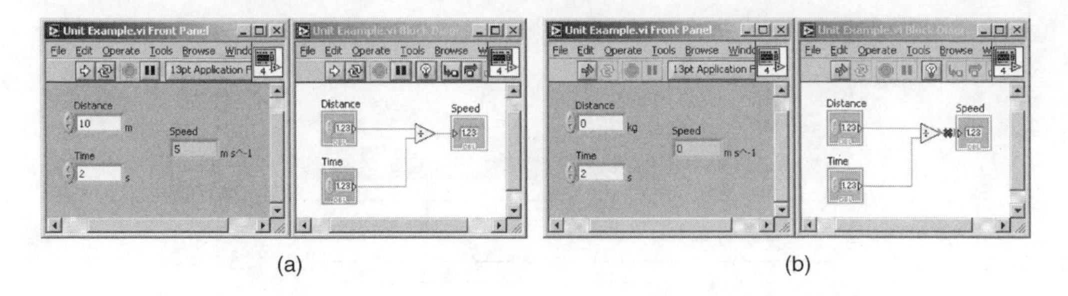

FIGURE 5.26 (a) Unit example OK; (b) unit example not OK.

associated with the node, all data to that node are converted to the unit specified, and all data from it bears its unit type. VIs that do not respect mathematical unit relationships are broken, and will not run. Figure 5.26(a) shows a VI where a distance (m) value is divided by a time (s) value, resulting in a speed (ms^{-1}) value. If the distance control's unit is changed to an incompatible type (e.g., kilogram in Figure 5.26(b)), the G development system reports a bad wire between the division primitive and the $msec^{-1}$ indicator, suggesting an incompatible unit.

The LabVIEW built-in functions, such as Add and Multiply, are polymorphic with respect to units, so they automatically handle different units. In order to build a subVI with the same polymorphic unit capability, one must create a separate daughter VI to deal with each unit configuration.

Data Coercion

When performing functions on data, it is possible to combine differing representations in the same structure. When this occurs, LabVIEW must decide on how to convert the incident types to a common format before executing the function. As shown in Figure 5.27, the widest data representation is chosen for the operation and subsequent display and/or manipulation.

The coercion of the 32-bit integer is demonstrated by the coercion dot on the input terminal of the function, indicating that the data type of the data input at this terminal is changed before the function is executed. Although in the example shown in Figure 5.27 no data are lost (the narrower data type is expanded), data coercion can lead to inefficient memory usage (storing numbers in a data format beyond what is required to accurately represent the physical data) and occasionally the loss of data (coercing data to a type narrower than the information encoded in it, thus clipping the data to its highest permitted value, or value wrapping when using signed/unsigned conversions). It is considered good form to hunt down and remove coercion dots from one's code, as they can represent coercion of data that are either beyond the software engineer's control and/or knowledge. Explicitly performing data coercion using the Conversion subpalette (Figure 5.28) of the Numerical function palette minimizes the incidence of poor block diagram comprehension.

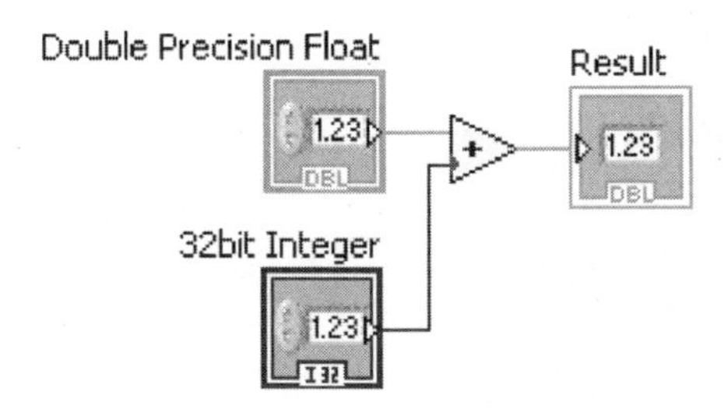

FIGURE 5.27 Data representation coercion.

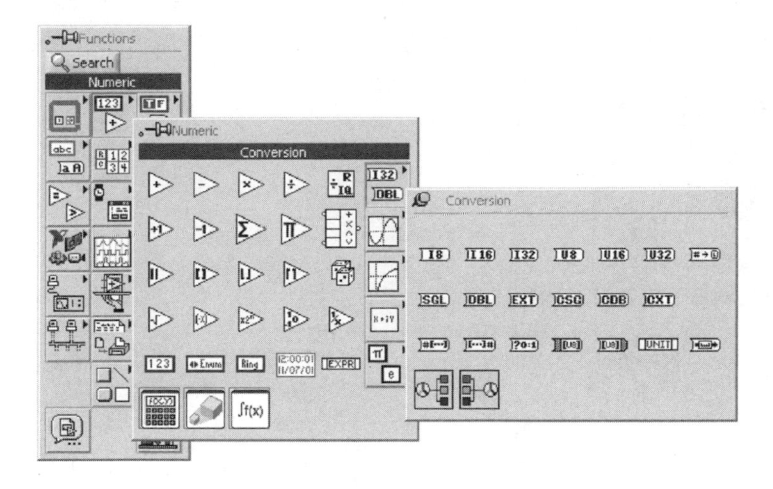

FIGURE 5.28 The Conversion subpalette.

Data coercion can be very important when considering application memory management. For example, if a floating point is inputted to the *N* node of a *for loop*, its data is coerced to a 32-bit integer format. If an upstream calculation causes the floating point to become *NaN* (not a number), it coerces to a very large number (on the order of 2×10^9), resulting in a large number of for loop iterations. LabVIEW will attempt to allocate an appropriate amount of memory to execute the loop (and handle any data inputs and outputs), and often crash trying. This issue may seem intermittent, as it will only occur when an upstream calculation fails. (This example was provided by Michael Porter, Porter Consulting, LLC.)

Error Handling

Writing VIs and subVIs that incorporate error handling is considered good form, not only to allow the user indication of abnormal software execution, but also to allow the software to make decisions based on the status of previous operations. Including error clusters in your code assists in troubleshooting, modularity, and user friendliness.

The Error Cluster

The error cluster is a special predefined LabVIEW cluster that is used to contain error status information (Figure 5.29 and Figure 5.30). The cluster contains the following three components:

Name	Data Type	Description
Status	Boolean	Indicates if an error has occurred (TRUE = error, FALSE = no error).
Code	32-bit integer	A standardized error code specific to the particular error. LabVIEW has a table of default error codes, although the user is able to define custom error codes. See below for more information.
Source	String	Textual information often describing the error, the VI it occurred within, and the call chain.

Usage

Although one of the most obvious methods of conditional code execution might be to unbundle the *Status* Boolean of the error cluster and feed it to the conditional terminal of a case structure (Figure 5.31(a)), the complete cluster can be wired to it instead (Figure 5.31(b)).

The functionality of the code in Figure 5.31(a) and (b) is identical, although its readability is vastly improved as the second example colors the case structure green for the *No Error* case, and red for the *Error* case. Wrapping the entire code of a subVI within a conditional case structure based on the error input allows VIs at higher levels to continue functioning, without executing code that could be useless or even dangerous when an error has occurred. Consider the simple report generation example shown in Figure 5.32.

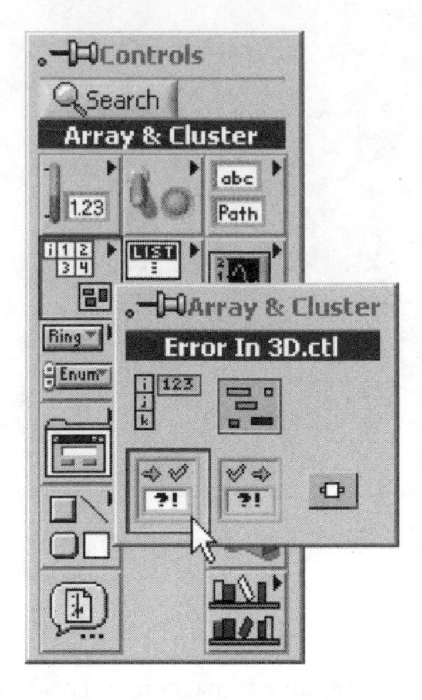

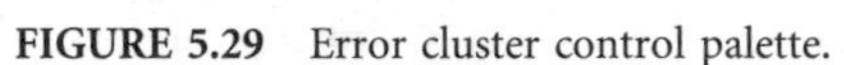
FIGURE 5.29 Error cluster control palette.

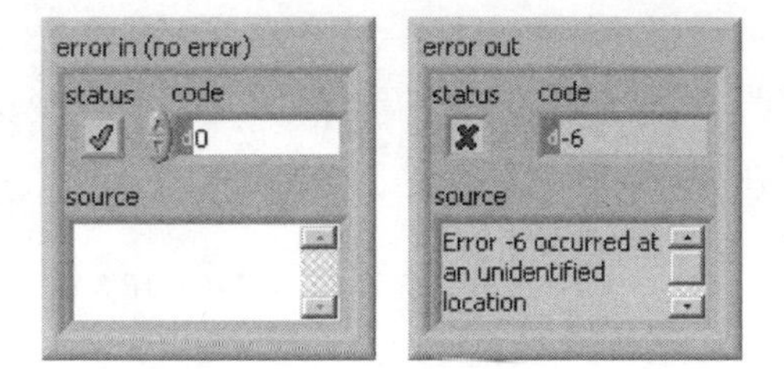

FIGURE 5.30 Front panel error clusters.

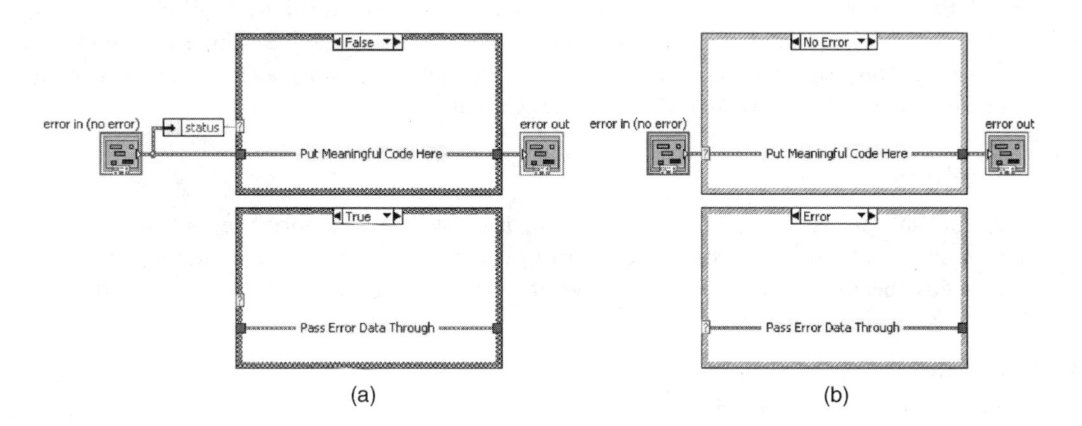

FIGURE 5.31 (a) Wire error cluster status into the conditional node 14; (b) wire error cluster directly into the conditional node.

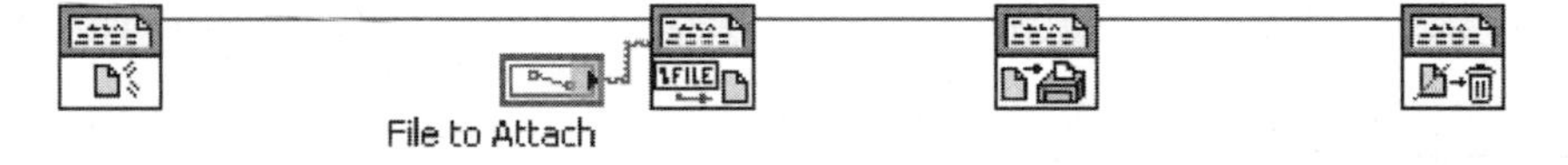

FIGURE 5.32 Create and print report without error handling.

A report is initially created, a file is then attached, the report is printed, and finally destroyed. The dataflow link between these subVIs is the report's reference number (*refnum*), which ensures each execute in a predefined order. If each of the subVIs execute without error, then the process completes successfully. Conversely, if one of the subVIs encounters an error, subsequent subVIs are unaware of the problem and attempt to execute regardless.

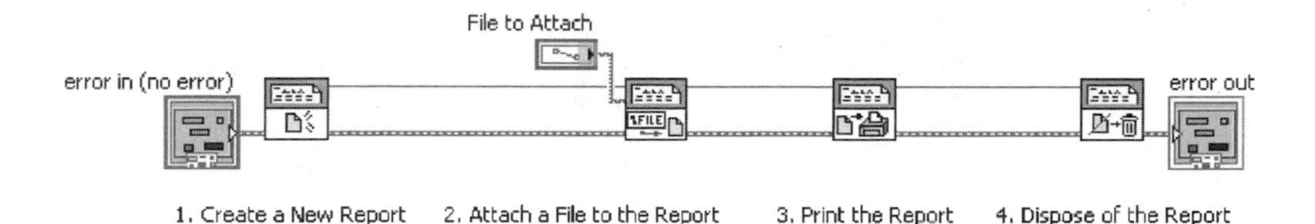

FIGURE 5.33 Create and print report with error handling.

In the example above, an error in the *Attach a File to the Report* subVI will not cause the *Print the Report* subVI to fail, resulting in a blank report print. If effective error handling is introduced (Figure 5.33), the Print the Report subVI will know if an error has occurred before its execution is requested. If the functional code inside the *Print the Report* subVI is enclosed within a conditional case structure based on the error input, the printing code is bypassed, and the data in the error cluster is passed on to the next subVI.

To attain a higher level of user interaction, standard subVIs exist to alert the user to an error on the error cluster, and prompt for conditional actions. The Simple Error Handler.vi (Figure 5.34) allows for a basic level of error cluster status reporting, displaying detected errors in a dialog box, and prompting the user for an action based on the *type of dialog* input (for example, OK, Cancel, Stop, etc.).

The Simple Error Handler.vi is a wrapper for the lower level General Error Handler.vi. The latter (Figure 5.35) is more configurable, and permits the dynamic definition of custom error codes, and error exception handling.

LabVIEW 7.0 brings with it an addition to the error handling function palette, Clear Errors.vi (Figure 5.36). This VI is simply an *error in* control and an *error out* indicator, which are not linked on the wiring diagram, causing any errors on the wired error link to be cancelled.

This VI can be useful when constructing custom error-handling VIs, including dialog boxes allowing user interaction that is not covered by the simple and general error-handling VIs, but should not be used alone. Although dumping the errors from the error cluster may be tempting, one *must* incorporate appropriate code to handle them.

Wiring Errors into a SubVI Connector Pane

As described above, subVIs have an associated connector pane, and the placement of error cluster inputs and output is generally in the lower quadrants (*error in* on the left, and *error out* on the right), with corresponding exclamation marks over the connectors on the subVI's icon (as shown in Figure 5.37).

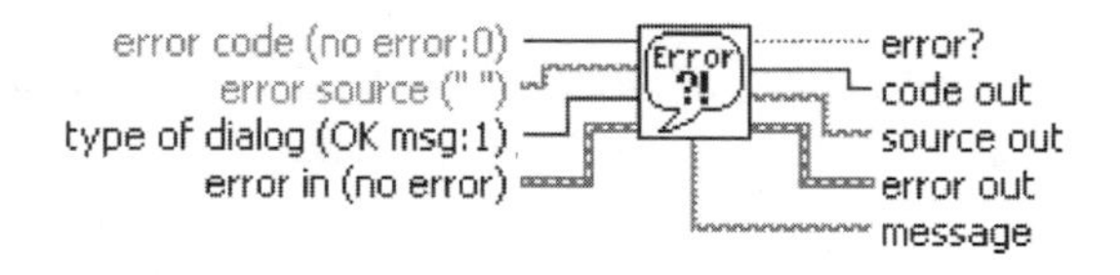

FIGURE 5.34 Simple error handler.

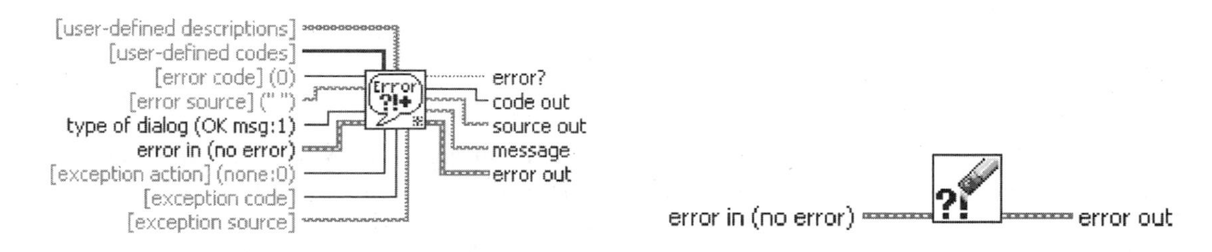

FIGURE 5.35 General error handler.

FIGURE 5.36 Clear errors.

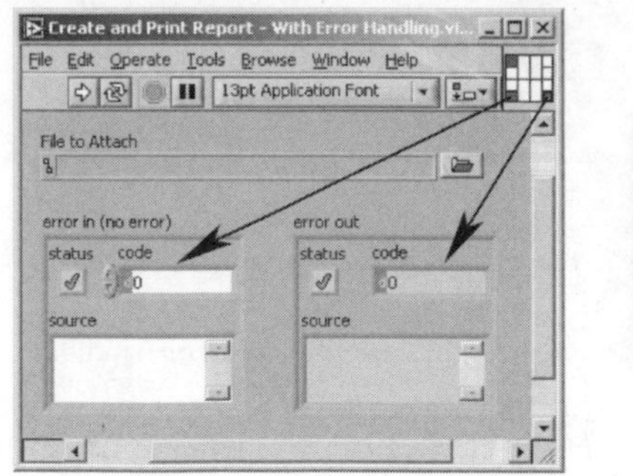

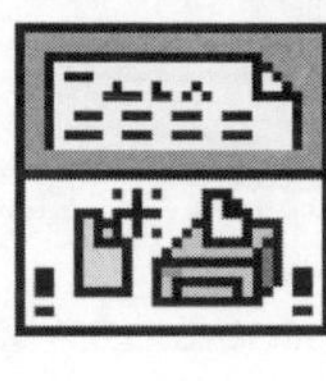

FIGURE 5.37 SubVI error cluster connector pane placement.

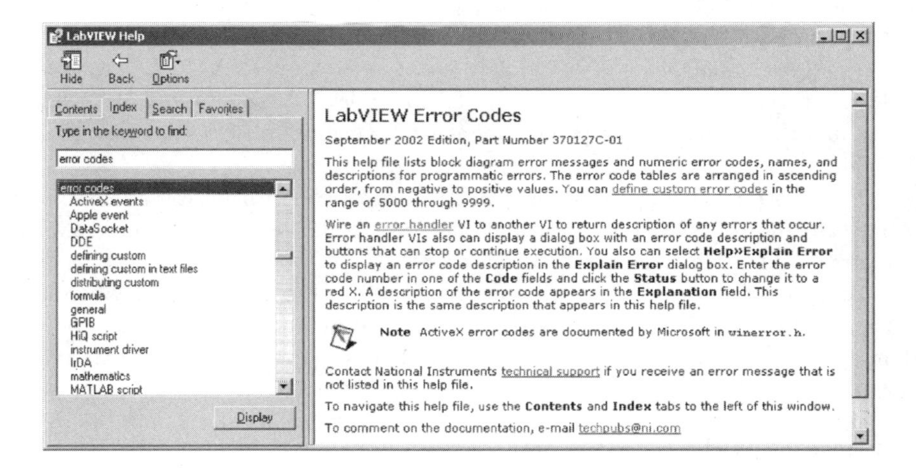

FIGURE 5.38 LabVIEW help error codes.

Default Error Codes

The LabVIEW execution system contains a large list of standard and specific errors, encouraging the reuse of generic codes across applications. A list of generic errors codes can be found under the LabVIEW *Help* menu (Figure 5.38).

Another method of parsing a small number of errors is to select the *Help*→ *Explain Error* menu item. This will launch an interface that allows the user to enter an error code, and a brief explanation is displayed (Figure 5.39). This interface is also accessible by right-clicking on a front panel error cluster, and selecting *Explain Error.*

Custom Error Codes

National Instruments has set several error codes aside for custom use. If an existing error code does not adequately describe the error condition, the user can define custom codes that are specific to the application. Codes between 5000 through to 9999 are available for use, and do not need to conform to any other application. Although General Error Handler.vi can be used to define custom error codes, one can also create an XML file in the labview\user.lib\errors directory that contains custom error codes and their

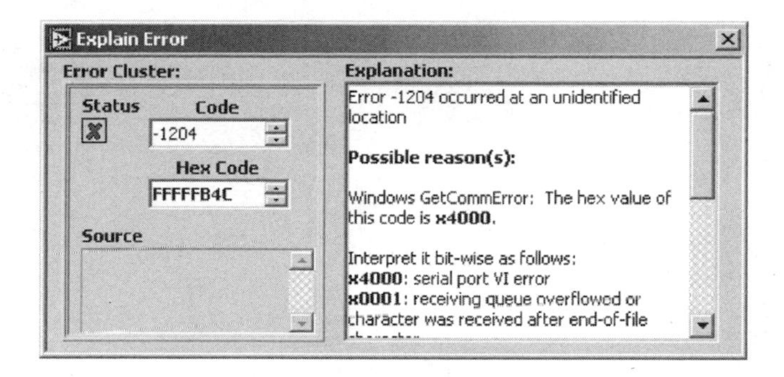

FIGURE 5.39 Explain error.

descriptions. This method is particularly useful if the user requires custom error codes to apply to several applications, or if the codes are used by several software engineers in a team or are to be distributed with an application.

For example, the XML filename must be in the format *-errors.txt (where * is user definable), and the internal file structure must adhere to the following format:

```
< ?XMLVersion = ''1.0'' >
< nidocument >
< nicomment >
This is a custom error code definition file for my application.
</nicomment >
< nierrorcode = ''5000'' >
User Access Denied!
Contact the Security Department to gain clearance to perform this function.
</nierror >
< nierrorcode = ''5001'' >
User Unknown.
Contact the People Development Department.
</nierror >
< nierrorcode = ''5100'' >
Driver Unable to Contact Instrument Database.
Contact the Software Engineering Department Helpdesk.
< /nierror >
< nierrorcode = ''5200'' >
Plug - In Module in R&D mode - not to be used in Production Environment.
Contact the New Product Development Group.
</nierror >
</nidocument >
```

As can be seen, a file comment can be created within the <nicomment> tag space. Each custom error is defined as an <nierror> with its associated error code, and its error message is then placed inside the <nierror> tag space. Although hand coding a custom error code XML file is possible, the Error Code File Editor (**Tools→Advanced→Edit Error Codes**) provides a simple GUI for file creation and editing (see Figure 5.40). Once custom error code files have been created and/or altered, LabVIEW must be restarted for the changes to take effect.

It is often useful to define error code bands during the project planning stage, setting aside bands for specific related error groups.

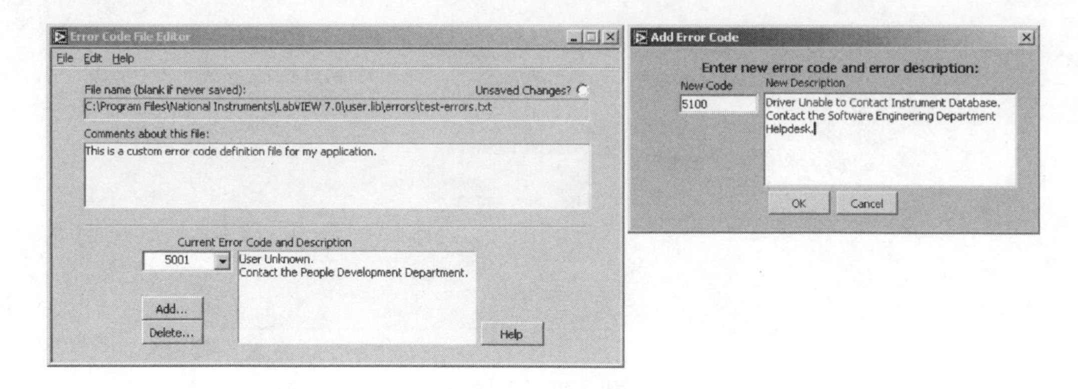

FIGURE 5.40 Error code file editor.

Shortcuts

Keyboard Shortcuts[1]

Most developers soon realize that their mouse or pointing device is not the only way to perform tasks; in fact, some actions can only be achieved through keyboard sequences (or *shortcuts*). Once committed to memory, keyboard shortcuts are often a faster way to achieve tasks that might otherwise take several mouse maneuvers. Appearing below are most of the common and some of the obscure keyboard shortcuts that LabVIEW offers. Occasionally the only way to achieve a task is to use the keyboard in combination with the mouse, and these cases have also been included for completeness.

LabVIEW offers the developer a wealth of useful keyboard shortcuts. The shortcuts presented here refer to LabVIEW installed on the Windows operating system. Substitutions for the Ctrl key apply for other operating systems, as detailed in Table 5.6.

The most commonly encountered tasks faced by a LabVIEW programmer focus on constructing and wiring the block diagram of a VI, while the next most common set of tasks is the manipulation of objects on the front panel. Switching between the front panel and the block diagram is a regular task. A shortcut to achieve panel/diagram switching is generally at the top of a shortcut enthusiast's "commonly used" list (assuming the enthusiast has mastered the automatic tool selection mode, and is therefore not continually switching tools with Space or Tab). Pressing Ctrl-E will change the focus between the block diagram and the front panel of the currently selected VI.

Tool Palette Shortcuts

An automatic tool selection tool palette mode was introduced with LabVIEW 6.1, where the active tool automatically changes to a selection that the development system considers the most useful as the cursor is moved over different parts of the front panel or block diagram. For the LabVIEW programmer who is accustomed to manually selecting the appropriate tool (whether by using the Tools Palette, or a keyboard shortcut), this takes some familiarization. Committing certain keyboard shortcuts to memory will enhance the automatic tool selection mode, making it a more useful (and less frustrating!) aid.

When automatic tool selection is enabled:

- Shift will temporarily switch to the positioning tool.
- Shift-Ctrl while cursor over panel or diagram space switches to the scroll tool.
- Double-click label text or constant values to edit them with the labeling tool.
- Ctrl while the cursor is over an object will switch to the next most useful tool. This is useful when the mouse pointer is over a wire, allowing the user to switch quickly between the positioning and wiring tools.

[1]This information on shortcuts was provided by Peter Badcock, engineering consultant, Australia.

TABLE 5.6 Control Key Substitutions across LabVIEW-Supported Platforms

Operating System	Control Key
Windows™	Ctrl
Macintosh™	Option or Command (context dependent)
Sun™/UNIX®	Meta
Linux™/HP-UX™	Alt

Note that Shift-Tab enables and disables the automatic tool selection mode.
When automatic tool selection is disabled:

- Tab selects the next tool on the tools palette.
- Space toggles between the positioning tool and the scrolling tool on the front panel, or the positioning tool and the wiring tool on the block diagram.

Miscellaneous Front Panel and Block Diagram Shortcuts

To create additional space in the selection, Ctrl-click (for operating systems other than Windows, use Shift+Ctrl+Click) from a clear point on the panel or diagram and select an area. The cursor keys (←, ↑, →, ↓) nudge selections 1 pixel in the direction chosen, whereas simultaneously holding down Shift while moving a selection with a cursor key increases the distance moved to 8 pixels. Other miscellaneous shortcuts include those listed in Table 5.7.

General Shortcuts

A complete list of keyboard shortcuts for the main pull-down menus can be found on the LabVIEW Quick Reference Card (shipped with LabVIEW and accessible in the online help). Some commonly used keyboard shortcuts include those shown in Table 5.8.

GOOP

G is well known for its speed of code development that provides engineers with a rapid prototyping advantage. This advantage is particularly evident when working with small projects with flat structures. However, as project complexity grows, initial stages of software architecture planning become vitally important.

GOOP (graphical object-oriented programming) is a method for developing object-oriented code, and is created using an external object model (often referred to as "LabVIEW external object" oriented programming, or LEO). Using GOOP has three main advantages to application development: code maintainability, scalability, and reusability. GOOP is the most common form of OOP with LabVIEW, and has been used successfully in many commercially available applications developed by G software engineers.

By implementing GOOP classes, you can take advantage of standard OOP analysis and design tools, including Microsoft Visual Modeler, and apply principles that describe object-oriented design and

TABLE 5.7 Other Miscellaneous Shortcuts

Shortcut	Description
Ctrl-double click	On a clear point, places text (otherwise known as a free label)
Shift-right click	Displays the tool palette
Ctrl-double click	On a sub VI, opens its block diagram
Ctrl-click-drag	An object with the positioning tool to duplicate it
Shift-click	The block diagram to remove the last wiring point
Esc	Cancels a wire route (dashed)
Ctrl-B	Removes broken wires (Beware: nonvisible broken wires may exist)
Drag-space	Activate autowiring when moving an element on the block diagram (Autowiring only occurs when first placing an element, or a copy of an element, on the block diagram)

TABLE 5.8 Common Shortcuts

Shortcut	Description	Comments
Ctrl-S	Saves the currently selected VI	
Ctrl-Q	Quits LabVIEW	The user is prompted to save any open unsaved VIs
Ctrl-C	Copy a selection to the clipboard	
Ctrl-X	Cut a selection and place it on the clipboard	
Ctrl-V	Paste the data from the clipboard	Pasting data from a previous LabVIEW session will insert an image representing the data, and not the data itself
Ctrl-F	Find object or text	
Ctrl-R	Run the currently selected VI	
Ctrl-	Aborts a running VI	Only available when Show Abort Button option in VI Properties»Windows AppearanceShow» Abort Button is selected
Ctrl-E	Toggle focus between the front panel and block diagram	
Ctrl-H	Display context help	
Ctrl-W	Close the current window.	The block diagram is automatically closed when a front panel is closed using this shortcut
Ctrl-Z	Undo the last action	

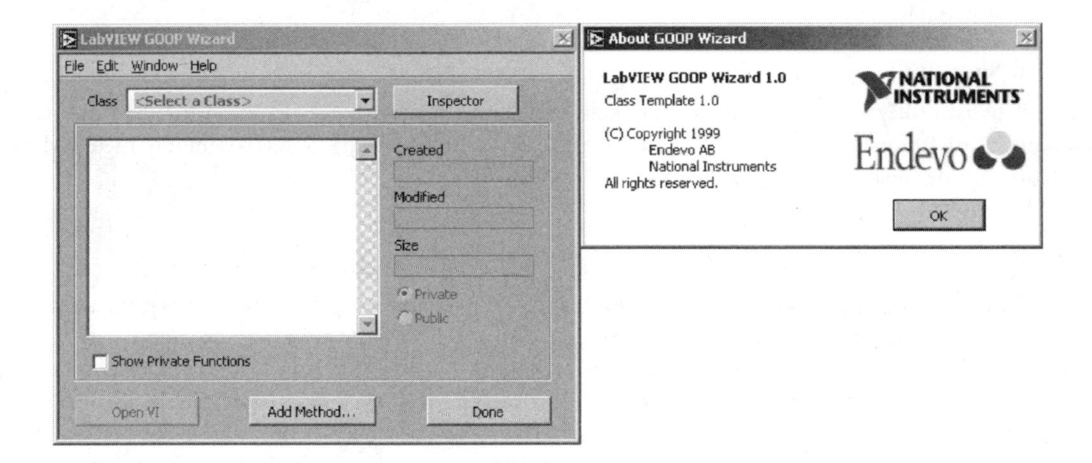

FIGURE 5.41 GOOP wizard.

development. The OOP component-based development approach to developing applications enhances the traditional data-flow programming paradigm used in G applications, and using tools including the GOOP Wizard (access *www.ni.com*, and enter "GOOP" in the Search box for more information) allows you to create and manage OOP classes easily (Figure 5.41).

Once the fundamental concepts are understood, GOOP is easy to use, allows encapsulation, and permits you to create, control, and destroy as many objects as required. Both functions and data can be accessed using LabVIEW refnums, which simplifies wiring diagrams and encourages dynamic and modularized code.

Code Distribution

Distributing code to encourage multiple programmer input and commercial reward can be an important part of software development, and hence should not be considered only in the final moments of a project. Depending on the purpose of distribution, the package format created can vary significantly.

llbs

A VI library (*.llb) is a National Instruments proprietary file that can contain several VIs and some of their settings. Files that are saved into an llb are lightly compressed, and can be set as *top level* (denotes which VIs should be launched when their respective llb is opened) or *companion*. Other than that, an llb is formless; all of the files reside at one level (i.e., you cannot create subdirectories or sub-llbs in a VI library). Although a library has a flat structure, it is possible to assign one of two levels to a VI in a library. A top-level VI will launch automatically when opened from your operating system's file explorer, whereas a normal-level VI will only open if explicitly opened from within the library. (A new feature to LabVIEW 7.0 allows Windows Explorer to navigate inside G libraries, effectively bypassing top-level assignments.) It is also acceptable to assign more than one VI in a library as top level, although this can make window negotiation difficult, as they all will be launched when the library is opened. Figure 5.42 demonstrates a library with one top-level VI.

Development Distribution Library

A development distribution library contains all custom VIs and controls that have been created in the project, so that it can be successfully opened and executed on a PC with a similar LabVIEW configuration installed. VIs from vi.lib and add-on toolkits are not included in a development library, as it is assumed that environments used for subsequent openings of the library will have these installed.

Application Distribution Library

An application distribution library is an llb file that contains all of the VIs listed in a development library, and all others that are used in the application. VIs from vi.lib and toolkits are included, as are all custom VIs and controls. Distributing an application library is useful when archiving an application, including all of the components used to execute it.

Diagram Access

Altering a user's access to a VI's diagram can minimize code theft and ensure that the VIs are opened with an appropriate version of LabVIEW. Setting a password to a VI's block diagram prevents users from accessing the code diagram and understanding hierarchical dependencies between modules. To change a VI's status, access the Security VI property (Figure 5.43) and select one of the settings shown in Table 5.9.

An extreme method of code protection is to remove the block diagram altogether, and can be achieved by performing a custom save (Figure 5.44), using File → Save with Options.

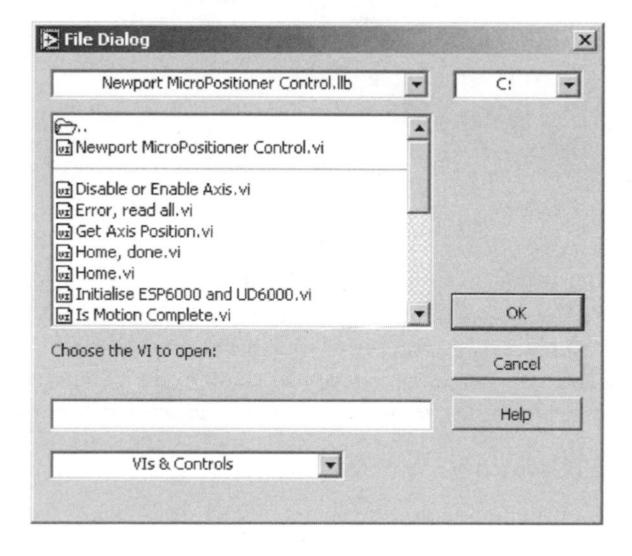

FIGURE 5.42 A library with a top-level VI.

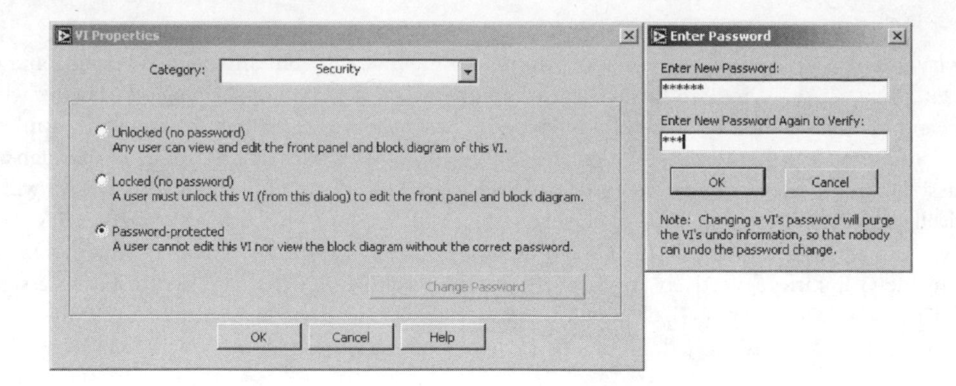

FIGURE 5.43 Set block diagram password.

TABLE 5.9 Block Diagram Security Access Levels

Security Level	Description
Unlocked (no password)	The default for a new VI. Permits read/write access to the block diagram
Locked (no password)	Access to the block diagram is prohibited until the user changes the security to *Unlocked*. A password is not required to change security settings
Password protected[a]	The highest level of block diagram security; access is prohibited unless the user enters the correct password

[a]Due to the nature of LabVIEW VIs, the password is not recoverable from the file. If you forget a password, you are unable to parse the file to "crack" it.

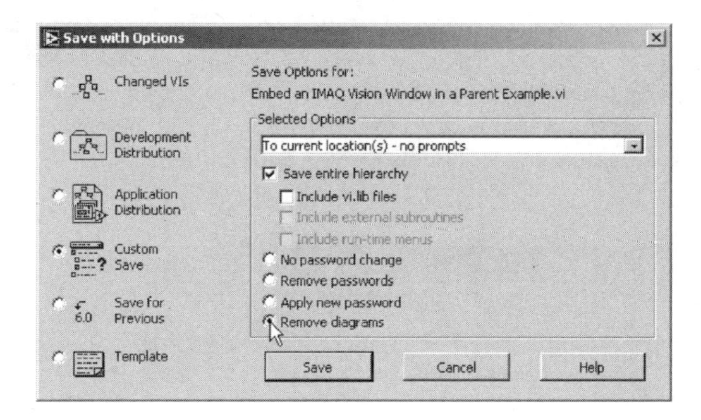

FIGURE 5.44 Remove diagrams.

When upgrading a VI from a previous version of LabVIEW, the diagram is recompiled; therefore, removing the diagrams from your VIs will prevent them from being opened with a version of LabVIEW other than the version used to create the VI. This minimizes conversion errors that may occur between versions (e.g., if your VI uses functions from vi.lib), and enhances commercial code control (limiting the lifetime of a VI to a particular version of LabVIEW, requiring users to obtain new versions when migrating between major versions of LabVIEW).

Application Building (Creating Executables)

Often left to the last minute in application development, building stand-alone executable code may not be as straightforward as one might expect. External code libraries, target operating systems, engines, and licenses must be considered before attempting to build an application.

The Runtime Engine (RTE)

Built executables require elements of the LabVIEW RTE to execute. The RTE should be distributed with your applications, as the target PC may not have it installed, and your applications will therefore fail to execute. The location of the RTE installed on a LabVIEW development PC is:

```
..\National Instruments\shared\LabVIEW Run – Time\Version\
```

and the following redistributable version is located on the LabVIEW installation CD-ROM:.

```
..\LVRun TimeEng\
```

Although manual distribution of the RTE is possible, it can be automated when distributing your built software, by using an installer as detailed below. In some cases, the installation of the RTE is not necessary. (This method is not authorized or supported by National Instruments and does not support DataSocket, NI-Reports, or 3D Graphs.) If an executable is a simple one, it may not need the RTE to be installed on the target machine; all one needs to do is include some of the engine's files with the exe for it to work. To determine whether this method will work with a particular built executable, copy the following files and folders into the folder containing the exe:

```
..\National Instruments\shared\nicontdt.dll.
..\National Instruments\shared.dll.
..\National Instruments\shared\LabVIEWRun – Time\ver\*
  (including all subdirectories)
```

Using the LabVIEW 6.1 development system as an example, the exe directory would look something like the following:

```
\AppDirectory.exe.
..\AppDirectory.ini.
..\AppDirectory\My_Apps_DLLs(if_any).
..\AppDirectory\nicontdt.dll.
..\AppDirectory\nicont.dll.
..\AppDirectory\lvapp.rsc.
..\AppDirectory\lvjpeg.dll.
..\AppDirectory\lvpng.dll.
..\AppDirectory\lvrt.dll.
..\AppDirectory\mesa.dll.
..\AppDirectory\serpdrv.
..\AppDirectory\models\*.
..\AppDirectory\errors\*.
..\AppDirectory\script\*
```

When the executable is launched on a PC without the RTE installed, it should find all of the RTE files it requires in the application's root directory, and execute normally. This method can be particularly useful when distributing autorun presentations on CD-ROMs.

Reverse Engineering Built Executables. As built executables have a similar structure to VI libraries, it is possible to extract and use the diagramless VIs within. Simply change the extension of the executable file to llb, and open the library within LabVIEW. One should be careful when designing the architecture of a commercial application, as this G executable characteristic can allow users to reverse engineer an executable, effectively accessing the functionality of the SubVIs within the executable.

Run Time Licenses (RTLs)

Distributing a simple executable to the world is free; the software engineer developed the code, so he or she may sell and distribute the resulting code desired. When the software contains specialist code that the software engineer did not write, then the users may need to pay the author a small amount for each instance of their code that is on-sold as a portion of the application. Products that currently require the inclusion of a runtime license include the National Instruments Vision toolkit, meaning that any applications released that use Vision VIs must be accompanied by an official NI Vision toolkit RTL, available from NI. Always check with the vendor of any software tools that you are planning to incorporate in an application, indicating the RTL costs at the project proposal stage.

Installers

Rather than providing a single executable file to customers, it is almost always preferable to pack your application into an installer. An installer is a mechanism that encourages the simple installation of the developer's application, support files (including RTEs is required), registration of external components (ActiveX controls, DLLs, documentation, links to web pages, etc.), and manipulation of the operating system (registry alteration). Installers provide intuitive graphical user interfaces that assist end users to customize your application installation to their needs (including the selection of components, installation destination locations, readme file display, etc.) and provide a professional finish to your product. Modern installers also have automatic support for damaged installations, and a facility to uninstall your product cleanly, returning the end user's system to a state comparable to that before installation. The NI LabVIEW Application Builder contains a simple installer that is often sufficient for small applications that do not require advanced operating system alterations, whereas there are several commercially available installers (Figure 5.45). One such installer, Setup2Go, fulfills many of the advanced installation requirements and has a very simple interface to package your software product (more information on Setup2Go can be found at *http://dev4pc.com/setup2go.html*).

Open Source G: Distributed Development

One of the most powerful tools available to software engineers today is open source project development. Unlike other engineering branches (including structural, electrical, etc.), software engineering projects can be

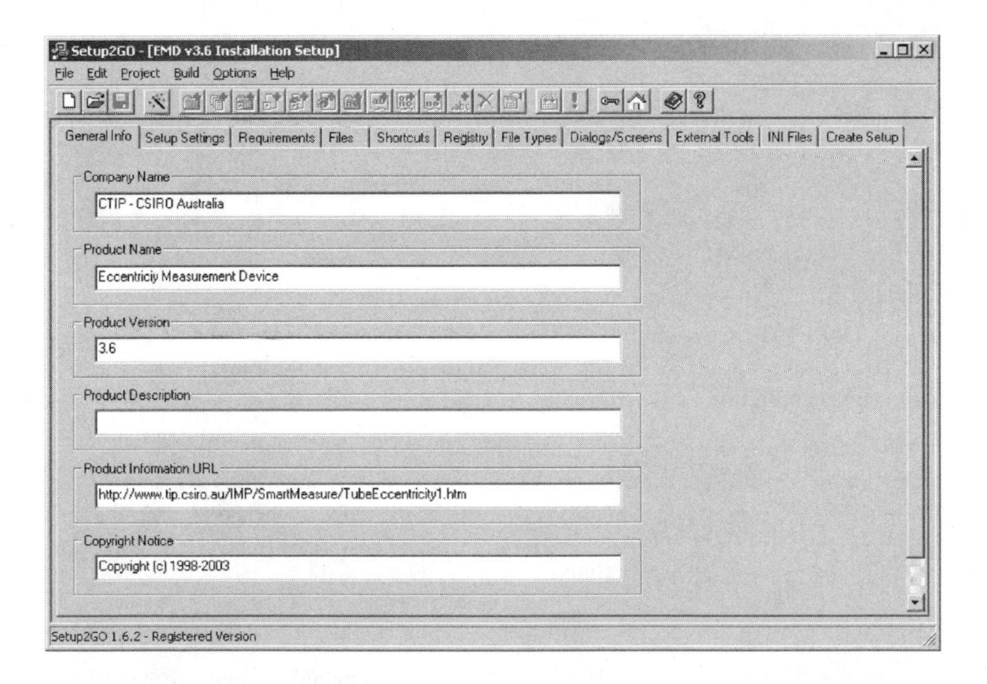

FIGURE 5.45 Custom installer Setup2Go.

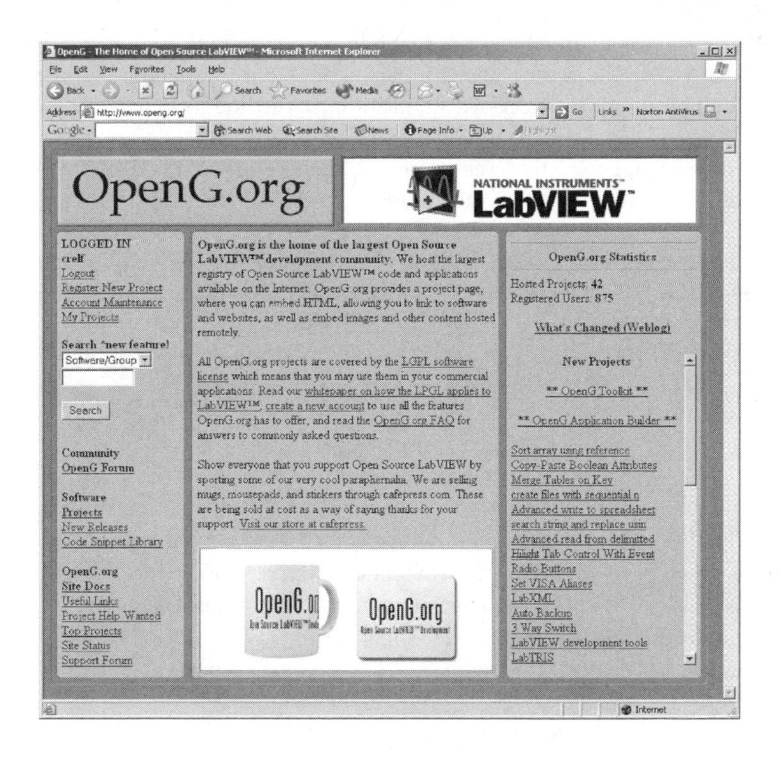

FIGURE 5.46 OpenG website.

easily transported to all corners of the earth in seconds using the Internet. Using this unique ability, projects can be developed at many different sites by several professionals simultaneously, ultimately leading to better tested software with extended features and more robust code. Sharing the burden of developing a software project allows engineers a much wider range of experience and expertise, and thus a more stable and useful application.

As you might imagine, coordinating such projects can be time intensive and legally difficult, which is why the OpenG community has been created. Spearheaded by the longtime LabVIEW expert Jim Kring, *OpenG.org* (Figure 5.46) is the home of our Open Source LabVIEW development community, hosting the largest registry of Open Source LabVIEW code and applications available on the Internet. OpenG.org is a not-for-profit venture, and provides each project a web page, where you can embed HTML, allowing you to link to software and websites, as well as embed images and other content hosted remotely.

All OpenG.org projects are covered by the *LGPL software license*, which protects source code, so that it remains Open Source, but it allows using protected code in commercial, proprietary, closed applications. Most people using LabVIEW are using it directly in commercial or industrial applications and systems that are sensitive because they contain intellectual property in the form of valuable trade secrets. The ideals of the OpenG community promote the adoption of open source everywhere that LabVIEW is used.

More information on the OpenG project, and how to develop software using open source principles is available at the OpenG website (*www.openg.org*) (Figure 5.46).

Defining Terms

Block (wiring) diagram: The coding portion of a VI, where the software engineer writes the G code.

Data type: The format the G development system uses to store a piece of information in memory. Using appropriate data types decreases application execution time, decreases memory footprint, and eradicates coercion errors.

Error cluster: A special cluster containing an error code, a Boolean indicating if an error has occurred, and the source of that error. The error cluster format is consistent throughout the G development system.

Front panel: The graphical user interface of a VI, including a method in which data are passed to and from the VI.

G: The programming language used to develop applications using the LabVIEW Development System.

Installer: Software that facilitates the automatic installation, upgrade, repair, or uninstallation of third-party software.

LabVIEW: The development system used to develop code in the G programming language.

Polymorphic VI: A collection of VIs with identical missions, operating on differing data types. A polymorphic VI exists on disk as a special form of a VI library.

Runtime engine (RTE): The system under which compiled G code runs, without the presence of the G development system.

Runtime license (RTL): A "user pays" system of charging for code portion development.

Unit: An attribute associated with a numerical value, giving it physical significance.

Further Information

National Instruments, *www.ni.com/labview* (G development system vendor)
National Instruments Alliance Members (system integrators), *www.ni.com/alliance*
The LabVIEW Zone, *www.ni.com/labviewzone* (developer forum)
OpenG—Open Source G Development, *www.openg.org* (developer forum)
InfoLabVIEW Mailing List, *www.info-labview.org* (developer forum)
LabVIEW Technical Resource, *www.ltrpub.com* (journal)

6

Reliability Engineering

6.1 Introduction 6-1
6.2 Terms and Definitions 6-2
6.3 Bathtub Hazard-Rate Concept 6-2
6.4 Important Formulas 6-3
Reliability • Mean Time to Failure • Hazard Rate
6.5 Reliability Networks 6-5
Series Network • Parallel Network • *k*-out–of-*m* Network
6.6 Reliability Evaluation Methods 6-8
Failure Modes and Effect Analysis • Fault-Tree Analysis • The Markov Method
6.7 Human Reliability 6-13
Classification and Causes of Human Errors • Human Reliability Measures • Modeling Human Operation in a Fluctuating Environment
6.8 Robot Reliability 6-16
Robot Failure Classifications and Causes • Robot Reliability Measures

B.S. Dhillon
University of Ottawa

6.1 Introduction

Reliability is an important consideration in the planning, design, and operation of engineering systems. The benefits of reliable systems are enormous and include a reduction in unexpected failures, lower maintenance costs, lower life-cycle costs, improved safety, less need for in-process inventory to cover downtime and more consistent quality [1,2]. Prior to World War II, the concept of reliability had been intuitive, subjective, and qualitative. Today, it is a well-recognized discipline with many specialized areas, including that of human reliability, robot reliability, software reliability, and mechanical reliability.

The reliability field is generally regarded as having started before World War II, with the development of V1 and V2 rockets in Germany. In 1950, the U.S. Department of Defense established an ad-hoc committee on reliability, and in 1952 it became known as the Advisory Group on the Reliability of Electronic Equipment (AGREE). In 1957, AGREE released a report that helped specificy the reliability of military electronic equipment [3,4].

In 1951, W. Weibull developed a statistical distribution that has played an important role in the development of the reliability field [5]. The first book on reliability, titled *Reliability Factors for Ground Electronic Equipment*, was published in 1956 [6]. Since then, more than 100 books on reliability have been published, as well as thousands of articles. Today, many scientific journals are totally or partially devoted to the reliability field. Refs. [7,8] provide a comprehensive list of publications on reliability and associated topics.

This chapter presents some important aspects of reliability.

6.2 Terms and Definitions

There are many terms and definitions in the reliability discipline and most can be found in Refs. [9–11]. Some commonly used terms and definitions are as follows [12–14]:

- **Reliability:** The probability that an item will conclude its mission satisfactorily for the stated period when used under the specified conditions.
- **Failure:** An item's inability to perform within the defined guidelines.
- **Hazard rate:** The quantity of the rate of change for the failed items over the number of survived items at time *t*.
- **Mean time to failure (exponential distribution):** The sum of the operating time of given items over the total number of failures.
- **Availability:** The probability that an item is available for use when required.
- **Redundancy:** The existence of two or more means for performing a required function.
- **Human error:** The failure to perform a specified task (or the performance of a forbidden action) that could disrupt scheduled operations or damage equipment or property.
- **Steady-state condition (statistical):** The condition where the probability of being in a certain state is independent of time.
- **Random failure:** A failure that cannot be predicted.
- **Repair rate:** A figure-of-merit that measures repair capability. In the case of exponential distribution, it is the reciprocal of mean time to repair.

6.3 Bathtub Hazard-Rate Concept

This concept often is used when performing a reliability analysis of engineering items, primarily for electronic parts. In this case, one assumes that an item's hazard rate or time-dependent failure rate follows a curve resembling the shape of a bathtub. A bathtub hazard-rate curve is shown in Figure 6.1. The curve in the figure can be divided into three parts: infant mortality period, useful life period, and wear-out period. In the infant-mortality period, the hazard rate decreases over time. Other names to describe this period are "burn-in period," "debugging period", and "break-in period." Causes for failures in this period include inadequate test specifications, ineffective quality control, marginal components, unsatisfactory manufacturing processes or tooling, overstressed parts, improper use procedures, inadequate materials, and improper handling or packaging [15].

During the useful life period, the hazard rate remains constant. Failures during this period are known as "random failures" because they occur unpredictably. Failures during the useful life period can be caused by inadequate design margins, wrong applications, and usage in the wrong environment.

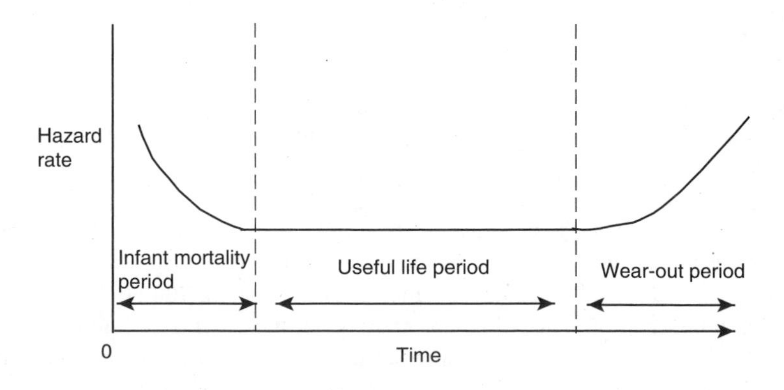

FIGURE 6.1 A bathtub hazard-rate curve.

In the wear-out period, the hazard rate increases over time and starts when an item has ended its useful life. Wear-out failures can be caused by material wear, unsatisfactory or improper preventative maintenance, scratching, misalignments, aging, limited-life parts, loose hardware, or incipient stress.

The following function can represent the bathtub hazard-rate curve [16]:

$$\lambda(t) = k\lambda n t^{n-1} + (1-k)bt^{b-1}\theta e^{\theta t^b} \quad \text{for} = \theta, n, b, \lambda > 0;\ 0 \leqslant k \leqslant 1;\ t \geqslant 0 \qquad (6.1)$$

where $\lambda(t)$ is the hazard rate (i.e., failure rate at time t), λ and θ are the scale parameters, and b and n are the shape parameters.

At $n = 0.5$ and $b = 1$, Equation (6.1) gives the bathtub hazard-rate curve. The hazard-rate functions of exponential, Rayleigh, Weibull, Makeham, and extreme-value distributions are special cases of Equation (6.1).

6.4 Important Formulas

Reliability work includes many frequently used mathematical formulas. This section presents formulas for achieving reliability, mean time to failure and an item's hazard rate.

Reliability

This is defined by

$$R(t) = 1 - \int_0^t f(t)\mathrm{d}t \qquad (6.2)$$

or

$$R(t) = e^{-\int_0^t \lambda(t)\mathrm{d}t} \qquad (6.3)$$

or

$$R(t) = \int_t^\infty f(t)\mathrm{d}t \qquad (6.4)$$

where $R(t)$ is reliability at time t, $f(t)$ is the probability or failure-density function, and $\lambda(t)$ is the hazard or time-dependent failure rate.

Example 1

Assume that the failure rate of a manufacturing system is 0.0004 failures per hour. Calculate the system reliability for a 10-hour mission.

By substituting the given data into Equation (6.3), we get

$$\begin{aligned} R(t) &= e^{-\int_0^t (0.0004)\mathrm{d}t} \\ &= e^{-(0.0004)t} \\ &= e^{-(0.0004)(10)} \\ &= 0.9960 \end{aligned}$$

The result is a 99.6% chance that the manufacturing system will not fail during the specified period.

Mean Time to Failure

An item's mean time to failure (MTTF) can be calculated by using any of the following three formulas:

$$\mathrm{MTTF} = \int_0^\infty R(t)\mathrm{d}t \tag{6.5}$$

or

$$\mathrm{MTTF} = \int_0^\infty tf(t)\mathrm{d}t \tag{6.6}$$

$$\mathrm{MTTF} = \lim_{s \to 0} \mathrm{R(s)} \tag{6.7}$$

where s is the Laplace transform variable and $R(s)$ is the Laplace transform of $R(t)$.

Example 2

In Example 1, find the mean time to failure of the manufacturing system.

By using the data in Equation (6.3) we find:

$$R(t) = \mathrm{e}^{-(0.0004)t} \tag{6.8}$$

Inserting Equation (6.7) into Equation (6.5) yields:

$$\begin{aligned}\mathrm{MTTF} &= \int_0^\infty \mathrm{e}^{-(0.0004)t}\mathrm{d}t \\ &= \frac{1}{0.0004} \\ &= 2{,}500\,\mathrm{hours}\end{aligned}$$

The mean time to failure of the manufacturing system is 2500 h.

Hazard Rate

This can be defined as

$$\lambda(t) = \frac{f(t)}{R(t)} \tag{6.9}$$

or

$$\lambda(t) = \frac{f(t)}{\int_t^\infty f(t)\mathrm{dt}} \tag{6.10}$$

or

$$\lambda(t) = \frac{f(t)}{1 - \int_0^t f(t)\mathrm{d}t} \tag{6.11}$$

or

$$\lambda(t) = -\frac{1}{R(t)}\frac{dR(t)}{dt} \tag{6.12}$$

Example 3

Assumc that the time to failure for a machine tool is described by the following probability density function:

$$f(t) = \lambda e^{-\lambda t} \tag{6.13}$$

where λ is the distribution parameter.

Obtain an expression for the machine-tool hazard rate.

By substituting Equation (6.13) into Equation (6.4), we get:

$$R(t) = \int_t^\infty \lambda e^{-\lambda t} dt = e^{-\lambda t} \tag{6.14}$$

Using Equation (6.13) and Equation (6.14) in Equation (6.9) yields:

$$\lambda(t) = \frac{\lambda e^{-\lambda t}}{e^{-\lambda t}} = \lambda \tag{6.15}$$

The abovc cxpression is used to find the machine-tool hazard rate and is independent of time. Usually, the hazard rate under this condition is known as the failure rate.

6.5 Reliability Networks

In reliability analysis, engineering systems can form various networks or configurations. Some commonly occurring configurations are that of series, parallel, and k-out-of-m. Each of these configurations is discussed below.

Series Network

In this case, if any n unit fails, the system fails. All system units must work normally for the system to succeed. Figure 6.2 shows the block diagram of a series network.

For independent units, the reliability of the series network is given by:

$$R_s = R_1 R_2 R_3 \ldots R_n \tag{6.16}$$

where R_s is the series system reliability and R_i is the unit i reliability; for $i = 1, 2, 3, \ldots, n$.

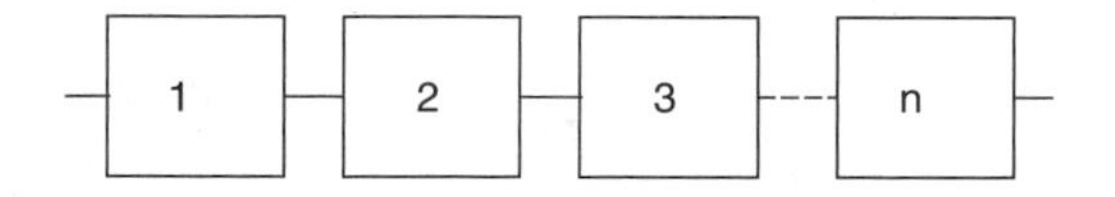

FIGURE 6.2 An n-unit series network.

For constant failure rate of unit i, i.e., $\lambda_i(t) = \lambda_i$, the unit i reliability from Equation (6.3) is

$$R_i(t) = e^{-\lambda_i t} \tag{6.17}$$

where $R_i(t)$ is the unit i reliability at time t and λ_i is the unit i failure rate.

For constant failure rates of all series units, by substituting Equation (6.17) into Equation (6.16), we get the following expression for the series-system, time-dependent reliability:

$$R_s(t) = e^{-\lambda_1 t} e^{-\lambda_2 t} e^{-\lambda_3 t} \ldots e^{-\lambda_n t} \tag{6.18}$$

where $R_s(t)$ is the series system reliability at time t.

Using Equation (6.18) in Equation (6.5), we get the following expression for the series-system mean time to failure:

$$\begin{aligned} \text{MTTF}_s &= \int_0^\infty e^{-\sum_{i=1}^{n} \lambda_1 t} dt \\ &= \frac{1}{\sum_{i=1}^{n} \lambda_i} \end{aligned} \tag{6.19}$$

Example 4

Assume that an aircraft has two independent engines and both of them must operate normally for the aircraft to fly successfully. The reliabilities of engines 1 and 2 are 0.95 and 0.98, respectively. Calculate the reliability of the aircraft with respect to the engines.

Substituting the given data into Equation (6.16) yields:

$$\begin{aligned} R_s &= (0.95)(0.98) \\ &= 0.9310 \end{aligned}$$

There is a 93.1% chance that the aircraft will fly successfully.

Parallel Network

In this case, all units are active, and at least one must operate normally for the system to succeed. The parallel-network block diagram is shown in Figure 6.3.

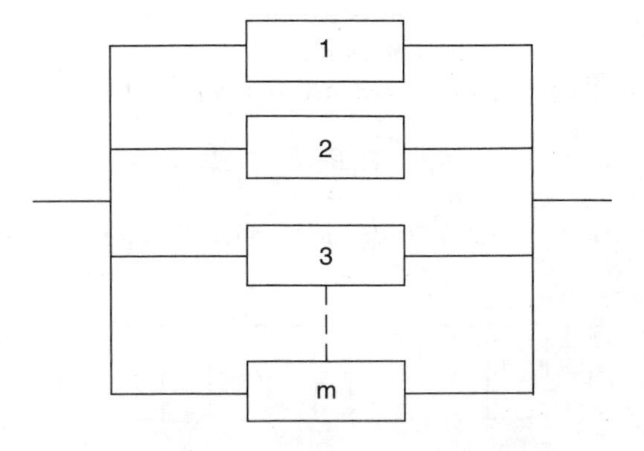

FIGURE 6.3 An m-unit parallel system.

For independent units, the parallel-network reliability is

$$R_p = 1 - (1 - R_1)(1 - R_2)\ldots(1 - R_m) \tag{6.20}$$

where R_p is the parallel-network or system reliability, m is the number of units in parallel, and R_i is the unit i reliability; for $i = 1, 2, 3, m$.

For constant-unit failure rates, using Equation (6.17) in Equation (6.20), we obtain

$$R_p(t) = 1 - (1 - e^{-\lambda_1 t})(1 - e^{-\lambda_2 t})\ldots(1 - e^{-\lambda_m t}) \tag{6.21}$$

where $R_p(t)$ is the parallel-network reliability at time t and λ_i is the unit i failure rate; for $i = 1, 2, 3, \ldots, m$.

For identical units, Equation (6.21) simplifies to:

$$R_p(t) = 1 - (1 - e^{-\lambda t})^m \tag{6.22}$$

where λ is the unit failure rate.

By inserting Equation (6.22) into Equation (6.5), we get the following expression for the parallel-network mean time to failure:

$$\begin{aligned} \mathrm{MTTF}_p &= \int_0^\infty [1 - (1 - e^{-\lambda t})^m]dt \\ &= \frac{1}{\lambda}\sum_{i=1}^{m}\frac{1}{i} \end{aligned} \tag{6.23}$$

where $\mathrm{MTTF_p}$ is the parallel-network or system mean time to failure.

Example 5

Assume that an aircraft has two independent and identical engines. At least one engine must operate normally for the aircraft to fly successfully. The engine failure rate is 0.0007 failures/hour. Calculate the reliability of the aircraft with respect to engines for a 12-h mission.

By substituting the given data into Equation (6.22), we get:

$$\begin{aligned} R_p(12) &= 1 - [1 - e^{-(0.0007)(12)}]^2 \\ &= 0.999 \end{aligned}$$

There is a 99.99% chance that the aircraft will fly successfully during its specified mission period.

k-out–of-*m* Network

In this case, the network is composed of m number of active units, and at least k must work normally for the system to succeed. Series and parallel networks are the special cases of this network, at $k = m$ and $k = 1$, respectively.

For independent and identical units, the k-out-of-m network reliability is given by

$$R_{k/m} = \sum_{i=k}^{m}\binom{m}{i}R^i(1 - R)^{m-i} \tag{6.24}$$

where $R_{k/m}$ is the k-out-of-m unit network reliability and R is the unit reliability:

$$\binom{m}{i} \equiv \frac{m!}{(m-i)!i!} \tag{6.25}$$

For constant failure rates of units, Equation (6.24) becomes

$$R_{k/m}(t) = \sum_{i=k}^{m} \binom{m}{i} e^{-i\lambda t}(1 - e^{-\lambda t})^{m-i} \tag{6.26}$$

where $R_{k/m}(t)$ is the k-out-of-m unit network reliability at time t.

Substituting Equation (6.26) into Equation (6.5) yields:

$$\begin{aligned} \mathrm{MTTF}_{k/m} &= \int_0^\infty \left[\sum_{i=k}^{m} \binom{m}{i} e^{-i\lambda t}(1 - e^{-\lambda t})^{m-i} \right] dt \\ &= \frac{1}{\lambda} \sum_{i=k}^{m} \frac{1}{i} \end{aligned} \tag{6.27}$$

where $\mathrm{MTTF}_{k/m}$ is the k-out-of-m unit network mean time to failure.

Example 6

Assume that a manufacturing system consists of three independent and identical units and at least two units must work normally for its successful operation. The unit failure rate is 0.0005 failures/hour. Calculate the manufacturing-system mean time to failure.

Substituting the given data into Equation (6.27) yields:

$$\begin{aligned} \mathrm{MTTF}_{2/3} &= \frac{1}{(0.0005)} \left(\frac{1}{2} + \frac{1}{3} \right) \\ &= 1666.67 \text{ hours} \end{aligned}$$

The mean time to failure of the manufacturing system is 1666.67 h.

6.6 Reliability Evaluation Methods

From the inception of the reliability field, many evaluation methods and techniques have been developed. The three most widely used methods and techniques are failure modes and effect analysis (FMEA), fault-tree analysis (FTA), and the Markov method [17].

Failure Modes and Effect Analysis

This has become a widely used method to analyze engineering systems. It can simply be described as a technique to conduct analysis of each potential failure mode in a system and is used to examine the results or effects of failure modes on that system [10]. FMEA originally was developed in the early 1950s to analyze flight-control systems. A comprehensive list of publications on the technique is presented in Ref. [18].

The steps associated with FMEA are as follows:

- Define system boundaries and associated requirements in detail.
- Establish ground rules.
- List system components and subsystems.

- List important failure modes, describing and identifying the component in question.
- Assign failure rate/probability to each component failure mode.
- Document each failure mode effect on the subsystem/system/plant.
- Enter remarks for each failure mode.
- Review and identify critical failure modes and take corrective measures.

Assigning criticalities or priorities to failure-mode effects is known as failure modes, effects and criticality analysis (FMECA). FMECA has some important characteristics:

- It is an upward approach that starts from the detailed level.
- By evaluating the failure effects of each component, the entire system is screened.
- It offers an effective approach to identify weak spots in system design, indicating areas for detailed analysis or corrective measures.
- It is useful to improve communication among design-interface personnel.

This approach is described in detail in Ref. [17].

Fault-Tree Analysis

This is another widely used method in the industrial sector to perform reliability analysis for engineering systems. The method was developed in the early 1960s at the Bell Telephone Laboratories to analyze the Minuteman launch control system. A comprehensive list of publications on the technique is presented in Ref. [7]. Four basic symbols used to perform FTA are shown in Figure 6.4.

The following steps are used in performing FTA:

- Define the system and assumptions associated with the analysis.
- Identify the undesirable or top-fault event to be investigated.
- Thoroughly understand the system under study.
- Using fault-tree symbols, identify all the possible causes for the occurrence of the top event.
- Develop the fault tree to the lowest level required.
- Conduct an analysis of the completed fault tree.
- Identify corrective actions.
- Document the FTA and review corrective measures taken.

Example 7

A windowless room contains one switch and two light bulbs. The switch only can fail to close. Develop a fault tree for the top event, "dark room."

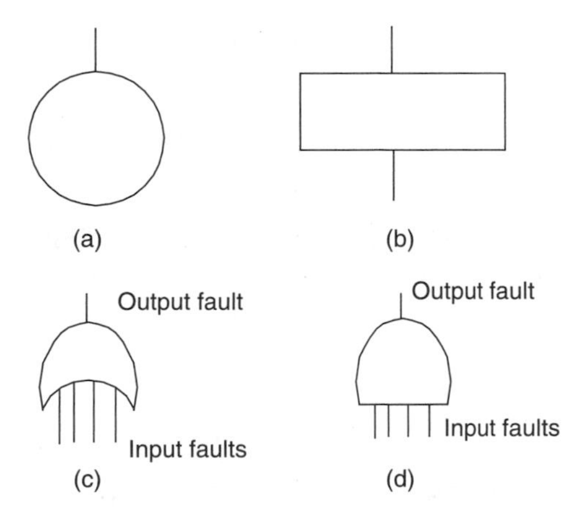

FIGURE 6.4 Fault tree basic symbols: (a) basic fault event, (b) resultant fault event, (c) OR gate, and (d) AND gate.

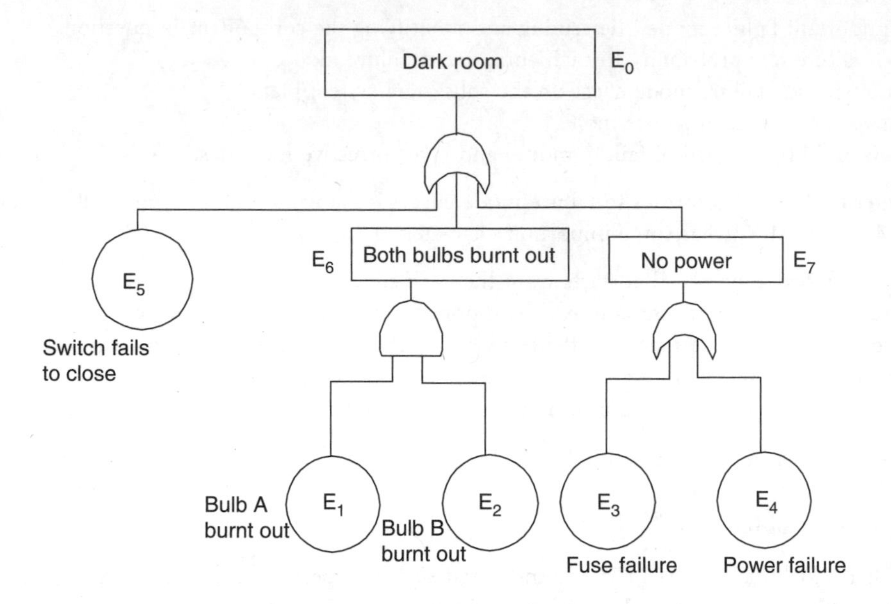

FIGURE 6.5 A fault tree for the top event "dark room."

A fault tree for this example is shown in Figure 6.5. Each fault event in the figure is labeled E_0, E_1, E_2, E_3, E_4, E_5, E_6, and E_7.

Probability Evaluation

For independent fault events, the probability of occurrence for the top event can be evaluated by applying basic rules of probability. In the case of the Figure 6.5 fault tree, we have:

$$P(E_6) = P(E_1)P(E_2) \tag{6.28}$$

$$P(E_7) = P(E_3) + P(E_4) - P(E_3)P(E_4) \tag{6.29}$$

$$\mathrm{P}(E_0) = 1 - \{1 - P(E_5)\}\{1 - P(E_7)\}\{1 - P(E_6)\} \tag{6.30}$$

where $P(E_i)$ is the probability of occurrence of fault event E_i; for $i = 0, 1, 2, \ldots, 7$.

Example 8

In Figure 6.5, assume that the probability of occurrence of fault events E_1, E_2, E_3, E_4, and E_5 are 0.1, 0.05, 0.02, 0.04, and 0.03, respectively. Calculate the probability of occurrence of the top event, "dark room."

By substituting the given values into Equation (6.28) to Equation (6.30) we get

$$\begin{aligned} P(E_6) &= (0.1)(0.05) = 0.005 \\ P(E_7) &= (0.02) + (0.04) - (0.02)(0.04) = 0.0592 \\ \text{and } P(E_0) &= 1 - (1 - 0.03)(1 - 0.0592)(1 - 0.005) = 0.0920 \end{aligned}$$

There is 9.2% chance of having "dark room."

Advantages and Disadvantages of FTA

As in the case of other evaluation methods, FTA has both advantages and disadvantages. Some advantages of FTA are as follows:

- It provides insight into the system behavior.
- It easily can work with complex systems.
- It ferrets out failures deductively.
- It requires analysts that thoroughly understand the system under study.
- It offers a useful visibility tool to justify design changes and to conduct trade-off studies.
- It provides an option for performing either a qualitative or quantitative reliability analysis.

Similarly, some disadvantages of performing FTA are as follows:

- It can be costly and time-consuming.
- End results are difficult to check.
- It is difficult to manage a component's partial failure states.

The Markov Method

This method, named after a Russian mathematician, is another frequently used method to perform a reliability analysis for engineering systems. Like the others, it can work with repairable systems and systems with partial failure states. The following assumptions are part of this approach:

- The transitional probability from one state to the other in the finite time interval Δt is given by $\lambda \Delta t$, where λ is the failure or repair rate associated with Markov states.
- All occurrences are independent of each other.
- The probability of more than one transition occurrence in time interval Δt from one state [U8] to the next state is small.

The following example demonstrates this method:

Example 9

A manufacturing system's state-space diagram is shown in Figure 6.6. The manufacturing system either can be in its operating state or its failed state. Appling the Markov method, develop expressions for the manufacturing system's reliability and unreliability if its failure rate is λ. Numerals in the Figure 6.6 diagram denote system states.

By applying the Markov method, we write the following two equations for the Figure 6.6 diagram:

$$P_0(t + \Delta t) = P_0(t)[1 - \lambda \Delta t] \tag{6.31}$$

$$P_1(t + \Delta t) = P_1(t) + \lambda \Delta t P_0(t) \tag{6.32}$$

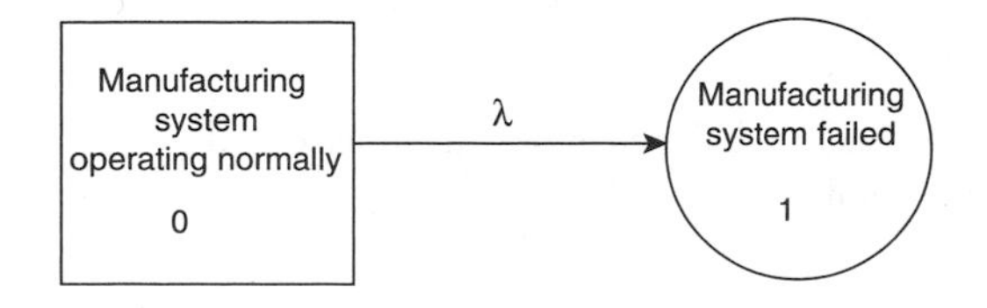

FIGURE 6.6 Manufacturing system state-space diagram.

where $P_i(t)$ is the probability that the manufacturing system is in state i at time t; for $i = 0$ (operating normally), $i = 1$ (failed), $P_i\,(t + \Delta t)$ is the probability that the manufacturing system is in state i at time $t + \Delta t$; for $i = 0$ (operating normally), $i = 1$ (failed), $\lambda \Delta t$ is the probability of failure in time Δt, and $(1 - \lambda \Delta t)$ is the probability of no failure in time Δt when the manufacturing system is in state 0.

In the limiting case, Equation (6.31) to Equation (6.32) becomes

$$\lim_{\Delta t \to 0} \frac{P_0(t + \Delta t) - P_0(t)}{\Delta t} = \frac{dP_0(t)}{dt} = -\lambda P_0(t) \tag{6.33}$$

$$\lim_{\Delta t \to 0} \frac{P_1(t + \Delta t) - P_1(t)}{\Delta t} = \frac{dP_1(t)}{dt} = -\lambda P_0(t) \tag{6.34}$$

At time $t = 0$, $P_0(0) = 1$ and $P_1(0) = 0$.

Solving Equation (6.33) and Equation (6.34) by using Laplace transforms, we obtain:

$$P_0(s) = \frac{1}{s + \lambda} \tag{6.35}$$

$$P_1(s) = \frac{\lambda}{s(s + \lambda)} \tag{6.36}$$

where s is the Laplace transform variable, $P_i(s)$ is the Laplace transform of the probability that the manufacturing system is in state i; for $i = 0$ (operating normally), $i = 1$ (failed).

Taking the inverse Laplace transforms of Equation (6.35) and Equation (6.36), we get:

$$P_0(t) = e^{-\lambda t} \tag{6.37}$$

$$P_1(t) = 1 - e^{-\lambda t} \tag{6.38}$$

Thus, from Equation (6.37) and Equation (6.38), the reliability and unreliability of the manufacturing system are

$$R_m(t) = P_0(t) = e^{-\lambda t} \tag{6.39}$$

and

$$F_m(t) = P_1(t) = 1 - e^{-\lambda t} \tag{6.40}$$

where $R_m(t)$ is the manufacturing-system reliability at time t and $F_m(t)$ is the manufacturing-system unreliability or failure probability at time t.

Example 10

Assume that the failure rate of a manufacturing system is 0.001 failures per hour. Calculate the system unreliability for a 200-h mission.

By inserting the given data into Equation (6.40), we have:

$$\begin{aligned} F_m(200) &= 1 - e^{-(0.001)(200)} \\ &= 0.1813 \end{aligned}$$

There is a 18.13% chance that the manufacturing system will fail during the specified period.

6.7 Human Reliability

As human links connect numerous engineering systems, reliability is an important factor in the successful operation of such systems. In the late 1950s, Williams [19] recognized the problem of human reliability in engineering systems and wrote that the reliability of the human element must be incorporated. Various studies subsequently have indicated that at least 10% of system failures are caused by human error [17,20].

The first book on human reliability appeared in 1986 [21]. Today, many other texts are available on the subject. A comprehensive list of publications on human reliability is presented in Ref. [7].

Classification and Causes of Human Errors

Human errors can be classified as follows [22]:

- Design errors
- Operator errors
- Maintenance errors
- Fabrication errors
- Inspection errors
- Handling errors
- Contributory errors

Human errors can be caused by a poor work environment (inadequate lighting, crowded workspaces, high noise levels), inadequate or poorly worded equipment operating and maintenance procedures, poor equipment design, wrong or inadequate work tools, complex tasks, poor work layout, low skill levels or inadequate worker training and unmotivated employees [21–23].

Human Reliability Measures

The following two equations can estimate human reliability:

$$\mathrm{HR} = 1 - \frac{E}{n} \tag{6.41}$$

and

$$R_{\mathrm{h}}(t) = e^{-\int_0^t \lambda_{\mathrm{h}}(t)\,dt} \tag{6.42}$$

where HR is human reliability, n is the total number of times the certain task was performed, E is the number of times the task was performed incorrectly, $R_{\mathrm{h}}(t)$ is the human reliability at time t, and $\lambda_{\mathrm{h}}(t)$ is the time-dependent human error rate.

Equation (6.42) is used to compute the reliability of time-continuous tasks such as scope monitoring, aircraft maneuvering, and operating an automobile. The following two examples demonstrate the application of Equation (6.41) and Equation (6.42).

Example 11

A person performed a task 200 times. It was performed incorrectly 15 times. Calculate the human reliability.

The specified data in Equation (6.41) yields:

$$\begin{aligned} \mathrm{HR} &= 1 - \frac{15}{200} \\ &= 0.9250 \end{aligned}$$

In this case, the value of human reliability is 92.50%.

Example 12

A person performed a time-continuous task, and the error rate was 0.004 errors per hour. Calculate the person's reliability over an 8-h period.

Substituting the given data into Equation (6.42), we get:

$$\begin{aligned} R_{\mathrm{h}}(8) &= \mathrm{e}^{\int_0^{-8} (0.004)\mathrm{d}t} \\ &= \mathrm{e}^{-(0.004)(8)} \\ &= 0.9685 \end{aligned}$$

The person's reliability is 96.85%.

Modeling Human Operation in a Fluctuating Environment

This model represents situations where the human operator performs a time-continuous task under alternating environments, both normal and abnormal. Two examples of such situations are operating a vehicle in normal and heavy traffic and piloting an aircraft in normal and extreme weather. The operator can make mistakes in both normal and abnormal conditions, but their occurrence rates could differ [24].

This model can calculate operator reliability and mean time to human error. The model state-space diagram is shown in Figure 6.7. The numerals in Figure 6.7 boxes and circles denote system states. The following symbols were used to develop equations for the model: $P_i(t)$ is the probability of the human operator being in state i at time t; for $i = 0, 1, 2, 3$, λ_1 is the human-operator error rate from state 0, λ_2 is the human-operator error rate from state 2, α is the transition rate from a normal to an abnormal state, and β is the transition rate from an abnormal to a normal state.

Applying the Markov method, we get the following equations for the Figure 6.7 state-space diagram [24]:

$$\frac{\mathrm{d}P_0(t)}{\mathrm{d}t} + (\lambda_1 + \alpha)P_0(t) = P_2(t) = P_2(t)\beta \tag{6.43}$$

$$\frac{\mathrm{d}P_1(t)}{\mathrm{d}t} = P_0(t)\lambda_1 \tag{6.44}$$

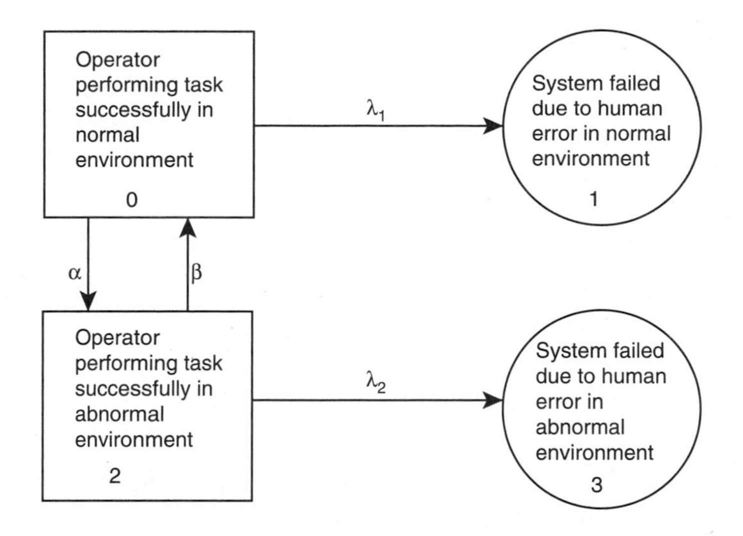

FIGURE 6.7 State-space diagram for the human operator under fluctuating stress environment.

$$\frac{dP_2(t)}{dt} + (\lambda_2 + \beta)P_2(t) = P_0(t)\alpha \tag{6.45}$$

$$\frac{dP_3(t)}{dt} = P_2(t)\lambda_2 \tag{6.46}$$

At time $t = 0$, $P_0(0) = 1$, and $P_1(0) = P_2(0) = P_3(0) = 0$.

Solving the above equations, we get the following expression for the human-operator reliability:

$$\begin{aligned} R_h(t) &= P_0(t) + P_2(t) \\ &= (x_2 - x_1)^{-1}[(x_2 + \lambda_2 + \beta]e^{x_2 t} - (x_1 + \lambda_2 + \beta)e^{x_1 t} + \alpha(e^{x_2 t} - e^{x_1 t})] \end{aligned} \tag{6.47}$$

where

$$x_1 = \frac{-b_1 + \sqrt{b_1^2 - 4b_2}}{2} \tag{6.48}$$

$$x_2 = \frac{-b_1 - \sqrt{b_1^2 - 4b_2}}{2} \tag{6.49}$$

$$b_1 = \lambda_1 + \lambda_2 + \alpha + \beta \tag{6.50}$$

$$b_2 = \lambda_1(\lambda_2 + \beta) + \alpha\lambda_2 \tag{6.51}$$

By integrating Equation (6.47) over the time interval 0 to ∞, we get:

$$\begin{aligned} \text{MTTHOE} &= \int_0^\infty R_h(t)\mathrm{d}t \\ &= (\lambda_2 + \alpha + \beta)/b_2 \end{aligned} \tag{6.52}$$

where MTTHOE is the mean time to human-operator error.

6.8 Robot Reliability

Though the idea of a functional robot can be traced to the writings of Aristotle in the fourth century B.C., the programmable device developed by George Devol in 1954 is regarded as the first industrial robot [25,26]. Today, robots are an important component of manufacturing systems.

In the early 1980s, robot reliability began to attract serious attention. In 1987, a comprehensive list of publications was first published on robot reliability and safety [27]. In 1991, a book titled *Robot Reliability and Safety* covered the subject in considerable depth [28]. Since then, many publications on robot reliability have been published.

Robot Failure Classifications and Causes

There are various failure types associated with robots and they can be classified into four categories [29,30]:

1. Random component failures
2. Systematic hardware faults
3. Software faults
4. Human errors

Random component failures occur unpredictably during the useful life of a robot. Reasons for their occurrence include low safety factors, undetectable defects, and unavoidable failures. Systematic hardware faults are the result of unrevealed mechanisms in the robot's design.

Software faults in robots occur due to embedded software or the controlling and application software. As with any other engineering system, human error also can occur during design, manufacturing, testing, operation, and maintenance of a robot.

There are various causes for robot failures. Frequent ones are servo value malfunctions, oil-pressure valve problems, circuit board problems, and human error. Nonetheless, some past studies [31,32] have indicated that robot problems occur in the following order:

- Control-system problems
- Jig and other tool incompatibility
- Robot body problems
- Programming and operation errors
- Welding-gun problems and problems with other tooling parts
- Deterioration and precision deficiency
- Runaway
- Other problems

Robot Reliability Measures

Several parameters measure robot reliability, including mean time to robot failure (MTRF), reliability, and mean time to robot-related problems (MTRP). Each is presented below.

Mean Time to Robot Failure (MTRF)

This can be defined in two ways:

$$\text{MTRF} = (\text{RPH} - \text{DTDRF})/\text{N} \tag{6.53}$$

where N is the total number of robot failures; RPH is the robot production time, expressed in hours; and DTDRF is downtime due to robot failures, expressed in hours, or:

$$\text{MTRF} = \int_0^\infty R_b(t)\mathrm{d}t \tag{6.54}$$

where $R_b(t)$ is the robot reliability at time t.

Example 13

Assume that total number of production hours for a robot system was 6000 h, with downtime due to robot failure of 200 h. If there were 10 robot failures during this period, calculate the robot mean time to failure.

By inserting the given values into Equation (6.53), we obtain:

$$\begin{aligned}\text{MTRF} &= (6,000 - 200)/10 \\ &= 580\,\text{hours}\end{aligned}$$

On average, the robot failed after every 580 h of operation.

Robot Reliability

This is defined by:

$$R_r(t) = \exp\left[\int_0^{-t} \lambda_r(t)\mathrm{d}t\right] \tag{6.55}$$

where $R_r(t)$ is the robot reliability at time t and $\lambda_r(t)$ is the robot hazard rate or time-dependent failure rate.

Example 14

A robot failure rate is 0.0005 failures per hour. Calculate robot reliability during a 200-h mission.

Substituting the above data into Equation (6.55) yields:

$$R_r(200) = \exp\left[-\int_0^{200} (0.0005)\mathrm{d}t\right] = \mathrm{e}^{-(0.0005)(200)} = 0.9048$$

There is a 90.48% chance that the robot will not fail during the 200-h mission.

Mean Time to Robot-Related Problems (MTRP)

This is defined by

$$\text{MTRP} = \frac{\text{RPH} - \text{DTDRP}}{\text{M}} \tag{6.56}$$

where M is the total number of robot-related problems and DTDRP is downtime due to robot-related problems, expressed in hours.

Example 15

The total number of production hours of an industrial robot was 8000 h, including downtime due to robot-related problems of 500 h. In addition, there were 20 robot-related problems. Calculate the mean time to robot-related problems.

Using the data in Equation (6.56), we get:

$$\text{MTRP} = \frac{8{,}000 - 500}{20} = 375\,\text{hours}$$

The mean time to robot-related problems is 375 h.

References

1. B.S. Dhillon and C. Singh, *Engineering Reliability: New Techniques and Applications*, New York: Wiley, 1981.
2. *Reliability and Maintainability Guideline for Manufacturing Machinery and Equipment*, Warrendale, PA: Society of Automotive Engineers, Inc., M-110.2, 1999.
3. AGREE Report, *Reliability of Military Electronic Equipment*, Washington, D.C.: Department of Defense, 1957.
4. MIL-R-25717 (USAF), *Reliability Assurance Program for Electronic Equipment*, Washington, D.C.: Department of Defense, 1957.
5. W. Weibull, "A statistical distribution function of wide applicability," *J. Appl. Mech.*, vol. 47, pp. 293–297, 1951.
6. K. Henney, Ed., *Reliability Factors for Ground Electronic Equipment*, New York: McGraw-Hill, 1956.
7. B.S. Dhillon, *Reliability and Quality Control: Bibliography on General and Specialized Areas*, Gloucester, ON: Beta Publishers, 1992.
8. B.S. Dhillon, *Reliability Engineering Applications: Bibliography on Important Application Areas*, Gloucester, ON: Beta Publishers, 1992.
9. J.J. Naresky, "Reliability definitions," *IEEE Trans. Reliab.*, vol. 19, pp. 198–200, 1970.
10. T.P. Omdahl, Ed., *Reliability, Availability, and Maintainability (RAM) Dictionary*, Milwaukee, WI: ASQC Quality Press, 1988.
11. T. McKenna and R. Oliverson, *Glossary of Reliability and Maintenance*, Houston, TX: Gulf Publishing Company, 1997.
12. B.S. Dhillon, *Reliability Engineering in Systems Design and Operation*, New York: Van Nostrand Reinhold Company, 1983.
13. W.H. Von Alven, Ed., *Reliability Engineering*, Englewood Cliffs, NJ: Prentice-Hall, 1964.
14. B.S. Dhillon, *Mechanical Reliability: Theory, Models and Applications*, Washington, D.C.: American Institute of Aeronautics and Astronautics, 1988.
15. W. Grant Ireson and C.F. Coombs, Eds., *Handbook of Reliability Engineering and Management*, New York: McGraw-Hill, 1988.
16. B.S. Dhillon, "A hazard rate model," *IEEE Trans. Reliab.*, vol. 29, p. 150, 1979.
17. B.S. Dhillon, *Design Reliability: Fundamentals and Applications*, Boca Raton, FL: CRC Press, 1999.
18. B.S. Dhillon, "Failure modes and effect analysis: bibliography," *Microelectron. Reliab.*, vol. 32, pp. 729–731, 1992.
19. H.L. Williams, "Reliability evaluation of the human component in man-machine systems," *Electr. Manuf.*, pp. 78–82, 1958 (April).
20. E.W. Hagen, Ed., "Human reliability analysis," *Nucl. Safety*, vol. 17, pp. 315–326, 1976.
21. B.S. Dhillon, *Human Reliability with Human Factors*, New York: Pergamon Press, 1986.
22. D. Meister, "The problem of human-initiated failures," *Proc. Eighth Natl. Symp. Reliab. Qual. Contr.*, pp. 234–239, 1962.

23. J.I. Cooper, "Human-initiated failures and man-function reporting," *IRE Trans. Human Factors*, vol. 10, pp. 104–109, 1961.
24. B.S. Dhillon, "Stochastic models for predicting human reliability," *Microelectron. Reliab.*, vol. 22, pp. 491–496, 1982.
25. E. Heer, "Robots in modern industry," in *Recent Advances in Robotics*, G. Beni and S. Hackwood, Eds., New York: Wiley, pp. 11–36, 1985.
26. M.I. Zeldman, *What Every Engineer Should Know about Robots*, New York: Marcel Dekker, 1984.
27. B.S. Dhillon, "On robot reliability and safety," *Microelectron. Reliab.*, vol. 27, pp. 105–118, 1987.
28. B.S. Dhillon, *Robot Reliability and Safety*, New York: Springer, 1991.
29. K. Khodabandehloo, F. Duggan, and T.F. Husband, "Reliability of industrial robots: a safety viewpoint," *Proc. 7th Br. Robot Assoc. Annu. Conf.*, pp. 233–242, 1984.
30. K. Khodabandehloo, F. Duggan, and T.F. Husband, "Reliability assessment of industrial robots," *Proc. 14th Int. Symp. Ind. Robots*, pp. 209–220, 1984.
31. K. Sato, "Case study of maintenance of spot-welding robots," *Plant Maint.*, pp. 14–28, 1982.
32. N. Sugimoto and K. Kawaguchi, "Fault tree analysis of hazards created by robots," *Proc. 13th Int. Symp. Ind. Robots*, pp. 9.13–9.28, 1983.

II

Biomedical Systems

7 **Bioelectricity** *J.A. White, A.D. Dorval II, L.A. Geddes, R.C. Barr, B.K. Slaten, F. Barnes, D.R. Martinez, R.A. Bond, M.M. Vai* 7-1
Neuroelectric Principles • Bioelectric Events • Biological Effects and Electromagnetic Fields • Embedded Signal Processing

8 **Biomedical Sensors** *M.R. Neuman* 8-1
Introduction • Physical Sensors • Chemical Sensors • Bioanalytical Sensors • Applications

9 **Bioelectronics and Instruments** *J.D. Bronzino, E.J. Berbari* 9-1
The Electro-encephalogram • The Electrocardiograph

10 **Tomography** *M.D. Fox* 10-1
Computerized Tomography • Positron Emission Tomography • Single Photon Emission Computed Tomography • Magnetic Resonance Imaging • Imaging

7

Bioelectricity

John A. White
Boston University

Alan D. Dorval II
Boston University

L.A. Geddes
Purdue University

R.C. Barr
Duke University

Bonnie Keillor Slaten
University of Colorado

Frank Barnes
University of Colorado

David R. Martinez
MIT Lincoln Laboratory

Robert A. Bond
MIT Lincoln Laboratory

M. Michael Vai
MIT Lincoln Laboratory

7.1 Neuroelectric Principles 7-1
Introduction • Electrochemical Potential • Action Potentials • Synaptic Transmission • Dynamic Clamp • Models of Extracellular Stimulation • Application: Deep Brain Stimulation

7.2 Bioelectric Events 7-13
Origin of Bioelectricity • Law of Stimulation • Recording Action Potentials • The Electrocardiogram (ECG) • Electromyography (EMG) • Electro-encephalography (EEG) • Magnetic (Eddy-Current) Stimulation • Summary and Conclusion

7.3 Biological Effects and Electromagnetic Fields 7-33
Introduction • Biological Effects of Electric Shock • Will the 120-V Common Household Voltage Produce a Dangerous Shock? It Depends! • Other Adverse Effects of Electricity • Biological Effects of Low Level, Time-Varying Electromagnetic Fields (EMF) from Power Lines • Exposures • Epidemiological Studies • Animal Studies • Cellular Studies • EMF from Cell Phones and Base Stations • Exposures • Epidemiological Studies • Animal Studies (*In vivo*) • Cellular Studies • Standards and Guidelines • Conclusion

7.4 Embedded Signal Processing 7-55
Introduction • Generic Embedded Signal Processing Architecture • Embedded Digital Signal Processor (DSP) • Software: Run-Time and Development Environment • Programmable DSP Technology Trends • Application-Specific Hardware • Summary

7.1 Neuroelectric Principles

John A. White and Alan D. Dorval II

Introduction

In the nervous system, signaling on fast time scales (10^{-4} to 10^{-1} sec) is electrical in nature. Neurons (nerve cells), the basic functional units of the nervous system, continually expend energy to maintain electrochemical gradients across their cell membranes. In response to an appropriate stimulus, neurons allow ions (mostly Na^+ and K^+) to run down their potential energy gradients. This charge movement leads to a brief, 100-mV change in membrane potential, known as the **action potential**. Action potentials are typically generated near the cell body and propagate down specialized processes (axons) to target nerve and muscle cells. Neuroelectric activity is studied by measuring electrical events both intracellularly and extracellularly. Recent technical advances allow basic researchers to mimic ion channels in living neuronal membranes. Applied scientists have used electrical stimulation of the nervous system to great clinical effect, but the specific mechanisms being exploited are still an object of active study.

Figure 7.1 shows an image of a neuron that has been filled with a light-opaque dye. Inputs are collected by the dendrites; integration of received input occurs in the cell body; when action potentials are generated (initially, at or near the soma), they propagate down the axon to the synaptic terminal, at which point the signal is communicated (usually chemically) to a number of so-called postsynaptic nerve or muscle cells.

The human body contains over 10^{11} neurons, each playing a specialized role. For example, specialized neurons associated with the five senses transduce photonic, mechanical, or chemical energy into the electrochemical "language" of the nervous system. Motor neurons of the brainstem and spinal cord are specialized to drive voluntary and involuntary muscular contractions. Within the brain itself, large populations of densely interconnected neurons interact to subserve language, learning and memory, and consciousness.

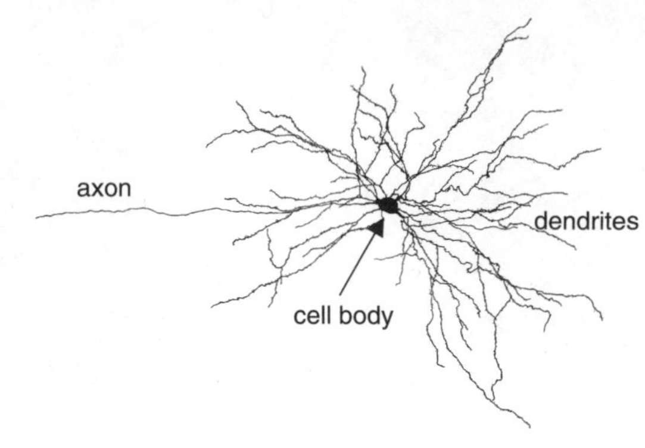

FIGURE 7.1 Anatomy of a neuron, highlighting the dendrites, which receive inputs from other neurons; the cell body, which integrates inputs; and the axon, which generates and propagates digital output pulses called action potentials. (Data courtesy of B. Burton and G.J. Lee.)

Electrochemical Potential

The mechanistic bases of electrical signaling in neurons can be understood by considering a simple spherical cell (Figure 7.2(a)) with a membrane that is *semi-permeable* (i.e., a membrane that passes ions, but only slowly, so that the internal and external concentrations of the ions can be assumed constant). Two factors influence the movement of ion X through the membrane. First, any concentration gradient of X across the membrane will drive a diffusive flux, according to Fick's first law. Second, because the ion has charge, its movement will be influenced by any electrical field across the membrane. The *Nernst equation* describes the equilibrium condition for ion X, in which these two sources of ionic flux cancel each other out, resulting in zero net flux:

$$E_x = \frac{RT}{z_x F} \ln\left(\frac{[X]_{\text{out}}}{[X]_{\text{in}}}\right) \tag{7.1}$$

In Equation (7.1), E_x is the equilibrium or Nernst potential, the value of membrane potential (inside minus outside, by convention) at which this single-ion system is at equilibrium. R is the molar gas constant, 8.31 J/(mol K). T is absolute temperature in degrees Kelvin. z_x is the valence of X (+1 for Na^+ and K^+). F is Faraday's constant, 96,500 C/mol. $[X]_{\text{out}}$ and $[X]_{\text{in}}$ are the external and internal concentrations of X, typically

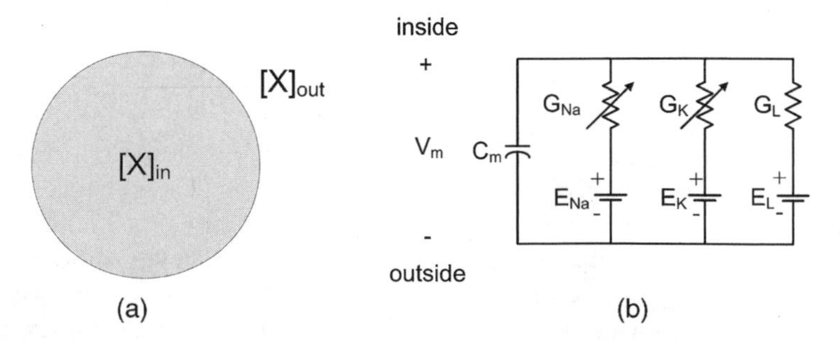

FIGURE 7.2 Simple electrical models of a spatially restricted neuron. (a) The equation for equilibrium potential for ion X can be derived by treating external and internal concentrations of X as fixed. (b) An equivalent electrical circuit describing a patch of neural membrane, or an electrically excitable neuron that can be considered isopotential, with voltage-gated Na^+ and K^+ conductances.

expressed in m*M*. It is often more convenient to convert the Nernst equation to $\log_{10}$, and to assume a value of temperature. At 37°C, the Nernst equation reduces to

$$E_x \approx \frac{61}{z_x} \log_{10}\left(\frac{[X]_{\text{out}}}{[X]_{\text{in}}}\right) \tag{7.2}$$

where E_x has units of mV.

As noted above, Na^+ and K^+ are crucial for neuroelectric signaling. In mammalian nerve and muscle cells, the external concentration of Na^+ is approximately an order of magnitude greater than the internal concentration, leading to an Na^+ Nernst potential $E_{Na} \approx +60$ mV. In contrast, the internal concentration of K^+ is more than an order of magnitude greater than the external concentration, giving a K^+ Nernst potential $E_{K}v \approx -80$ mV.

The disparate values of E_{Na} and E_K imply that these two ions cannot be in equilibrium simultaneously. In fact, neither Na^+ nor K^+ is typically in equilibrium. The simple electrical model shown in Figure 7.2(b) is commonly used to describe small patches of neuronal membrane that are permeant to both Na^+ and K^+ (along with other ions). In this model, C_m represents membrane capacitance, generated by the relatively poorly conducting cell membrane between the highly conductive intracellular and extracellular fluids. G_{Na} and G_K represent membrane conductances that specifically pass Na^+ and K^+, respectively. Note that these conductances are, in general, nonlinear. G_L represents the so-called "leak" conductance. This conductance represents the flow of multiple ions through linear membrane conductances. The battery E_L represents the Thevenin equivalent combination of the Nernst potentials of all of the ions flowing through the linear conductance. In the steady state, membrane potential V_m is given by the equation:

$$V_m = \frac{G_{Na}E_{Na} + G_K E_K + G_L E_L}{G_{Na} + G_K + G_L} \tag{7.3}$$

This simple equation has the important implication that V_m is bounded between E_{Na} (+60 mV) and E_K (−80 mV). (E_L lies between these bounds.) Thus, neurons have an operating range of slightly more than 100 mV. Under steady-state conditions, G_K is typically significantly larger than G_{Na} or G_L, consistent with typical resting values of $V_m \approx -65$ mV.

Because both Na^+ and K^+ are out of equilibrium at rest, there is a constant inward trickle of Na^+ (because $V_m < E_{Na}$) and outward trickle of K^+ (because $V_m > E_K$). Over time-scales of minutes to hours, this trickle would be sufficient to "run down" the concentration gradients in Na^+ and K^+, thus causing E_{Na} and E_K to approach zero. Nerve cells expend energy to continually pump Na^+ out and K^+ in, thus maintaining nearly constant values of E_{Na} and E_K throughout life.

Action Potentials

Neurons make use of their nonequilibrium conditions for purposes of signaling. Figure 7.3 shows results from a hypothetical experiment in which an electrode has been inserted into a neuron. Parameters match those from the "giant axon" of the squid, in which the mechanisms underlying action potentials were first elucidated (see below). The left panels show responses of this *gedanken* neuron to a square pulse of current (duration = 1 msec, amplitude = 5 μA/cm^2, onset at $t = 0$ msec). This stimulus induces only a small deflection in membrane potential. Both G_{Na} and G_K remain very near their resting values. For stimuli of this size, the cell is well approximated by the circuit of Figure 7.2(b), with ohmic conductances.

The situation changes dramatically for larger stimuli (Figure 7.3, right panels). Such stimuli induce a voltage deflection with amplitude roughly 100 mV. This is the action potential. To a first approximation, the action potential is all-or-nothing; large stimuli generate a stereotypical action potential like that in the upper-right panel of Figure 7.3, whereas weak stimuli generate no action potential at all. For a fixed duration of the current pulse, there is a sharply defined threshold for action potential generation.

The lower-right panel of Figure 7.3 gives insight into the mechanisms underlying the action potential. The sharp rise in V_m near $t = 1$ msec, often referred to as the *depolarizing* phase of the action potential, is driven by

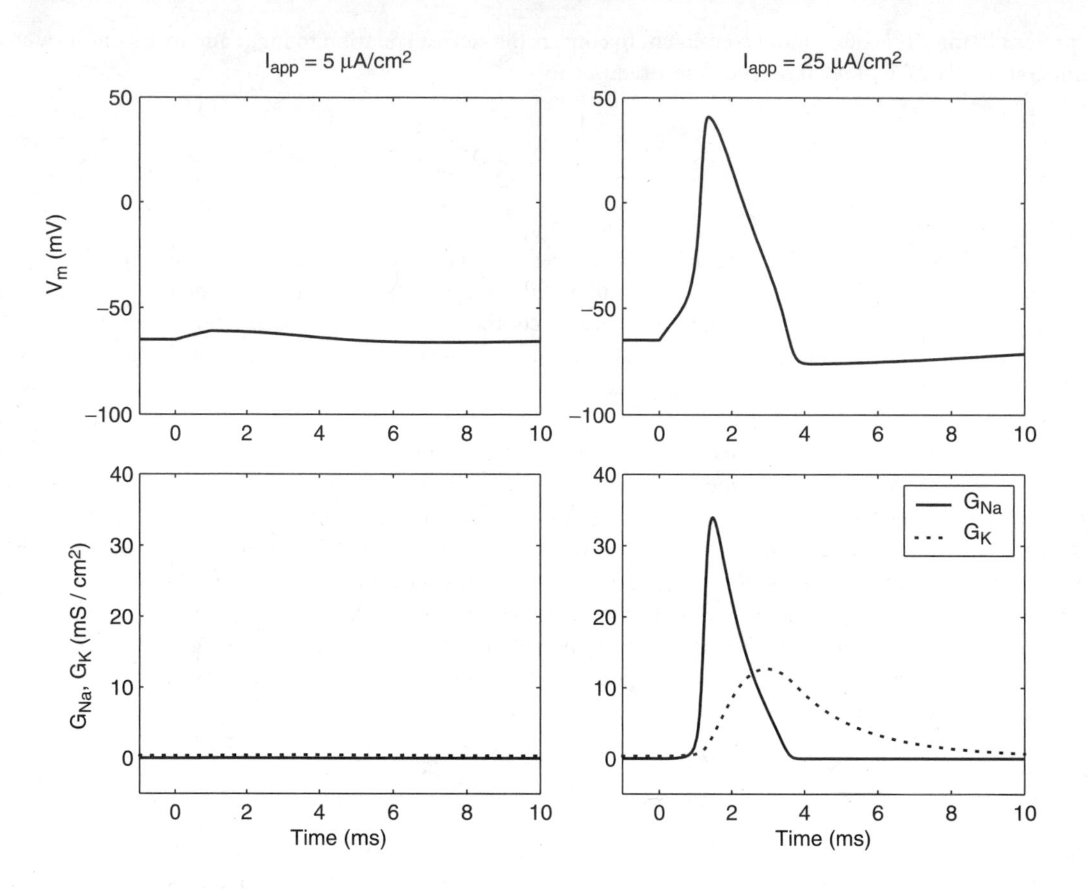

FIGURE 7.3 Intracellular responses of a modeled excitable neuron to subthreshold (left column) and suprathreshold (right column) pulses of intracellularly applied current. Top traces show membrane potential V_m vs. time. Bottom traces show the values of the two voltage-gated conductances.

an enormous increase in G_{Na}. As we would expect from the circuit model in Figure 7.2(b) and Equation (7.3), this increase in G_{Na} will pull membrane potential toward E_{Na}. Two factors drive the subsequent *repolarizing* phase of the action potential (around $t = 2$ to 4 msec), during which V_m falls below its resting value. First, G_{Na} begins to turn off near $t = 2$ msec. Second, G_K increases substantially during the repolarizing phase. Both of these factors drive V_m to a value near E_K. The repolarizing phase corresponds closely to the neuron's *absolute refractory period*, during which a second action potential cannot be induced.

The repolarizing phase is followed by a gradual return of G_{Na} and G_K to their resting values (around $t =$ 4 to 10 msec). During this phase, the membrane potential is generally below resting potential (because the membrane is more G_K-dominated than at rest). The neuron can generate an action potential during this phase, the *relative refractory period*, but only with a larger stimulus than under resting conditions. At around $t = 10$ msec, G_{Na}, G_K, V_m, and threshold have all returned to their resting values.

The Nobel Prize-winning work of Hodgkin and Huxley (1952), culminating in an accurate model of the action potential in the squid giant axon, still stands as one of the great achievements in quantitative biology. Prototypical bioengineers, Hodgkin and Huxley utilized techniques from applied mathematics, instrumentation and biology to achieve this goal. Three major, interrelated technical innovations made their work possible. First, they were able to slide a fine wire down the center of the squid giant axon. This wire effectively short-circuited the inside of the axon, meaning that the entire axon was **space-clamped** (isopotential) and described well by the electrical circuit model in Figure 7.2(b). Second, they reasoned that the nonlinear behavior of G_{Na} and G_K was likely to depend on membrane potential V_m. Improving on the work of Kenneth Cole, Hodgkin and Huxley constructed and used feedback circuitry that allowed them to switch V_m, nearly instantaneously, from one constant value to another, and measure the resulting current fluxes through G_{Na} and G_K. The **voltage-clamp** technique remains one of the most valuable tools used by cellular electrophysiologists. Third, Hodgkin and Huxley had the mathematical prowess to develop a relatively simple set of four nonlinear differential equations that could be parameterized simply using voltage-clamp data, and solved numerically to describe the action potential in the space-clamped axon. The full Hodgkin–Huxley equations are described elsewhere (e.g., Weiss, 1996; White, 2002). The first of the four equations is simply Kirchoff's current law applied to the circuit of Figure 7.2(b):

$$C_m \frac{dV_m}{dt} = -G_{Na}(V_m, t)[V_m - E_{Na}] - G_K(V_m, t)[V_m - E_K] - G_L[V_m - E_L] \tag{7.4}$$

The second and third Hodgkin–Huxley equations (not shown) describe the processes by which G_{Na} *activates* (i.e., turns on to generate the depolarizing phase of the action potential) and *inactivates* (i.e., turns off during the repolarizing phase of the action potential). Both processes depend nonlinearly on membrane potential V_m. The fourth Hodgkin–Huxley equation describes V_m-dependent activation of G_K.

Two features of the Hodgkin–Huxley model are crucial to account for the action potential:

1. G_{Na} rapidly activates in response to depolarization of the membrane (i.e., positive excursions of V_m). This property implies that G_{Na}, once activated, is prone to destabilization via positive feedback: a small depolarization partially activates G_{Na}, which in turn further depolarizes the membrane, further activating G_{Na}, an so on. This destabilizing positive feedback gives rise to the depolarizing phase of the action potential.
2. In response to depolarization, G_{Na} eventually inactivates and G_K activates, but these processes are an order of magnitude slower than the activation of G_{Na}. Both of these processes contribute to the repolarizing phase of the action potential. Once the action potential is complete, these processes return to their resting values over the course of several milliseconds. During the repolarizing phase, and immediately afterward, G_{Na} is nearly fully inactivated. Thus, the positive feedback mechanism cannot be triggered, and the membrane is absolutely refractory. After the absolute refractory period comes the relative refractory period, during which G_{Na} is still partially inactivated and G_K is partially activated. Consequently, a larger depolarization than normal is required to trigger an action potential.

The greatest achievement of Hodgkin and Huxley was that their equations, parameterized under voltage- and space-clamped conditions, accurately described the details of propagation of the action potential when these conditions were relaxed. In simple bare axons (e.g., squid giant axon and small axons of the human nervous system), called *unmyelinated* axons, the action potential propagates simply because the "spiking" region of the axon depolarizes adjacent regions, causing those regions to spike as well. In the wake of the propagating action potential lies a region of refractory (unexcitable) membrane. Mathematically, this situation is described by a nonlinear partial differential equation, the nonlinear cable equation (Hodgkin and Huxley, 1952; Weiss, 1996):

$$\begin{aligned}\frac{1}{2\pi a(r_i + r_o)} \frac{\partial^2 V_m}{\partial z^2} = {} & C_m \frac{\partial V_m}{\partial t} + G_{Na}(V_m, t)[V_m - E_{Na}] + G_K(V_m, t)[V_m - E_K] \\ & + G_L[V_m - E_L]\end{aligned} \tag{7.5}$$

where a is the axonal radius; r_i and r_o are the internal and external resistances per unit length of axon, respectively; and z is distance along the cylindrical axon. Note that V_m in Equation (7.5) is a function of both z and t.

Large axons of the human body are usually *myelinated*: most of the axon is covered by an insulating sheath, with periodic patches of bare axon called *nodes of Ranvier*. In myelinated axons, nonlinear ionic fluxes occur only at the nodes. Excitation of one node is sufficient to rapidly depolarize and excite adjacent nodes. The resulting "saltatory" conduction of the action potential is faster, for large axons, than the continuous conduction seen in unmyelinated axons (Weiss, 1996). A number of serious neurological conditions, including multiple sclerosis and chronic inflammatory demyelinating polyneuropathy (CIDP), involve disruption of axonal myelination.

More recent work on action potentials has revealed the molecular mechanisms underlying voltage-gated membrane conductances. Most notably, two Nobel Prizes have been granted in this area. Sakmann and Neher won the 1991 Nobel Prize in Physiology or Medicine for their conclusive, direct recordings of ion flow through single ion channels (see Sakmann and Neher, 1995). To a great degree, the problems solved by Sakmann and Neher were engineering problems. In particular, they took a number of steps to dramatically improve the signal-to-noise ratio of their recordings, eventually managing to obtain clean recordings of the single-channel currents (on the order of pA). MacKinnon won the 2003 Nobel Prize in Chemistry for obtaining and interpreting high-resolution x-ray-crystallographic images of voltage-gated ion channels. Using these images, MacKinnon explained the mechanism by which an individual ion channel can pass K^+ but exclude Na^+, an ion with very similar chemical properties but much different effects on membrane potential (Doyle et al., 1998).

Synaptic Transmission

Action potentials generated in an individual neuron influence each other via either chemical or electrical *synapses*. In chemical synapses, the axonal action potential triggers release of small vesicles of chemically active substances called *neurotransmitters*, which diffuse across the small synaptic cleft to an adjacent neuron. Chemically gated ion channels respond to these neurotransmitters by opening or closing, leading to effects that can be understood electrically using simple elaborations of Figure 7.2(b). Chemical neurotransmitters can also trigger a wide-ranging set of biochemical effects that operate on a slower time scale than the direct electrical effects.

Electrical synapses, formed by so-called *gap junctions* between physically adjacent neurons, are perhaps less prevalent in the nervous system than in the heart, but they still serve as important lines of communication between neurons. From an electrical perspective, electrical synapses can be modeled as resistors connecting multiple compartments of the form seen in Figure 7.2(b). Linear (ohmic) electrical synapses seem to be more prevalent than nonlinear electrical synapses, but both kinds have been observed.

Dynamic Clamp

For decades, cellular electrophysiologists have relied upon two intracellular recording techniques: current-clamp recordings (e.g., Figure 7.3), in which electrical current is passed into the cell and resulting changes in V_m are observed; and voltage-clamp recordings, in which V_m is manipulated and the resulting membrane currents are measured. More recently, a third recording technique, termed the **dynamic clamp** or *conductance clamp* technique, has been developed (Prinz et al., 2004). The dynamic clamp allows the neurophysiologist to introduce *virtual membrane conductances* into the neuronal membrane. Thus, the user has the newfound ability to introduce realistic virtual chemical synaptic inputs into the neuron; to couple two recorded neurons via virtual electrical and/or chemical synapses, or to construct hybrid neuronal networks, consisting of biological and artificial neurons that are coupled in realistic, user-defined ways.

The dynamic clamp method is inherently more complex than the current clamp or voltage clamp techniques. Figure 7.4 shows schematic circuitry for current clamp (Figure 7.4(a)), voltage clamp (Figure 7.4(b)), and two forms of dynamic clamp (Figure 7.4(c) and (d)). In typical current-clamp circuitry (Figure 7.4(a)), membrane potential is recorded with a resistive electrode (R_e) and buffered. A copy of the V_m signal is summed with the command potential V_c. (Here and throughout, we assume that circuit components have a gain of 1.) This summed signal serves as a source of current through a feedback resistor. This circuit ensures that the current flowing through the feedback resistor, and thus into the neuron, is proportional to V_c and independent of V_m (Sherman-Gold, 1993). The flaw in this design is that the measured value of V_m is distorted by the current passing through the electrode resistance R_e. Current-clamp amplifiers use modern equivalents of Wheatstone bridges to cancel the effects of R_e (Sherman-Gold, 1993).

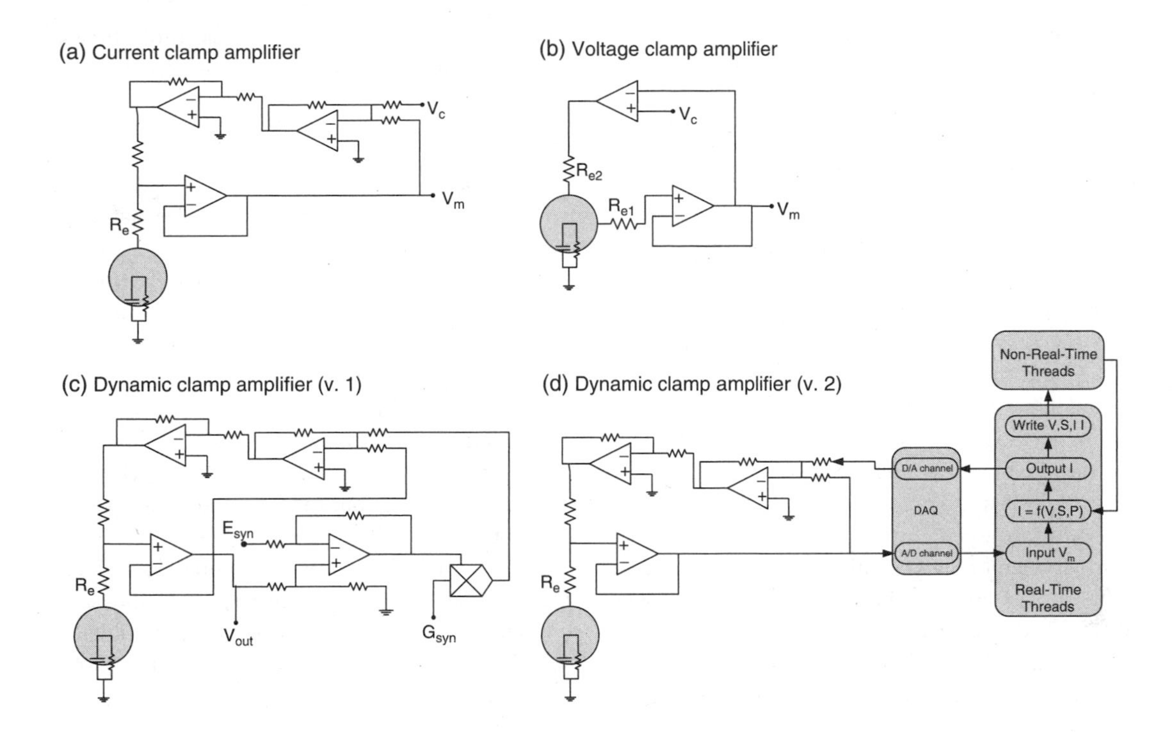

FIGURE 7.4 Intracellular recording configurations. (a) In current clamp, the experimenter injects a controlled amount of current into the neuron and records the resulting changes in membrane potential V_m. (b) In voltage clamp, an amplifier passes sufficient current through one electrode to hold membrane potential at a user-controlled value. (c) Hardware-based dynamic clamp systems can be used to introduce artificial synaptic conductances into neurons. (d) Software-based dynamic clamp systems can be used to introduce artificial voltage-gated conductances into neurons, or to immerse living neurons into artificial neuronal networks that run in real time.

Figure 7.4(b) depicts a voltage-clamp circuit. In this example, two electrodes (R_{e1} and R_{e2}) are inserted into the cell. A buffer records V_m via R_{e1}. A copy of this signal is sent to one input terminal of a high-gain operational amplifier; the other input terminal receives the command signal V_c. Within the limits of capacity and bandwidth (not discussed here), the op-amp will pass current through the second electrode (R_{e2}) to "clamp" V_m at the value $V_m = V_c$ (Sherman-Gold, 1993).

Figure 7.4(c) shows the simplest form of dynamic clamp circuit, capable of injecting a current signal $I_{syn} = G_{syn}\ (V_m - E_{syn})$, where G_{syn} is a user-supplied, time-dependent conductance signal and E_{syn} is the associated constant synaptic reversal potential. In this case, E_{syn} is subtracted from the signal V_m via a differential amplifier, and this difference is multiplied by G_{syn}. This conditioned signal, along with V_m itself, is passed to the current-clamp section of the amplifier.

The circuit in Figure 7.4(c) works well as long as two conditions hold. First, it is crucial that the experimentalist compensate for electrode series resistance R_e; otherwise, induced current flow through R_e will distort measurements of V_m and hence I_{syn}. Second, this circuit is useful only if the applied conductance G_{syn} does not depend on V_m itself. For many applications (e.g., applying artificial synaptic inputs to a cell), this condition holds. However, if one wishes to mimic *voltage-gated* conductances, one must also model the differential equations that describe how conductance depends on V_m.

The simplest and most flexible way to model conductances that are voltage dependent is to use a data acquisition card (DAQ) to digitize V_m, so that gating equations can be solved digitally in real time

(Figure 7.4(d)). The user interacts with the real-time thread via a GUI and other non-real-time threads (Dorval et al., 2001). A number of systems of this type have been created and used to model even the fastest conductance events in neurons (Prinz et al., 2004).

Models of Extracellular Stimulation

Thus far we have discussed intrinsic neuronal activation and the techniques used to examine naturally occurring neuronal activity. We now turn our attention to external neuronal stimulation, a much older but less thoroughly understood field. In 1791, Luigi Galvani publicized what he deemed "animal electricity," supposedly generated by probing frog motor neurons with bimetallic rods. Two years later, Allessandro Volta showed that Galvani's animal electricity was actually a discharge of static electricity from the rod that activated the nerve, and the field of extracellular stimulation was born. Little theoretical progress was made however, until Hodgkin and Huxley elucidated the mechanisms of neuronal excitability in 1952. As stated previously, the all-or-nothing action potential described by Hodgkin and Huxley initiates when the potential difference across the membrane depolarizes to some threshold. This threshold-achieving depolarization is typically generated via synaptic input coupling with membrane-intrinsic conductances, but can be achieved artificially with a well-positioned electrode delivering an appropriate stimulus.

Consider membrane potential V_m as the difference between the intrinsic neuronal potential V_i and the potential just external to the neuron V_e, both varying in time and space, defined with respect to the same distant ground somewhere within the extracellular space: $V_m(z,t) = V_i(z,t) - V_e(z,t)$. Under physiological conditions, the extracellular space is primarily isopotential but stimulation via a point electrode in an isotropic extracellular space can shape $V_e(z,t)$ according to:

$$V_e(z,t) = [\rho_e I_s(t)]/[4\pi x] \tag{7.6}$$

where ρ_e is the resistivity of the extracellular space (typically ~300 Ω cm), x is the distance between the electrode and the axon at location z, and $I_s(t)$ is the current applied through the electrode. From first principles, Equation (7.6) can be extended to anisotropic, inhomogeneous media and more complex electrode geometries.

To understand extracellular axonal stimulation, we revisit Equation (7.5) with the knowledge that the axoplasm is isopotential except during action potentials or stimulation. Hence, under normal conditions, the second spatial derivative of extracellular potential (along the length of the axon) drives axonal activation, and is often referred to as the **activating function,** $\partial^2 V_e/\partial z^2$. When the axon is at rest, $\partial V_m/\partial t$ must be positive for the membrane to approach threshold. From Equation (7.5), we can deduce that positive deflections of the activating function depolarize the membrane potential (Rattay, 1986). As an example, we consider a stimulating electrode placed 1.0 mm from an infinitely long Hodgkin–Huxley axon. Figure 7.5(a) shows the extracellular potential and activating function along an axon, in response to the minimum amplitude cathodic and anodic stimuli capable of eliciting action potentials when applied for 0.1 msec. Action potential initiation depends on the duration of the applied stimulus and the amplitude of the positive portion of the activating function. Since cathodic stimulation yields a larger positive region of the activating function in response to a smaller external field (and thus less applied current), cathodic stimulation initiates action potentials more efficiently. Figure 7.5(b) depicts action potential propagation in the Hodgkin–Huxley model in response to cathodic stimulus. Note that the action potential propagates in both directions from the site of origin.

Not all stimuli are strong enough to elicit an action potential. Figure 7.6(a) shows membrane potential vs. time for a patch of axonal membrane at $z = 0$, in response to four different cathodic stimuli. Electrode and model configuration are the same as in the previous figure. In general, the smaller the stimulus amplitude, the longer it must be applied for an axon to reach threshold. Some stimuli are so small, however, that even if they were applied forever they would not elicit an action potential. The smallest amplitude stimulus capable of generating a response is known as the **rheobase**. The **chronaxie** is the required duration to generate an action potential using a stimulus whose amplitude is twice the rheobase. Rheobase and chronaxie vary greatly across experimental conditions: electrode size and position, axon radius, conductance distributions, and the presence

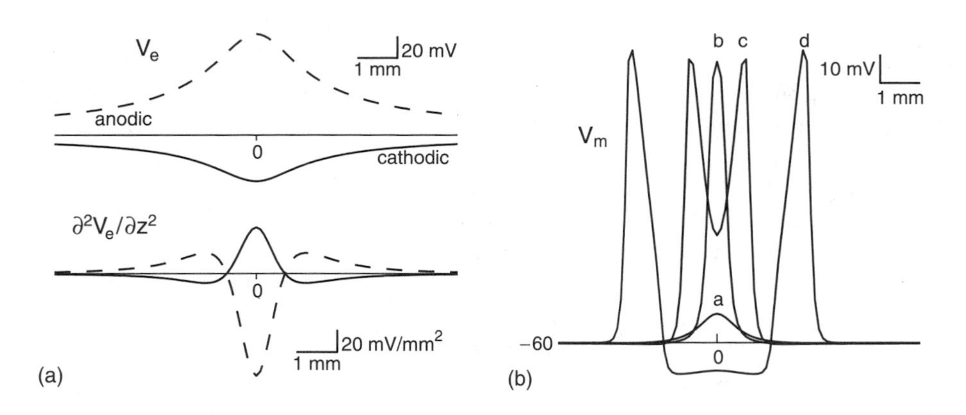

FIGURE 7.5 Extracellular stimulation of an infinitely long, 1-μm diameter Hodgkin–Huxley axon, in a homogenous, isotropic medium, from an electrode 100 μm away, at $z = 0$. (a) Cathodic stimuli yield action potentials at smaller amplitudes. *Top*: Extracellular potential as a function of space. *Bottom*: Activating function along the axon. The amplitude of the positive region of the activating function determines action potential initiation. (b) Action potential initiation and bidirectional propagation following a 100-μsec cathodic stimulation at $t = 0$. Waveforms are membrane potential as a function of space at $t =$ (a) 1.0 msec, (b) 2.5 msec, (c) 4.0 msec, and (d) 8.0 msec.

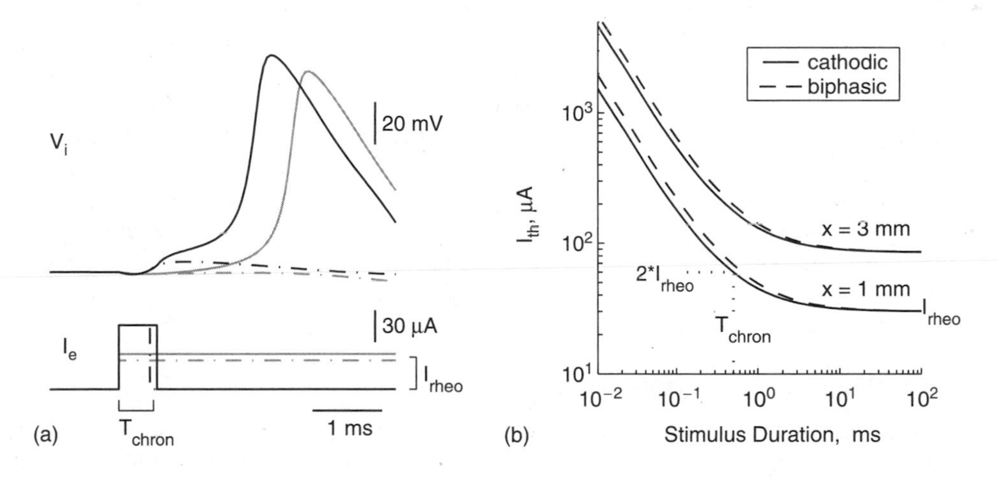

FIGURE 7.6 Action potential thresholds in an infinitely long, 1-μm diameter Hodgkin–Huxley axon, in a homogenous, isotropic medium. (a) Extracellularly applied currents are shown on bottom, resulting potentials are shown on top. Gray lines illustrate action potential threshold with respect to the rheobase, I_{rheo}. Solid and dotted lines are from stimuli of amplitude 1.1 I_{rheo} and 0.9 I_{rheo}, respectively. Black lines illustrate threshold with respect to the chronaxie, T_{chron}. Solid and dotted lines are from stimuli of duration 1.1 T_{chron} and 0.9 T_{chron}, respectively. (b) Strength–duration curves (i.e., threshold I_{th} vs. duration), illustrating the relationships between rheobase and chronaxie, and between cathodic and biphasic stimulation. Bottom two traces are with the electrode placed 1 mm from the axon; top two traces are with the electrode placed 3 mm from the axon.

of a myelin sheath all affect these parameters. In experimental or clinical situations, it is difficult to accurately predict either rheobase or chronaxie, but they are relatively easy to measure. Once measured, rheobase and chronaxie can be used to determine strength–duration curves. The classic strength–duration relationship is described by functions of the form (Weiss, 1901):

$$I_{\text{th}}(T) = [1 + T_{\text{chron}}/T]I_{\text{rheo}} \tag{7.7}$$

where T is the stimulus duration, I_{th} is the minimum applied current required to induce an action potential, T_{chron} is the chronaxie, and I_{rheo} is the rheobase. The solid lines of Figure 7.6b display strength–duration curves for a Hodgkin–Huxley axon stimulated by electrodes at two distances from the axon.

The monophasic stimulation discussed so far is often unsuitable for clinical use because it encourages charge buildup on the electrode upon repeated bouts of stimulation. To reduce charge buildup, cathodic pulses are often followed by equal-amplitude–anodic pulses to create biphasic stimulation that delivers no net charge through the electrode. The rheobase for biphasic stimuli is the same as for monophasic cathodic because the action potential occurs during the cathodic stimulation in either case. For stronger but shorter applied currents (e.g., at the chronaxie) action potentials actually occur after the cathodic stimulus has ended. In the biphasic stimulus case, the anodic phase interacts with membrane potential before action potential generation. Hence, for short-duration stimuli, biphasic currents require slightly larger amplitudes than monophasic currents (compare dashed and solid lines in Figure 7.6(b)).

In living organisms, axons rarely exist in isolation. Axons of various sizes are typically bound together in a nerve bundle that travels between brain regions or from the brain to elsewhere in the body. Hence, *in vivo* considerations of extracellular stimulation focus on the recruitment of multiple axons within a nerve. That is, for a given amplitude stimulus, a certain number of axons within a nerve will be recruited, or fire action potentials. For a larger amplitude stimulus, a larger number of axons will be recruited. Axonal diameter and distance from the electrode will determine which axons are recruited and in what order. As demonstrated by Figure 7.6(b), a couple of millimeters can make a large difference in axonal excitability.

Unlike the neurons thus far examined, living axons are not perfect cylinders residing in homogenous, isotropic media. Thus, any consideration of *in vivo* extracellular stimulation must include details about the organism that we have heretofore overlooked. For real systems, extracellular resistivity ρ_e varies as a function of space. For example, the extracellular medium is likely to be more conductive in the direction of a bundle of nerves, and more resistive perpendicular to the bundle. Anisotropies of this type change the extracellular potential experienced by any local axon, and thus modify the susceptibility to electrical stimulation. In many cases these differences alter the qualitative behavior of the system (e.g., the order in which axons in a nerve are recruited depends on subtle differences in the extracellular resistivity anisotropy). These modifications can be worked out analytically for some configurations, but are beyond the scope of this chapter (see Grill, 1999).

Application: Deep Brain Stimulation

While the details of neural activation via extracellular stimulation continue to be elucidated, the underlying principles described in the previous section have been understood for decades. With this knowledge, researchers and physicians have devised a number of ways that extracellular stimulation can be used to treat medical conditions. Some of these techniques have been used clinically since the 1970s, others are relatively new, and many more are still being developed. Like many medical technologies, extracellular stimulation has practical complications unrelated to a scientific understanding of the problem, which pose obstacles for clinical implementation (Davis, 2002).

Clinical applications of electrical stimulation can be divided into three categories:

1. Neural output activation involves electrical stimulation of nerves that control some output function of the nervous system. For example, stimulation of peripheral nerves is used to provide some skeletal muscle control to quadriplegics and other individuals afflicted with motor deficits (Sinkjaer et al., 2003). Direct stimulation of the spinal cord is now being used to return bladder and sphincter control to paraplegics and patients suffering from incontinence (Jezernik et al., 2002).
2. Neural input activation is used to bypass defective sense organs. By electrically stimulating the auditory nerve, cochlear implants provide a sense of hearing sufficient for previously deaf individuals to understand speech (Skinner, 2003). On a more experimental frontier, retinal implants have had some success restoring sight to the visually impaired by electrically stimulating retinal neurons at the back of the eye (Hetling and Baig-Silva, 2004).

3. Central nervous system processing activation treats diseases located more centrally within the nervous system than the previous two classes. Electroconvulsive therapy, in its current form, is often an effective treatment for individuals suffering from severe depression (Reisner, 2003). Deep brain stimulation (DBS), a more recent and less controversial form of brain stimulation, lessens the debilitating effects of Parkinson's disease, and shows promise as a treatment for a number of other diseases of the central nervous system.

As an example of extracellular stimulation in use clinically, we briefly explore DBS. This clinically effective treatment reduces the symptoms of many motor disorders, including Parkinson's disease, essential tremor, and multiple sclerosis. For DBS, a chronic electrode is placed in some brain region — typically the thalamus or basal ganglia for treatment of motor disorders. High-frequency (100 to 250 Hz) current is passed through the electrode to the surrounding neural tissue. Amazingly, signs of malfunction such as rigidity or tremor are reduced. Exactly how stimulation of certain regions reduces these symptoms is poorly understood. In fact, exactly what populations of neurons are excited by electrical stimulation is still largely unknown.

The stimulating electrode is placed in a heterogeneous region of the brain that consists of neuronal cell bodies and axons of passage (axons just passing through the region). Since local cells and axons of passage can project to widely different brain regions, it is of utmost importance to know which group is stimulated. As we know from the previous section, electrical stimulation excites infinitely long, cylindrical axons at the positive peak of the relatively simple activating function (Figure 7.5). Not surprisingly, the effects of stimulation are more complicated for finite, noncylindrical membranes. Geometric differences between cell bodies and axons lead to widely varying stimulus–duration curves. In some cases, simple knowledge of the rheobases and chronaxies may allow for the differential excitation of either axons or cell bodies simply by delivering modified stimulus waveforms (Grill and McIntyre, 2001).

From models and experiments we know that DBS inhibits cell bodies near the electrode but excites the output axons of those cells. How this complex activity translates to improved motor function is still largely unknown. One model of DBS suggests that stimulation causes an over-excitation of axons leaving the region. This over-excitation actually leads to decreased action potential generation via a mechanism known as *depolarization blockade*. Another model suggests that DBS works primarily by exciting inhibitory neurons which then suppress the cells to which they project. In contrast to these excitation-vs.-inhibition approaches, newer models incorporate action potential firing times into a theory of DBS function (Grill et al., 2004). Clinical data and continued modeling will soon determine which of these approaches accurately models the mechanisms of DBS. For more details on recent developments in deep brain stimulation, see McIntyre (2004).

The mechanisms by which DBS (and other stimulation techniques) benefits patients are slowly being elucidated. Theoretical results from the basic understandings laid out in this section are likely to be incorporated into experimental and clinical work. As understanding of electrical stimulation grows, so does ubiquity of use and the number of conceivable clinical applications.

Glossary of Terms

Action potential: The all-or-nothing electrical impulse used to communicate information between neurons and from neurons to muscle fibers.

Activating function: The second spatial derivative of extracellular potential determines where a neuron will be excited to produce an action potential.

Activation: A term referring to the time- and voltage-dependent growth of a membrane's conductance after membrane depolarization.

Chronaxie: The minimum duration of time required for a stimulus twice the amplitude of the rheobase to induce an action potential.

Current clamp: An experimental protocol in which transmembrane current is controlled, usually at a series of constant values, and resulting transmembrane potentials are measured.

Dynamic clamp: An experimental protocol in which circuitry, often along with a real-time computer program, is used to mimic membrane conductances.

Inactivation: The time- and voltage-dependent decline of the Na^+ conductance, which follows shortly after its activation.

Ligand-gated ion channels: Transmembrane proteins that open in response to changes in the extracellular concentration of a particular neurotransmitter (ligand).

Membrane potential: The voltage difference across the neural membrane.

Refractory period: The period immediately after an action potential, in which it is difficult or impossible to induce a second action potential.

Rheobase: The minimum current, when provided for an infinite duration, capable of inducing a neuron to fire an action potential.

Space clamp: The condition in which membrane potential is the same throughout the spatial extent of the cell.

Voltage clamp: An experimental protocol in which membrane potential is controlled, usually in a stepwise fashion, and resulting transmembrane currents are measured.

Voltage-gated ion channels: Transmembrane proteins that open in response to changes in membrane potential, allowing a particular ionic species to cross the membrane.

References

R. Davis, "Twenty-eight years of clinical experience with implantable neuroprostheses for various applications," *Artif. Organs*, 26, 280–283, 2002.

A.D. Dorval, D.J. Christini, and J.A. White, "Real-time linux dynamic clamp: a fast and flexible way to construct virtual ion channels in living cells," *Ann. Biomed. Eng.*, 29, 897–907, 2001.

D.A. Doyle Morais, J. Cabral, R.A. Pfuetzner, A. Kuo, J.M. Gulbis, S.L. Cohen, B.T. Chait, and R. MacKinnon, "The structure of the potassium channel: molecular basis of K+ conduction and selectivity," *Science*, 280, 69–77, 1998.

W.M. Grill Jr., "Modeling the effects of electric fields on nerve fibers: influence of tissue electrical properties," *IEEE Trans. Biomed. Eng.*, 46, 918–928, 1999.

W.M. Grill, Jr. and C.C. McIntyre, "Extracellular excitation of central neurons: implications for the mechanisms of deep brain stimulation," *Thalamus Relat. Sys.*, 1, 269–277, 2001.

J.R. Hetling and M.S. Baig-Silva, "Neural prostheses for vision: designing a functional interface with retinal neurons," *Neurol. Res.*, 26, 21–34, 2004.

A.L. Hodgkin and A.F. Huxley, "A quantitative description of membrane current and its application to conduction and excitation in nerve," *J. Physiol.*, 117, 500–544, 1952.

S. Jezernik, M. Craggs, W.M. Grill, G. Creasey, and N.J. Rijkhoff, "Electrical stimulation for the treatment of bladder dysfunction: current status and future possibilities," *Neurol. Res.*, 24, 413–430, 2002.

C.C. McIntyre, M. Savasta, B.L. Walter, and J.L. Vitek, "How does deep brain stimulation work? Present understanding and future questions," *J. Clin. Neurophysiol.*, 21, 40–50, 2004.

A.A. Prinz, L.F. Abbott, and E. Marder, "The dynamic clamp comes of age," *Trends. Neurosci.*, 27, 218–224, 2004.

F. Rattay, "Analysis of models for external stimulation of axons," *IEEE Trans. Biomed. Eng.*, 33, 974–977, 1986.

A.D. Reisner, "The electroconvulsive therapy controversy: evidence and ethics," *Neuropsychol. Rev.*, 13, 199–219, 2003.

B. Sakmann and E. Neher, *Single-Channel Recording*, 2nd ed., New York: Plenum Press, 1995.

R. Sherman-Gold, Ed., *The Axon Guide*, Foster City, CA: Axon Instruments, Inc., 1993.

T. Sinkjaer, M. Haugland, A. Inmann, M. Hansen, and K.D. Nielsen, "Biopotentials as command and feedback signals in functional electrical stimulation systems," *Med. Eng. Phys.*, 25, 29–40, 2003.

M.W. Skinner, "Optimizing cochlear implant speech performance," *Ann. Otol. Rhinol. Laryngol. Suppl.*, 191, 4–13, 2003.

G.G. Weiss, "Sur la possibilité de rendre comparables entre eux les appareils: à l'excitation," *Arch. Ital. Biol.*, 35, 413–445, 1901.

T. Weiss, *Cellular Biophysics*, Cambridge, MA: MIT Press, 1996.

J.A. White, "Action potential," in *Encyclopedia of the Human Brain*, V.S. Ramachandran, Ed., San Diego, CA: Academic Press, 2002, pp. 1–12.

7.2 Bioelectric Events

L.A. Geddes (revised by R.C. Barr)

Bioelectric signals are exploited for the diagnostic information that they contain. Such signals are often used to monitor and guide therapy. Although all living cells exhibit bioelectric phenomena, a small variety produce potential changes that reveal their physiological function. The most familiar bioelectric recordings are the electrocardiogram (ECG) (which reflects the excitation and recovery of the whole heart); the electromyogram (EMG) (which reflects the activity of skeletal muscle); and the electroencephalogram (EEG) (which reflects the activity of the outer layers of the brain, the cortex). The following paragraphs will describe (1) the origin of all bioelectric phenomena; (2) the nature of the electrical activity of the heart, skeletal muscle, and the brain; and (3) some of the characteristics of instrumentation used to display these events.

Origin of Bioelectricity

Cell membranes are thin lipid bilayers that resemble charged capacitors operating near the dielectric breakdown voltage. Assuming a typical value of 90 mV for the transmembrane potential and a membrane thickness of 100 Å, the voltage gradient across the membrane is 0.9×10^5 V/cm. A typical value for membrane capacitance is about 1 μF/cm^2, while membrane resistance may be 10,000 ohm cm^2.

The transmembrane charge is the result of a **metabolic process** that creates ionic gradients with a high concentration of potassium ions (K^+) inside and a high concentration of sodium ions (Na^+) outside. Ions cross membranes through specialized structures called channels, which may be ion-selective. There are concentration gradients for other ions, the cell wall being a semipermeable membrane that obeys the Nernst equation (60 mV/decade concentration gradient for univalent ions). The result of the ionic gradient is the transmembrane potential that, in the cells referred to earlier, is about 90 mV, the interior being negative with respect to the exterior. Figure 7.7 illustrates this concept for a cylindrical cell.

The transmembrane potential is stable in inexcitable cells, such as the red blood cell. However, in excitable cells, a reduction in transmembrane potential (either physiological or induced electrically) results in excitation, characterized by a transmembrane ion flux, resulting from a membrane permeability change. When the transmembrane potential is reduced by about one third, Na^+ ions rush in; K^+ ions exit slightly later while the cell depolarizes, reverse polarizes, then repolarizes. The resulting excursion in transmembrane potential is a propagated action potential that is characteristic for each type of cell. In Figure 7.8, the action potentials of (a) a single cardiac ventricular muscle cell, (c) a skeletal muscle cell, and (e) a nerve cell, are shown. In (b) and (d), the ensuing muscular contractions are shown. An important property of the action potential is that it is

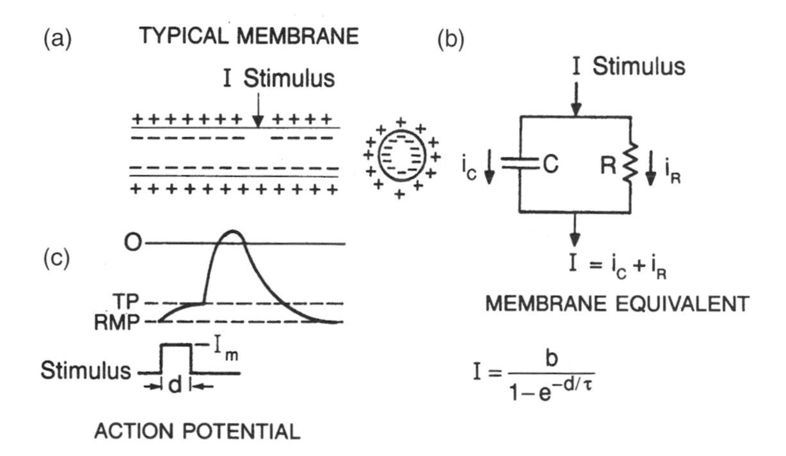

FIGURE 7.7 (a) Typical charged membrane, (b) its equivalent circuit, and (c) action potential resulting from a stimulus *I* of duration *d*.

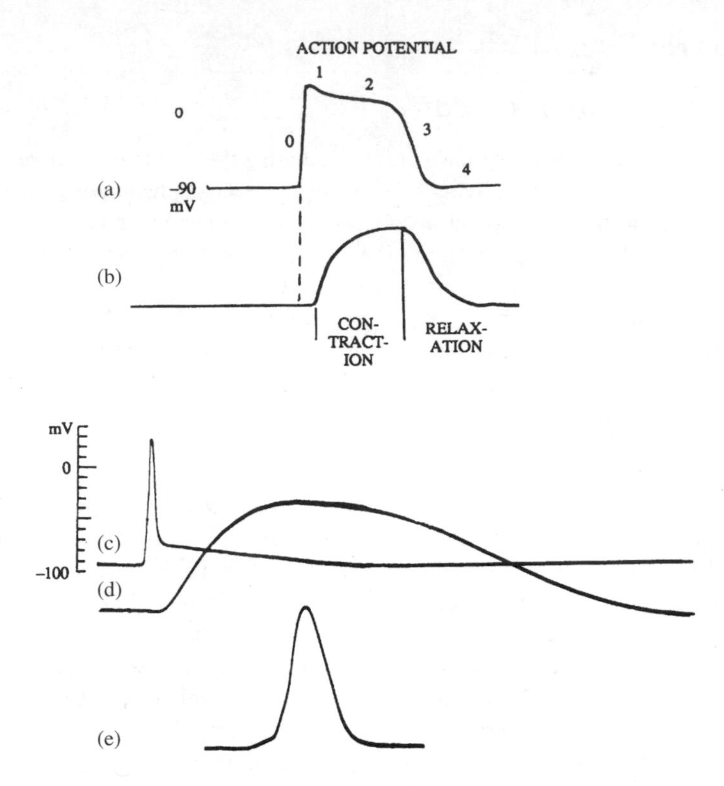

FIGURE 7.8 The action of (a) cardiac muscle and (b) its contraction, (c) skeletal muscle, and (d) and its contraction. The action potential of nerve is shown in (e).

propagated without decrement over the entire surface of the cell, the depolarized region being the stimulus for adjacent polarized regions. Action potentials may move from cell to cell through intracellular electrical connections (connexons) located at points where cells touch. In contractile cells it is the action potential that triggers release of mechanical energy as shown in Figure 7.8(b) and (d). The movement of action potentials, while having some wave-like aspects, is better pictured as a kind of chain reaction, with each element of the membrane supplying its own energy and then triggering the next. (The energy comes from drawing down the ionic concentration differences across the membrane.)

Law of Stimulation

Although action potentials are generated physiologically, excitable cells also respond to the application of a negative pulse of sufficient current density (I) and duration (d). Such a current triggers an action potential by reducing the transmembrane potential to a critical value by removing charge, thereby reducing the membrane potential to the threshold potential (TP), as shown in Figure 7.7. The law of stimulation is $I = b/(1-e^{-d}/\tau)$, where b is the threshold current density for an infinitely long-duration pulse and τ is the cell membrane time constant, being different for each type of excitable tissue. The equation is empirical, usually holding well over a certain range of values of d. Constant b is chosen experimentally to reflect electrode size and position as well as tissue responsiveness. Figure 7.9 is a plot of the threshold current (I) vs. duration (d) for mammalian cardiac muscle, sensory receptors, and motor nerve. This relationship is known as the *strength–duration curve.*

Recording Action Potentials

Action potentials of single excitable cells are recorded with transmembrane electrodes (micron diameter) by optical responses to laser illumination mostly for research studies. When action potentials are used for

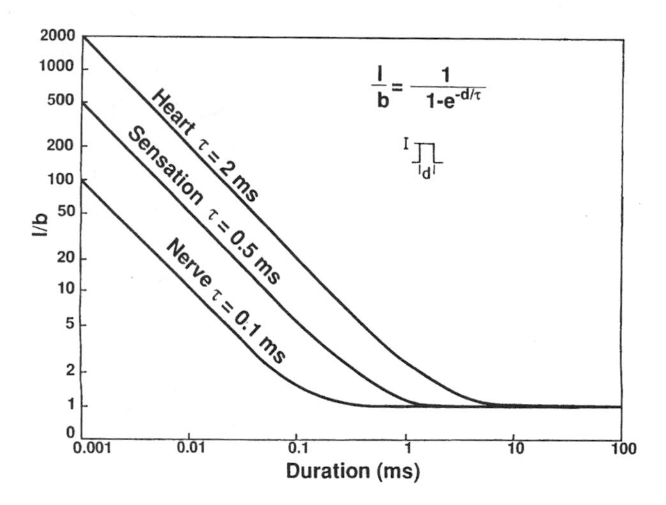

FIGURE 7.9 The strength–duration curve for heart, sensory receptors, and motor nerve. I is the stimulus current, b is the rheobasic current, and τ is the membrane time constant. The stimulus duration is d.

diagnostic purposes, usually extracellular electrodes are used. Often these electrodes are distant from the population of cells which become active and recover. The electrodes also are much larger than individual cells. The depolarization and repolarization processes send small currents through the conducting environmental tissues and fluids, resulting in a time-varying potential field throughout the conducting medium formed by the body volume. Appropriately placed electrodes allow sampling of this field and thus recording the electrical activity of the bioelectric generators. The waveforms of such recordings are vastly different from those of the transmembrane action potentials shown in Figure 7.8. By using cable theory, it is possible to show that such extracellular recordings resemble the second derivative of the excursion in transmembrane potential (Geddes and Baker, 1989). Despite the difference in waveform, extracellular recordings identify the excitation and recovery processes very well, especially their timing.

The rising edge of an action potential is its fastest phase and takes place over a few tenths of a millisecond. Often interest focuses on the action potential's wave shape and on the first and second time derivatives. Sampling rates as high as 50 kHz are necessary. Other bioelectric signals derive from action potentials, so this value forms an upper limit. Most of the time, the signals present at a particular anatomical location are spatial averages of action potentials arising from many cells simultaneously. Because of this averaging, waveform transitions are slower, and good fidelity may be present with sampling rates as low as 1 kHz. Even lower sampling rates, such as 250 Hz, are often sufficient to distinguish whether or not a waveform is present (and thus a bioelectric event, such as a heartbeat, has occurred).

The Electrocardiogram (ECG)

Origin

The heart is two double-muscular pumps. The atria pump blood into the ventricles, then the two ventricles contract. The right ventricle pumps venous blood into the lungs, and the left ventricle pumps oxygen-rich blood into the aorta. Figure 7.10 is a sketch of the heart and great vessels, along with genesis of the ECG.

An ECG may be recorded between any two sites on the body surface, and will vary among sites chosen, from person to person, and from time to time within the same person. Thus there is no single or standard wave shape that is observed; rather, there seems to be unending variability. Extensive and detailed measurements from within the heart, with comparisons to waveforms observed simultaneously or under similar conditions, were performed through the 1900s, together with substantial theoretical development, so as to better tease out, understand, and classify the origins of the body surface observations. Over this same period, observations

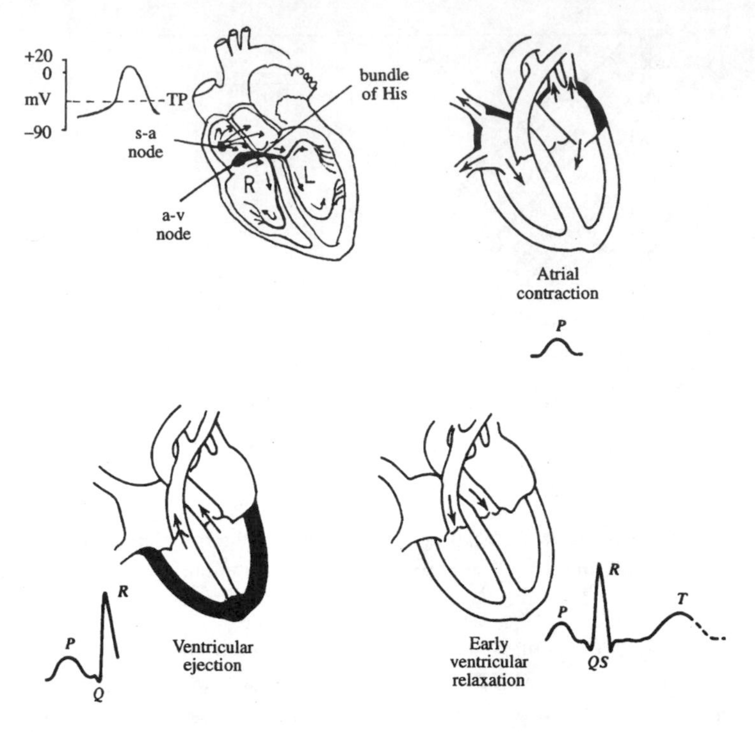

FIGURE 7.10 Genesis of the ECG. The SA node is the pacemaker, setting the rate. Excitation is propagated from the atria to the AV node, then to the bundle of His, and to the ventricular muscle via the Purkinje fibers. The SA node has a decreasing membrane potential that reaches the threshold potential (TP), resulting in spontaneous excitation (inset).

from thousands of patients were accumulated and carefully categorized according to the subject's age, status, or diagnosis, and the ease of use of ECG recording equipment advanced greatly. Such systematic research led to standardized systems of measurement and standard nomenclature, and showed that systematic and reproducible conclusions could be drawn from ECG observations. Because ECGs can be obtained simply and relatively inexpensively, at present millions of ECG recordings are obtained from patients each year. More information on ECG data and theory is given by Nelson and Geselowitz (1985), a reference that additionally includes an excellent early history by Johnson and Flowers.

The ECG arises from two parts of the heart: the electrical activity of the atria and that of the ventricles. Both components have an excitation wave and a recovery wave. Within the right atrium is a specialized node of modified cardiac muscle, the sinoatrial (SA) node, that has a spontaneously decreasing transmembrane potential which reaches the threshold potential (TP), resulting in self-excitation (Figure 7.10, upper left). Therefore, the SA node is the cardiac pacemaker, establishing the heart rate. The SA node action potential stimulates the adjacent atrial muscle, completely exciting it and giving rise to the first event in the cardiac cycle, the P wave, the trigger for atrial contraction. Atrial excitation is propagated to another specialized node of tissue in the base of the ventricles, the atrioventricular (AV) node, through which activation travels very slowly, thus allowing time for blood movement from the atria to the ventricles. From the AV node activation travels to the ventricles, the main pumping chamber, first through the bundle of His and the Purkinje fibers, and then to the ventricles. This sequence allows all the ventricular muscle to contract nearly simultaneously (within about 80 msec in a normal human heart), thus increasing pumping effectiveness. It is electrical propagation of excitation over the ventricular muscle that gives rise to the QRS, or simply the R wave, which triggers ventricular contraction. Meanwhile during the QRS wave, the atria recover, giving rise to the T_p wave, following which the atria relax. The T_p wave is not ordinarily seen in the ECG because it is obscured by the ventricular QRS wave. During the QRS wave, the ventricles contract, then relax following their recovery potential, the T wave; Figure 7.10 summarizes this sequence.

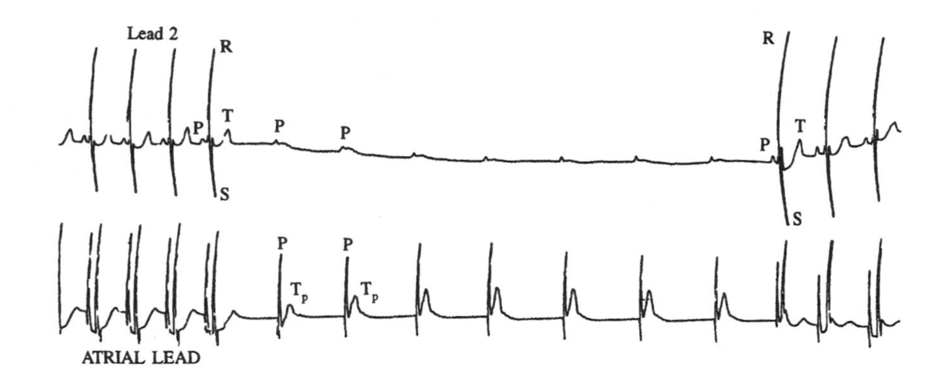

FIGURE 7.11 Lead 2 ECG and an atrial lead. In the center of the record AV block was produced, showing the P waves in lead 2 and the P and T_P waves in the atrial lead.

Ordinarily, the T_P wave is not visible. However, if the propagation of excitation from the atria to the ventricles is blocked, the T_P wave can be seen. Figure 7.11 is a record of the ECG from a limb lead and a recording from a lead within the right atrium in a subject with transient AV block. Note that the sharp P wave in the atrial lead coincides with the P wave in the limb recording and that the atrial lead shows both P and T_P waves, easily identified during AV block.

Clinical Significance

From the foregoing it can be seen that the ECG is effective as a timing signal. There may also be dynamic information in its amplitude or wave shape, with the latter normally determined by historical comparison to previous groups of subjects or patients. By observing the orderly P–QRS–T sequence both as to timing and wave form it is possible to determine if the excitatory and recovery processes in the heart are functioning normally.

Disturbances in the orderly timing of the cardiac cycle are elegantly displayed by the ECG. For example, each atrial excitation may not be delivered to the AV node. AV block exists when there is less than a 1/1 correspondence between the P and QRS complexes (Figure 7.11).

Figure 7.12(1) shows a normal ECG and Figure 7.12(2) illustrates a 2/1 AV block with two P waves for each QRS–T complex. Complete AV block exists when none of the atrial excitations reach the AV node, as shown in Figure 7.12(3). In this case the ventricles developed their own rhythm, which was slow; cardiac output is low, and in such a situation an artificial pacemaker must be implanted.

For many reasons, the atria develop a rapid rate called *atrial tachycardia* or *supraventricular tachycardia.* A very rapid atrial rate is designated *atrial flutter* (Figure 7.12(4)). With both atrial tachycardia and flutter, the atrial contractions are coordinated, although the ventricular pumping capability is reduced owing to inadequate filling time. The ventricles are driven at a rapid rate, and cardiac output is low.

Atrial fibrillation is an electrical dysrhythmia in which all the atrial muscle fibers are contracting and relaxing asynchronously and there is no atrial pumping. This dysrhythmia (Figure 7.12(5)) causes the ventricles to be excited at a very rapid and irregular rate. Cardiac output is reduced, and the pulse is rapid and irregular in force and rate.

If the propagation of excitation in the ventricles is impaired by damage to the bundle of His, the coordination of excitation and contraction is impaired and reveals itself by a widening of the QRS wave, and often a notch is present; Figure 7.12(6) illustrates right (RBBB) and left (LBBB) bundle-branch block. These waveforms are best identified in the chest (V) leads.

All parts of the heart are capable of exhibiting rhythmic activity, there being a rhythmicity hierarchy from the SA node to the ventricular muscle. In abnormal circumstances, the atria and ventricles generate spontaneous beats. Such ectopic excitations do not propagate through the structures of the heart in the same sequence, so the ECG waveforms are different. Figure 7.12(7) illustrates ventricular **ectopic beats** in which the

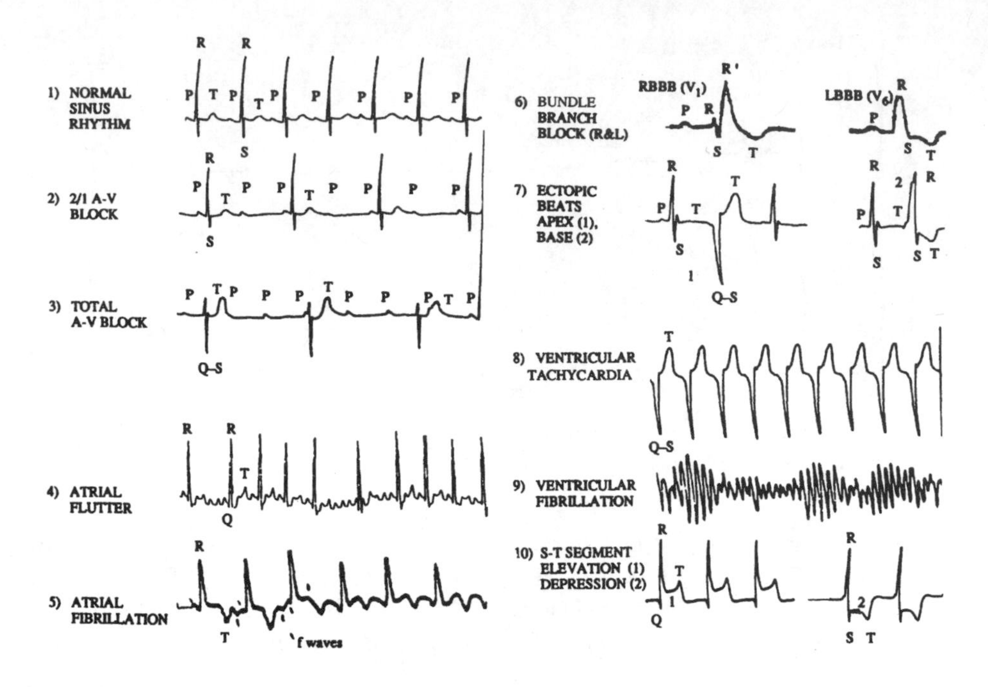

FIGURE 7.12 ECG waveforms.

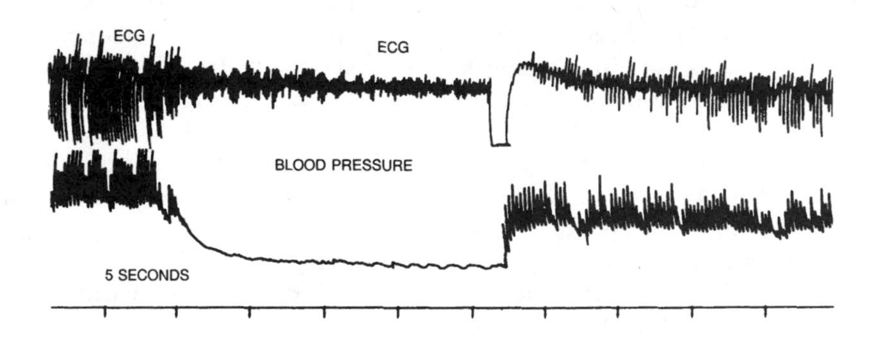

FIGURE 7.13 The electrocardiogram (ECG) and blood pressure during ventricular tachycardia (left), which progressed to ventricular fibrillation (center). A strong transchest shock was applied to defibrillate the ventricles that resumed pumping with the tachycardia returning (right).

first (1) Q–S,T wave arose at the apex and the second (2) R–S,T wave arose at the base of the ventricles. The coupled (bigeminus) beat usually produces no arterial pulse because of inadequate time for filling of the ventricles and poor coordination of the contraction.

The ventricles may become so excitable that they develop a rapid rhythm called *ventricular tachycardia*, as shown in Figure 7.12(8). In this situation, the pumping capability is diminished owing to the high rate that impairs filling and to impaired coordination of contraction. Ventricular fibrillation is a condition in which all of the ventricular muscle fibers contract and relax independently and asynchronously. Pumping ceases and cardiac output falls to zero. The ECG (Figure 7.12(9)) exhibits rapid oscillations of waxing and waning amplitude at a rate of 800 to 1500 per minute because it is the composite record of currents generated at many sites within the ventricles. Ventricular fibrillation is lethal unless the circulation is restored within a few minutes, first by cardiopulmonary resuscitation (CPR) and then by electrical defibrillation. The latter technique employs the delivery of a substantial pulse of current through the heart applied directly or with transchest electrodes. Recent years have seen the development of sophisticated external and even implanted automatic defibrillators. Figure 7.13 illustrates ventricular tachycardia (left), ventricular fibrillation (center), and defibrillation (right), with the restoration of pumping.

When a region of the ventricles is deprived of its coronary artery blood supply, the cells in this region lose their ability to generate action potentials and to contract. These cells remain depolarized. Sustained currents flowing within the heart between such cells and the remaining normal cells produce a sustained abnormal current within the heart and throughout the body volume. On the body surface, these currents are most readily visible as a displacement from the baseline in the time period of the ECG between the S and T waves, i.e., there is an S–T segment shift after ventricular excitation. This is one sign of a **myocardial infarction** (heart attack). It often is accompanied by chest pain (angina pectoris). Figure 7.12(10) illustrates the ECG in myocardial infarction. Whether the S–T segment displacement is up (1) or down (2) depends on the region of the ventricles injured and the lead used (that is, the position of the electrodes) to record the ECG.

ECG Leads

The spread of excitation and recovery over the atria and ventricles varies in direction with time. Therefore, the aggregate current generated by excitation or recovery flows preferentially in specific directions, changing with time. To a first approximation it is as if there was a single current-generating electrical dipole creating the currents seen on the body surface (though latter careful mapping of the potentials on the body surface shows many nondipolar observations). Thus, the location of body-surface electrodes relative to the heart determines the amplitude and wave shape that is measured. Historically, tremendous confusion was possible since electrodes at any two sites produced a different amplitude and waveshape, even for the same heartbeat in the same person, preventing systematic comparisons. As a consequence, standard electrode sites were adopted, as shown in Figure 7.14. Measurements between prescribed sites using a defined polarity are called "leads." There are three standard limb leads, three augmented (a) limb leads, and six chest (V) leads, the latter being called "monopolar." The reference for the monopolar chest leads is the centerpoint of three resistors (r), each joined to one of the limb electrodes. The right leg may be used to ground the subject to diminish noise from electrical interference. Each lead "sees" a different region of the heart. Observations from a set of nine to twelve leads allow a quick approximation of the overall direction of propagation of excitation (and recovery) by inspecting the amplitudes of the waveforms in the various leads. If excitation (or recovery) travels orthogonal to a lead axis, the net amplitude will be zero or very small. If excitation (or recovery) travels parallel to a lead axis, the amplitude of the wave will be a maximum. Figure 7.14 illustrates the amplitudes of the P, QRS, and T waves for the 12 ECG leads. Note that leads 1, 2, 3, aVR, aVL, and aVF identify the vector projections in the frontal plane. Leads V_{1-6} identify the vector components in a quasi-horizontal plane. There are normal values for the amplitudes and durations for the P, QRS, and T waves as well as their vectors. Cardiologists often inspect waveforms visually, though automated computer programs are also widely used, or used with over-reading to prevent gross errors. The interested reader can find more on ECG interpretation in the many handbooks on this subject, such as those by Chou (1991) and Phillips and Feeney (1990). Basicmechanisms of cardiac impulse propagation and associated arrhythmias are reviewed by Kleber and Rudy (2004).

Instrumentation

Standards of performance address issues of patient safety, interference, measurement accuracy, and measurement standardization. Safety standards take into account the fact that ECG electrodes, well coupled to the patient, may provide a path for electric shock, while the need for ECG measurements to be obtained from the critically ill requires measurements to be taken from patients with other equipment simultaneously functioning, including catheters directly in the heart. Noise sensitivity, especially to power line and some RF sources, is increased because of the high input impedance of ECG equipment, necessary because of the high skin-electrode resistance of many electrodes.

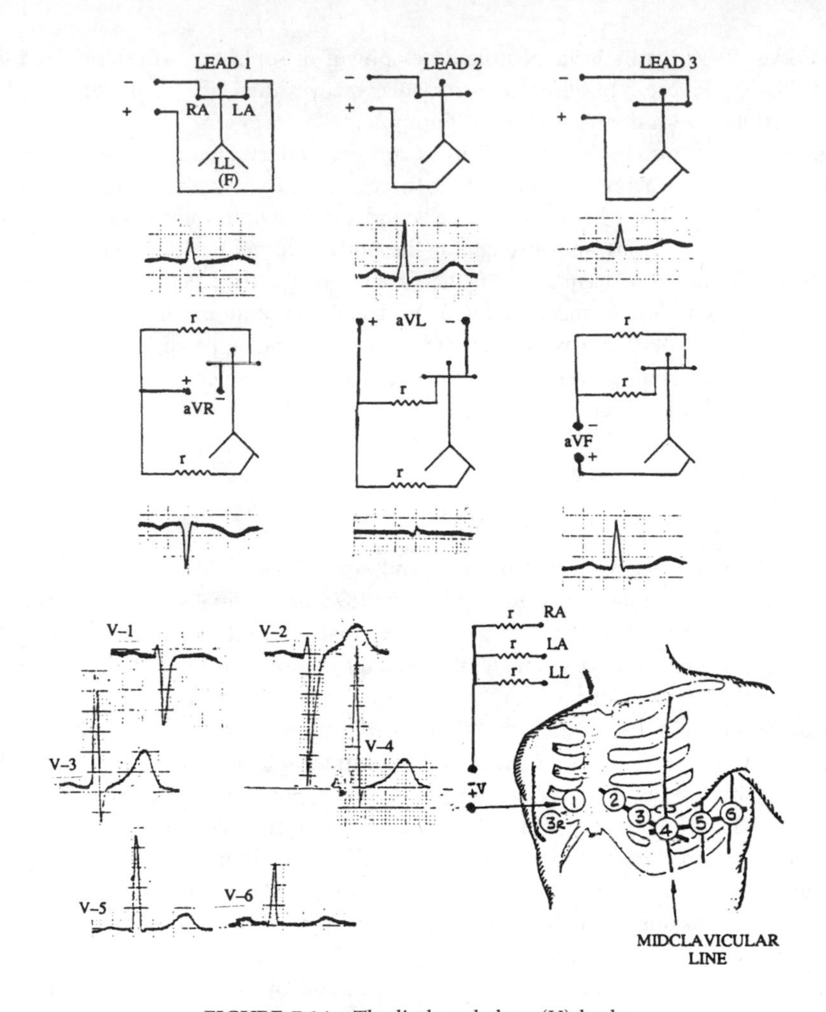

FIGURE 7.14 The limb and chest (V) leads.

Current standards evolved from recommendations by the American Medical Association in 1950 and the American Heart Association in 1954 and 1967. These recommendations have been collected and expanded into an American National Standard, published by the Association for the Advancement of Medical Instrumentation (AAMI) (1991, 1998, 2000). The title of the document is "Diagnostic Electrocardiographic Devices." This document lists performance and labeling requirements and also provides useful information on testing ECGs, as well as on special aspects such as portable devices and electrode leads.

A few highlights of the standard will be presented here. In considering the following, one must bear in mind that today's standards evolved from a time when ECGs were displayed by a direct-writing pen that employed a stylus writing on special paper. The standards are carried forward today with the terminology of pen and paper often continuing to be used even as the actual pen and paper have become replaced by virtual devices created by a computerized data acquisition system and modern displays. The standard provides that the ECG be written with two chart speeds, 5 and 50 mm/sec. The rulings on the paper represent 40 ms when the standard speed (25 mm/sec) is used. The amplitude sensitivity is 10 mm for a 1-mV input signal. The sinusoidal frequency response extends from 0.05 to 100 Hz for the 30% attenuation points. The input stage is a differential amplifier with an input impedance in excess of 2.4 MΩ The common-mode rejection ratio (CMRR) is measured with a 20-V (rms) 60-Hz generator with an output impedance of 51,000 Ω connected in series with a 10-pF capacitor. (Common mode interference is high since the subject becomes an antenna.) The 60-Hz CMRR should be in excess of 5000. The maximum dc leakage current through any patient electrode is 0.2 μA.

Recordings Taken Directly from the Heart

When electrocardiograms are taken directly from the heart, they are usually called "electrograms," to distinguish them from signals recorded from electrodes on the torso surface. Electrograms are several times larger in amplitude and include more rapid waveform deflections, both because they are closer to the sources (and thus do not reflect as much spatial averaging) and because electrograms may include visible deflections arising from the cardiac conduction system. Recordings taken directly from the heart come from clinical studies, where catheters are employed to move lead wires to within the cardiac chambers, and are employed by cardiac pacemakers, which analyze the cardiac excitation sequence, as judged from cardiac electrograms, and provide stimuli only when judged necessary. More information about cardiac electrograms and their interpretation is given by Biermann et al. (in Shenasa et al., 2003). The signal content of pacemaker leads and other pacemaker design information is given by Webster (1995).

Electromyography (EMG)

The electrical activity of skeletal muscle is monitored to assess the integrity of the motor nerve that supplies it and to evaluate recovery of the motor nerve following injury to it. The EMG is also characteristically altered in many degenerative muscle diseases. Although muscle action potentials can be detected with skin-surface electrodes, a monopolar or bipolar needle electrode is used in clinical EMG. The electrical activity is displayed on an oscilloscope screen and monitored aurally with a loudspeaker.

Contraction of Skeletal Muscle

The functional unit of the muscular system is the motor unit, consisting of a nerve cell located within the spinal cord, its axon (nerve fiber), and the group of muscle fibers that it innervates, as shown in Figure 7.15. Between the nerve fiber and the muscle fibers is the myoneural junction, the site where acetylcholine is liberated and transmits excitation to the muscle fibers. The number of muscle fibers per nerve fiber is called the innervation ratio, which ranges from 1:1 to about 1000:1; the former ratio is characteristic of the extraocular muscles, and the latter is typical for the postural muscles.

A single stimulus received by the nerve fiber physiologically, or a single stimulus delivered to it electrically, will cause all the innervated muscle fibers to contract and relax; this response is called a *twitch*. Figure 7.8(c) and (d) illustrate the relationship between the muscle action potential and twitch. Note that the action potential is almost over before contraction begins and the contraction far outlasts the duration of the action potential.

If multiple stimuli are delivered to a single motor-nerve fiber with an increasing frequency, the twitches fuse into a sustained (tetanic) contraction whose force is much more than that of a twitch. This occurs because

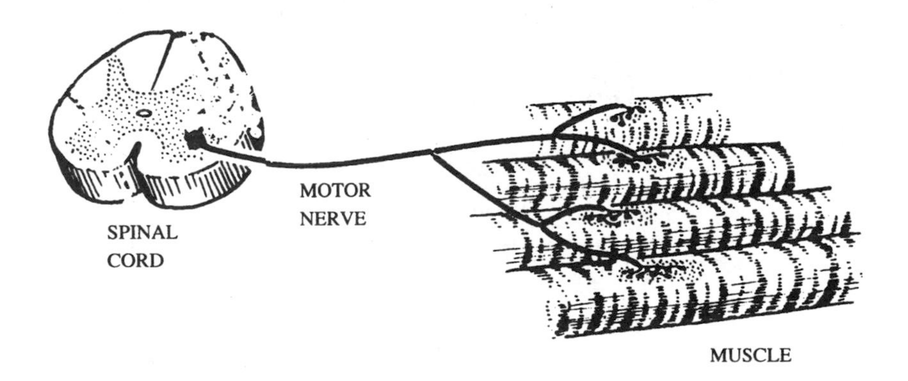

FIGURE 7.15 The functional unit of the muscular system, the motor unit, consisting of a nerve cell located within the spinal cord, its axon, and the muscle fibers that it innervates.

each action potential liberates contractile energy. The critical fusion frequency depends on the type of muscle, but in general it is about 25 to 40 per second.

The force developed by a whole muscle consisting of thousands of motor units is graded in two ways: (l) by the frequency of nerve impulses in each nerve fiber and (2) by the number of motor units that are activated.

Clinical EMG

When the electrical activity of skeletal muscle is examined for diagnostic purposes, an insulated needle electrode, bare only at the tip (Figure 7.16(a)), is inserted into the muscle and paired with a skin-surface electrode. Another skin-surface electrode is used to ground the subject. Occasionally a coaxial needle electrode (Figure 7.16(b)) or a bipolar hypodermic needle electrode (Figure 7.16(c)) is used. In the latter case the outer sleeve is used as the ground. A high-gain, differential amplifier, oscilloscope, and loudspeaker are used, as shown in Figure 7.16(d).

In a normal subject at rest, the electrical activity monitored during insertion of the needle electrode consists of a short burst of muscle action potentials displayed on the oscilloscope and heard in the loudspeaker. These action potentials are called insertion potentials and subside quickly in the normal muscle. When the muscle is at rest, there is no electrical activity (electrical silence). If the muscle is contracted voluntarily, the frequency of action potentials increases with the force developed by the muscle. However, there is no linear or constant relationship between these two events. Each action potential, called a *normal motor-unit* potential, lasts a few milliseconds to the first zero crossing, as shown in Figure 7.16(e).

There is considerable art associated with placing the exploring electrode. If the electrode tip is not adjacent to contracting muscle fibers, the sound of the action potential is muffled and electrode adjustment is required. The same is true for detecting fibrillation potentials (see below).

If the nerve cell in the spinal cord or the nerve fiber supplying a muscle is damaged, the muscle cannot be contracted voluntarily or reflexly (by tapping the tendon) and is therefore paralyzed. In the absence of therapeutic intervention and with the passage of time, the nerve beyond the damaged site dies and the muscle fibers start to degenerate. In about 2 1/2 to 3 weeks in humans, the individual muscle fibers start to contract and relax spontaneously and randomly, producing short-duration, randomly occurring action potentials called *fibrillation* potentials (Figure 7.16(f)), which are displayed on the oscilloscope screen and heard as clicks

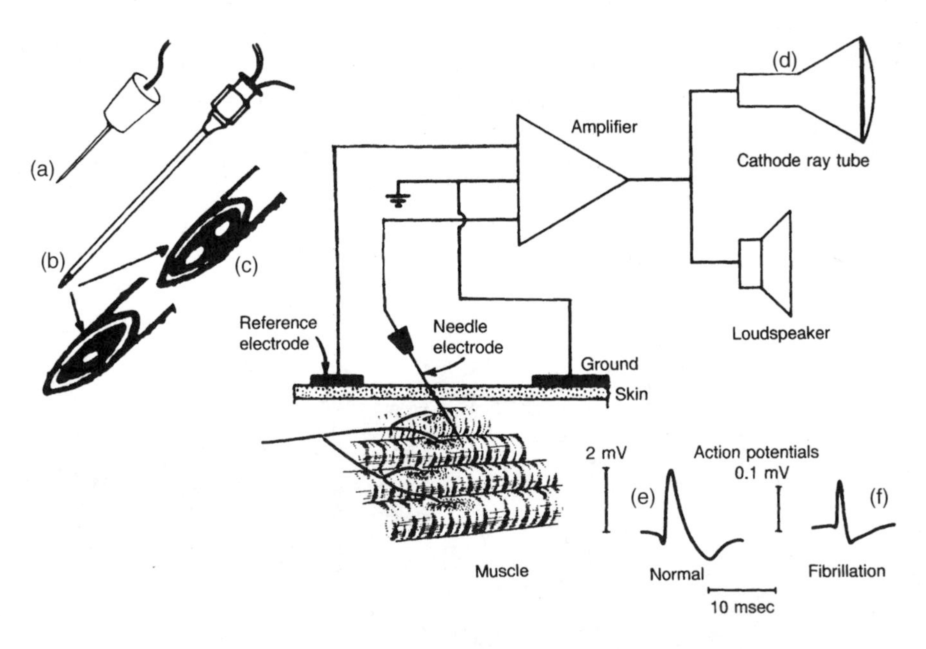

FIGURE 7.16 Equipment used for electromyography. (a) Needle electrode; (b) hypodermic monopolar and (c) bipolar electrodes; (d) the recording apparatus; (e) skeletal muscle action potential; and (f) fibrillation potential.

in the loudspeaker. Although there is electrical activity, the muscle develops no net force. The fibrillation potentials persist as long as there are viable muscle fibers. In such a denervated muscle, insertion of the needle electrode elicits a vigorous train of short-duration insertion potentials that resemble fibrillation potentials with a frequency of about 1 to 10 per second. If the damaged ends of the nerve are brought together surgically, the central end of the nerve will start to grow slowly and reinnervate the muscle. Gradually, the fibrillation potentials disappear, although the muscle is still not able to be contracted. Long before there is visible evidence of muscle contraction, if the subject is presented with the EMG display and asked to contract the affected muscle, primitive muscle action potentials can be elicited. With the passage of time, the fibrillation potentials disappear and there is electrical silence at rest and primitive (nascent) motor-unit activity occurs with voluntary contraction. Later when reinnervation is complete, only normal motor-unit potentials are present with voluntary contraction and electrical silence at rest.

The EMG is also used to diagnose some degenerative muscle and related nerve disorders. *Myotonia* is a degenerative disease of muscle fibers in which the muscle relaxes poorly. Insertion of the needle electrode elicits an intense burst of insertion potentials that sound like a thunderstorm in the loudspeaker. A similar response is obtained by tapping the muscle. When relaxation does occur, there is electrical silence. Voluntary contraction produces normal action potentials along with shorter-duration action potentials from the diseased muscle fibers.

Myasthenia gravis is a disease in which there is impairment of transmission of acetylcholine across the myoneural junctions to the muscle fibers. As a result, muscle contraction cannot be sustained. Because the muscle fibers are normally innervated, there are no fibrillation potentials. With voluntary contraction, normal action potentials occur, and if the disease is severe, the action potentials decrease in frequency as the force of contraction decreases and soon sustained muscle contraction cannot be maintained.

Muscular dystrophy is a degenerative disease of muscle fibers in which there is atrophy of some fibers, swelling in others, and an increase in sarcolemmal and connective tissue with the deposition of fat. Insertion of the needle electrode elicits a vigorous burst of short-duration, high-frequency action potentials. Typically at rest there are no fibrillation potentials. With voluntary contraction, the action potentials are short in duration, high in frequency, and produce a whirring sound in the loudspeaker. As fatigue supervenes, the frequency and amplitude decrease.

The reader who is interested in obtaining more information on EMG will find it in books by Oh (2003), Kimura (2001), and Preston and Shapiro (1998). All contain a wealth of clinical information.

Instrumentation

As yet there is no American National Standard for EMG, although steps are being taken in this direction. As shown in Figure 7.16, the EMG is displayed in two ways: (1) visually with an oscilloscope and (2) aurally with a loudspeaker. Both are needed to enable acquisition and analysis of the EMG.

Buchtal et al. (1954) stated that the principal frequency components for the human EMG require a bandwidth of 1 Hz to 10 kHz. It has been found that a time constant of about 50 msec is satisfactory, which corresponds to a low-frequency –3-dB point of 3 Hz. For needle electrodes with a tip diameter of 0.1 mm or larger, the input impedance (one side to ground) should not be lower than that of a 500-kΩ resistor in parallel with less than 25-pF capacitance.

Smaller-area electrodes require a higher input impedance (Geddes et al., 1967). The cable used to connect the needle electrode to the amplifier should not add more than 250 pF to the input capacitance. The common-mode rejection ratio (CMRR) should be in excess of 5000.

Electro-encephalography (EEG)

The electrical activity of the brain can be recorded with electrodes on the scalp, on the exposed brain, or inserted into the brain. The major advantage of the EEG is its simplicity, while its major limitation is poor spatial resolution (as evaluated by Purves et al., 1997, p. 500). EEGs are sometimes interpreted in conjunction with magnetic reasonance imaging (MRI), a recent imaging methodology that provides good spatial localization (within 1 mm) of active regions of the brain (Purves et al., 1997, p. 22). The EEG has been particularly valuable for research and clinical studies of sleep physiology and of epilepsy. When recordings are made with brain-surface (cortex) electrodes, the recording is called an electrocorticogram (ECoG). With scalp electrodes, the recording is designated an electroencephalogram (EEG) that is displayed by direct-inking pens using a chart speed of 3 cm/sec. Typically, eight to twelve channels are recorded simultaneously.

Although the brain consists of about 10^{14} neurons, the EEG reflects the electrical activity of the outer layer, the cortex, which is the seat of consciousness. The type of electrical activity depends on the location of the electrodes and the level of alertness. The frequency and amplitude are profoundly affected by alertness, drowsiness, sleep, hyperventilation, anesthesia, the presence of a tumor, head injury, and epilepsy. The clinical correlation between cerebral disorders and the voltage and frequency spectra is well ahead of the physiological explanations for the waveforms.

Recording Technique

Both bipolar (Figure 7.17(a)) and monopolar (Figure 7.17(b)) techniques are used. With monopolar recording, one side of each amplifier is connected to a reference electrode, usually on the earlobe. With bipolar recording, the amplifiers are connected between pairs of scalp electrodes in a regular order. With both types of recording, one-half the number of channels is connected to electrodes on the opposite side of the head. In this way, the electrical activity from homologous areas of the brain can be compared at a glance.

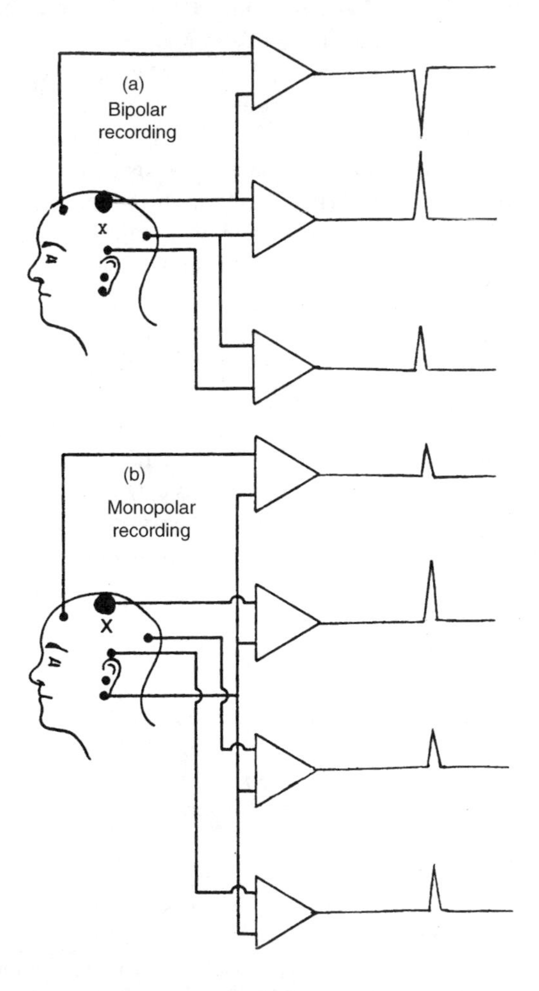

FIGURE 7.17 Methods of recording the EEG. (a) The bipolar and (b) the monopolar method. Note how abnormal activity under electrode X is revealed by the two techniques.

With the bipolar method illustrated in Figure 7.17(a), abnormal activity located under electrode X will be revealed as a phase reversal in adjacent channels. With monopolar recording using the earlobe reference electrode (Figure 7.17(b)) the abnormal activity under electrode X will be largest in the channel connected to that electrode and smaller in the adjacent channels.

In clinical EEG, 21 electrodes are applied to the scalp in what is known as the 10-20 system. This array was established by the International Federation of EEG Societies in 1958. The 10-20 system employs skull landmarks as reference points to locate the electrodes.

The Normal EEG

In the normal resting adult, the EEG displays a fluctuating electrical activity having a dominant frequency of about 10 Hz and an amplitude in the range of 20 to 200 μV. This activity is called the *alpha rhythm* and ranges in frequency from about 8 to 12 Hz, being most prominent in the **occipital** and **parietal** areas. It may occupy as much as half the record. The alpha rhythm increases in frequency with age from birth and attains its adult form by about 15 to 20 years. The alpha rhythm is most prominent when the eyes are closed and in the absence of concentration. Opening the eyes, engaging in patterned vision, or performing such cerebral activity as mental arithmetic diminishes or abolishes the alpha rhythm. Figure 7.18 presents a good example of this phenomenon.

Although the alpha rhythm is the most prominent electrical activity, other frequencies are present. For example, there is a considerable amount of low-voltage, high-frequency (beta) activity ranging from 18 to 30 Hz. It is usually found in the frontal part of the brain. However, the normal electroencephalogram contains waves of various frequencies (in the range of 1 to 60 Hz) and amplitudes, depending on the cerebral state. To establish communication among electroencephalographers, a terminology has been developed to describe waveforms and their frequencies; Table 7.1 presents a glossary of these terms.

Drowsiness and sleep affect the normal EEG profoundly. Figure 7.19 illustrates the typical changes that occur as a subject goes to sleep. With drowsiness, the higher-frequency activity which is associated with alertness or excitement, and the alpha rhythm that dominates the waking record in the relaxed state, are replaced by a characteristic cyclic sequence of changes which constitute the focus of a new specialty devoted to sleep physiology, in which the EEG is used to identify different stages of sleep.

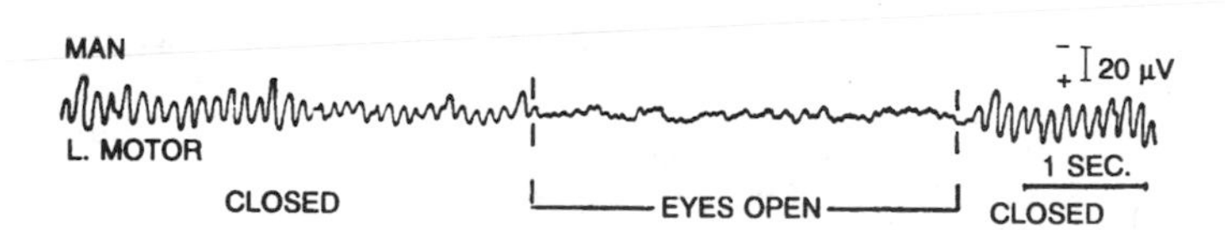

FIGURE 7.18 The EEG of a relaxed human subject with eyes closed and open. Note that the record is dominated with alpha rhythm (8 to 12 Hz) when the eyes are closed. (*Source:* Derived in part from M.A.B. Brazier, *The Electrical Activity of the Nervous System*, London: Sir Isaac Pitman & Sons, Ltd., 1951. With permission.)

TABLE 7.1 EEG Waveform Terminology

Waveform	Frequency (Hz)	Conditions
Alpha	8–12	Parietal-occipital, associated with the awake and relaxed subject, prominent with eyes closed
Beta	18–30	More evident in frontal-parietal leads, seen best when alpha is blocked
Delta	1–3.5	Associated with normal sleep and present in children less than 1 year old, also seen in organic brain disease
Theta	4–7	Parietal-temporal, prominent in children 2 to 5 years old
Sleep spindle (sigma)	12–14	Waxing and waning of a sinusoidal-like wave having the envelope that resembles a spindle, seen during sleep
Lambda	Transient	Visually evoked, low-amplitude, occipital wave, resulting from recognition of a new visual image
Spike and wave	ca. 3	Sharp wave (spike) followed by rounded wave associated with petit mal epilepsy

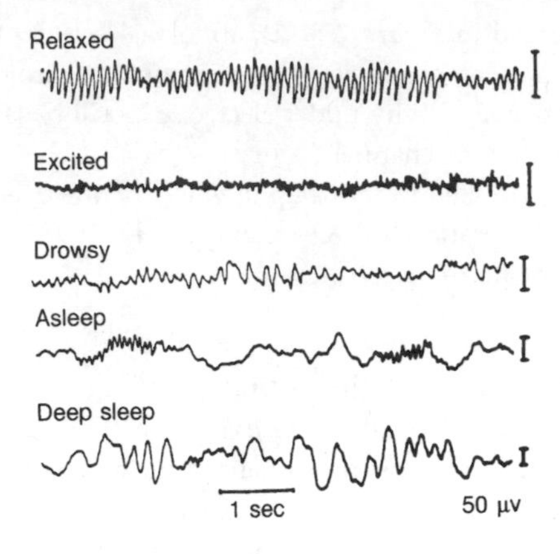

FIGURE 7.19 The EEG of a subject going to sleep. (*Source:* H. Jasper, in *Epilepsy and Cerebral Localization*, W.G. Penfield and T.C. Erickson, Eds., Springfield, IL: Charles C Thomas, 1941. With permission.)

Rapid, deep breathing (hyperventilation) at a rate of 30 per minute for about 3 min reduces the partial pressure of carbon dioxide in the blood, which reduces cerebral blood flow. A typical EEG response consists of large-amplitude, bilaterally synchronous, frontally prominent waves with a frequency of 4 to 7 per second. The frequency usually decreases with increasing hyperventilation. The lack of bilateral symmetry is an indication of abnormality.

Anesthesia dramatically alters the EEG in a manner that depends on the type and amount of anesthetic given. Despite differences among anesthetic agents, some important similarities accompany anesthesia. The first change is replacement of the alpha rhythm with low-voltage, high-frequency activity that accompanies the analgesia and delirium stages. Thus, the EEG resembles that of an alert or excited subject, although the subject is not appropriately responsive to stimuli; usually the response is excessive and/or inappropriate. From this point on, the type of EEG obtained with deepening anesthesia depends on the type of anesthetic. However, when a deeper level of anesthesia is reached, the EEG waveform becomes less dependent on the type of anesthetic. Large-amplitude low-frequency waves begin to dominate the record, and with deepening anesthesia their frequency is reduced and they begin to occur intermittently. With very (dangerously) deep anesthesia, the record is flat (i.e., isoelectric). Complicating interpretation of the EEG in anesthesia are the effects of **hypoxia**, **hypercapnia**, and hypoglycemia, all of which mimic deep anesthesia.

Clinical EEG

The EEG plays a valuable role in identifying intracranial pathology. The clinical utility relies on recognition of patterns of frequency, voltage, and waveform. Localization of abnormal areas is provided by the multiple scalp electrodes and recording channels.

The EEG has its greatest value as an aid in the diagnosis and differentiation of the many types of epilepsy, a condition in which groups of neurons in the brain become hyperexcitable and, depending on their location, produce sensory, motor, and/or **autonomic** manifestations. The epilepsies associated with cortical lesions are often detected by the scalp EEG. The EEG in epileptics is usually abnormal between, as well as during, attacks. The EEG provides information on the location of the area (or areas) of abnormal neuronal activity.

Petit mal epilepsy is characterized by a transient loss (few to 20 sec) of conscious thought, although motor activity may continue. Often there are eye movements and blinking. The EEG shows a characteristic 3 per second spike-and-wave pattern (Figure 7.20(a)). Psychomotor epilepsy is characterized by sensory hallucinations and abnormal thoughts, often with stereotyped behavior. During the attack, the subject is stuporous and the EEG (Figure 7.20(b)) has a characteristic pattern. Jacksonian, or motor, epilepsy starts in a specific area of the motor cortex and is preceded by an aura, a characteristic sensation perceived by the subject.

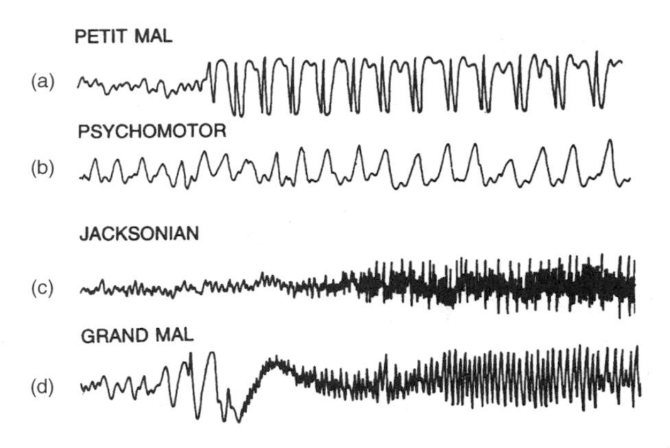

FIGURE 7.20 EEG waveforms in epilepsy: (a) petiti mal, (b) psychomotor, (c) Jacksonian, and (d) grand mal. (*Source:* Derived from F.A. Gibbs and E.L. Gibbs, *Atlas of Encephalography*, London: Addison-Wesley, 1952. With permission.)

The convulsion starts with localized muscle twitching that often starts in the face, hand, arm, then spreads over the entire body as a generalized convulsion; Figure 7.20(c) shows the onset of a convulsion. Consciousness is lost during and for a short time after the fit. The EEG provides information on the origin of the abnormal discharge in the motor cortex. Grand mal epilepsy is characterized by a contraction of all the muscles (tonic phase), then jerking (clonic phase). Consciousness is lost, and the subject is in a coma for some time following the attack. The EEG (Figure 7.20(d)) shows high-voltage, high-frequency waves that progress over the entire cortex.

Traumatic epilepsy results from injury to the brain. It is believed that contraction of scar tissue acts as a stimulus to adjacent nerve cells which discharge rhythmically, the excitation spreading to a grand mal convulsion. The EEG provides information on the origin of the abnormal discharge.

Tumors are associated with low-frequency (delta) waves. However, other intracranial lesions also produce slow waves. Although the EEG can identify the location of tumors, usually it cannot differentiate between brain injury, infection, and vascular accident, all of which produce low-frequency waves. Interpretation of the EEG always includes other clinical information.

For those wishing to delve deeper into EEG, clinical applications are presented by Niedermeyer and DaSilva (1993).

Instrumentation

The American EEG Society (1986) published guidelines for the performance of EEG machines. The guidelines recommended a minimum of eight channels. Chlorided silver disks or gold electrodes, adhered to the scalp with collodion, are recommended; needle electrodes are not. A chart speed of 3 cm/sec is standard, and a recording sensitivity of 5 to 10 μV/mm is recommended. The frequency response extends from 1 to 70 Hz for the –3-dB points.

Evoked Potentials

With the availability of signal averaging using a digital computer, it is possible to investigate the integrity of the neural pathways from peripheral sense organs to the cortex by using appropriate stimuli (e.g., clicks, light flashes, or current pulses). Usually the stimulus consists of a few hundred to about 1000 pulses, averaged to produce the somatosensory-evoked potential (SSEP). Likewise, it is possible to evaluate the integrity of the neural pathways from the motor cortex to peripheral muscles by applying multiple short-duration current pulses to scalp electrodes and recording nerve and/or muscle action potentials with skin-surface electrodes.

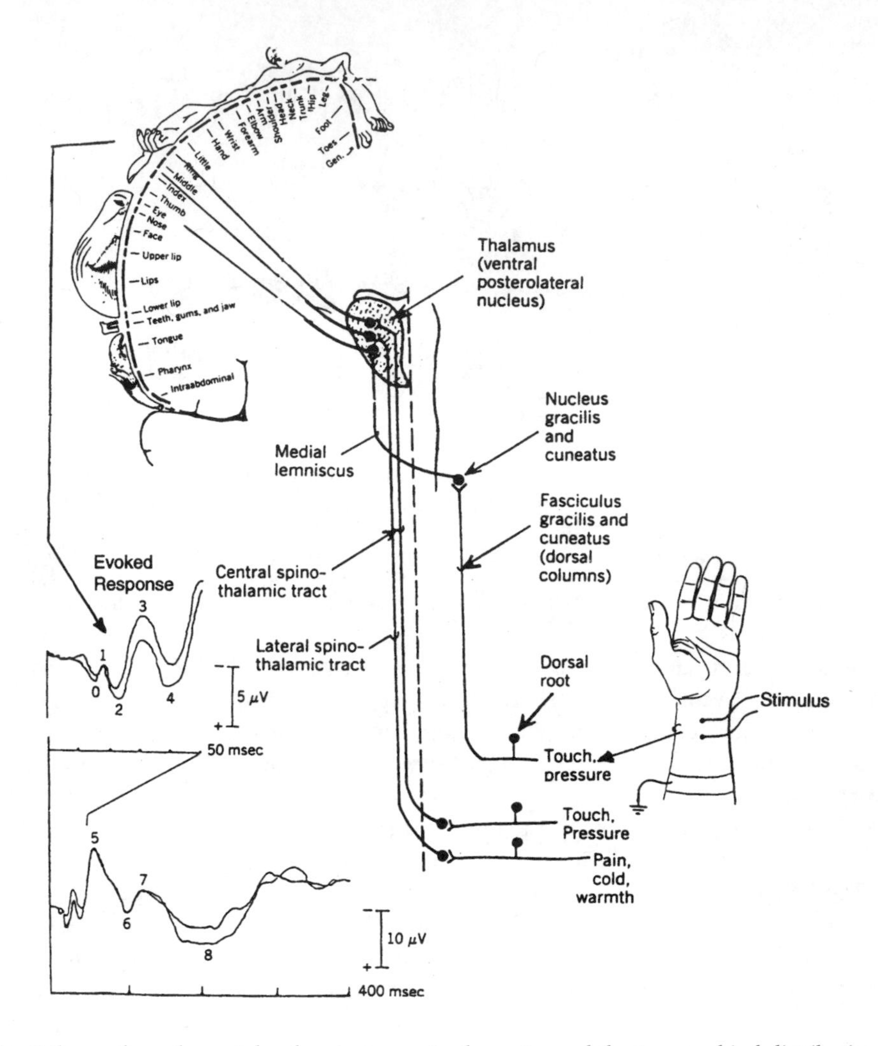

FIGURE 7.21 Pathways from the peripheral sense organs to the cortex and the topographical distribution of sensation along the cortex with Penfield's homunculus. Also shown are the stimulating electrodes on the wrist and the SSEPs recorded from the contralateral cortex. (*Source:* SSEPs redrawn from T. W. Picton, "Evoked cortical potentials, how? what? and why?," *Am. J. EEG Technol.*, vol. 14, no. 4, 1974, pp. 9–44. With permission.)

Such recordings are called motor-evoked potentials (MEPs). With both SSEPs and MEPs, the largest responses appear on the opposite side of the body from the stimulus.

Because the responses are in digital form, they can be written out in hard-copy format. With SSEPs, the response consists of many waves occurring at various times after the stimulus. To permit close examination of the various waveforms, several displays are presented, each with a different time axis. Figure 7.21 presents a sketch of the neural pathways from the periphery to the cortex, showing the topographic distribution of sensation along the cortex using the homunculus created by Penfield, described in detail in 1968. Also shown in Figure 7.21 is a typical SSEP obtained by stimulating the median nerve with skin-surface electrodes connected to an isolated (i.e., not grounded) stimulator output circuit. Note the remarkably low amplitude of the responses that were obtained by averaging the response to 240 stimuli. Note also that the first display showed the responses from 0 to 50 msec and the second display presented the responses in the 0- to 400-msec interval.

Figure 7.22 shows the motor pathways from the motor cortex to a typical muscle. The cortical motor areas are represented by Penfield's homunculus. A train of 240 stimuli were applied between electrodes on the scalp

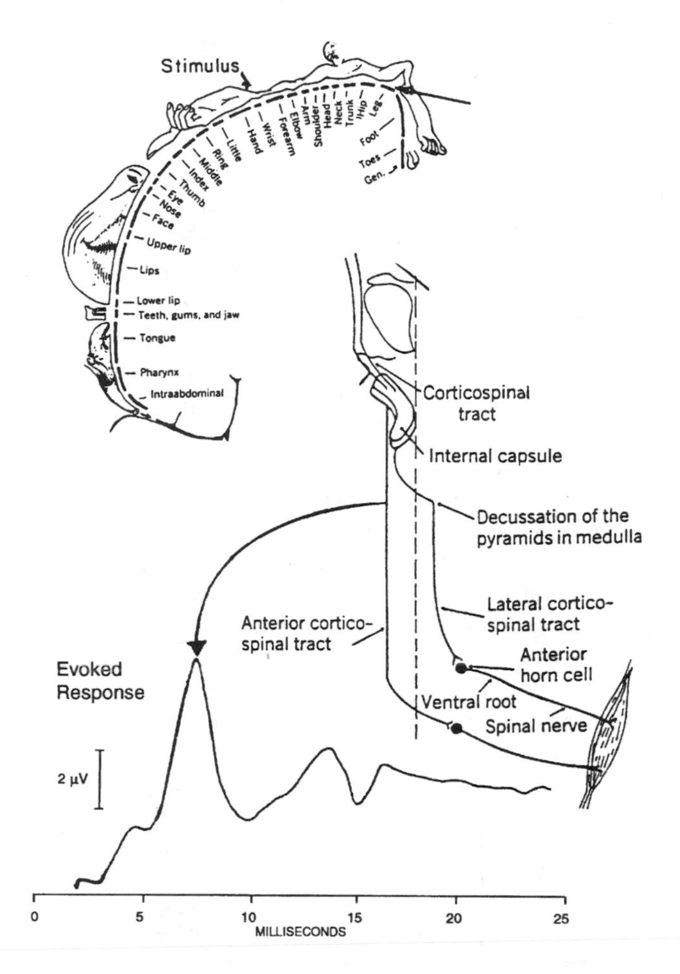

FIGURE 7.22 Neural motor pathways from the cortex to a typical muscle. The motor areas are represented by Penfield's homunculus. A train of 240 stimuli delivered to the motor cortex provided the average MEP detected with electrodes placed over the spinal column in this patient to whom a muscle paralytic drug was given; therefore the MEPs are from the spinal cord. (*Source:* Redrawn from Levy et al., 1984, and Penfield and Rasmussen, 1968.)

and in the mouth. The motor-evoked potentials were recorded with skin-surface electrodes over the spinal column. The MEP of a patient in whom the muscles were paralyzed is also shown in Figure 7.22. Because the muscles were paralyzed, the MEPs shown in the figure represent action potentials in the spinal cord. Note the prominent peaks at 7 and 14 msec. These peaks provide information on the path taken by the nerve impulses initiated in the motor cortex. Although there is no ANSI standard for evoked-potential recording, the American EEG Society (1986) published guidelines for equipment performance and recording techniques. This information should be consulted by those contemplating entry into this field.

Magnetic (Eddy-Current) Stimulation

When scalp electrodes are used to stimulate the brain, there is considerable skin sensation under the electrodes owing to the high perimeter current density (Overmeyer et al., 1979). It has been found that sufficient eddy current can be induced in living tissue by discharging an energy-storage capacitor into an air-cored coil placed on the skin. This mode of stimulation is almost without skin sensation; by some it is called "ouchless stimulation" and it can be used to stimulate the brain, peripheral nerves, and the heart. The parameters associated with eddy-current stimulation are kiloamperes, Teslas/sec, milliohms, microhenries, microseconds, and low damping. Because the forces on the coil conductors are very large, special care is required in fabricating such coils.

Stimulators

With **magnetic** (eddy-current) **stimulation**, three circuits and two coil geometries are used. The simplest circuit is illustrated in Figure 7.23, which shows a capacitor (C) being discharged into the stimulating coil (L). The induced current (i) is proportional to the rate of change (di/dt) of the coil current (i). The resistance (R) in the entire circuit is low and the coil current is an underdamped sinusoid. The tissue is stimulated by the induced current density J = k(de/dx)/r, where de/dx is the induced voltage gradient, r is the tissue resistivity, and k is a constant that depends on coil geometry and target distance. The effective stimulus duration (d) is from the onset of the induced current to the first zero crossing as shown in Figure 7.23. Typical durations (d) range from 20 to 200 μsec. When the damping is low, the multiple pulses of induced current can elicit responses, providing the period is longer than the refractory period of the tissue being stimulated. Note that the capacitor voltage falls to zero and the capacitor must be recharged to deliver the next stimulus.

The second type of eddy-current stimulator employs energy recovery and is shown in Figure 7.24. The charged capacitor (C) is discharged into the stimulating coil (L) by triggering a silicon-controlled rectifier (SCR). By placing a diode across the SCR as shown, some of the energy stored in the magnetic field can be recovered to recharge the capacitor. In this way, the power supply need only deliver a modest amount of current to restore the charge on the capacitor.

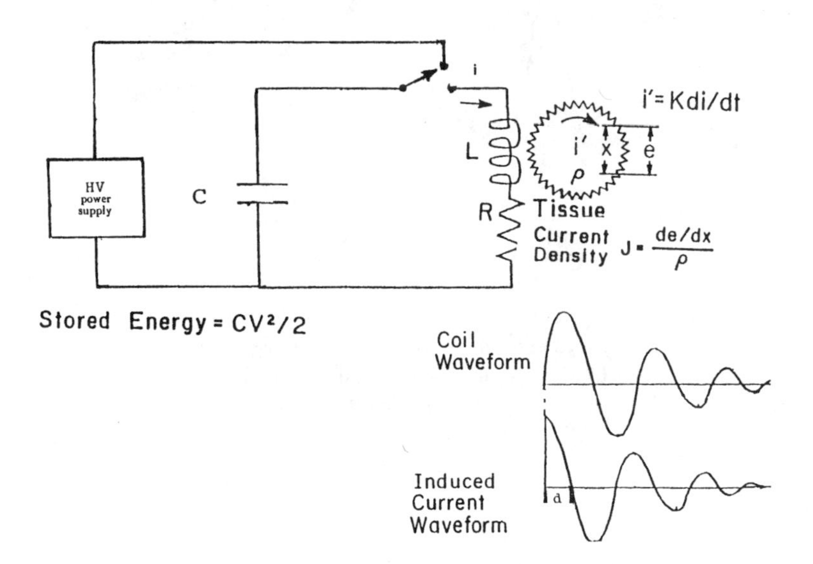

FIGURE 7.23 Simplest type of magnetic (eddy-current) stimulator and coil and induced current waveforms.

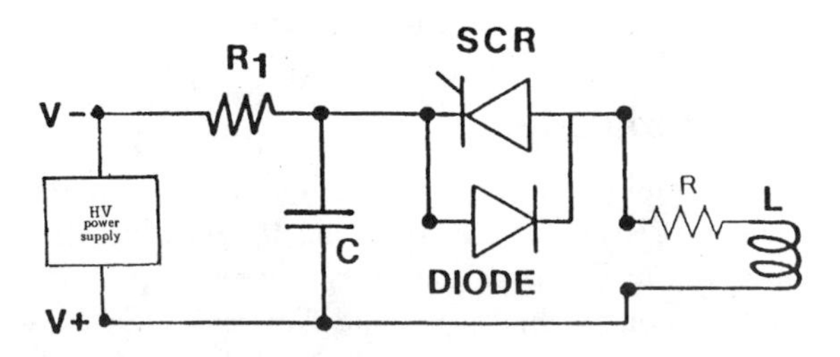

FIGURE 7.24 Magnetic (eddy-current) stimulator that recovers energy stored in the magnetic field.

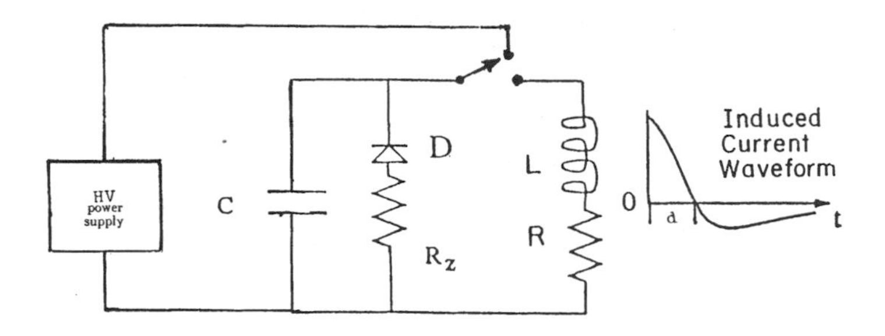

FIGURE 7.25 Method of using a diode (D) and current-limiting resistor (Rz) to avoid reverse polarity on the energy-storage capacitor (C).

With the circuits shown in Figure 7.23 and Figure 7.24, it is necessary to use non-polarized capacitors. When a long-duration pulse is desired, it is more practical to employ electrolytic capacitors because of their high energy storage per unit of weight. When employing electrolytic capacitors, it is necessary to prevent reverse charging. To achieve this goal, a diode (D) and a series current-limiting resistor (Rz) are placed across the capacitor, as shown in Figure 7.25. The resulting induced current waveform is shown on the right.

Cardiac muscle has also been stimulated to contract with single pulses of eddy current. The first to achieve this feat was Bourland et al. (1990), who applied a coplanar coil to the left chest of an anesthetized dog. Blood pressure and the electrocardiogram were recorded and the heart was stopped by right vagal stimulation, during which time a pulse of current was delivered to the coplanar coils and a ventricular contraction was produced, showing an inverted QRS wave in the ECG and a blood-pressure pulse.

That it is difficult to stimulate the heart with a pulse of eddy current can be assessed by the parameters of the stimulator used by Bourland et al. (1990) which employed a 682 μF capacitor, charged to 9900 volts, and discharged into the 220 μH coplanar coil assembly. The peak current was 17,000 amps and the stored energy was 33,421 joules. The duration of the induced current pulse was 690 μsec. This stimulator was used by Mouchawar et al. (1992), who reported mean current and energy thresholds for cardiac stimulation in the range of 9200 amps and 11,850 joules.

From the foregoing it is clear that the ventricles can be caused to contract with pulses of eddy current. However, if it is desired to pace at 60/min (1/sec), the power needed is 11.85 kW, hardly a practical value for domestic or hospital use.

Summary and Conclusion

Although eddy-current stimulation of excitable tissue is quite popular now, the first report was by d'Arsonval (1896), who reported seeing bright flashes in the visual field (phosphenes) when the head was placed in a coil carrying 30 amperes of 42 Hz current (see Geddes translation, 1991). It is now known that stimulation of the retinal receptors in the eye produces such phosphenes. A similar phenomenon is sometimes reported by subjects undergoing magnetic resonance imaging (MRI).

Magnetic stimulation is largely used to excite nerve cells in the brain and spinal cord. The diagnostic information is contained in the time between the stimulus and the response (action potential). The same measure is used when a peripheral nerve is stimulated.

A major advantage of magnetic stimulation is that no electrodes are required and the skin need not be exposed to apply the stimuli. However, the main advantage is that the skin sensation is very mild. A major disadvantage is the high energy needed to induce sufficient eddy current density to achieve stimulation. When repetitive pulses are required, the power drawn by the magnetic stimulator may require a 60-Hz AC energy source of 220 or 440 volts. Moreover, with repetitive stimulation, coil heating becomes a problem. The availability of magnetically permeable materials that saturate at several orders of magnitude above presently available materials would be of benefit to the field of magnetic (eddy-current) stimulation.

This section has focused only on the three most prominent bioelectric events, those of the heart, skeletal muscle, and brain. The eye, ear, sweat glands, and many types of smooth muscle produce action potentials that are used for their diagnostic value, as well as being the subject of ongoing research. The reader interested in delving deeper into this field can find such information in a book by Geddes and Baker (1989).

Defining Terms

Atrophy: Wasting of cells deprived of nourishment.

Autonomic: That part of the nervous system that controls the internal organs.

Ectopic beat: A heart beat that originates from other than the normal site.

Hypocapnia: A condition of reduced carbon dioxide in the blood.

Hypoxia: A reduced amount of oxygen.

Magnetic stimulation: Eddy-current stimulation.

Metabolic process: The method by which cells use oxygen and produce carbon dioxide and heat.

Myocardial infarction: A heart attack in which a region of the heart muscle is deprived of blood and soon dies.

Occipital: The back of the brain.

Parietal: The side of the brain.

References

American EEG Society, "Guidelines in EEG and evoked potentials," *Am. J. Clin. Neurophysiol.*, 3, Suppl., 1986.

Association for the Advancement of Medical Instrumentation (AAMI), Diagnostic ECG Devices, ANSI-AAMI Standard EC-101-1991.

J.D. Bourland, G.A. Mouchawar, J.A. Nyenhuis, et al., "Transchest magnetic (eddy-current) stimulation of the dog heart," *Med. Eng. Comput.*, March, pp. 196–198, 1990.

F. Buchtal, C. Guld, and P. Rosenflack, "Action potential parameters of normal human muscle and their dependence on physical variables," *Acta Physiol. Scand.*, 32, pp. 200–220, 1954.

T-C. Chou, *Electrocardiography in Clinical Practice*, 3rd ed., Philadelphia, PA: W.B. Saunders, 1991.

H.L. Cohen and F. Brumlik, *Manual of Electromyography*, New York: Hoeber Medical Division, Harper & Row, 1969.

A. d'Arsonval, "Dispositifs pour la mesure des courants alternatifs de toutes frequences," *C.R. Soc. Biol. (Paris)*, 2, pp. 450–451, 1896.

L.A. Geddes, "The history of magnetic stimulation," *J. Neurophysiol.*, vol. 8, no. 1, pp. 3–9, 1991.

L.A. Geddes, L.E. Baker, and M. McGoodwin, "The relationship between electrode area and amplifier input impedance in recording muscle action potentials," *Med. Biol. Eng. Comput.*, vol. 5, pp. 561–568, 1967.

L.A. Geddes and L.E. Baker, *Principles of Applied Biomedical Instrumentations*, 3rd ed., New York: Wiley, 1989.

J. Kimura, *Electrodiagnosis in Diseases of Nerve and Muscle: Principles and Practice*, Oxford: Oxford University Press, 2001.

A.G. Kleber and Y. Rudy, "Basic mechanisms of cardiac impulse propagation and associated arrhythmias," *Physiol. Rev.*, 84, pp. 431–488, 2004.

International Federation of EEG Societies, J. Knott, Chairman, *EEG Clin. Neurophysiol.*, 10, pp. 378–380, 1958.

International Federation for Electroencephalography and Clinical Neurophysiology, *EEG. Clin. Neurophysiol.*, 10, pp. 371–375, 1958.

W.J. Levy, D.H. York, M. McCaffery, and F. Tanzer, "Evoked potentials from transcranial stimulation of the motor cortex in humans," *Neurosurgery*, vol. 15, no. 3, pp. 287–302, 1983.

G.A. Mouchawar, J.D. Bourland, and J.A. Nyenhuis et al., "Closed-chest cardiac stimulation with a pulsed magnetic field," *Med. Biol. Eng. Comput.*, March, pp. 162–168, 1992.

S. Nelson, D.B. Geselowitz, and C.V. Nelson, *The Theoretical Basis of Electrocardiology*, Oxford: Oxford University Press, 1985.

E. Niedermeyer and F. L. DaSilva, *Electroencephalography, Basic Principles, Clinical Applications, and Related Fields*, Baltimore, MD: Williams & Wilkins, 1993.

S.J. Oh, *Clinical Electromyography: Nerve Conduction Studies*, Philadelphia, PA: Lippincott Williams & Wilkins, 2003.

K.M. Overmeyer, J.A. Pearce, and D.P. DeWitt, "Measurement of temperature distributions at electrosurgical dispersive electrode sites," *Trans. ASME, J. Biomech. Eng.*, 101, pp. 66–72, 1979.

W. Penfield and T. Rasmussen, *The Cerebral Cortex of Man*, New York: Hafner, 1968.

R.E. Phillips and M.K. Feeney, *The Cardiac Rhythms: A Systematic Approach to Interpretation*, 3rd ed., Philadelphia, PA: W.B. Saunders, 1990.

T.W. Picton, "Evoked cortical potentials, how? what? and why?," *Am. J. EEG Technol.*, vol. 14, no. 4, pp. 9–44, 1974.

D.C. Preston and B. E. Shapiro, *Electromyography and Neuromuscular Disorders: Clinical-Electrophysiologic Correlations*, London: Butterworth–Heinemann, 1998.

D. Purves, G.J. Augustine, D. Fitzpatrick, L.C. Katz, A.S. LaMantia, and J.O. McNamara, *Neuroscience*, Sunderland, MA: Sinauer Associates, Inc. 1997

M. Shenasa, M. Borggrefe, and G. Breithardt, Eds., *Cardiac Mapping*, 2nd ed., Mount Kisco, NY: Futura Pub. Co., 2003.

J. Webster, Ed., *Design of Cardiac Pacemakers*, New York: IEEE Press, 1995.

7.3 Biological Effects and Electromagnetic Fields

Bonnie Keillor Slaten and Frank Barnes

Introduction

The purpose of this section is to provide the electrical professional with information on the biological effects of electric and magnetic fields at levels ranging from those that result in shock, to the low-level time-varying electromagnetic fields (EMF) from power lines. Additionally, we will review some of the current data on biological effects, at higher frequencies, from cell phones and base stations. The effects of electric shock are probably the best understood and a cause–effect relationship has been established. The biological effects of EMF from power lines, cell phones, and base stations to a population are more problematic, as a cause–effect relationship has not been established for these exposures. Intermediate levels have shown therapeutic effects for the repair of broken bones and modifications of cell growth rates. The potential of biological effects of EMF from power lines, cell phones, and base stations has been in the public eye and has become quite controversial. The data on health effects continues to be inconclusive, and the setting of standards reflects the differing philosophies with respect to incomplete understanding of the thresholds and nature of the biological effect of EMF. This section attempts to provide some of the background on these controversies.

The first subsection discusses the biological effects of electric shock. The second subsection is a discussion of the biological effects of EMF from power lines. A short discussion of exposure is presented and a review of the epidemiological studies follows. Reviews of animal and cellular studies of EMF from power lines are also presented. The third subsection is a discussion of the biological effects of EMF from cell phones and base stations. Exposure is discussed, followed by a review of epidemiological and cellular studies. Standards and guidelines are presented, as well as a discussion on risk.

Biological Effects of Electric Shock

The biological effects of an electrical shock are a function of the duration, magnitude, frequency, and path of the current passing through the body, as well as skin moisture. Electric current damages the body in three different ways:

1. It harms or interferes with proper functioning of the nervous system and heart.
2. It subjects the body to intense heat.
3. It causes the muscles to contract.

The nervous system is an electrical network that uses extremely low currents. Even very low-current electric shock can disrupt the normal functioning of muscles—most significantly, the heart. Electric shock also produces violent muscle contractions, which is why a person receiving a shock is frequently unable to "let go." It may also cause the heart to lose its coordination or rhythm. Even currents that produce no noticeable heating of tissue or visible injury can cause these effects (Jefferson Lab, 2004).

Electrical shock can also produce rapid and destructive heating of body tissue. Seemingly minor external effects (specifically burns) may be indicative of much more extensive internal injury and there can potentially be delayed effects.

Alternating current (ac) is more dangerous than direct current (dc), and 60-cycle current is more dangerous than high-frequency current. ac is said to be four to five times more dangerous than dc because ac causes more severe muscular contraction. In addition, ac stimulates sweating that lowers the skin resistance. Humans and animals are most susceptible to frequencies at 50 to 60 Hz because the internal frequency of the nerve signals controlling the heart is approximately 60 Hz (Electric Shock Precautions, 2004).

The National Electrical Code (NEC) in the United States considers 5 mA (0.005 amps) to be a safe upper limit for children and adults; hence the 5-mA Ground Fault Interrupter (GFI) circuit breaker requirement for wet locations (Bass Associates, 2004). The values in Table 7.2 should be used as a guide instead of absolute data points. For instance, 99% of the female population have a "let go" limit above 6 mA, with an average of 10.5 mA; while 99% of the male population have a "let go" above 9 mA, with an average of 15.5 mA (Bass Associates, 2004).

Ventricular fibrillation can occur at current levels as low as 30 mA for a 2-year-old child and 60 mA for adults. Most adults will go into ventricular fibrillation at hand-to-hand currents below 100 mA (0.1 amp) (Bass Associates, 2004).

Typically, if touching a 120-V circuit with one hand, a person can escape serious shock if he has insulating shoes that prevent a low-resistance path to ground. This fact has led to the common "hand in the pocket" practice for engineers and electrical workers. If they keep one hand in their pocket when touching a circuit, they are less likely to have the kind of path to ground that will result in a serious shock (Nave and Nave, 1985).

TABLE 7.2 Physiological Effects of Shock

Electric Current (1 sec contact)	Physiological Effect	Voltage Required to Produce the Current with Assumed Body Resistance	
		100,000 Ω	1,000 Ω
1 mA	Threshold of feeling, tingling sensation	100 V	1 V
5 mA	Accepted as maximum harmless current	500 V	5 V
10–20 mA	Beginning of sustained muscular contraction ("can't let go" current)	1,000 V	10 V
100–300 mA	Ventricular fibrillation, fatal if continued Respiratory function continues	10,000 V	100 V
6 A	Sustained ventricular contraction followed by normal heart rhythm (defibrillation) Temporary respiratory paralysis and possibly burns	600,000 V	6,000 V

Source: C.R. Nave and B.C. Nave, *Physics for the Health Sciences*, 3rd ed., Philadelphia: W.B. Saunders, 1985.

Will the 120-V Common Household Voltage Produce a Dangerous Shock? It Depends!

If your body resistance is 100,000 Ω, then the current which would flow would be:

$$I = \frac{120\,\mathrm{V}}{100,000\,\Omega} = 0.0012\,\mathrm{A} = 1.2\,\mathrm{mA}$$

This is just about at the threshold of perception, so it would only produce a tingle.

If you had just played a couple of sets of tennis, and were sweaty and barefoot, then the resistance to ground might be as low as 1,000 Ω. Then the current would be:

$$I = \frac{120\,\mathrm{V}}{1000\,\Omega} = 0.12\,\mathrm{A} = 120\,\mathrm{mA}$$

This is a lethal shock, capable of producing ventricular fibrillation and death! The severity of shock from a given source will depend upon its path through the body (Nave and Nave, 1985).

Table 7.3 shows some of the typical human body resistances to electrical current. Barring broken skin, body-circuit resistance, even in contact with liquid, will probably be not less than 500 Ω. However, the current flow at this resistance and 120 V is 240 mA—over twice that required to cause death (Jefferson Lab, 2004).

The path through the body has much to do with the shock danger. A current passing from finger to elbow through the arm may produce only a painful shock, but that same current passing from hand to hand or from hand to foot may well be fatal.

A burn from electrocution is much different than a burn from scalding or fire. Fleshy tissue is destroyed at 122°F and the vascular tissue serving the nerves suffers damage at considerably lower temperatures. Victims of industrial high-voltage accidents will display obvious thermal destruction at the skin contact points. The extremities may be slightly swollen but otherwise without visible surface damage. Yet beneath the involved skin, the skeletal muscle will often be in a state of severe unrelenting spasm or rigor. There will frequently be marked sensory and motor nerve malfunction. Within the first week after injury, many victims will undergo sequential surgical procedures to remove damaged nonviable skeletal muscle, resulting in a weak, stiff extremity that is often anesthetic because of nerve damage, and cold because of poor circulation. Under these circumstances, the patient is better off undergoing amputation and then receiving a prosthetic extremity (R. Lee, 1991).

In general, muscle and nerve appear to be the tissues with the greatest vulnerability to injury by electrical current. There is a characteristic skeletal muscle tissue injury pattern in victims of high-voltage electrical shock that is relatively unique to shock victims. Muscle adjacent to the bone and joints is recognized clinically to be the most vulnerable to electrical trauma. In addition, muscle cells located in the central region of the muscle may also be vulnerable and nerves seem to have a lower threshold for damage than muscle (R. Lee, 1991).

In conclusion, if the contact to the source of the shock is brief, nonthermal mechanisms of cell damage may be most important. If the contact is much longer, heat damage will be most destructive and if heat damage predominates, then the injury may not be limited just to the plasma membrane but to other cell membranes as well, and this is unlikely to be reversible (R. Lee, 1991).

TABLE 7.3 Typical Human Body Resistance to Electrical Current

Body Area	Resistance (Ω)
Dry skin	100,000–600,000
Wet skin	1,000
Internal body (hand to foot)	400–600
Ear to ear	~100

Source: C.R. Nave and B.C. Nave, *Physics for the Health Sciences*, 3rd ed., Philadelphia: W.B. Saunders, 1985.

Other Adverse Effects of Electricity

Electrical Arc Flash

When an electrical arc occurs, it can produce temperatures up to 35,000°F. This melts and vaporizes the constituents of the conductor, rapidly heating the surrounding air—with potentially explosive force. One cubic inch of copper, for example, produces 1.44 cubic yards of vapor. This is comparable to the expansion rate of dynamite. Electrical explosions can be fatal within 10 ft of the arc, and can cause burns up to 40 ft away (Jefferson Lab, 2004).

Biological Effects of Low-Level, Time-Varying Electromagnetic Fields (EMF) from Power Lines

The effects of electric fields on biological systems have been studied since the discovery of electricity, and electricity has been used to treat a wide variety of illnesses including depression and broken bones. It is relatively recently that the general population has become concerned that weak magnetic fields, those that are less than a tenth of the Earth's magnetic field, may cause adverse biological effects. The possibility that the time varying magnetic field from power lines might be associated with the incidence of childhood cancer was first raised by Wertheimer in an epidemiological study in 1979 (Wertheimer et al., 1995). Since that time a large number of studies have been carried out and more than 37,000 papers written on the biological effects of electric and magnetic fields. The results of many of these studies are controversial for a number of reasons; the primary reason being the inability to establish a cause–effect relationship at the weak field levels that are generally associated with exposures from power lines.

It is well established that there are biological effects of electric and magnetic fields at high levels of exposure. As presented earlier, currents at lower levels, of the order of 10 mA, are large enough to produce an electric shock. Current densities of microamperes per centimeter squared are about the same intensity as the currents that flow naturally in the human body and are large enough to modify growth processes. The current densities that are typically induced by the time-varying fields from power lines that are in the range from 0.1 to 10 μT (1 to 100 mG) at 60 Hz are estimated to result in current densities significantly less than 0.04 μA cm^{-2}. As these currents are considerably smaller than the naturally flowing currents in the human body, it is not clear whether or not they are biologically significant. Biological systems are typically highly nonlinear and have thresholds. Thus, a small current injected into the heart's natural pacemaker cell may have little or no effect on its firing rate, whereas a current of the same intensity at a different time or one that is two or three times larger may either stop the firing altogether or speed it up. The biological effect of the current depends on the direction of the current and when it is applied during the cell's firing cycle.

Additionally, biological systems have a large number of feedback loops that tend to cancel out undesirable changes. Thus, one can have changes in a biological system as a result of small currents or small concentrations of chemicals that are corrected by the body and do not result in adverse health effects. For example, exercise may dissipate four or five times as much metabolic energy as rest. This could be expected to raise the body temperature. However, the result of such exercise causes you to sweat and your body temperature remains nearly constant. To make things even more complex, some effects like stress can be either positive or negative depending on the circumstances and past history. Stress reactions like the release of heat shock proteins can protect the body against elevated temperature; however, prolonged stress can deplete the body's ability to respond a new stress.

The net result of these complexities is that the scientific community is not in a position to say that any given exposure level is safe. However, it is equally true that data are not available to say that the magnetic fields in the ranges that are associated with power lines are harmful.

Exposures

Both electric and magnetic fields are associated with power lines. The electric fields are proportional to the voltage and typically decrease rapidly with distance. The voltage rating on power lines in Colorado, ranges from 340 kV to 110 V to ground and 220 V between lines into the house (Thompson, 2003). These electric fields are relatively easy to reduce by metal shields from the typical values of 5 to 10 kV m^{-1} under power lines to levels less than 100 to 200 V m^{-1}, which is typical for peak values in normal households. Average values for electric fields in houses are typically about 10 V m^{-1}.

The magnetic fields are proportional to the current flowing in the wires and also decrease rapidly with distance. The intensity of these fields at a distance typically increases with the spacing between the wires and decreases as the distance from the wires increases at a rate that is greater than one over the distance cubed (1 D^{-3}). It should be noted that currents flowing in low-voltage lines, and thus the magnetic fields, might be as large as those in high-voltage lines. However, transmission lines tend to have higher average currents as the power is delivered to a wide variety of customers with peak power demands at different times. As the required power increases, the power companies typically raise the voltage in order to reduce the losses in the transmission lines that are proportional to the square of the current. It often occurs that when the transmission lines are upgraded and the voltages are raised, the currents and the magnetic fields are reduced.

Burying the transmission lines primarily means that the lines are out of sight. The fields typically decrease more rapidly with distance, as the spacing between the wires is smaller. However, the distance to places where people might be exposed usually decreases, as power lines are not buried nearly as far below the surface as they are suspended in the air and the fields in the right-of-way may increase. Burying power lines is much more expensive than suspending them in the air.

It should also be noted that the largest source of magnetic fields in a home may be the plumbing. Metal plumbing is often used as a ground and current, though it can generate magnetic fields that decrease as one over the distance (1 D^{-1}) rather than one over the distance cubed (1 D^{-3}) as it does for a pair of wires. The current in the plumbing may be generated either by the difference in the current between the two halves of the circuit feeding the house or by similar currents in adjacent homes that are returning to the pole via a lower-resistance connection than others in the neighborhood. These fields are often larger than exposure from nearby power lines.

The following sections review a few of the more than 37,000 papers that have been published on this subject. The first group of these papers addresses epidemiological studies. There are more than 40 studies and approximately half of these show a weak effect and the other half show no statistically significant effects. The second group of studies to be reviewed includes animal studies where the electric and magnetic field exposures can be carefully controlled. The third group of studies covers cellular studies.

Epidemiological Studies

In the early 1980s, health research on EMF began to shift from general health concerns to cancer.

In the 1970s, Wertheimer and Leeper conducted an exploratory study in Denver, Colorado, which was the first to identify 60-Hz magnetic fields as a possible risk factor for childhood cancer. Their study found statistically significant associations between child cancer mortality and proximity of children's homes to high-current electric power lines. The results seemed surprising because of the weakness of the fields. They said their findings appeared to relate to current rather than voltages, and therefore, magnetic instead of electric fields were of interest. Additionally, the study suggested that weak 60-Hz magnetic fields of only 0.2 to 0.3 μT, or 2 to 3 mG, and above, might in some way affect cancer development. It is of note that some measurements of magnetic field were made but they were not used in the analysis of cancer data. Wertheimer and Leeper suggested that the main sources of magnetic fields include power lines and currents on water pipes (Wertheimer et al., 1995).

The Denver study was criticized for a number of reasons. The results seemed even more problematic after another study a year later in Rhode Island failed to find similar results (Fulton et al., 1980) There were apparent biases in the Rhode Island study and the next studies that were conducted did find statistically significant associations between power line types and child cancer (Wertheimer et al., 1995, Tomenius and Savitz et al., 1998). The research by Savitz et al. was done in Denver and researchers used newer child cancer cases. Savitz et al. concluded that the results of their research were generally consistent with Wertheimer and Leeper's study (Savitz et al., 1998) A re-examination of the second Denver study showed statistically significant associations that were stronger than originally reported in the 1988 paper. Savitz and Kaune (1993) used a three-level code to classify homes near power lines, and they found statistically significant risks for total child cancer (odds ratio=1.9), leukemia (odds ratio = 2.9), and for brain cancer (odds ratio = 2.5)[1] (Savitz et al., 1998).

Another reassessment of the study by Savitz et al. found a statistically significant threefold increase in child cancer risk for homes in Denver with metal pipes compared to homes with nonconductive pipes (Wertheimer et al., 1995). Non-conductive or polyvinylchloride (PVC) pipes do not conduct electric grounding current so they do not generate a magnetic field. Additional studies followed, and in 1996 there were 19 studies of power lines and child cancer conducted in ten different countries. The newer epidemiologic studies have generally enrolled larger numbers of subjects and these focused on childhood leukemia and to a lesser degree, brain and nervous system tumors. Earlier methodological shortcomings were addressed and these studies increasingly collected data on a broader range of additional, possibly confounding, factors.

The study by Feychting and Ahlbom (1995) of all children in Sweden who lived on property within 300 m (984 ft) of transmission lines has received considerable attention. "Among the findings was a fourfold increase in leukemia for children living in dwellings where the calculated magnetic field near the time of cancer diagnosis was $\geq$0.3 μT (3 mG). There was also evidence of dose-response for magnetic fields and cancer" (J. Lee, 1996).

The Oak Ridge Associated Universities (ORAU) Panel in 1993 concluded that the study by Feychting and Ahlbom (1995) was not compelling because of inconsistencies with an earlier Swedish study by Tomenius and because no significant associations with cancer were found when present-day magnetic field measurements were analyzed (ORAU, 1993).

Some researchers conclude that factors other than magnetic fields are more likely causes of the observed associations between power lines and child cancer. Others suggest that power-line classifications or calculated magnetic fields near the time of cancer diagnosis may provide more meaningful estimates of past exposure than present-day magnetic field measurements (Feychting and Ahlbom, 1995 and Savitz and Loomis, 1995).

Differences in residential mobility and in the age of residences between cases and controls have been suggested as reasons to believe that the cancer-magnetic field association in the Denver study is false (Jones et al., 1993; Jones, 1993 and Jones et al., 1994). In the Denver study, cases and controls differed on the basis of residential mobility (controls were more residentially stable). Jones found that in Columbus, Ohio, residents near high-current-carrying power lines moved more often than those near low-current lines (Jones, 1993).

Linet et al. (1997) published a large U.S. case–control study (638 cases and 620 controls) to test whether childhood acute lymphoblastic leukemia is associated with exposure to 60-Hz magnetic fields. In this study magnetic field exposures were determined using 24-h time-weighted average measurements in the bedrooms and 30-sec measurements in various other rooms. Measurements were taken in homes in which the child had lived for 70% of the five years prior to the year of cancer diagnosis, or the corresponding period for the controls. A computer algorithm assigned wire-code configuration of nearby power lines to the subjects rsquo; main residences (for 416 case patients and 416 controls). The study concluded that the results provided little evidence that living in homes characterized by high measured time-weighted average magnetic-field levels or by the highest wire-code category increases the risk of acute lymphoblastic leukemia.

An association may or may not exist but a cause–effect relationship has definitely not been proven.

Animal Studies

Just as childhood cancer and EMF research has prompted numerous studies; the effect of EMF on animals has produced an even greater volume of studies. This very large volume of research extends back to the 1960s where *in vivo* studies were mostly intended to provide data to help assess the potential for adverse effects of EMF on people.

[1]Exposures of cases and controls are compared by calculating an odds ratio (OR). The OR is the proportion of cases exposed to some factor (e.g., strong magnetic fields), divided by the proportion of controls exposed to the factor. It gives the odds that the cases were exposed compared to the controls. An OR of 1.00 means that there was no difference between the cases and controls in the proportions that were exposed to the factor (i.e., there was no association between exposure and the disease). An OR of 2.00 means that the cases were exposed to the factor were twice as likely as the controls to show a positive association between exposure to the factor and the disease.

TABLE 7.4 Summary of Epidemiological Studies

Subjects/Exposure	Selected Results	References
344 child cancer deaths compared to two groups of controls. Exposure by size and number of power lines and distance to home	Excess of height-current configuration power lines found near homes of child cancer cases. ∓ Leukemia, OR = 3.00*, 1.78–5.00; lymphoma, OR = 2.08, 0.84–5.16; CNS OR = 2.40*, 1.15–5.01; total cancer, OR = 2.23*, 1.58–3.13	Wertheimer and Leeper (1979) U.S., CO
Lines within 150 m of homes of 716 child cancer cases and 716 controls were mapped. Magnetic fields measured at front door	For total homes and fields ≥3 mG; leukemia OR = 0.3; CNS OR = 3.7*, $p<0.05$; lymphoma, OR = 1.8; total cancer, OR = 2.1*, $p<.05$. In this study analyses were based on case and control homes, not on persons	Tomenius (1986) Sweden
Power lines were classified and mapped near homes of 356 child cancer cases and 278 controls. EMF were measured in homes	For high vs. low current lines: OR = 1.54, 0.90–2.63; brain cancer, OR = 2.04*, 1.11–3.76; total cancer OR = 1.53, 1.04–2.26. For ≥2 mG leukemia, OR = 1.93, 0.67–5.56; total cancer, OR = 1.35, 0.63–2.90.	Savitz et al. (1988), U.S., CO
142 child cancer cases within 300 m of 220–400 kV lines. Exposure defined as residence within 50 m of a power line. ENM	For all dwellings ≥3 mG: total cancer OR = 1.3, 0.6–2.7 (10 cases); leukemia OR = 3.8*, 1.4–9.3 (7 cases); CNS cancer OR = 1.0, 0.2–3.9 (2 cases). For all dwelling within 50 m: total cancer OR = 1.0, 0.5–2.2, leukemia OR = 2.9, 1.0–7.3	Feychting and Ahlbom (1993), Sweden
638 cases and 620 controls to test whether childhood acute lymphoblastic leukemia is associated with exposure to 60-Hz magnetic fields. Measurements were taken in homes in which the child had lived for 70% of the 5 years prior to the year of cancer diagnosis	Results provided little evidence that living in homes characterized by high measured time-weighted average magnetic-field levels or by the highest wire-code category increases the risk of acute lymphoblastic leukemia	Linet et al. (1997)

OR = odd ratio, ENM = EMF not measured, * = statistically significant, ∓ odds ratios were not included in Wertheimer and Leeper (1979) but they can be calculated from data in their paper.

In a review of EMF animal cancer research by Löscher and Mevissen (1994), the researchers concluded that there is accumulating evidence that magnetic fields induce a carcinogenic response in laboratory animals. However, they stated that the existing evidence was insufficient to differentiate a cause–effect relationship. A different review, by Anderson and Sasser (1995) concluded that the results of the animal tumor promotion studies are mixed, and the strongest evidence is in the area of mammary carcinogenesis. They also believed that the studies with animals had not yet confirmed the results of the epidemiologic studies that in some instances suggest a slight association between EMF and cancer.

Animal carcinogenic studies of EMF were done at levels of exposure generally much higher and having greater uniformity in frequency and intensity than would appear in environmental settings. These experimental conditions were chosen to maximize the ability of a researcher to detect an effect, if one exists, for a clearly defined exposure (Olden NIH Publication No. 99-4493).

The effects of EMF exposure on the immune system were investigated in multiple animal models including baboons and rodents, and there is no consistent evidence in experimental animals for effects from EMF exposure. Reports of effects in baboons were not confirmed when the study was repeated (Murthy et al., 1995). Some studies had methodological difficulties making interpretation of the findings difficult (Mevissen et al., 1996).

Each summer during 1977 to 1981, cattle behavior was studied near the Boneville Power Administration 1200-kV prototype line (Rogers et al., 1982). Each year five different steers were placed in a pasture where the animals could range both beneath and away from the line. The location of the cattle throughout the day was monitored with time-lapse cameras. Forage, salt, and water consumption were also measured. The line was alternately turned on and off at times during the study. The animals showed no reluctance to graze or drink beneath the line, which produced a maximum electric field of 12 kV m^{-1} (the test line carried no load so there was no magnetic field). A refined statistical analysis of the 1980 to 1981 data indicated the cattle spent slightly more time near the line when it was turned off. This may indicate a reaction of the cattle to audible noise from corona, or to the electric field. During the 1980 study of the 1200-kV line, one steer died of a bacterial infection. The other cattle studied remained healthy and no abnormal conditions developed (J. Lee, 1996).

Cellular Studies

Many areas of research also include studies of cells and tissues conducted outside the body, or *in vitro* studies. These studies are typically used to obtain information on how EMF interacts with biological processes and structures. An area of research currently being pursued is EMF and gene expression. "Gene expression is the process for making proteins from information in DNA within genes. During *transcription*, information in DNA is transferred out of the nucleus by mRNA. *Translation* occurs in the cytoplasm on ribosomes where information on mRNA is used to construct specific proteins" (J. Lee, 1996).

At the 1996 annual meeting of the Bioelectromagnetics Society, several papers on gene expression were presented. Goodman et al. (1996) summarized their past research and suggested that many lines of evidence indicate that 60-Hz magnetic fields increase transcripts for stress genes in cells from humans, flies, and yeast (Goodman et al.). Other researchers have reported that they were unable to find effects of 50- or 60-Hz magnetic fields on gene expression (Mattsson et al., 1996; Buthod et al., 1996; Hui et al., 1996; Owen et al., 1996; Thurston and Saffer, 1996) or on protein synthesis (Shi et al., 1996).

In recent years, researchers have been studying the gene expression leading to protein synthesis of the stress response. The cell membrane is currently thought to be the primary region for sensitivity to electric and magnetic fields (Lin et al., 1997). When cells are exposed to a problematical environment such as heavy metals, chemical toxins, heat or EMF they produce stress proteins, called heat shock proteins (HSPs). When the cell is under stress, the production of HSPs is a programmed response through the induction of the heat shock gene expression. These HSPs bind to other molecules to protect them against the stress.

Miyakawa et al. (2001) reported that low-frequency magnetic fields had an influence on stress response, growth retardation and small body size in adulthood, and low brood number. Importantly, they examined responses of the heat shock protein gene, *HSP*-16 in transgenic *Caenorhabidities elegans* exposed to magnetic fields at 60 Hz with a peak flux density of 0.5 T, and their results are comparable to others.

Junkersdorf et al. (2000) made a clear point that weak low-frequency magnetic fields act as a second stress factor in addition to a mild heat stress on the expression of a *lacZ* reporter gene under the control of HSP16 or HSP70 in *C. elegans*.

Mevissen et al., (1998) reported that with a second stress factor, chemical carcinogen DMBA, the (50 μT, 50 Hz) magnetic field-exposed group showed more tumors than groups without exposure.

The signaling pathway of the stress response is a two-part process; the stress detection in cytoplasm by the heat shock transcription factors (HSFs) and the gene expression in the nucleus by the heat shock elements (HSEs). Although there are not many molecular mechanisms that can describe how electromagnetic fields affect biological structures, one research group has studied the relation between gene expression and electromagnetic fields. Blank and Soo (1998) postulated that magnetic fields may interact on one part of the signaling pathway of the stress response because there may be magnetic-field–sensitive sites in the genes. When these sites were deleted, no magnetic sensitivity was found. They found that 60-Hz magnetic fields below 0.5 μT accelerated the oxidation of cytochrome C and presumed that the magnetic fields interact directly with moving electrons in DNA, which in turn stimulate the stress response. These magnetic field sensitive sites within the genes could explain some of the biological effects of EMF at the cellular level. Other studies have shown effects including bone healing that seem to be related to the induced current density at the levels of microamperes per square centimeter. Still other studies indicate a stress response at magnetic fields of 21 μT or 210 mG (J. Lee, 1996).

The lack of consistent, positive findings in animal or mechanistic studies for these low-level fields weakens the belief that this association is actually due to EMF. However, the epidemiological findings cannot be

TABLE 7.5 Stress Response of Magnetic Field (MF) Exposure with Second Stress Factors

Author	Exposure	Target	Results	Second stress factor
Blank et al. (1998)	60 Hz magnetic fields below 0.5 μT		Accelerated the oxidation of cytochrome C and presumed that the magnetic fields interact directly with moving electrons in DNA by which stimulate the stress response	
Miyakawa et al. (2001)	MF 60 Hz 0.5 T (peak)	Transgenic nematode, *C. elegans*	Stress response: heat shock proteins gene expression induced at 26°C in 80% of the exposed nematodes (without exposure 80% animals responded at 29°C)	Mild heat increase up to 26°C
Junkersdorf et al. (2000)	MF 50 Hz, 100 μT	Transgenic nematode, C. elegans	Stress response: heat shock proteins gene expression; the 86.9% of stained nematodes at 29°C (without exposure 39.9% of stained nematodes at 29°C)	Mild heat of 29°C
Mevissen et al. (1996)	MF 50 Hz 50 μT	Rats	More tumors in MF-exposed rats than sham-exposed after 8 weeks (in both cases with DMBA treatment)	Chemical stressor: carcinogen, DMBA*

*2-Dimethylbenz[a]anthrancene.

completely discounted. The National Institute of Environmental Health Sciences (NIEHS) in the U.S. concluded that EMF exposure cannot be recognized as entirely safe because of weak scientific evidence that exposure may pose a leukemia hazard. Since the scientific evidence for a leukemia hazard is weak, the NIEHS found it insufficient to warrant aggressive regulatory concern (EMF RAPID, 1995).

EMF from Cell Phones and Base Stations

The most rapidly growing source of RF exposure is that of cell phone use. In the U.S. there are currently more than 193,689,404 wireless subscribers (CTIA, 2005) and the industry predicts that there will be as many as 1.6 billion mobile phone subscribers worldwide in 2005 (Electromagnetic Fields and Public Health, Mobile Telephone and Their Base Stations, Fact Sheet N193).

Cellular communications systems in the United States use frequencies in the 800 to 900 MHz portion of the radiofrequency (RF) spectrum, which were formerly used for UHF-TV broadcasting. Transmitters in the Personal Communications Service (PCS) use frequencies in the range of 1850 to 1990 MHz. In the United Kingdom, cellular mobile phone services operate within the frequency ranges of 872 to 960 MHz and 1710 to 1875 MHz.

Paging and other communications antennae such as those used by fire, police, and emergency services operate at similar power levels as cellular base stations, and often at a similar frequency. In many urban areas television and radio broadcast antennae commonly transmit higher RF levels than do mobile base stations.

Primary antennae for cellular and PCS transmissions are usually located on elevated structures and the combination of antennae and associated electronic equipment is referred to as a cellular or PCS "base station" or "cell site." Typical heights for base station towers are 50 to 200 ft. A typical cellular base station may utilize several "omni-directional" antennae that look like poles or ships, 10 to 15 ft in length. PCS (and also many cellular) base stations use a number of "sector" antennae that look like rectangular panels. The dimensions of a sector antenna are typically 1 ft. × 4 ft. Antennae are usually arranged in three groups of three with one antenna in each group used to transmit signals to mobile units (car phones or handheld phones). The other two antennae in each group are used to receive signals from mobile units (Cleveland, Jr. et al., 1995).

Vehicle-mounted antennae used for cellular communications normally operate at a power level of 3 watts or less. The cellular antennae are typically mounted on the roof, on the trunk, or on the rear window of a vehicle. Studies have shown that in order to be exposed to RF levels that approach the safety guidelines, it would be necessary to remain very close to a vehicle-mounted cellular antenna.

Exposures

Mobile phones and base stations emit RF nonionizing radiation. In both instances, levels of exposure generally reduce with increasing distance from the source. For mobile phones, exposure will be predominantly to the side of the head for hand-held use, or to parts of the body closest to the phone during hands-free use.

For base-station emissions, exposures of the general population will be to the whole body but typically at levels of intensity many times lower than those from handsets.

At a cell site, the total RF power that could be transmitted from each transmitting antenna at a cell site depends on the number of radio channels (transmitters) that have been authorized and the power of each transmitter. The FCC permits an effective radiated power (ERP) of up to 500 watts per channel (dependant on the tower height). The majority of the cellular base stations in urban and suburban areas operate at an ERP of 100 watts per channel or less. An ERP of 100 watts corresponds to an actual radiated power of 5 to 10 watts, depending on the type of antenna used. As dividing cells (i.e., adding additional base stations) expands the capacity of a system, lower ERPs are normally used. In urban areas, an ERP of 10 watts per channel (corresponding to a radiated power of 0.5 to 1 watt) or less is commonly used (Cleveland, Jr. et al., 1995).

For cellular base station transmitters, at a frequency of 869 MHz (the lowest frequency used), the FCC's RF exposure guidelines recommend a maximum permissible exposure level of the general public (or exposure in "uncontrolled" environments) of about 580 microwatts per square centimeter (μW cm^{-2}), as averaged over any 30-min period. This limit is many times greater than RF levels typically found near the base of typical cellular towers or in the vicinity of other, lower-powered cellular base station transmitters (Cleveland, Jr. et al., 1995).

The FCC's exposure guidelines, and the ANSI/IEEE and NCRP guidelines upon which they are based, specify limits for human exposure to RF emissions from hand-held RF devices in terms of specific absorption rate (SAR). For exposure of the general public, e.g., exposure of the user of a cellular or PCS phone, the SAR limit is an absorption threshold of 1.6 W kg^{-1}, as measured over any one gram of tissue (Cleveland, Jr. et al., 1995).

Measurements and computational analysis of SAR in models of the human head and other studies of SAR distribution using hand-held cellular and PCS phones have shown that, in general, the 1.6 W kg^{-1} limit is unlikely to be exceeded under normal conditions of use (Cleveland, Jr. et al., 1995).

Epidemiological Studies

Since the late 1970s, there have been numerous epidemiological studies undertaken to investigate a link between higher-frequency EMF and a myriad of conditions such as decreased motor functions and cancer. Most of these studies show no effect, or replications fail to confirm the original results, indicating an increased hazard for exposures to low levels of radiation from sources like TV stations and radar. A weakness of many of these studies is poor data on the difference between exposure levels for the exposed and control populations. A recent NRC study of the PAVE PAWS radar with better but still inadequate exposure data indicates a non-statistically significant decrease in cancer incidence for residents within line of sight of the radar and exposure levels averaging less than 1 μW cm^{-2} (National Research Council Report, Jan. 13, 2005). Three epidemiological studies are noteworthy in reporting results that appear to be deserving of further investigation. The first study investigated motor function, memory, and attention of school children living in the area of the Skrunda Radio Location Station (RLS) in Latvia. The Skrunda RLS is a pulse radar station that operates at frequencies of 154 to 162 MHz. The duration of pulses is 0.8 ms and time between pulses is 41 msec, i.e., the pulses occur at a frequency of 24.4 Hz (Kolodynski 1996). The investigators found that children living in front of the Skrunda RLS had less-developed memory and attention, slower reaction times and decreased endurance of neuromuscular apparatus. Children living in the exposed zone in front of Skrunda RLS performed worse in psychological tests than the children living behind the RLS, and even worse when compared with the control group. The authors stated that "the validity of a statement that the radio frequency EMF at Skrunda has caused these differences can only be claimed with continuous and accurate assessment of dose, and close to exact standardization of subjects." The measurement of dose is problematic since the children move in and out of the radiation zone and the temporal changes in intensity are high. The correlation between performance and distance to the RLS suggests that this path of research is worthwhile and that further study should be undertaken.

The next two studies were undertaken by Hardell et al. The first included a case-control study of 1617 patients of both sexes, aged 20 to 80 years, with brain tumor diagnosis between January 1, 1997 and June 30, 2000. The subjects were alive at the study time and had histopathologically verified brain tumors. One match control to each case was selected from the Swedish Population Register. The study area was the Uppsala-Örebro, Stockholm, Linköping, and Göteborg regions of Sweden. Exposure was assessed by a questionnaire that was answered by 1429 (88%) cases and 1470 (91%) controls. In total, use of analog cellular telephones gave an increased risk with an odds ratio (OR) of 1.3 (95% confidence interval [CI] 1.02 to 1.6). With a tumor induction period of >10 years, the risk increased further, to OR 1.8 (95% CI 1.1 to 2.9). No clear association was found for digital or cordless telephones. With regard to the anatomical area of the tumor and exposure to microwaves, the risk was increased for tumors located in the temporal area on the same side of the brain that was used during phone calls; for analog cellular the OR was 2.5 (95% CI 1.3 to 4.9). Use of a telephone on the opposite side of the brain was not associated with an increased risk for brain tumors. The highest risk for different tumor types was for acoustic neurinoma (OR 3.5, 95% CI 1.8 to 6.8) among analog cellular telephone users (Hardell et al.). The study does not imply cause and effect, but rather an increased risk for brain tumors among users of analog cellular phones.

The second study undertaken by Hardell et al. used the database from the case–control study (the above analysis) and further statistical analysis was carried out. The second study showed an increased risk for brain tumors among users of analogue cellular telephones. In total, use of analogue cellular telephones gave an increased risk with odds ration (OR) = 1.3, 95% confidence interval (CI) = 1.04 to 1.6, whereas digital and cordless phones did not overall increase the risk significantly. Ipsilateral exposure increased the risk significantly. Cordless phones yielded significantly increased risk overall with a >5-year latency period (Hardell et al.). Additional studies, such as those by Hardell et al. need to be undertaken using digital cell phones and latency periods of greater than 15 years.

Epidemiological studies undertaken by R.P. Gallagher et al., S. Slevin, Johansen, and Inskip et al. showed no significant increases or negative results.

TABLE 7.6 Summary of Epidemiological Studies

Model	Exposure Conditions	Results	References
Children living near radar station	Pulse radar at 154–162 MHz; pulse is 0.8 msec; time between pulses is 41 msec; pulses occur at 24.4 Hz	Less developed memory and attention functions of school children. Reaction time for exposed children was slower and endurance was decreased.	Kolodynski
Case control of 1617 patients with brain tumor diagnosis	Analog cellular telephone use; 800–900 MHz; 2450 MHz	A significant increased risk for analog telephone use. No significant increase for digital or cordless telephone use.	Hardell et al.
Case control of 1617 patients with brain tumor diagnosis	Analog cellular telephone use; 800–900 MHz; 2450 MHz	Further statistical analysis carried out from previous study. Increased risk for brain tumors with use of analog phones. Significant risk for cordless phones, if tumor induction period was >5 years.	Hardell et al.
Cell phone users from 1982 to 1995	900–1800 MHz	No significant increase in cancer.	Johansen
Cell phone users; short-term use	Cell phone users from 1994 to 1998	No significant increase in brain tumors.	Inskip et al.

Animal Studies (*In Vivo*)

In vivo studies offer an approach that may be used in cases where experimental animals and conditions can be controlled so that specific variables can be tested and exposure levels measured accurately. A considerable amount of data has been generated to evaluate the impact of both thermal and nonthermal effects of RF exposure on laboratory animals. It is beyond the scope of this section to list all the studies but rather the goal is to emphasize the most significant studies.

Modak et al. (1981) reported that RF exposure caused a decrease in the concentration of the transmitter acetylcholine in the mouse brain, but they employed a very intense 2.45-GHz single pulse, causing a 2 to 4°C rise in temperature. The rate-limiting step in the synthesis of acetylcholine is the uptake of choline by nerve cells. In an extensive series of experiments, Lai and colleagues (1987, 1989a,b, 1990, 1991, 1994) have reported that 20 min of exposure of rats to pulsed 2.45-GHz radiation at low intensities causes an increase in choline uptake and a reduction in the concentration of acetylcholine receptors, whereas exposure for 45 min had the opposite effect. Although the average intensities used in these studies were relatively low, the findings might depend on thermal effects, especially since acetylcholine is known to be involved in transmission in the parts of the hypothalamus responsible for temperature regulation, which is acutely sensitive to temperature change. The studies by Lai et al. used radar-like pulses of quite high peak intensity that are capable of eliciting auditory responses in animals, which themselves might have behavioral effects (W. Stewart, 2000).

In contrast to the above, Baranski et al. reported a decrease in the activity of acetylcholinesterase in guinea pigs exposed to pulsed RF fields at high power densities, but they attributed this to thermal effects (W. Stewart, 2000).

Chou et al. (1992) exposed 100 rats aged 2 to 27 months to low-level pulsed 2.45-GHz fields. The total number of benign tumors in the adrenal medulla was higher in the exposed group compared to the control group, although not particularly higher than that reported elsewhere for this strain of rat. When the

TABLE 7.7 Summary of Animal Studies (*In Vivo*)

Model	Exposure Conditions	Results	References
Mouse brain	2.45 GHz single pulse	Decrease in acetylcholine	Modak et al. (1981)
Rat brain	2.45 GHz pulsed; 2 μsec pulses at 500 ppsec; 0.6 W kg^{-1}	Exposure for 45 min decreased choline uptake and concentration of acetylcholine receptors. Exposure for 20 min opposite effect seen. Effects blocked with naltrexone	Lai et al. (1987, 1989a,b, 1990, 1991, 1994)
Guinea pig	3 GHz CW or pulsed; 400 ppsec (no pulse width specified); 35–250 W m^{-2}	Decrease in acetylcholinesterase activity	Baranski et al. (1972)
Sprague–Dawley rats	2.45 GHz pulsed; 10 μsec pulses at 800 ppsec, pulse modulated at 8 ppsec; whole body SAR of 0.4–0.15 W kg^{-1} for up to 25 months	No increase in individual cancers; fourfold increase in primary malignancies	Chou et al. (1992)
Lymphoma-prone Eμ-*Pim1* transgenic mice	900 MHz pulsed (GSM); 600 μsec; 217 ppsec; whole-body SAR; 0.008–4.2 W kg^{-1}; 1 h per day; 18 months	Twofold increase in lymphoma incidence	Repacholi et al. (1997)
Mammary tumor prone C3H/HeA mice	435 MHz pulsed; 1-μsec pulses at 1000 ppsec; whole-body SAR of 0.32 W kg^{-1}; 21 months	No effect	Toler et al. (1997)
Mammary tumor prone c2H/HeA mice	2.45 GHz; whole-body SAR 0.3–1.0 W kg^{-1}; 18 months	No effect	Frei et al. (1998a,b)

occurrence of primary malignant lesions was pooled without regard to site or mode of death, the exposed group had a significantly higher incidence compared to the control group (W. Stewart, 2000).

The most positive evidence, as yet unreplicated, of an effect of exposure to RF similar to that used by digital mobile phones was reported by Repacholi et al. (1997) using E*μ-Pim 1* transgenic mice. Experimental transgenic rodents have genetic material added to their DNA to predispose them to the endpoint being investigated. The mice, which were moderately susceptible to the development of lymphoblastic lymphomas, were exposed or sham-exposed for 1 h per day for 18 months to pulse-modulated 900-MHz radio frequencies. The exposure conditions were a whole-body SAR of 0.008 to 4.2 W kg^{-1} for 1 h per day for 18 months. The authors reported an increase in the incidence of all lymphomas in the exposed mice (43% compared to 22% in the controls). However, lymphoma incidence was rapidly increasing in both exposed and sham-exposed animals when the study was terminated; in addition, only moribund animals were examined histopathologically. Replication of this study and extension with more complete follow-up and improved dosimetry would be useful and is currently underway in Australia (W. Stewart, 2000).

Still other researchers, such as Toler et al. (1997) and Frei et al. (1998a,b), have reported a lack of effect of RF exposure on cancer incidence in mice prone to mammary tumors (W. Stewart, 2000).

Cellular Studies

As stated earlier, many areas of research also include *in vitro* studies. These studies are typically used to obtain information on how RF interacts with biological processes and structures.

Most observations of sister chromatic exchange *in vitro* have failed to detect any effect of RF exposure, even at high intensities (Lloyd et al., 1984; 1986; Wolff et al., 1985; Maes et al., 1993; 2000) on human lymphocytes; (Wolff et al., 1985; Meltz et al., 1990; Ciaravino et al., 1991) on hamster ovary cells. Maes et al. (1997) described a very small increase (statistically significant in two out of four samples) in sister chromatid exchange in human lymphocytes exposed to 935.2 MHz at a SAR of 0.3 to 0.4 W kg^{-1}. Khalil et al. (1993) observed a clear increase in sister chromatid exchange in isolated human lymphocytes after exposure to 167 MHz at 55 W m^{-2}. This study was described as preliminary, and may have been compromised by the fact that the control cultures were kept in the stable environment of an incubator while the experimental samples were brought out for exposure (W. Stewart, 2000).

TABLE 7.8 Summary of Cellular Studies

Model	Exposure Conditions	Results	References
Human lymphocytes in hypothermic or midly hyperthermic conditions	2.45 GHz; up to 200 W kg^{-1}; 20 min	No effect on sister chromatid exchange	Lloyd et al. (1984; 1986)
Human lymphocytes and Chinese hamster ovary cells during MRI	100 MHz pulsed; 330 μsec pulses; 100 ppsec; static magnetic field of 2.35 Tesla	No effect on sister chromatid exchange	Wolff et al. (1985)
Chinese hamster ovary cells with or without chemical mutagen; mildly hyperthermic	2.45 GHz pulsed; 10-μsec pulses; 25×10^3 ppsec; 33.8 W kg^{-1}; 2 h	No effect of RF on SCE frequency; no effect on mutagen-induced SCE frequency	Ciaravino et al. (1991)
Human lymphocytes	167 MHz; 55 W $m^{-2;}$ up to 72 h	Increased frequency of SCE	Khalil et al. (1993)
Human lymphocytes maintained at 36.1°C	2.45 GHz; 75 W kg^{-1}; 30 or 120 min	No effect on sister chromatid exchange	Maes et al. (1993)
Human lymphocytes with or without chemical mutagen (Mitomycin C)	935.2 MHz CW; 0.3–0.4 W kg^{-1}; 2 h	Little or no effect of RF alone on SCE frequency; slight enhancement of effects of the mutagen	Maes et al. (1997)

Many studies have not detected obvious chromosomal aberrations in isolated animal cells after exposure to low-power RF radiation (see Alam et al., 1978; Lloyd et al., 1984, 1986; Wolff et al., 1985; Meltz et al., 1987, 1989, 1990). However, a similar number of studies have reported increased chromosomal aberration (Yao and Jiles, 1970; Chen et al., 1974; Yao, 1976, 1982; Garaj-Vrhovac et al., 1990a, 1991, 1992; Khalil et al., 1993; Maes et al., 1993, 1995). In those studies with positive results in which the stimulus intensity was properly documented, it was generally rather high and therefore thermal effects cannot be ruled out (W. Stewart, 2000).

Standards and Guidelines

The purpose of this section is to review the current standards for exposure to electric and magnetic fields as set by various international groups as well as U.S. entities.

Table 7.9 originates from the Institute of Electrical and Electronics Engineers, Inc. The IEEE-SA Standards Board approved the C95.6 standard in September of 2002.

The C95.6 standard falls within the category of short-term effects such as an electric shock. Exposure limits defined in the C95.6 standard are not based on low-level time-varying electromagnetic fields for long-term exposure such as those near a transmission power line.

The table from the IEEE C95.6 standard lists the maximum electric field in terms of the undisturbed (absent a person) environmental field, *E*. It is assumed that the undisturbed field is constant in magnitude, direction, and relative phase over a spatial extent that would fit the human body.

The IEEE set a standard for short-term effects because "... there is not sufficient, reliable evidence to conclude that long-term exposure to electric and magnetic fields at levels found in communities or occupational environments are adverse to human health or cause a disease, including cancer. In addition, there is no confirmed mechanism that would provide a firm basis to predict adverse effects from low-level, long-term exposure" (C.95.6 IEEE, 2002).

Presently, there are no national standards in the United States for exposure to 60-Hz electric or magnetic fields. Other countries in the international community and certain states in the U.S. have set exposure standards for this type of low-level time-varying EMF. The states that have set standards did so during regulatory proceedings for proposed transmission lines.

Exposure standards do not provide a line in the sand delineation, above which adverse health effects occur and below which no adverse health effects occur. What exposure standards attempt to provide, is an overall guide for the average population, a level at which adverse effects are not expected according to the present scientific data.

Exposure standards are set using the best available scientific data showing the threshold at which adverse health effects are first observed. Different groups have different philosophies with respect to how standards

TABLE 7.9 IEEE C95.6 Environmental Electric Field Maximum Permissible Exposures (MPEs), Whole Body Exposure

General Public		Controlled Environment	
Frequency Range (Hz)	*E*–rms* (V/m)	Frequency Range (Hz)	*E* –rms* (V/m)
1–368[c]	5000[a,d]	1–272	20,000[b,e]

[a] Within power line rights-of-way, the MPE for the general public is 10 kV/m under normal load conditions.
[b] Painful discharges are readily encountered at 20 kV/m and possible at 5–10 kV/m without protective measures.
[c] Limits below 1 Hz are not less than those specified at 1 Hz.
[d] At 5 kV/m induced spark discharges will be painful to approximately 70% of adults (well-insulated individual touching ground).
[e] The limit of 20,000 V/m may be exceeded in the controlled environment when a worker is not within reach of a grounded conducting object. A specific limit is not provided in this standard.
*rms = root mean square.

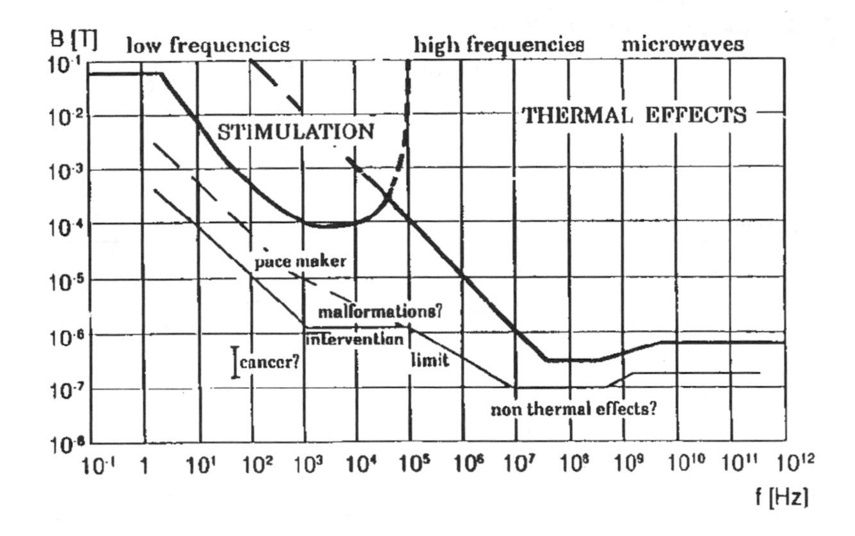

FIGURE 7.26 Thresholds of magnetic field effects. (*Source:* J. Bernhart.)

should be set by using differing interpretations of the levels at which biological changes are observed. In the United States, standards have typically been set by finding the level where clearly demonstrated and reproducible damage is known to first occur, and then multiplying by a safety factor. Typical safety factors are in the range of 10 to 50. Figure 7.26 and Figure 7.27 show levels at which effects are observed in electric and magnetic fields. Some groups include exposure data that indicate that biological changes may occur, but where clearly reproducible hazards have not been demonstrated. This often leads to significantly lower exposure limits. The Soviet Union had standards that were approximately 1000 times lower than the U.S. standards for radio frequency exposures and the enforcement of these standards was also very different. Therefore, it does not automatically follow that, above a given limit, exposure is harmful.

In 2001, an expert scientific working group of WHO's International Agency for Research on Cancer (IARC) reviewed studies related to the carcinogenicity of static and extremely low-frequency (ELF) electric and magnetic fields. Using the standard IARC classification that weighs human, animal, and laboratory evidence,

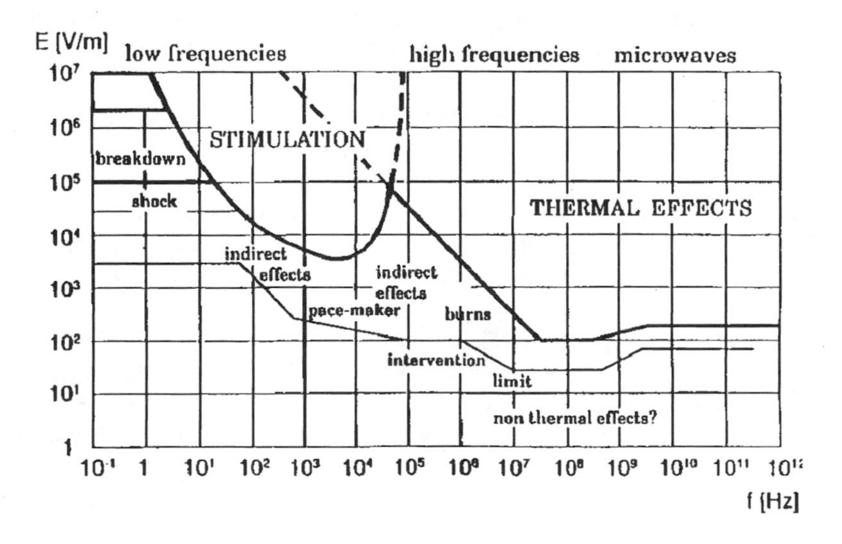

FIGURE 7.27 Thresholds of electrical field effects. (*Source:* J. Bernhart.)

TABLE 7.10 Summary of the ICNIRP Exposure Guidelines for European Power

	European Power Frequency	
Frequency	50 Hz	50 Hz
	Electric field (V m^{-1})	Magnetic field (μT)
Public exposure limits	5,000	100
Occupational exposure limits	10,000	500

Source: World Health Organization, 2003.

ELF magnetic fields were classified as *possibly carcinogenic to humans* based on epidemiological studies of childhood leukemia (WHO, 2002). An example of a well-known agent classified in the same category is coffee, which may increase risk of kidney cancer, while at the same time be protective against bowel cancer. "Possibly carcinogenic to humans" is a classification used to denote an agent for which there is limited evidence of carcinogenicity in humans and less than sufficient evidence for carcinogenicity in experimental animals. While the classification of ELF magnetic fields as possible carcinogenic to humans has been made by the IARC, it remains possible that there are other explanations for the observed association between exposure to ELF magnetic fields and childhood leukemia (WHO, 2002).

Table 7.10 is exposure standards from the International Commission on Non-Ionizing Radiation Protection (ICNIRP) and it pertains to European power at 50 Hz.

Many countries in the international community set their own national standards for exposure to electromagnetic fields. However, the majority of these national standards draw on guidelines set by ICNIRP. This non-governmental entity, formally recognized by the World Health Organization (WHO), evaluates scientific results from all over the world. Based on an in-depth review of the literature, ICNIRP produces guidelines recommending limits on exposure. These guidelines were last updated in April 1998 (WHO, 2002).

Not all standards and guidelines throughout the world have recommended the same limits for exposure to cell phones and base stations. For example, some published exposure limits in Russia and some eastern European countries have been generally more restrictive than existing or proposed recommendations for exposure developed in North America and other parts of Europe (Cleveland, Jr. et al., 1995).

The exposure limits adopted by the Federal Communications Commission (FCC) in 1996, based on the ANSI/IEEE and NCRP guidelines, are expressed in terms of electric and magnetic field strength and power density for transmitters operating at frequencies from 300 kHz to 100 GHz are shown in Table 7.11.

The FCC also adopted limits for localized ("partial body") absorption in terms of specific absorption rate (SAR), shown in Table 7.12, that apply to certain portable transmitting devices such as hand-held cellular telephones (Cleveland et al., 1995).

In 1998 the ICNIRP published its own guidelines covering exposure to RF radiation. These were based on essentially the same evidence as that used by the National Radiation Protection Board (NRPB), and for workers the limits of exposure are similar. However, under the ICNIRP guidelines, the maximum levels of exposure of the public are about five times less than those recommended for workers. The reason for this approach was the possibility that some members of the general public might be particularly sensitive to RF radiation. However, no detailed scientific evidence to justify the additional safety factor was provided (Stewart report).

The ICNIRP guidelines for the public have been incorporated in a European Council Recommendation (1999), which has been agreed to in principle by all countries in the European Union, including the U.K. In Germany, the ICNIRP guidelines have been incorporated into a statute (Stewart report).

The ICNIRP guidelines are presented with *reference levels* and these reflect the factor of five differences between the public and occupational basic restrictions. The ICNIRP public reference levels for the frequencies used by mobile phones are shown in Table 7.14. Reference levels for mobile communications in the frequency range 800 to 1000 MHz are from 4 to 5 W m^{-2} and for 1800 to 1900 MHz from 9 to 9.5 W m^{-2} (ICNIRP, 1998a).

TABLE 7.11. FCC Limits for Maximum Permissible Exposure (MPE)

Frequency Range (MHz)	Electric Field Strength (H) (V/m)	Magnetic Field Strength (H) (A/m)	Power Density (S) (mW/cm^2)	Averaging Time $\|H\|^2 \cdot \|H\|^2$ or S (min)
	(A) Limits for Occupational/Controlled Exposure			
0.3–3.0	614	1.63	(100)*	6
3.0–30	$1842/f$	$4.89/f$	$(900/f^2)$*	6
30–300	61.4	0.163	1	6
300–1500			$F/300$	6
1500–100,000			5	6
	(B) Limits for General Population/Uncontrolled			
0.3–1.34	614	1.63	(100)*	30
1.34–30	$824/f$	$2.19/f$	$(180/f^2)$*	30
30–300	27.5	0.073	0.2	30
300–1500			$f/1500$	30
1500–100.000			1	30
f = frequency in MHz				

Source: OET Bulletin 56, 4th ed., 08/1999, FCC.
*Plane-wave equivalent power density.

TABLE 7.12 FCC Limits for Localized (Partial-Body) Exposure Specific Absorption Rate (SAR)

Occupational/Controlled Exposure (100 kHz to 6 GHz)	General Uncontrolled/Exposure (100 kHz to 6 GHz)
$<$0.4 W kg^{-1} whole-body	$<$0.08 W kg^{-1} whole-body
$\leq$0.08 W kg^{-1} partial-body	$\leq$1.6 W kg^{-1} partial-body

Source: OET Bulletin 56, 4th ed., 08/1999, FCC.

TABLE 7.13. ICNIRP Basic Restrictions on Occupational Exposure and General Public Exposure (in parentheses) in the Frequency Range 10 MHz to 10 GHz

Tissue Region	SAR Limit (W kg^{-1})	Mass (g)	Time (min)
Whole body	0.4 (0.08)	—	6
Head, trunk	10 (2)	10	6
Limbs	20 (4)	10	6

Source: ICNIRP, 1998.

TABLE 7.14 ICNIRP Reference Levels for Public Exposure at Mobile Telecommunications Frequencies

Frequency (MHz)	Electric Field Strength (V/M)	Magnetic Field Strength (A m^{-1})	Power Density (W m^{-2})
400–2000	$1.375f^{1/2}$	$0.0037f^{1/2}$	f/200
2000–3000	61	0.16	10

f is the frequency in MHz.
Source: ICNIRP, 1998.

Risk

There is growing movement throughout the world to adopt precautionary approaches for management of health risks in the face of scientific uncertainty and the assessment of potential health risks from EMF includes numerous uncertainties. "The Precautionary Principle is a risk management policy applied in circumstances with a high degree of scientific uncertainty, reflecting the need to take action for a potentially serious risk without awaiting the results of scientific research."[1]

On February 2, 2000, the European Commission approved guidelines for the application of the Precautionary Principle and these guidelines should be:

- Tailored to the chosen level of protection
- Nondiscriminatory in their application, i.e., they should treat comparable situations in a similar way
- Consistent with similar measures already taken, i.e., they should be comparable in scope and nature to measures already taken in equivalent areas in which all scientific data are available
- Based on an examination of the potential benefits and costs of action or lack of action (including, where appropriate and feasible, an economic cost/benefit analysis)
- Provisional in nature, i.e. subject to review in the light of new scientific data
- Capable of assigning responsibility for producing the scientific evidence necessary for a more comprehensive risk assessment[1]

"People are disturbed, not by things, but by their view of them."

—Epictetus

In trying to understand people's perception of risk, it is important to distinguish between a health hazard and a health risk. A *hazard* can be an object or a set of circumstances that could potentially harm a person's health. Risk is the likelihood, or probability, that a person will be harmed by a particular hazard. Driving a car is a potential *health hazard*. Driving a car fast presents a *risk*. The higher the speed, the more risk is associated with the driving (WHO, 2002).

The *nature of the risk* can lead to different perceptions. The more factors that are added to the public's perception of risk, the greater the potential for concern. The following pairs of characteristics of a situation generally affect risk perception:

- Familiar vs. Unfamiliar Technology

  Familiarity with a given technology or a situation helps reduce the level of the perceived risk. The perceived risk increases when the technology or situation, such as EMF, is new, unfamiliar, or hard-to-comprehend (WHO, 2002).

- Personal Control vs. Lack of Control over a Situation

  If people do not have any say about installation of power lines and mobile telephone base stations, especially near their homes, schools, or play areas, they tend to perceive the risk from such EMF facilities as being high (WHO, 2002).

- Voluntary vs. Involuntary Exposure

  People feel much less at risk when the choice is theirs. Those who do not use mobile telephones may perceive the risk as *high* from the low RF fields emitted from mobile telephone base stations. However, mobile telephone users generally perceived the risk as *low* from the much more intense RF fields of their voluntarily chosen handsets (WHO, 2002).

- Dreaded vs. Not Dreaded Outcome

  Some diseases and health conditions, such as cancer, or severe and lingering pain, are more feared than others. Thus, even a small possibility of cancer, especially in children, from a potential hazard such as EMF exposure receives significant public attention (WHO, 2002).

[1]Electromagnetic Fields and Public Health Cautionary Policies, 2000.

- Direct vs. Indirect Benefits

  If people are exposed to electric and magnetic fields from a high-voltage transmission line that does not provide power to their community, they may not perceive any direct benefit from the installation and are less likely to accept the associated risk (WHO, 2002).

- Fair vs. Unfair Exposure

  Issues of social justice may be raised because of unfair EMF exposure. If facilities were installed in poor neighborhoods for economic reasons (e.g., cheaper land), the local community would perceive the potential risks as being an unfair burden (WHO, 2002).

The risk of developing cancer or being in an automobile accident is described in several ways, the most common being lifetime risk and relative risk. Lifetime risk is the probability that an individual will develop cancer or be involved in an auto accident sometime between birth and death. For example, the lifetime risk of breast cancer in American women is now one in eight (i.e., one woman in eight can expect to develop breast cancer sometime in her life). This may seem like a frightening number but it is also misleading because the risks are really very different for different age groups, particularly for pre- and postmenopausal women. The lifetime risk for death from an automobile accident is 1 in 70.

The risk of developing a cancer is usually described in terms of relative risk. Relative risk is calculated by dividing the incidence rate of disease in a group exposed to a suspected carcinogen or risk factor by the incidence of disease in a non-exposed group. The relative risk for average smokers developing lung cancer is 9.9. This means that smokers are about ten times more likely to develop lung cancer relative to nonsmokers (Risk and Cancer, 2003). A relative risk of 1.0 indicates a risk no greater than that of the comparison group used in a study. A relative risk of less than 1.0 indicates lower risk, or a protective effect. Many relative risks are in the range of 1.3 or 1.5, meaning that the exposed person has a 30% or 50% greater chance of developing the disease than an unexposed person (Risk and Cancer, 2003). The following table shows some relative risk factors for various cancers.

Monson (1980) characterized the significance of relative risk levels as follows:

Relative Risk	Strength of Association
1.0–1.2	None
1.2–1.5	Weak
1.5–3.0	Moderatc
3.0–10.0	Strong
Above 10.0	Infinite

It has been suggested by epidemiologists that cause-and-effect associations are only clearly established when relative risks are large (i.e., five or more) and when data from epidemiological studies are consistent.

Risk of developing cancer from exposure to a carcinogen is also evaluated by excess lifetime cancer risk. The EPA uses this terminology in regulating some chemicals, and remediating Superfund sites. The EPA uses a

TABLE 7.15 Relative Risk Factors for Disease Factors

Factor (Cancer Type)	Relative Risk	References
Smoking (lung cancer)	10–40	Wynder and Hoffman (1982)
Benzene, occupational exposure (leukemia)	1.5–20	Sandler and Collman (1987)
Asbestos, occupational exposure (lung cancer)	2–6	Fraumeni and Blot (1982)
Prenatal x-ray exams (childhood cancer)	2.4	Harvey et al. (1985)
Hair dye (leukemia)	1.8	Cantor et al. (1988)
Powerlines (childhood cancer)	1.5–3	Wertheimer and Leeper (1979), Savitz et al. (1988)
Saccharin (bladder cancer)	1.5–2.6	IARC (1987)
Excessive alcohol (oral cancer)	1.4–2.3	Tuyns (1982)
Coffee (bladder cancer)	1.3–2.6	Morrison and Cole (1982)

Source: J. Lee, Bonneville Power Administration.

target level of one in a million (10^{-6}) excess lifetime cancer risk from long-term exposure. This is the probability that at a specific exposure level in a population, one extra person out of a million will develop cancer in their lifetime. This is considered a *de minimus* risk because it is many times below other risks which people face every day, and pales in comparison to the about one in four chance that an American has of developing cancer in their lifetime.

Reducing the perceived risk involves countering the factors associated with personal risk. Members of communities feel they have a right to know what is proposed and planned with respect to the construction of EMF sources that, in their opinion, might affect their health. They need to have some control and be part of the decision-making process. New EMF technologies will be mistrusted and feared unless an effective system of public information and communication among stakeholders is established.

Conclusion

The purpose of this section was to provide the electrical professional with information on the biological effects of electric and magnetic fields. Effects from electric shock are the best understood and a cause-and-effect relationship is known. Burns from electric shock are different from other kinds of burns and the destruction is most venerable to muscle and nerve tissue. The biological effects of EMF from power lines, cell phones, and base stations are more problematic as a cause–effect relationship has not been proven. These issues are also very controversial and the data on health effects from power lines, cell phones, and base stations continues to be inconclusive. Guidelines and standards differ vastly due to differing philosophies with respect to the incomplete understanding of the thresholds and mechanisms of the biological effect of EMFs. Finally, the controversy surrounding health effects from power lines, cell phones, and base stations is due to the perception of risk and the more factors that are added to the public's perception of risk, the greater the potential for concern.

Reference

L.E. Anderson and L.B. Sasser, "Electromagnetic fields and cancer: laboratory studies," *Electromagnetic Fields Biological Interactions and Mechanisms: Advances in Chemistry Series 250*, Washington, DC: American Chemical Society, pp. 225–234, 1995.

Bernhart, J., personal communication.

Jefferson Lab, "Biological Effects of Electric Shock," 2003, *Jefferson Lab EH&S*, 2004, <http://www.jlab.org/ehs/manual/EHSbook-404.html>.

M. Blank and R. Goodman, "Electromagnetic fields may act directly on DNA," *J. Cell Biochem.*, 75, 369–374, Dec. 1999.

M. Blank, and L. Soo, "Enhancement of cytochrome oxidase activity in 60 Hz magnetic fields," *Bioelectrochem. Bioenerg.*, 253–259, 1998.

J.L. Buthod, W. Engdahl, J.R. Gauger, and W.R. Adey, "Influence of 60 Hz magnetic fields and 12-0-tet radecanoylphorbol-13-acetate on expression of c-myc in HL-60 cells, Abstract P-209A," presented at the 18th Annual Meeting of the Bioelectromagnetics Society, Victoria, BC, Canada, 1996, p. 179.

"C95.6, IEEE standard for safety levels with respect to human exposure to electromagnetic fields, 0–3 kHz," *IEEE Stand. Coordinating Comm., 28*, 2002 (approved September 12).

Cleveland, Jr., Robert F., and Jerry L. Ulcek. "Questions and answers about biological effects and potential hazards of radiofrequency electromagnetic fields," *OET Bulletin 56. Fed. Commun. Comm.*, 1999, pp. 1–36.

R. Cleveland, D.M. Sylvar, J.L. Ulcck, and E.D. Mantiply, "Measurement of radiofrequency fields and potential exposure from land-mobile paging and cellular radio base station antennae. Abstracts," 17th Annual Meeting of the Bioelectromagnetics Society, Boston, MA, 1995, p. 188.

Draft National Research Council Report on PAVE PAWS Radar, 1/13/05.

"Electric Shock Precautions," 2004, <http://pchem.scs.uiuc.edu/pchemlab/eletric.htm.

"Electromagnetic Fields and Public Health Cautionary Policies," March 2000, WHO Backgrounder, World Health Organization, <http://www.who.int/docstore/peh-emf/publications/facts_press/EMF-Precaution.htm>, 2004.

"Electromagnetic Fields and Public Health, Mobile Telephone and Their Base Stations, Fact Sheet N193," June 2000, http://www.who.int/docstore/peh-emf/publications/facts-press/efact/World Health Organization, 2004

EMF RAPID, "EMF electric and magnetic fields associated with the use of electric power: questions and answers," prepared by the National Institute of Environmental Health Sciences, National Institutes of Health, sponsored by the NIEHS/DOE EMF RAPID Program, 1995.

WHO, "Establishing a dialogue on risks from electromagnetic fields," *Radiation and Environmental Health*, Geneva, Switzerland: Department of Protection of the Human Environment, World Health Organization, 2002.

M. Feychting and A. Ahlbom, "Childhood leukemia and residential exposure to weak extremely low frequency magnetic fields," *Environ. Health Perspect.*, Suppl. 2, 59–62, March 1995.

J.P. Fulton, S. Cobb, L. Preble, L. Leone, and E. Forman, "Electrical wiring configuration and childhood leukemia in Rhode Island," *Am. J. Epidemiol.*, 111, 292–296, March 1980.

R. Goodman, H. Lin, M. Jin, and M. Blank, "The cellular stress response is induced by electromagnetic fields. Abstract A-4-1," presented at the 18th Annual Meeting of the Bioelectromagnetics Society, Victoria, BC, Canada, p. 13.

S.W. Hui, G.P. Jahreis, Y.L. Zhao, and P.G. Johnson, "Effect of 60 Hz magnetic field on proto-oncogene transcription. Abstract P-213A," Presented at the 18th Annual Meeting of the Bioelectromagnetics Society, Victoria, BC, Canada, 1996.

ICNIRP, "Guidelines for limiting exposure to time-varying electric, magnetic and electromagnetic fields (up to 300 GHz)," *Health Phys.*, vol. 74, no. 4, pp. 494–522, April 1998.

T.L. Jones, "Magnetic fields and cancer (correspondence)," *Environ. Health Perspect.*, vol. 101, no. 5, pp. 368–369, 1993.

T.L. Jones, C.H. Shih, D.H. Thurston, B.J. Ware, and P. Cole, "Selection bias from differential residential mobility as an explanation for associations of wire codes with childhood cancer," *J. Clin. Epidemiol.*, 46, 546–548, 1993.

T.L. Jones, C.H. Shih, D.H. Thurston, B.J. Ware, and P. Cole, "Response to: bias in studies of electromagnetic fields (letter to the editor)," *J. Clin. Epidemiol*, vol. 47, p. 1083, 1994.

B. Junkersdorf, H. Bauer, and H.O. Gutzeit, "Electromagnetic fields enhance the stress response at elevated temperatures in the nematode *Caenorhabditis elegans*," *Bioelectromagnetics*, vol. 21, pp. 100–106, 2000.

J. Lee, K. Semple Pierce, C. Spiering, R.D. Stearns, and G. VanGinhoven, *Electrical and Biological Effects of Transmission Lines: A Review*, Portland, Oregon: Bonneville Power Administration, December 1996.

R.C. Lee, "Physical mechanisms of tissue injury in electrical trauma," *IEEE Trans. Educ.*, vol. 34, pp. 223–230, 1991.

H. Lin, M. Opler, M. Head, M. Blank, and R. Goodman, "Electromagnetic field exposure induces rapid transitory heat shock factor activation in human cells," *J. Cell Biochem.*, 66, 482–488, 1997.

M. Linet, E. Hatch, R. Kleinerman, L. Robison, W. Kaune, D. Friedman, R. Severson, C. Haines, C. Hartsock, S. Niwa, S. Wacholder, and R. Tarone, "Residential exposure to magnetic fields and acute lymphoblastic leukemia in children," *New Engl. J. Med.*, July, 1–7, 1997.

W. Löscher and M. Mevissen, "Animal studies on the role of 50/60-Hertz magnetic fields in carcinogenesis," *Life Sci.*, vol. 54, pp. 1531–1543, 1994.

M.O. Mattson, K.H. Mild, and U. Valtersson, "Are there transcriptional effects in Jurkat cells exposed to a 50-Hz magnetic field? Abstract P-81A," 18th Annual Meeting of the Bioelectromagnetics Society, Victoria, BC, Canada, 1996, p. 127.

M. Mevissen, M. Haussler, M. Szamel, A. Emmendorffer, S. Thun-Battersby, and W. Löscher, "Complex effects of long-term 50 Hz magnetic field exposure *in vivo* on immune functions in female Sprague-Dawley rats depend on duration of exposure," *Bioelectromagnetics*, vol. 19, pp. 259–270, 1998.

M. Mevissen, W. Löscher, and M. Szamel, "Exposure of DMBA-treated Female Rats in a 50-Hz 50 μT magnetic field: effects on mammary tumor growth, melatonin levels, and T lymphocyte activation," *Carcinogenesis*, vol. 17, no. 5, pp. 903–910, 1994.

T. Miyakawa, S. Yamada, S. Harada, T. Ishimori, H. Yamanoto, and R. Hosono, "Exposure of caenorhabditis elegans to extremely low frequency high magnetic fields induces stress responses," *Bioelectromagnetics*, vol. 22, pp. 333–339, 2001.

R.R. Monson, *Occupational Epidemiology*, 2nd ed., Boca Raton, FL: CRC Press, 1990, p. 94.

K.K. Murthy, W.R. Rogers, and H.D. Smith, "Initial studies on the effects of combined 60 Hz electric and magnetic field exposure on the immune system of nonhuman primates," *Bioelectromagnetics*, Suppl. 3, 93–102, 1995.

National Research Council, "An Assessment of Potential Health Effects from Exposure to PAVE Paws Low-Level Phased-Array Radiofrequency Energy," National Research Council Report, January 2005.

C.R. Nave and B.C. Nave, *Physics for the Health Sciences*, 3rd ed., Philadelphia, PA: W.B. Saunders, 1985.

D. Olden, "NIEHS report on health effects from exposure to power-line frequency electric and magnetic fields," National Institute of Environmental Health Sciences, National Institutes of Health, NIH Publication No. 99-4493.

ORAU Panel on Health Effects of Low-Frequency Electric and Magnetic Fields, "EMF and cancer (letter)," *Science*, 260, 13–16, 1993.

R.D. Owen, L.W. Cress, A.B. Desta, H.E. Sprehn, and D.P. Thomas, "ELF–EMF replication studies: gene expression and enzyme activity. Abstract P-229A," Presented at the 18th Annual Meeting of the Bioelectromagnetics Society, Victoria, BC, Canada, 1996, p. 189.

Bass Associates Inc., "The Physical Effects of Electricity," Electrocution Thresholds for Humans, February 2004, <http://www.bassengineering.com/E_Effect.htm>.

"Risk and Cancer," November 2003, <http://www.acs.ohio-state.edu/units/cancer/handbook/risk.pdf>.

L.E. Rogers, N.R. Warren, K.A. Hinds, R. E. Gano, R.E. Fitzner, and G.F. Piepel, "Environmental studies of a 1100-kV prototype transmission line: an annual report for the 1981 study period," Prepared by Battelle Pacific Northwest Laboratories for Bonneville Power Administration, 1982.

D.A. Savitz, H. Wachtel, F.A. Barnes, E.M. John, and J.G. Tvrdik. "Case-control study of childhood cancer and exposure to 60-Hz magnetic fields," *Am. J. Epidemiol.*, 128, 21–38, 1988.

D.A. Savitz and W.T. Kaune, "Childhood cancer in relation to a modified residential wire code," *Environ. Health Perspect.*, 101, 76–80, 1993.

D.A. Savitz and D.P. Loomis, "Magnetic field exposure in relation to leukemia and brain cancer mortality among electric utility workers," *Am. J. Epidemiol.*, 141, 123–134, 1995.

B. Shi, R.R. Isseroff, and R. Nuccitelli, "Twenty and 60 Hz 80 gauss electromagnetic fields do not enhance the rate of protein synthesis in human skin fibroblasts. Abstract P-227A," presented at the 18th Annual Meeting of the Bioelectromagnetics Society, 1996, p. 187.

W. Stewart, "Mobile Phones and Health," 11 May 2000, Independent Expert Group on Mobile Phones, 2004, <http://www.iegmp.org.uk/report/text.htm>.

R. Thompon, *Siting and Land Rights*, Minneapolis, MN: Xcel Energy Inc., 2003.

S.J. Thurston and J.D. Saffer, "Cellular effects of weak electromagnetic fields. Abstract P-215A," Presented at the 18th Annual Meeting of the Bioelectromagnetics Society, Victoria, BC, Canada, 1996, p. 182.

N. Wertheimer and E. Leeper, "Electrical wiring configuration and childhood cancer," *Am. J. Epidemiol.*, 109, 273–284, 1979.

N. Wertheimer and E. Leeper, "Re: electrical wiring configurations and childhood leukemia in Rhode Island," *Am. J. Epidemiol.*, 16, 461–462, 1980.

N. Wertheimer, D.A. Savitz, and E. Leeper, "Childhood cancer in relation to indicators of magnetic fields from ground current sources," *Bioelectromagnetics*, 16, 86–69, 1995.

World Health Organization, "What are Electromagnetic Fields?" 2003, http://www.who.int/peh-emf/about/WhatisEMF/en/print.html

CTIA, "WOW–COM World of Wireless Communications–CTIA," Cellular Telecommunications & Internet Associationm, January 2005, <www.wow-com.com>.

7.4 Embedded Signal Processing

David R. Martinez, Robert A. Bond, and M. Michael Vai

Introduction

The term *embedded signal processing* refers to the digital signal processing functionality that is part of a larger system. Embedded signal processing has been used in a broad range of applications, including consumer electronics, automotive, telecommunications, medical, and military. Among all these application domains, however, military systems continue to be one of the dominant users of high-performance embedded computing (HPEC). Although the technologies in military applications are drawn from commercial enablers, their usage is adapted to very demanding embedded systems.

The capabilities demanded by military systems differ from other industries in very distinct ways. One important difference is the often paramount requirement for small size, weight, and power (SWAP). Another important difference, which is shared by industrial and automotive control applications but is not always critical in other areas, is the need for hard real-time performance; this requirement emerges because the system must meet stringent system deadlines and cannot tolerate any failures in the middle of a military combat situation. A third distinction is a demand for low latencies to convert sensor data to information, to knowledge, and finally to understanding useful to the user. These capabilities are feasible only if the hardware can support them. In addition to demanding hardware capabilities, the software needed in these systems also becomes increasingly complex.

Throughout this section, the military sensor application of embedded signal processing is frequently drawn upon as a challenging example to illustrate the demands in computing, memory, and interconnects, as well as the requisite development techniques and standards. Therefore, let us begin by defining a representative military embedded signal processing system. Such a system will be part of a payload typically consisting of front-end sensing and other hardware (e.g., RF array, EO camera, receivers, sensor timing and control, etc.). The signal processing system starts at the output of the analog-to-digital converters (ADCs) and ends, for onboard computations in an unmanned vehicle or satellite application, at the input to a communication antenna connected to a wireless network.

In particular, our discussion focuses on a generic military embedded signal processing architecture representative of active electronically steered array (AESA)-based sensor systems, such as ground moving target indicator (GMTI) radar or synthetic aperture radar (SAR) (see section "Generic Embedded Signal Processing Architecture"). In the last ten years, there has been significant emphasis on advancing AESA sensor systems. Improvements in ADCs make it feasible and affordable to bring digital sampling closer to the antenna array, which simplifies the front-end analog electronics. Furthermore, recent advances in computing technologies make it affordable to exploit the flexibility of AESA antenna using very high performance embedded computers for signal and image processing.

These AESA systems will consist of hundreds to thousands of sensor channels, with data rates exceeding tens to hundreds of billion bytes per second (driven by the ADC sampling rates). The demands in computation will exceed tens of trillion of operations per second (TOPS). Even though there are special purpose processors with the ability to perform TOPS in computation, the large data rates demand that the computation be distributed across many parallel processors working on different portions of the incoming data. The challenge is to efficiently balance the input and output (I/O) with the holding memory (buffers to hold incoming data and intermediate data products) and the real-time computation. This balance must be accomplished with SWAP restricted to a size of a fraction of a cubic meter (or equivalently a few cubic feet[1]), power in the tens to hundreds of watts, and weight not exceeding tens of kilograms. These constraints can be seen to be quite severe when one considers that, for more challenging applications, the power efficiency needed approaches 100,000 million operations per second per watt (MOPS/W) and the required computing density is nearly 100,000

[1]This section uses a mix of metric and English units. All numbers expressed in ft^3 can be converted to m^3 by applying a 0.03 factor.

billion operations per second per cubic foot (GOPS/ft^3). Of course, the SWAP requirements vary depending on the specific applications. However, the most interesting and challenging applications are found with ground-based unmanned vehicles, airborne platforms, and space platforms.

The principal functions performed in the embedded systems consist of signal and image processing algorithms. These algorithms are primarily operating on the data to increase the signal-to-noise ratio (SNR) to permit the transformation of raw data into information useful to the user. The typical functions, described in more detail in the following subsection, represent operations such as digital filtering, fast Fourier transforms (FFT), matrix inversions, digital beamforming, target detections, and tracking. As the data are processed to improve the SNR, an important outcome is the reduction in data volume per unit time. This reduction allows inputs to be converted from hundreds of gigabytes per second at the output of the ADCs to a few megabytes per second, which is compatible with wireless data bandwidths necessary to transfer the processed data to the users for further processing off-board the embedded platforms.

The choice of implementation depends on the constraints imposed by the embedded platform. For example, space satellites are constrained to very low power and weight, as well as radiation tolerance. Increases in weight result in higher satellite payload launch costs. Unmanned air vehicles also demand very small SWAP. Therefore, there is no one best choice of computing technology. The options range from custom application-specific integrated circuits (ASICs) and field programmable gate arrays (FPGAs) to programmable digital signal processors (DSPs) and general-purpose processors (GPPs). ASICs and FPGAs offer higher levels of delivered performance at the expense of limited to no flexibility in programming. In contrast, DSPs and GPPs offer flexibility in software programming but typically deliver much lower performance relative to their peak throughput capabilities.

The next subsection addresses a generic architecture representing the typical processing functions demanding high performance embedded signal and image processing. This description will serve to better illustrate the embedded signal processing implementation options described in the later subsections. Later, several subsections present a detailed description of hardware and software technologies necessary to meet the demands of these embedded applications.

Generic Embedded Signal Processing Architecture

The most demanding computation on board an embedded platform happens soon after the received signals from the antenna are converted to digital streams, right after the ADCs. Figure 7.28 illustrates a generic processing architecture from the output of an assumed two-dimensional AESA antenna. The outputs of the antenna system must typically go through a front-end receiver to convert the carrier frequency signals into an intermediate frequency compatible with the ADC sampling rate. The example shown in Figure 7.28 is representative of future airborne and space-borne systems with the task of performing surface surveillance. However, the same generic processing flow is also applicable to many other applications of interest where signal and image processing must be performed to provide robustness against either intentional or

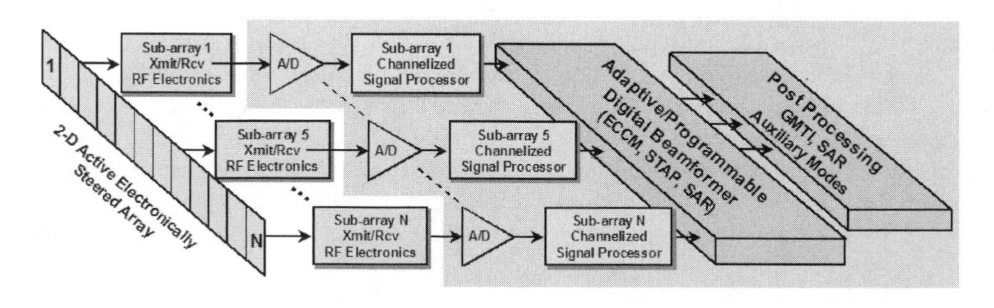

FIGURE 7.28 Generic embedded signal processing architecture.

unintentional interference, as well as the need to create images and pull signals of interest through post processing. So, here, this example is chosen as representative of demanding on-board embedded computing.

In order to quantify the signal processing drivers in I/O, memory, and computation, it is useful to work through a representative example. Since the signal of interest is buried in interference (e.g., jamming and clutter) the ADC must have sufficient number of bits to span the ratio of the largest interference levels to the intrinsic noise floor. Furthermore, the embedded system must maintain the signal bandwidth of interest. These two factors combined lead to ADCs sampling at approximately 1000 mega-samples per second and maintaining at least 8 bits in precision. Just a few tens of sensor channels combined with the ADC sampling leads to data rates after the ADC reaching tens of gigabytes per second. The processing following the ADC consists of digital filtering (data channelization to separate the signal into multiple subbands is an example of this type of processing), followed by adaptive digital beamforming and post processing. The adaptive digital beamforming serves to focus multiple sensor channels into a set of directed beams pointed in the direction of the signal (target) of interest while nulling interference. The post-processing allows the signal to be further extracted from the noise and to also form images (such as synthetic aperture radar images). Adaptive digital beamforming often involves matrix inversion and weight application (vector multiplications). Post-processing involves Doppler filtering (often implemented using FFTs) and cross-correlation, as well as threshold comparisons to isolate (detect) the target above the remaining background noise.

For the chosen tens of sensor channels, from the output of the ADCs to the output of the post-processing, the computation throughput often exceeds several trillions of operations per second. In embedded military applications, it is not only important to achieve the computation throughput but it is also important to process the incoming sensor signal channels with the lowest possible latency. The latency objective is one of the most demanding real-time constraints in order to achieve the expected mission goals. Embedded systems of interest require real-time performance with extremely low (tens of milliseconds) latency.

Since sensor data arrive in real-time in a continuous stream, memory buffers must be placed before and after every processing stage to provide holding areas for the data while waiting for the computation to complete. Aggregate memory existing in the embedded computing system is typically on the order of tens of gigabytes. Thus a typical processor to perform the functions illustrated in Figure 7.28 must achieve data rates of tens of gigabytes/sec, computation throughputs on the order of TOPS, and aggregate memory on the order of tens of gigabytes, while producing answers in tens of milliseconds. Since these computations are embedded in highly constrained platforms, these goals must be achieved within the available SWAP allotted for the platform payload. The combination of embedded computing characteristics together with constrained SWAP while keeping costs affordable makes this application quite different from what the commercial sector (for example, personal digital assistants, video game units, and cell phones) demands of today's processing systems.

There are several technologies available to build a system to meet the desired goals established earlier. The type of hardware will vary depending on the functions performed. The front-end processing, from the ADC through the digital filtering, requires very high computation throughput but can be accomplished with a limited amount of programmability. Most of the programmability (flexibility) comes from the need to download different filtering coefficients. However, the subsequent processing stages, adaptive digital beamforming and post-processing, require increasingly higher levels of programmability (more flexibility) in the algorithm implementation.

Figure 7.29 illustrates the embedded processing spectrum for different classes of embedded system applications and different digital computing technologies. The computing technologies range from programmable processors to full-custom VLSI multi-chip modules. The chart depicts different technologies and their respective delivered performance in GOPS/ft^3 versus MOPS/watt. The processing architecture shown in Figure 7.28 can be thought of consisting of front-end and back-end processing stages. The front-end signal processing can be performed using either ASICs or FPGAs to get the maximum throughput per unit power. For back-end processing the computing engines must be highly programmable, typically using commodity processors to allow for maximum flexibility. However, for some applications, for example for space-borne systems, the options are more limited. The requirements for the on-board signal processor are especially

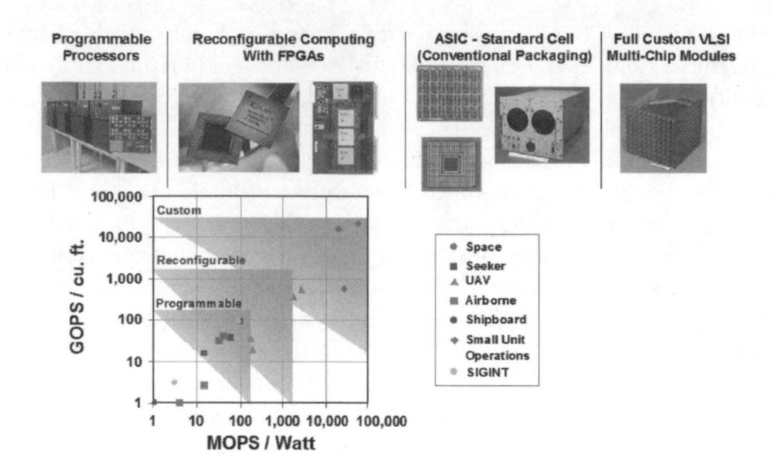

FIGURE 7.29 Embedded processing spectrum (applications vs. digital technology).

challenging because the processor must perform enough computation on the satellite to reduce the data throughput to a communication bandwidth compatible with the available data links. Today, that break point for a near-term space-borne radar payload occurs after adaptive digital beamforming and clutter suppression (space-time adaptive processing), which means that potentially several TOPS of computation must be performed on the satellite. The highly constrained payload in SWAP leads the designer to most likely choose a fully custom processor solution from the ADC through the on-board post processing.

It is useful to work through an example based on today's demonstrated computing capabilities. Table 7.16 below illustrates a hypothetical example of highly constrained embedded signal processing systems. They are both airborne systems to avoid issues beyond the scope of this discussion, such as radiation tolerance constraints. The first case is representative of an unmanned air vehicle. The second example is representative of a larger airborne platform. Both systems are assumed to be performing identical signal processing functions.

As mentioned earlier, full-custom ASICs offer the highest computation throughput at the lowest unit SWAP. FPGAs are another option but at about a factor of 30× less in throughput per watt compared to full-custom ASICs. DSP-based systems are about a factor of 100× to 400× worse than full-custom ASICs, depending on the levels of efficiency the programmers are able to achieve in the implementation of the algorithms. Figure 7.30 shows examples of demonstrated systems (ca. 2004) for three different classes of contemporary real-time signal processor technologies. The power consumption assumes that 50% is dedicated to peripherals, memory, and I/O. Another important observation is the fact that the throughput of the programmable DSP processor represents peak throughput and not delivered (sustained) throughput. The typical efficiency (after significant optimization) for these programmable processors is 25% of peak. Therefore, the more representative throughput is 0.125 GOPS/watt. This efficiency number is highly dependent on the algorithms and the complexity in the mapping of the algorithms over multiple processors.

For the different technologies shown in Figure 7.30 fixed to a common goal of 10 TOPS delivered performance, the total SWAP performance is shown in Table 7.17. The full-custom ASICs solution is able to meet the postulated airborne system goals in computation throughput and SWAP for both the small and large platforms. The FPGA solution meets the large platform goals. The programmable DSP processor does not meet any of the postulated goals. A system designer might consider using a small number of programmable

TABLE 7.16 Hypothetical System Goals for Two Classes of Systems

Example Platform	Computation Throughput (Peak TOPS)	Size (ft^3)	Weight (kg)	Power (W)
Small Airborne System	10	2	40	1000
Large Airborne System	10	10	200	5000

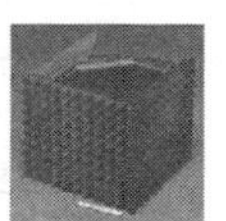
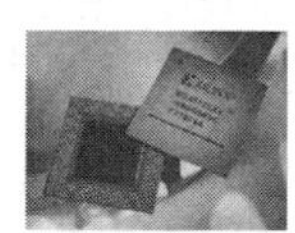
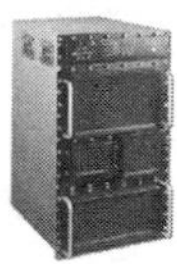

	Full Custom VLSI	Field Programmable Gate Array	Programmable DSP Processor
Throughput per chassis* (Total Power)	TERAOps (20 W)	1 TERAOps (700 W)	1 TERAOps (2 kW)
Computational density +	50 GOPS/W	1.5 GOPS/W	0.5 GOPS/W (Peak)
Processor type	Custom (1 GHz, 130 nm)	Virtex 8000 (400 MHz, 130 nm)	PowerPC 7447 (1 GHz, 130 nm)
Power per processor	2 Watts (100 GOPS/W)	20 Watts (3 GOPS/W)	8 Watts (1 GOPS/W peak)
Input control	Coefficients	Reconfigurable	Fully Programmable

* Power assumes 50% dedicated to peripherals, memory, and I/O
\+ Weights = Full Custom ~4 Kg; FPGAs ~25 Kg; Programmable System ~150 Kg

FIGURE 7.30 Real-time signal processor technologies (ca. 2004).

TABLE 7.17 Performance of Different Classes of Real-Time Signal Processor Systems (ca. 2004)

Example Platform	Computation Throughput (Peak TOPS)	Size (ft^3)	Weight (kg)	Power (W)	Performance
Full-custom ASICs	10	2	40	200	Meets small and large platform system goals
Field programmable gate array	10	20	250	7000	Meets large platform goals
Programmable DSP processor	10	100	1500	20,000	Does not meet goals for either platform

DSP computing engines to calculate, for example, the matrix inversion (typically less demanding in computation) but perform all the other functions (such as weight application) using ASICs or FPGAs, depending on the platform payload constraints. This approach offers computation throughput as well as programming flexibility.

The predictions are that the rate of advances in semiconductor feature size reductions will continue according to the 2003 report from the International Technology Roadmap for Semiconductors [1]. However, to get a 10× improvement in performance (according to Moore's law) will take 5 years at the current improvement rate of a 2× factor every 18 months. By looking at Table 7.17, it will take approximately 5 years before the programmable DSP system is able to meet the large platform system goals. This prediction assumes a continuing advancement in semiconductor performance, as experienced for the past several decades, and no de-rating in throughput due to inefficiencies in the algorithm performance relative to the peak throughput available in the system. Both of these assumptions are optimistic. In any case, these examples help to quantify the present system capabilities and the achievable performance. Assuming a more realistic de-rating by a factor of 4 (which reflects the typical 25% program execution efficiency) it would take 8 to 10 years before the programmable DSPs are able to meet the large platform SWAP goals. This generalization is not applicable to all cases, since there are cases where the system can be simplified to meet the available embedded signal processor performance by reducing the system capability. The embedded processors of tomorrow will run at 250 GHz and will contain 4.5 billion transistors by the year 2018 [1]. This transistor capacity will permit greater flexibility in system functionality. The bottleneck will be the communication of data into and out of the processors. In addition to the problems in memory access, the CPU will be unacceptably high in power consumption; and no end in sight is foreseen. The computing farm will likely be distributed across the platform and not localized at a single physical location, thereby permitting optimum use of the constrained space available.

The software complexity will significantly dominate the overall cost of the system. Today, one can purchase embedded system hardware for about $1/MFLOP (system based on PowerPC G4 CPUs and a significant amount of memory at each node). Therefore, a trillion operations per second embedded system can be procured for about $1M. However, the application software will consist of 200K to 1M software source lines of code (SLOC). Analysis of software development often equates 10 SLOCs to the cost of a single PC station; that is, 10 SLOCs cost about $500. Therefore, the cost of software development, for lines debugged and tested, can range from $10M to $40M (for 200K to 1M SLOCs, respectively)! It is important to clarify that these estimates are for a full software suite, including sensor timing, command, and control. For just signal processing, the software cost may be somewhat lower because of the more stream-like data flow dependency present in the algorithms.

The above costs only include the acquisition of the embedded system to the point where one is ready to integrate it with the remaining payload. Additional costs must be accounted for during the integration and testing of the embedded computing system with the sensor and overall payload package. These costs are directly dependent on the functionality expected of the platform system. Experience indicates that these costs can be a significant percentage of the total system cost. However, the integration and testing can be simplified if each respective part of the overall payload package is carefully tested independently, but verified end-to-end against a set of established "golden" test vectors and algorithms. These independent systems should also comply with open standards to allow easier hardware and software refresh as technology matures, and to allow for the reuse of hardware and software components. The following sections elaborate on implementation approaches and best practices to effectively develop high performance embedded signal processor systems.

Embedded Digital Signal Processor (DSP)

This subsection discusses the use of programmable processors in embedded digital signal processing. Today, programmable technologies find wide use in virtually every embedded signal and image processing domain. In the consumer electronics and telecommunications markets programmable implementations account for about 40% of the DSP market [2], and their market share is expected to grow. Programmable devices are employed in speech, video, multimedia applications, wired and wireless telecommunications, voice-over-IP and streaming video Internet, as well as short-range communications such as Bluetooth, EDCT, and DECT.[1] High-end consumer electronics such as HDTV and set-top boxes employ programmable DSPs. Programmable DSPs are used in multimedia applications that require support for multiple video compression techniques such as MPEG-2, MPEG-4, and H.264. The automotive industry now relies on programmable embedded computing for sensor processing and engine control. The medical industry employs programmable signal processing in sophisticated sensing and imaging applications such as MRI and ultrasound.

DSPs and GPPs have become widespread in modern military sensor signal processing applications such as sonar, radar, ladar, and passive optical sensors (cameras as well as optical and infrared CCD arrays). With the advent of the software radio, programmable processors are also becoming prevalent in military communications. They are found in virtually all military platforms of all sizes; submarines, ships, manned aircraft, UAVs (unmanned aerial vehicles), satellites, missiles, and torpedoes. They are used at practically all scales. A modern torpedo may use on the order of a dozen DSPs to perform its front-end active sonar signal processing. Modern radars and sonars often require programmable throughput in the range of 10 to 1000 billion FLOPS (GFLOPS) and employ tens to thousands of DSPs and GPPs.

Advantages of Programmable DSP

Programmable signal processing solutions have the principal advantages of increased flexibility and faster time-to-market. Changes in functionality can be rapidly accomplished through software changes.

[1]DECT is the Digital European Cordless Telephone reference design and EDCT is the U.S. Enhanced Digital Cordless Telephone reference design.

Design specification changes can be incorporated later in the development cycle and new applications can be implemented faster in software than with custom hardware designs. Thus, software implementations allow new capabilities to be specified later and to enter the marketplace sooner and thereby provide a competitive advantage. Moreover, software can more readily accommodate additional features, leading to product differentiation that can make the difference between success and failure in the highly competitive consumer marketplace. Finally, product fixes and upgrades can be made in the field, which allows for a cost-effective way to evolve product lines and serves to reduce development risks.

In the military domain, programmable solutions allow the military electronics industry to exploit advances in commercial-off-the-shelf (COTS) processor technologies. With moderate ruggedization, low-cost COTS processor chips, boards, and systems can be employed in many military sensor applications. This capability leads to reduced development and production costs and faster development time. It also avoids expensive, custom processor technology developments. However, the military use of COTS processors brings the need to deal with COTS technology refresh and obsolescence, as discussed later in section "Challenges of Programmable DSP".

Development and production costs figure prominently in the designer's choice between fixed function and programmable DSP approaches. Because of lower development costs programmable approaches are generally preferred for low production volumes, provided that SWAP constraints can be met. However, there are exceptions; for example, if the longest possible battery life is desired, low-power ASICs might be the best solution regardless of production volumes.

When larger production runs are involved, as in the case of consumer electronics products, the tradeoff can be complex. Both fixed-function and programmable technologies enjoy the Moore's law performance advancement trends of semiconductor process technology. However, the entry cost of chip fabrication has grown exponentially as feature sizes have continued to shrink. For example, as lithography sizes approach 90 nm, mask costs for ASICs are exceeding $1M per mask [2]. Thus, the unit production volume necessary to justify ASICs continues to grow exponentially as feature sizes shrink. However, popular commercial DSPs and GPPs are produced in large quantities (and used across multiple applications), so the up-front design and fabrication set-up costs are amortized across much larger unit volumes.

Challenges of Programmable DSP

Form-factor issues such as SWAP are the principal challenges facing programmable DSP implementations. In a custom, fixed-function hardware solution, the hardware performs the precise functionality required by the application. For a defined functional capability and a chosen technology, a fixed-function hardware design can be optimized to meet SWAP constraints. The designer is free to exploit the details of the computations to minimize resource utilization. However, programmable processors by their very nature are not as form-factor efficient as fixed-function hardware. Whether DSPs, GPPs, or media processors, the circuitry is less than 100% efficient on any specific algorithm, since the design is aimed at attaining generally high average efficiency over a larger set of applications. The key to effective use of programmable processors, therefore, is the efficient use of the hardware resources by the software program. Inefficient software implementations require more hardware resources to meet a given throughput and latency requirement. More hardware implies higher power consumption, heat generation, and cost, as well as larger size and greater weight. In form-factor constrained consumer applications, such as a handheld or mobile devices, inefficient software translates directly into reduced capability; either less functionality in the software, or shorter battery life, or larger size. In a military application, reduced capability may not be an option; demanding form-factor constraints consequently drive the design toward custom hardware solutions. This is especially the case in the front-end of a sensor system, where the signal processing tends to be better suited to custom hardware due to the simpler, more regular computations and the need for extremely high throughput.

Programmable processor technology improvements occur at a rapid pace. Within a specific processor family, new processors appear in the marketplace at 18-month to 2-year intervals. Once newer versions are available, production of the older versions is curtailed. Thus, applications and products using these earlier processors face the issue of hardware obsolescence. In military systems, the problem is exacerbated by the extremely long platform life cycles. It can take several years to design and develop a radar or sonar and once deployed these systems can remain in use for decades. Thus, several generations of COTS processor upgrades span the lifetime of these military systems. A strategy of lifetime buys of spare parts is occasionally employed, but at some point the growing requirements of the system outstrip the performance capabilities of the obsolete hardware, at which time a major hardware upgrade and a software re-implementation are needed. A better strategy is to build processor-independent software implementations at the outset that can be readily ported to new processors as they emerge in the marketplace. This permits a more regular, less disruptive COTS hardware refresh cycle. This approach is also attractive in the commercial domain. The ability to reuse intellectual property (IP) captured in software implementations allows developers to exploit new processor technologies for higher performance, which in turns allows new capabilities to be added to a product line. Being able to port the IP software to the new processor, rather than having to re-develop it, leads to faster time to market and reduced development costs. Thus, the key lifecycle challenge in embedded signal processing is to build portable, reusable software that is also highly efficient.

For large signal processing applications such as military radars or medical ultrasound products, the scale of the system is another key challenge. These systems often involve over 100,000 lines of highly optimized signal processing code. Not only must the software be designed for performance and portability, but it must also be designed to run on parallel processors consisting of tens or even thousands of processing units. Middleware, discussed below, is a key enabler of portability and scalability in high-end embedded signal processing systems.

Programmable DSP Hardware

Programmable DSPs emerged as a distinct class of processor in the late 1970s. They have evolved through several generations [3] and today range widely in both cost and performance. In general, programmable DSPs are designed to provide high throughput, low latency, power efficient programmable implementations of signal processing applications. To do this, they must address the key computational characteristics of typical signal processing algorithms. Signal processing computations are characterized by:

1. Continuous or long streams of digitized data samples that are acted on by signal processing functions. After a processing delay, the processed results are output continuously and concurrently with the input stream. This implies that a processor must have processing and I/O capabilities that are matched to the input data rates, the algorithm complexity, and the output data rates. Also, I/O and processing need to occur concurrently and continuously.
2. Multiplication, addition, and accumulation (summation) operations. Most basic signal processing functions, such as FIR, IIR, FFT, convolution, inner products, and others, are based on simple loops involving multiplies, adds, and accumulation of results. The FFT requires a butterfly operation, which consists of a special sequence of multiplies, sign changes, and additions.
3. Relatively simple and regular computation flow-of-control. Signal and image processing algorithms tend to proceed through a straightforward series of mathematical transformations. Looping is required to support vector and matrix mathematics, but complex program flows with irregular or global data memory accesses are rare.
4. Intrinsic data parallelism. Often, the same operation needs to be applied to different data, and dependencies from one sample, vector, or matrix to the next are weak. Thus, there are opportunities to apply operations in parallel across data sets.
5. Multidimensional datasets. For more complex applications, the data streams are often multidimensional. For example, in the AESA radar example discussed earlier, the data representing the returns from a transmitted waveform are digitized and input into the signal processor from each receiver channel (or, in some cases, from each analog beam of a sub-array). The waveform for each channel is divided into multiple pulse repetition intervals. Thus, each sample is multidimensional, representing the return for a particular pulse, channel, and range gate.

To handle signal processing efficiently, digital signal processors have the following features [3,4]:

1. High-speed data interfaces to handle input and output data streams. The interfaces are designed to minimize the need for main processor intervention and control. Typically, they have their own direct memory access (DMA) circuitry and interact with the main processor through low-overhead interrupts

and memory mapped control registers. Some DSPs, such as the SHARC ADSP21060, are designed to work in multi-processor configurations and have direct processor-to-processor communication ports.

2. Specially designed architectures referred to as Harvard[1] architectures. In Harvard architectures, separate buses are provided for data and instruction memory accesses. Usually, distinct data and instruction address spaces are provided, along with dedicated address generation hardware that can execute in parallel with the main processor unit. In a more conventional GPP architecture, the operands and the operation (program instruction) are accessed sequentially over a single bus, resulting in the need for multiple clock cycles per instruction. The main goal of the Harvard architecture is to remove this memory bottleneck. Data and instructions can be accessed concurrently, thereby permitting single-cycle instruction execution. Furthermore, through special auto-increment and address stride instructions, separate address generation hardware allows the next data to be accessed immediately after the current data are processed; the main unit does not need to pause to compute the new data locations.
3. Highly optimized, dedicated hardware for multiply-accumulate (MAC) operations. Additionally, some processors, such as the Analog Devices SHARC DSP, have specialized instructions and hardware for butterfly operations to support FFTs. Many DSPs also have parallel execution units, for example, dual MAC units as found in the Analog Devices TigerSHARC DSP.
4. On-chip instruction and data memories to allow complete datasets and programs to be "close" to the processing units. While general purpose microprocessors provide both data and instruction caches, the logic that controls cache contents is hardwired and designed for good average performance on general codes. DSPs provide programmable control over on-chip memories, so that programs can explicitly control the placement of highly optimized, repetitive inner loop codes, and the data that these code operate on, in the high speed, zero wait state on-chip memory.
5. Special data address increment and stride instructions as well as dedicated loop control hardware, to efficiently handle the short inner loops found in many signal processing kernels. Since DSP algorithms such as FIR, convolution, inner product, up and down sampling, etc., often involve short, computationally intensive inner loops, the loop control overhead must be kept to a minimum. In conventional processors, it often takes several instructions to implement a conditional loop or to calculate addresses for data striding. DSPs have dedicated hardware optimized to minimize this overhead.

Major DSP vendors include Lucent, Texas Instruments, Motorola, NEC, and Analog Devices. These vendors produce DSPs with most or all of the features described above. Sophisticated fourth-generation, high-end DSPs have recently entered the marketplace that provide additional enhancements and improved performance. For example, the VelociTI TMS320C62xx from Texas Instruments provides support for very-long-instruction-word (VLIW) processing. VLIW architectures achieve high performance through the parallel issuance and execution of multiple instructions [4]. Today, all major DSP vendors employ multiple-issue architectures for their highest performing DSPs. Although VLIW-based processors allow for very high performance, this benefit tends to come at the expense of lower code density (programs require more instruction memory) and higher power consumption.

DSP products either support just fixed-point or both fixed-point and floating-point arithmetic. Fixed-point processors provide the advantage that they can be very power efficient. However, fixed-point DSPs are more difficult to program than their floating-point counterparts. A typical fixed-point DSP has several different precision fixed-point representations: 8, 16, 32, and often 24 bits. The programmer must explicitly mix and match operations between these different precisions, and must handle arithmetic underflow, overflow, and finite-precision effects. In floating-point, there are typically single and double precision representations. Most applications can be implemented completely in single precision floating point, and checks for underflow and overflow are not required. A few modern applications, such as certain radar adaptive processing implementations, have such large dynamic ranges that double precision arithmetic is required. Nevertheless, underflow and overflow are generally not issues in floating-point arithmetic, whereas they are very relevant in fixed-point representations and require special programming considerations.

---

[1]Named for the work done at Harvard University in the 1940s under Howard Aiken.

DSPs, although they are designed explicitly for signal processing applications, are not the only technology choice for embedded programmable signal processing. GPPs, media processors, and application specific instruction-set processors (ASIPs) can also be used. GPPs are designed to provide high average efficiency for a wide class of applications and algorithms. To support general information processing algorithms, GPPs must accommodate complicated flows of control, arbitrary memory access patterns, and full-featured data manipulation capabilities. As such, their architectures are designed for this wider application space and are not optimized for signal processing.

Superscalar architectures are used in the more advanced processors. Superscalar processors analyze instruction dependencies dynamically to determine instruction-level parallelism. Then, they reorder instructions where legal to exploit maximum parallelism. Multiple execution units then process the reordered instructions in parallel. Although this results in significant performance enhancement compared to single-issue architectures (for a given instruction cycle time), the instruction reordering makes it difficult to predict execution time for code fragments. In fact, the same code can have a different latency depending on when it is executed; for example, the execution time for the first iteration through a loop can be different from subsequent iterations. This indeterminacy can make the use of these processors problematic for signal processing applications with extremely tight real-time budgets.

In recent generations, GPPs have begun to be enhanced with specialized instruction sets and supporting hardware for media processing applications. The Motorola PowerPC has been augmented with the AltiVec instruction set, a single-instruction-multiple-data (SIMD) instruction set that permits the execution of an instruction simultaneously on up to four samples. The design permits the simultaneous issue of up to two SIMD instructions, so that at peak rate eight floating point vector operations can be executed in parallel in a single clock cycle. Similarly, the MMX (multimedia extension) instruction set has been added to the Intel Pentium architecture to provide SIMD capabilities and performance. A comparison of FFT performance of these two GPPs and two modern DSPs is shown in Figure 7.31. Note that with these SIMD extensions, GPPs are still more power hungry than DSPs, but their power efficiency in terms of floating-point operations per second (FLOPS) per watt is competitive.

Multimedia processors, such as the Philips Nexperia PNX1300 and PNX1500 processors, are recent additions to the mix. They combine VLIW DSP and RISC (reduced instruction set computers) cores on a single chip. The Blackfin ADSP-BF5xx from Analog Devices provides a microcontroller embedded on the DSP chip [2]. This architecture is optimized for applications that require both signal processing as well as device control functions. Mobile communications products are a good example of the target marketplace for this type of processor. Multimedia applications have the general characteristics of the larger signal processing domain,

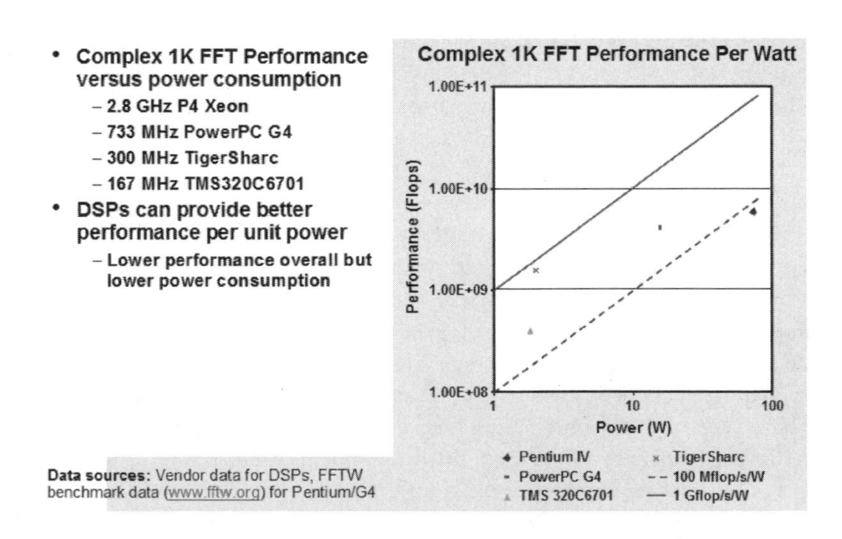

FIGURE 7.31 DSP and GPP FFT performance.

but they especially tend to involve repetitive, loosely coupled data parallel operations on data that can be represented with shorter word lengths. Many multimedia processors tend to have VLIW instruction set architectures. Newer architectures designed to exploit data parallelism and pipelining, for example, the Stanford Imagine processor, employ tiled chip architectures with multiple, interconnected processor units per chip,

Application-specific instruction set processors (ASIPs) fill the gap between commercial processors and fixed-function ASICs. Tensilica's Xtensa core is an example of a recent commercial ASIP core. Often, a company may elect to design in-house ASIPs for high production volume products to reduce production cost and power consumption. These processors can serve as the backbone for a product line. Developing efficient retargetable compiler technology for this class of processors is essential to provide C language programmability and code portability [5,6].

Larger signal processing applications, such as sonars and medical imaging systems, require multiprocessor implementations. Board-level vendors provide standard form-factor boards, for example boards conforming to the VME specification, with multiple DSPs or GPPs. A typical modern VME board is a very capable multiprocessor. It will have up to four DSPs or GPPs for a peak throughput of 4 to 16 GFLOPS, parallel and serial I/O ports, an Ethernet interface, 64 to 256 Mbytes of SDRAM as well as up to 32 Mbytes of L2 cache and flash memory. One of the principal limitations of these boards is the maximum amount of power that can be bused to a chassis slot on the backplane. For example, a standard 6U VME board is only rated for 55 W, but modern GPPs can consume 40 W or more. These boards are bundled with support software, including device drivers, signal processing libraries and real-time operating system options.

For even more demanding applications, such as AESA radars, parallel computers consisting of multiple multi-processor boards and high speed interconnection fabrics are required. Sky Computer and Mercury Computing Systems (MCS) are examples of leading manufacturers of these highly capable systems. Current embedded signal processors in this class are approaching 1 Tera-FLOPS peak throughput in a single, ruggedized chassis. The interconnect bandwidth afforded by a bus-based architecture is insufficient for the high-bandwidth, multi-channel signal applications targeted by these machines, so more advanced, crossbar-based interconnects are employed. Sky Computers employs the Infiniband switched fabric interconnect standard while Mercury uses the Parallel RapidIO switched fabric standard. The MCS PowerStream 7000, shown in Figure 7.32, is a representative state-of-the-art system in this class. It can be configured up to a peak throughput of nearly 1 TFLOPS. The architecture is based on the PowerPC 7447 GPP.

Bisection bandwidth, defined as the peak communication throughput (bytes/sec) across a bisection of the machine (half of the processors in each section), is an important figure of merit for these large multiprocessors. The PowerStream 7000, for example, has a 60 Gbytes/sec bisection bandwidth.

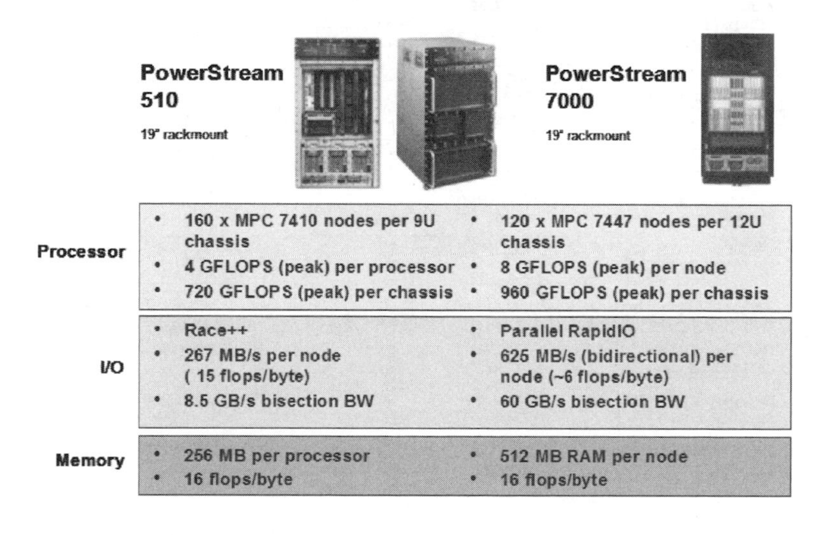

FIGURE 7.32 Two generations of MCS multicomputers.

Given the paramount importance of performance, it is not surprising that benchmarking is an important element in the embedded signal processor design process. Benchmarks can be carried out at several levels:

1. Compact applications: The most accurate benchmark is, of course, the application itself. This is usually impractical, though, since the application may not exist and the time and effort involved in coding the whole application may be prohibitive, especially if product deadlines are tight. Smaller codes, referred to as *compact applications*, are simplified facsimiles of an application or class of applications that can serve as surrogates for full applications. The key advantages of this approach are (a) complex interactions between computational stages can be captured in the compact application, thereby making performance results more accurate; and (b) a lower bound on code size can be established. For many embedded signal processing applications that must fit in memory constrained systems, code size is an important metric.
2. Application kernels: Quite often, an application is dominated by a few key computation kernels. For example, fast convolution, an important front-end signal processing task for many sensor applications, is dominated by the FFT (and IFFT). Therefore, programmable front-end signal processors require high throughput performance on FFTs. As discussed already, form factor issues often dictate technology choices in embedded applications. Consequently, computational power efficiency (throughput per unit power) is also a key metric. Figure 7.33 provides 1K complex FFT performance benchmarks executed in floating point arithmetic on modern DSPs and GPPs. The figure shows both effective throughput, in MFLOPS (million of floating point operations per second), and power efficiency in MFLOPS/watt.
3. Standard benchmark suites: In the signal processing domain, the BDTi benchmark suite serves the same role as SPECmarks do in the general purpose microprocessor domain. The BDTi benchmarks consist of a representative set of signal and image processing kernels, as shown in Figure 7.34. A composite figure of merit, called the BDTiMark, allows for a general, head-to-head, comparison of DSPs. Figure 7.34 also shows a recent BDTi benchmark result for a representative set of modern fixed-point DSPs. One of the unique aspects of the BDTi benchmarks is that they are developed and hand optimized for each benchmarked DSP by BDTi, as opposed to DSP vendors. This results in uniform, high quality implementations across all tested processors.

Blue denotes double precision

DEVICE	PEAK THROUGHPUT	% PEAK USED (1K CMPLX FFT)	TYPICAL POWER @ CORE VOLTAGE (DATE)	EFFICIENCY FOR COMPUTING FFT
Texas Memory Systems TM-44, 100 MHz	8.0 GFLOPS (32-bit)	80% (8 usec)	5.0W (11/01)	1280 MFLOPS/W
Analog Devices ADSP-TS201S Tiger SHARC, 500 MHz	3.0 GFLOPS (32-bit)	85% (20 usec, not verified)	2.4W @ 1.0V (9/03)	1070 MFLOPS/W
MIPS Technologies MIPS64 20Kc "Hard Core," 533 MHz, TSMC 0.13um	2.1 GFLOPS (64-bit)	50% (24 usec, est.)	1.4W @ 1.0V (11/01)	778 MFLOPS/W
Motorola PowerPC G4 MPC7457, 1 GHz, 0.13um	7.3 GFLOPS (32-bit)	64% (11 usec)	7.5W @ 1.0V (10/03)	623 MFLOPS/W
TI TMS320C6713, 225 MHz, 0.13um	1.35 GFLOPS (32-bit)	47% (80 usec)	1.2W @ 1.2V (6/02)	529 MFLOPS/W
PMC-Sierra MIPSIV RM9000x2, 1 GHz, 0.13um	4.0 GFLOPS (64-bit)	50% (26 usec, est.)	5.0W @ 1.2V (10/02)	400 MFLOPS/W
PMC-Sierra MIPSIV RM7000C, 600 MHz, 0.13um	1.6 GFLOPS (64-bit)	50% (64 usec, est.)	2.5W @ 1.3V (1/03)	320 MFLOPS/W
IBM PowerPC 750FX, 800 MHz, 0.13um	1.6 GFLOPS (32-bit)	58% (55 usec)	3.6W @ 1.4V (4/03)	260 MFLOPS/W
Honeywell RHPPC 603e, 133 MHz, 0.35um	200 MFLOPS (32-bit)	60% (431 usec)	2.6W @ 3.3V (11/01)	46 MFLOPS/W
BAE Systems RAD750, 133 MHz, 0.25um	266 MFLOPS (32-bit)	43-58% (448 usec SDRAM, 329 usec cache in future)	5.0W @ 2.5V (11/01)	23 (31) MFLOPS/W now (future)

FIGURE 7.33 Floating-point processor FFT performance (8 October 2003).

Manufacturer	Processor	Family Speed (MHz)	Architecture	MIPS	BDTImark2000
Texas Instruments	TMS320C1x	20	conventional	8.77	n/a
Hitachi	SH2-DSP	100	hybrid	100	280
Motorola	DSP563xx	150	hybrid	150	450
Analog Devices	ADSP-21xx	75	conventional	75	230
Texas Instruments	TMS320C54xx	160	enh. Conventional	160	500
Lucent Technologies	DSP16xx	170	enh. Conventional	170	810
LSI Logic	ZSP164xx	200	superscalar	400	n/a
Texas Instruments	TMS320C62xx	300	VLIW	2400	1920

Function	Description	BDTi Benchmark Suite	
Real Block	Finite impulse filter operating on real data.	Vector Add	Pointwise addition of two vectors resulting in third vector.
Complex Block FIR data.	FIR filter operating on complex	Vector Maximum	Locate the value of the maximum vector.
Real Single Sample FIR	FIR filter operating on single sample of real data.	Viterbi Decoding	Decode a block of convolutionally encoded bits.
LMS Adaptive Filter	Least mean square adaptive filter operating on single sample of real data.	256-Point-In-Place	Fast Fourier transform to convert time domain signal to frequency domain.
Two-Biquad IIR	Infinite impulse respone filter operating on single sample of real data.	Bit Unpack	Unpack variable length data from a bit stream.
Vector Dot Product	Sum of pointwise multiplication of two vectors.	Control	Sequence of control operations e.g. test, pop, push, branch and bit manipulation.

FIGURE 7.34 BDTi benchmarks for fixed-point DSPs.

Software: Run-time and Development Environment

DSPs are programmed almost exclusively in either C/C++ or assembly language. Assembly programming is still common practice in many commercial DSP applications for the simple reason that many such applications require maximum achievable performance. Hand-coded assembly programs that exploit processor-specific instruction sets are still capable of out-performing signal processing codes generated by the best C compilers. Typically, assembly codes will be 1.5 to 3 times faster than compiled C code, but can reach as much as 100 times faster [6]. Assembly code can also be made much more compact, which is an important goal in embedded applications with limited on-chip or secondary memory. On the negative side, assembly coding is labor intensive, requires programming expertise not readily available in the computer science mainstream, and tightly binds the implementation to the host DSP. Thus, performance is purchased at the cost of increased development time and lack of code portability. Upgrading an assembly-based application to a new processor requires a significant rewrite of the code. Also, since assembly coding is not a common expertise, it is often difficult to staff the development team.

The key benefits of C/C++ programming are greater programmer productivity, higher quality programs (fewer defects), the ability to develop very large applications, and code portability. C and C++ implementations dominate the large, high-end applications such as radars, sonars, and medical imaging systems. For these applications, which often exceed 100,000 SLOC, only higher level languages can handle the size and complexity of the programming task.

One approach to achieving the high performance of assembly code and the productivity of C/C++ programming is to embed (or "inline") into the C/C++ code assembly routines that provide highly optimized implementations of key DSP functions. Usually, the DSP manufacturer will provide a comprehensive library of such function calls. Often, the assembly routines are wrapped in C calls for programming convenience. Of course, the introduction of processor-specific assembly routines, whether wrapped in C code or not, reduces the portability of the implementation.

Ultimately, efficient compiler technology is the key challenge in the adoption of C/C++ for embedded signal processing. Compilers for embedded signal processors need to produce code that is both fast and compact. This is particularly difficult for DSP architectures, due to their shorter lifetimes relative to GPP architectures (such as the Pentium and PowerPC) and the numerous DSP architectural specializations. Efficient C compilers for DSP architectures is an active area of research, with recent work focused on the creation of retargetable compilers, that is, compilers capable of generating object and executable code for several different types of DSP [6]. Retargetable compilers rely on abstract representational languages to describe the target processor architectures. Using these representations, the compilers develop lower level optimizations tuned to specific processor architectures. These compilers enhance code portability and can be upgraded along with the evolving processor technology, thereby permitting very high performance compiler functionality to be developed and optimized incrementally over several processor generations.

Signal processing applications can also benefit from embedded, real-time operating systems (RTOS). Several operating system vendors, for example, Wind River, which offers VxWorks and VSPWorks, specialize in providing highly optimized RTOSs for DSPs and GPPs. The defining characteristic of a real-time OS is that it delivers deterministic or time-bounded performance. RTOSs need to provide a good balance between deterministic response, high speed, small footprint (code size), and useful feature sets. The capabilities offered by RTOSs include:

1. Multitasking and task scheduling: For smaller applications, the processor is dedicated to a single program and multitasking is not required. However, for applications that are multimodal or multipurpose, such as multifunction radar or multimedia applications, multitasking is often the preferred technical approach. This allows the designer to dedicate a separate task to each major system input and mode of operation. Background and periodic tasks can be interspersed with asynchronous, interrupt-driven tasks. The net result is a cleaner, more maintainable software architecture. In a real-time system, the important considerations are support for pre-emptive, priority-based scheduling, support for real-time scheduling approaches such as earliest-deadline-first (EDA), and fast, bounded, task context switch latency.
2. Interrupt services: Signals typically arrive from external sources over an input port that indicates data availability through an interrupt. Fast, deterministic interrupts servicing is an important characteristic of a real-time OS. The ability to disable other interrupt and tasks while an interrupt is being serviced is essential.
3. Timing services: In order to measure and optimize code performance, and to schedule periodic tasks, operating system time services are important.
4. Intertask communication, signaling, and synchronization: A signal processing application that requires multiple tasks will more than likely need to synchronize and communicate between tasks. A front end data conditioning task may operate at a faster rate than a down-stream task. The ability to communicate the data from one task to the next and signal the downstream task is needed. For example, in a radar application, the up-stream task of matched filtering and detection communicates target detection data to a downstream task that performs tracking. Although middleware libraries such as MPI are often used to perform data communications, especially for multiprocessor implementations, MPI relies on underlying OS support.
5. Device drivers: Embedded signal processors receive signals for processing from a variety of different devices and interfaces. Often, the device is custom-made for the application. An RTOS must provide a means for installing device drivers and accommodating custom device drivers.

Often, for small devices, the RTOS is left out altogether and the program executes "on the bare metal." There is, however, a general trend toward reliance on RTOSs as systems grow in complexity, memory becomes increasingly less expensive, and time-to-market becomes a primary driver. A principal advantage of an RTOS is that it can provide robust, commonly used, well-tested system-level functionality, thereby reducing the amount of code that needs to be developed and providing a degree of isolation between the application and underlying processor. In this way, an RTOS that is widely used provides a degree of portability across processor types.

Middleware is another important technology for providing code portability. Middleware is software that delivers high-performance functionality while isolating machine specific details into a lower level software layer. It provides a standard application programming interface (API) to the user application, so that the application can be ported with minimal changes to any processor platform that support the middleware. Computer vendors and third-party vendors can concentrate on providing implementations for several platforms, allowing an application programmer to program at a higher level of abstraction and in a machine-independent manner.

In a wider sense, the operating system can be thought of as middleware specifically designed to isolate computer operation details from the user program. Standard OS specifications such as POSIX and open software implementations such as Linux provide a uniform, standard API that promotes portability across processor families and generations. However, middleware is usually viewed as a software layer residing between the operating system and the application that provides a standard API for domain-specific functionality. The Vector, Signal, and Image Processing Library (VSIPL) [7] is an example of a C language middleware specification for military embedded signal processing. VSIPL has wide and growing support among embedded single board multiprocessor and large multicomputer vendors, and thereby provides signal processing portability across many COTS computer systems employed in military signal processing.

For high performance signal processing applications that require parallel processors, the data communication and reorganization between computation stages can be complex. To address this, many parallel applications use the Message Passing Interface (MPI) [8], a *de facto* messaging middleware standard developed for large-scale scientific computing. MPI is widely supported in the multiprocessor industry and provides a large set of primitives for both interprocessor point-to-point and collective communications. A later version, MPI2, provides enhanced features. MPI-real-time (MPI-RT) is a recent variant designed to support real-time quality-of-service. MPI-RT is not yet widely accepted; its API is quite different from MPI, since it employs early-binding of communication constructs to help ensure real-time performance. An open research issue in MPI for military and other high-reliability applications is fault-tolerant communications.

The Data Reorganization Interface (DRI) [9] has been developed for complex data reorganizations in parallel signal processor implementations. Typically, a multidimensional data set is organized in DSP memory so that the data for a chosen dimension reside in sequential locations. This permits highly efficient signal processing along that dimension. When the algorithm proceeds to the next dimension, the data (before any reorganization) are separated by a stride equal to the length of the first dimension. For DSPs that support strided accesses, such as the SHARC DSP, this is not a problem as long as the complete dataset can fit within local memory. Otherwise, the data must be reorganized to place the next dimension in sequential memory order. This reorganization is referred to as a corner turn. If the dataset is distributed across the processors in a parallel signal processor application, then the corner turn will involve a many-to-many interprocessor data movement. DRI provides a standard API for defining such data reorganizations on parallel architectures.

Often, a signal processing application such as a radar is embedded in a larger application, such as a military command and control or combat system. The overall application is often interconnected to the signal processor through a high-speed local area network. Communication of data, control, and status can be accomplished using various communication mechanisms: shared files, MPI, Unix-based sockets, and others. The Object Management Group's (OMG) Common Object Request Broker Architecture (CORBA) [10] standard provides applications with an open, vendor-independent specification for an architecture and infrastructure, so that services and client applications can work together over networks. A standard CORBA interface description language (IDL) allows applications (clients) and servers to describe their capabilities and needs to an object request broker (ORB). The ORB mediates service requests and responses in a manner that isolates the actual location of the service providers from the clients. This allows remapping of applications and provides portability in a distributed, networked architecture. Currently, the overhead of standard CORBA is not commensurate with high-performance real-time systems requirements, but real-time variants that avoid data copies are being developed to address the needs of the real-time community. A newer OMG standard, called the Data Distribution Standard (DDS), is being developed that is intended to address high throughput data communications for command and control applications. DDS is based on publish-subscribe semantics that facilitate data multicasting.

Programmable DSP Technology Trends

As compilers continue to improve, processors continue to increase in performance, and applications become more and more complex, assembly level programming is being phased out in favor of C programming. The role of assembly programming is becoming restricted to highly optimized library codes or applications that have extremely constrained code sizes. C programming, on the other hand, is giving way to C++ in high-end applications, where code complexity, programmer productivity, portability, and scalability are the driving concerns. VSIPL++, a C++ interface for the VSIPL standard library, has recently been specified and should emerge in products in the next few years. VSIPL++ uses advanced C++ expression template techniques to direct compiler optimizations of signal processing expressions [7].

Parallel DSP implementations, found in high end signal processing applications such as radar and sonar, must be able to scale up or down as the application functionality is increased or more capable processors become available. To deal with these high performance embedded applications, the military community has begun to adopt middleware technology that is both portable and scalable. Thus, a parallel processor variant of VSIPL++ is being developed to support high-end multiprocessor signal applications. Parallel VSIPL++ borrows and standardizes techniques from the scientific computing middleware POOMA [11] and the embedded processing middleware Parallel Vector Library [12].

Beyond the wider adoption of C and C++ and the emergence of middleware products, several other trends in software development tools and environments are evident. Graphical programming tools and products using the Unified Modeling Language (UML) for automatic code generation of object-oriented C++ programs have begun to be applied to embedded programming applications. Signal processing programs developed using the Mathworks MATLAB problem solving environment can now be translated to C/C++. Simulink, a graphical signal processing extension to MATLAB, can also generate C/C++ code. All of these developments are aimed at increasing programmer productivity. The major challenge these approaches face is the efficiency of the auto-generated C/C code.

In university research laboratories, there is renewed interest in special signal, image, and stream programming languages. These languages use stream processing constructs to make the communications patterns between signal processing functions explicit. This permits compilers to implement highly efficient mapping and scheduling techniques. For example, the StreaMIT language developed at MIT and the Brook language developed at Stanford are designed to produce efficient codes for the tiled, parallel processing chip architectures that are emerging out of the DARPA Polymorphous Computing Architectures (PCA) program.

Self-optimizing portable software libraries are also appearing. The Fastest Fourier Transform in the West (FFTW) developed at MIT is an FFT generator that designs and generates highly optimal, C-callable FFT routines on new processor architectures [13]. The ATLAS system [14] tunes signal processing libraries for high performance on new architectures. SPIRAL [15], another optimization technology, automatically designs high-performance routines for signal processing routines, such as the FFT, that can be expressed as sequences of tensor product factorizations.

Application-Specific Hardware

In the earlier sections, the need for application-specific hardware was justified for cases where programmable devices were not sufficient to meet the demanding needs of the embedded signal processing applications. Performance beyond the capability of general-purpose, software-programmable processors (DSPs and GPPs) can potentially be achieved by creating a processor specifically for the application. The performance gain of an application-specific processor comes from the elimination of overhead associated with more general-purpose processor architectures.

There are two types of application-specific devices: ASICs and FPGAs. An ASIC is an integrated circuit designed and manufactured to perform a specific function in a particular application. An FPGA contains a logic network that can be configured into an application-specific device after it is manufactured.

Figure 7.35 shows a typical design flow of a high performance application-specific signal processor. The development of a processor has to go through a modeling phase followed by a physical design phase. In the modeling phase, a floating-point simulation model, typically written with a high-level programming language (e.g., C, MATLAB, etc.), is used for algorithm simulation and verification. Despite the convenience of floating-point operations, their implementations are significantly more complicated than their fixed-point counterparts. The floating-point simulation model is thus converted into a fixed-point model in the precision analysis step to determine implementation requirements (e.g., word size, etc.). The fixed-point simulation model is often referred to as a "bit-true" model since it can be used to develop binary test vectors and output vectors.

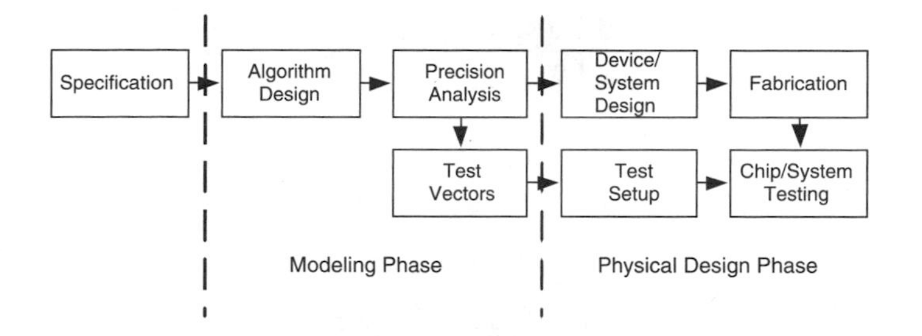

FIGURE 7.35 Typical design flow of an application specific signal processor.

The algorithm is developed into an architecture in the physical design phase. The device can be implemented with a number of different technologies, each of which has its own benefits and limitations. The rest of this section examines these technologies with the objective of enabling a proper technology selection for a high-performance embedded signal processor. Note that the adaptation of an application-specific device in a system will require the support of a printed circuit board (PCB), power supply, input/output, memory, control, etc. ASICs almost always require the development of custom boards. However, COTS FPGA boards are available, even though their capability must be carefully investigated before adaptation. Typically a COTS FPGA board would consist of one to three FPGAs, on-board memory, I/O interface, and host interface (e.g., VME or PCI). COTS FPGA board vendors usually also provide API libraries. In any case, the design and material costs of the support components thus have to be included, along with those of the device, in the budget.

Semiconductor Technology

Application-specific hardware devices are enabled by the semiconductor technology. Currently, almost all digital circuits are implemented with CMOS (complementary metal-oxide-semiconductor) technology, which employs transistors operating in complementary operating conditions to form low power and high density logic circuits. CMOS technology is characterized by its minimum feature size, which defines its minimum transistor size. A smaller feature size implies faster transistors and a higher circuit density. As of 2004, the state-of-the-art feature size is 90 nm (nanometer). Figure 7.36 shows the typical performance of CMOS applications developed with different feature sizes. As indicated in Figure 7.36b, the power consumption of a CMOS application is proportional to its switching frequency, so a device should be operated at the minimum clock frequency that meets the specifications to save power.

A set of physical masks has to be created for device fabrication. Figure 7.37 shows, as an example, the physical design of a NAND gate, called a layout, which represents the transistors and their connections. Each transistor in the layout is characterized by its channel width (W) and channel length (L), as indicated in Figure 7.37b. The transistor dimensions, as well as the interconnections between transistors, determine key IC performance factors such as chip area, operating speed, and power consumption. The techniques for IC layout

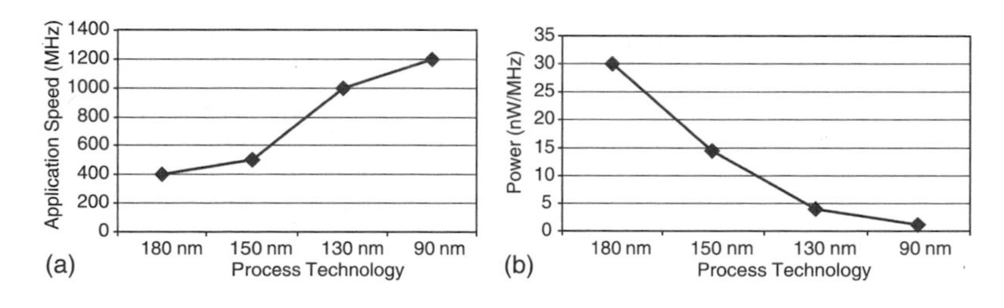

FIGURE 7.36 Typical performance of different CMOS processes: (a) operating speed, (b) power consumption.

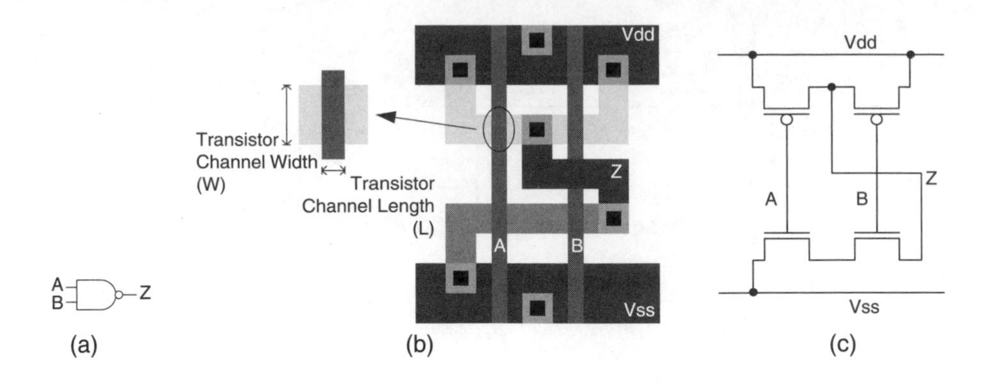

FIGURE 7.37 NAND gate design: (a) symbol, (b) layout, (c) schematic diagram.

design and optimization are beyond the scope of this handbook, so interested readers are referred to Ref. [16] for a more in-depth explanation of topics related to IC designs.

An embedded signal processor designer often has to balance between various competing objectives: development cost, production cost, performance (operation speed and power consumption), time-to-market, and volume expectation. It is very difficult, if not impossible, to optimize a design for all of these objectives. The constraints specific to an application should be used to select from available implementation technologies, which include full-custom ASICs, standard-cell ASICs, FPGAs, and structured ASICs.

Full-Custom ASIC

The layout of a module or even a complete IC can be manually created by specifying individual transistor dimensions, locations, and their connections. This approach is commonly referred to as the full-custom design. Potentially very high performance can be achieved in a full-custom design since the circuit is under the direct control of the designer. However, the performance benefit comes at the price of an extremely high design complexity. Usually, this design flow is only used to meet extremely high performance requirement with a high volume production so that the non-recurring engineering (NRE) cost can be divided among a large number of devices.

There are architectural properties that can be explored to facilitate a full-custom design. If a circuit has a high degree of regularity, then only a few types of cells need to be crafted. Another useful property is local communication between cells, which allows interconnections to be formed when cells are put together without the need for explicit routing. Cells can then be assembled using a process called tessellation, which is similar to laying the tiles on a bathroom wall.

Figure 7.38 shows the typical design flow of a full-custom ASIC. The layouts of the cells (i.e., building blocks) are created. In order to verify the cells, layouts are converted into circuit schematic diagrams in a process called extraction. The extracted schematics are compared to target schematics with a layout vs. schematic (LVS) tool. The function and performance of the cells are determined by simulation. A tessellation technique is used to assemble the cells into the final chip layout. The entire circuit is verified by LVS, design rule check (DRC), electric rule check (ERC), and simulation before it is delivered to a silicon foundry for

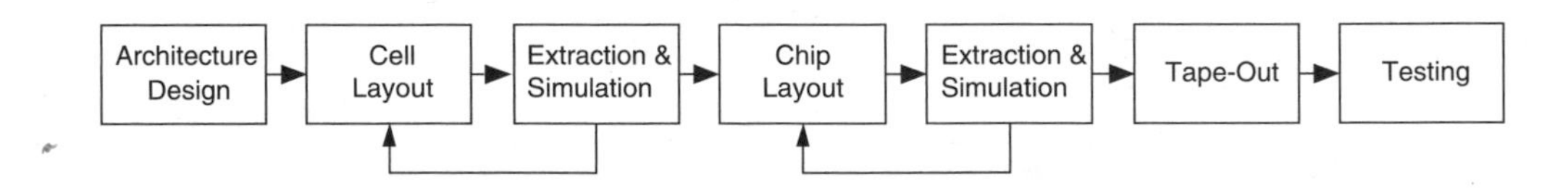

FIGURE 7.38 Full-custom ASIC design flow.

fabrication, which is commonly referred to as a tape-out. The ASICs are tested when they come back from the silicon foundry.

Standard-Cell ASIC

With millions of transistors involved, it is extremely difficult to manually lay out an entire IC. Another approach to creating an ASIC uses a library of basic building blocks, called standard cells. Standard-cell libraries are commercially available for specific fabrication processes. A library usually contains primary logic gates (e.g., inverter, NAND, NOR, etc.) as well as function blocks (e.g., adder, multiplier, memory, etc.). The quality of a library is a significant determining factor of the design performance, so choosing a library is critical to the success of a design.

A typical standard-cell ASIC design flow is shown in Figure 7.39. The device to be designed is described in a hardware description language (HDL) program, which can be simulated for verification and synthesized into a netlist of standard cells. Currently, the popular HDLs are (very high speed integrated circuit hardware description language (VHDL) and Verilog, which are programming languages specially designed to allow the description of circuits. However, SystemC, a language based on the context of C+ and enhanced with a class library of hardware-oriented constructs, is also gaining popularity. Advocates of SystemC claim that the use of an HDL originated as a general programming language can facilitate the design and verification of a system from concept to implementation in hardware and software.

The standard cells are then arranged on the available chip area with all the associated signals connected. The task of arranging the cells on the layout, called the placement process, attempts to determine the best location for each cell. The routing process takes the result of a placement and automatically completes the interconnections. A chip level verification (LVS, DRC, ERC, etc.) is performed before a tape-out.

FPGA Design

While ASICs have the potential of achieving the highest performance offered by a semiconductor process, their high design complexity (especially in the case of a full-custom design) and high fabrication cost often make them cost prohibitive. FPGA-based designs are appropriate for applications that do not require ASIC-like performance and can thereby benefit from much lower total development costs. As shown in the conceptual architecture of Figure 7.40, an FPGA is a fully manufactured device that contains an array of configurable logic blocks, memory blocks, arithmetic blocks, and interconnects that are designer controllable. Advanced FPGAs may have microprocessor hard cores embedded to implement functions that are more suitable for a programmable processor than a dedicated circuit, such as a controller. Alternatively, microprocessor soft cores are also available.

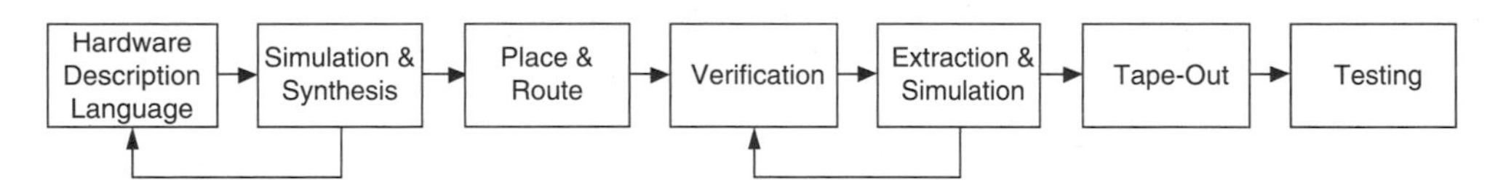

FIGURE 7.39 Standard-cell ASIC design flow.

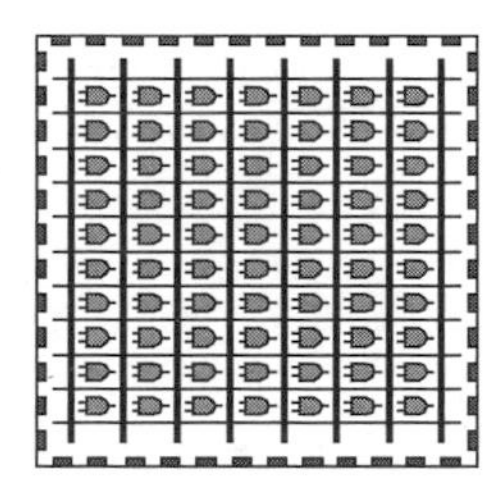

FIGURE 7.40 Conceptual FPGA architecture.

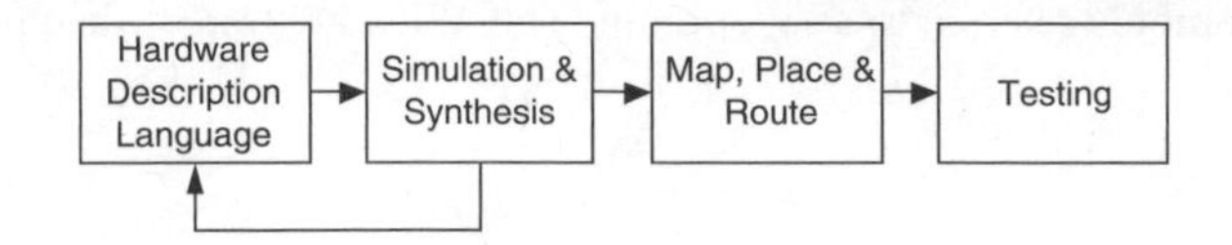

FIGURE 7.41 FPGA design flow.

The FPGA design flow is shown in Figure 7.41. Similar to the standard-cell ASIC design flow, a HDL program describing the circuit is created for simulation and synthesis. The resultant netlist is mapped, placed, and routed to create configuration data, which contain the information needed to configure the FPGA into an application-specific design.

There are three types of FPGAs. SRAM (static random access memory)-based FPGAs store configuration data in SRAMs so they are reprogrammable. However, the configuration is volatile since they are lost when the power is off. Anti-fuse-based FPGAs are one-time programmable and nonvolatile. Flash-based FPGAs use flash memories and are both reprogrammable and nonvolatile.

An FPGA is a good implementation platform for prototyping and low volume production. When the volume of a product warrants, it may be desirable to take an FPGA design and convert it into an ASIC. The most common reason for FPGA-to-ASIC conversion is to get better speed and lower power consumption since FPGAs are significantly more power hungry than their ASIC counterparts. While theoretically, the HDL program originally designed for an FPGA can be re-synthesized into a standard-cell ASIC, in reality, the design effort is close to a new design cycle. The re-synthesizing effort can be facilitated by targeting a gate-array style architecture designed to somewhat mimic an FPGA structure.

One approach for FPGA-to-ASIC conversion is to use a mask-programmed device with the same architecture as the FPGA to be replaced. Improved performance is a direct result of replacing programmable routing connections with metal customization. This approach has the advantage that the original FPGA designed for prototyping and early production can be extended into an ASIC without modifications. However, this is an FPGA-vendor-supplied solution.

Structured ASIC

A new kind of semi-custom mask-programmable device, the structured ASIC, can be viewed as a technology located on the spectrum between FPGAs and ASICs. The structured ASIC appears to have the potential to achieve close to ASIC level performance without high non recurring engineering (NRE) costs, long design cycles, and high risk factors. Structured ASIC devices typically provide pre-manufactured logic components, routing fabric and a number of commonly used functional blocks (e.g., high-speed I/O, memory, microprocessors, etc.). The devices are manufactured except for a few metal layers, which are used to customize the final devices for a specific design.

The advantages of a structured ASIC over an ASIC are lower design, manufacturing, testing, and integration costs. Compared with FPGAs, structured ASICs offer higher performance with lower power consumption and a smaller footprint.

Intellectual Property

Design reuse contributes to both risk mitigation and a reduction in development time. The most direct use of this principle is the use of functions from a previous product. The intellectual property (IP) core approach extends the concept to the use of functions designed by another party. IP cores are available for a large variety of functions, ranging from adders to microprocessors.

There are three types of IP cores: soft, firm, and hard. A soft IP core is represented with HDL at the register transfer level (RTL). Users will be required to perform the typical steps (synthesis, place and route, and verification) in the design flow following HDL development. Since the IP representation is provided in HDL, it is relatively technology independent. A firm IP core moves a bit closer to the physical side by delivering the IP design in a netlist of generic logic cells. No synthesis is required. The responsibility of the user is to perform the physical designs steps (place and route, verification). There is an assumption that the generic logic cells are available in most cell libraries. Firm IP possesses a certain degree of technology dependence, but remains relatively generic. On the extreme end of the spectrum, a hard IP core can be delivered as a layout in the form of a drop-in module. The user only needs to perform verification. Since the IP is in a physical form, it is technology dependent.

Summary

This section has addressed the embedded signal processing technologies needed to meet demanding system applications. The principal examples chosen were drawn from military sensor applications, since this application area represents a very good case of hard real-time, low-latency performance in a very limited size, weight, and power form factor. However, similar technologies are equally applicable to other commercial applications with similar signal processing functions from the analog-to-digital converters through to output data products. Several technologies were covered including embedded programmable devices (e.g., DSPs and GPPs) and application-specific hardware. The former is most often used where flexibility in programming is critical. The latter is most prevalent for applications where high-throughput performance per unit SWAP is necessary. In many applications, a combination of both technologies is often employed.

Acknowledgment

This work was sponsored by DARPA ATO under Air Force Contract F19628-00-C-0002. Opinions, interpretations, conclusions, and recommendations are those of the authors and are not necessarily endorsed by the Department of Defense.

References

International Technology Roadmap for Semiconductor (http://public.itrs.net), 2003.

The Rise of Embedded Media Processing, Analog Devices, Inc. (http://www.analog.com/processors).

E.J. Tan and W.B. Heinzelman, "DSP architectures: past, present, and future," *ACM SIGARCH Comput. Archit. News*, vol. 31, no. 3, 2003.

J. Eyre and J. Bier, "The evolution of DSP processors," *IEEE Signal Process. Mag.*, March 2000.

G. Goosens, J. Van Praet, D. Lanneer, W. Geurts, A. Kifli, C. Liem, and P.G. Paulinr, "Embedded software in real-time signal processing systems: design technologies," *Proc. IEEE*, vol. 85, no. 3, 1997.

R. Leupers, "Code Generation for Embedded Processors," *ACM ISS 2000*, Madrid, Spain, 2000.

The VSIPL Forum (http://www.vsipl.org).

The MPI Forum (http://www.mpi-forum.org).

The Data Reorganization homepage (http://www.data-re.org).

The Object Management Group (http://www.corba.org).

The POOMA homepage (http://www.codesourcery.com/pooma/pooma).

J. Kepner and J. Lebak, "Software technologies for high performance parallel signal processing," *MIT Lincoln Lab. J.*, vol. 14, no. 2, pp. 181–198, 2003.

The FFTW homepage (http://www.fftw.org).

R.C. Whaley and J.J. Dongarra, "Automatically tuned linear algebra software," *Conference on High Performance Networking and Computing; Proceedings of the 1998 ACM/IEEE Conference on Supercomputing*, San Jose, CA, 1998, pp. 1–27.

A. Gacic, J. Moura, and M. Pueschel, "High-performance code generation for FIR filters and the discrete wavelet transform using SPIRAL," *Proceedings of the Seventh Annual High Performance Embedded Computing (HPEC) Workshop*, September 2003.

M. Vai, *VLSI Design*, Boca Raton, FL: CRC Press, 2001.

Credits

Figure 7.29 courtesy of Xilinx Inc. and Annapolis Micro Systems, Inc. Xilinx and Virtex wordmarks and logomarks are registered trademarks protected by copyright. With permission.

Figure 7.30 courtesy of Xilinx Inc. and Mercury Computer Systems, Inc. Xilinx and Virtex wordmarks and logomarks are registered trademarks protected by copyright. With permission.

Figure 7.32 courtesy of Mercury Computer Systems, Inc. With permission.

8

Biomedical Sensors

Michael R. Neuman
Michigan Technological University

8.1 Introduction 8-1
8.2 Physical Sensors 8-2
8.3 Chemical Sensors 8-6
8.4 Bioanalytical Sensors 8-9
8.5 Applications 8-10

8.1 Introduction

Any instrumentation system can be described as having three fundamental components: a sensor, a signal processor, and a display and/or storage device. Although all these components of the instrumentation system are important, the sensor serves a special function in that it interfaces the instrument with the system being measured. In the case of biomedical instrumentation, a biomedical sensor (which in some cases may be referred to as a biosensor) is the interface between the electronic instrument and the biological system. There are some general concerns that are important for any sensor in an instrumentation system regarding its ability to effectively carry out the interface function. These concerns are especially important for biomedical sensors because the sensor can affect the system being measured and the system can affect the sensor. Sensors must be designed so that they minimize their interaction with the biological host. It is important that the presence of the sensor does not affect the variable being measured in the vicinity of the sensor via interaction between the sensor and the biologic system. If the sensor is placed in a living organism, that organism will probably recognize it as a foreign body and react to it. This may change the quantity being sensed in the vicinity of the sensor so that the measurement reflects a reaction to the foreign body rather than a central characteristic of the host.

Similarly, the biological system can affect the performance of the sensor. The foreign body reaction might cause the host's system to attempt to break down the materials of the sensor in order to remove it. This may, in fact, degrade the sensor package so that it can no longer perform in an adequate manner. Even if the foreign body reaction is not strong enough to affect the measurement, just the fact that the sensor is in a warm, aqueous environment may cause water to eventually invade the package and degrade its function. Finally, as will be described below, sensors that are implanted in the body are not accessible for calibration. Thus, they must have extremely stable characteristics so that frequent calibrations are not necessary.

Biomedical sensors can be classified according to how they are used with respect to the biological system. Table 8.1 shows that sensors can range from noninvasive to invasive as far as the biological host is concerned. The most noninvasive of biomedical sensors do not even contact the biological system being measured. Sensors of radiant heat or sound energy coming from an organism are examples of noncontacting sensors. Noninvasive sensors can also be placed on the body surface. Skin surface thermometers, biopotential electrodes, and strain gauges placed on the skin are examples of noninvasive sensors. Indwelling sensors are those that can be placed into a natural body cavity that communicates with the outside. These are sometimes referred to as minimally invasive sensors and include such familiar sensors as oral–rectal thermometers, intrauterine pressure transducers, and stomach pH sensors. The most invasive sensors are those that need to be surgically placed and

TABLE 8.1 Classification of Biomedical Sensors According to Their Interface with the Biologic Host

Degree of Invasion	Sensor Classification
Isolated	Noncontacting
Noninvasive	Body surface
Minimally invasive	Indwelling
Invasive	Implanted

that require some tissue damage associated with their installation. A needle electrode for picking up electromyographic signals directly from muscles; a blood pressure sensor placed in an artery, vein, or in the heart itself; or a blood flow transducer positioned on a major artery are all examples of invasive sensors.

We can also classify sensors in terms of the quantities that they measure. **Physical sensors** are used in measuring physical quantities such as displacement, pressure, and flow, while **chemical sensors** are used to determine the concentration of chemical substances within the host. A sub-group of the chemical sensors that are concerned with sensing the presence and the concentration of biochemical materials in the host are known as **bioanalytical sensors** or biosensors.

In the following paragraphs we will look at each type of sensor and present some examples as well as describe some of the important issues surrounding these types of sensors.

8.2 Physical Sensors

Physical variables associated with biomedical systems are measured by a group of sensors known as physical sensors. A list of typical variables measured by these devices and examples of sensors used to measure them are given in Table 8.2. These quantities are similar to physical quantities measured by sensors for nonbiomedical applications, and the devices used for biomedical and nonbiomedical sensing are, therefore, quite similar. There are, however, two principal exceptions: pressure and flow sensors. The measurement of blood or other fluid pressure and flow in humans and other animals is problematic. Direct pressure measurement refers to the evaluation of the pressure using a sensor that is in contact with the blood or another fluid being measured, or contacts it through an intermediate fluid such as a physiologic saline solution. Direct pressure sensors are invasive in that there needs to be a physical connection between the sensor and the circulating blood or fluid being measured. This means that a needle or surgical approach to the fluid compartment being measured is necessary. Indirect pressure measurement involves a sensor that does not actually contact the fluid being measured. An indirect pressure sensor measures a quantity, such as the tension in a vessel wall, that is related to the desired pressure and allows the sensor to be separated from the fluid being measured. The most familiar indirect pressure measurement involves the determination of arterial blood pressure using a sphygmomanometer cuff. This is the method that is usually used in medical examinations. It is a noninvasive instrument and the measurement is easily performed. Often, however, it is less accurate than the direct measure of blood pressure, and it provides only a sample in time rather than a continuous record as is possible with the direct measurement technique.

TABLE 8.2 Physical Variables Measured by Biomedical Sensors

Displacement (linear and angular)
Velocity
Acceleration
Temperature
Force (torque, weight, and mass)
Pressure
Sound
Flow
Radiant energy

Until recently, the primary sensor used for direct blood pressure measurement was the unbonded strain gauge pressure transducer shown in Figure 8.1. The basic principle of this device is that a differential pressure seen across a diaphragm will cause that diaphragm to deflect. This deflection is then measured by a displacement transducer. In the unbonded strain gauge sensor a closed chamber is covered by a flexible diaphragm. This diaphragm is attached to a structure that has four fine-gauge wires drawn between it and the chamber walls. A dome with the appropriate hardware for fluid coupling to a pressure source covers the diaphragm on the side opposite the chamber and wires such that when the pressure in the dome exceeds the pressure in the chamber, the diaphragm is deflected into the chamber. This causes two of the fine wires to

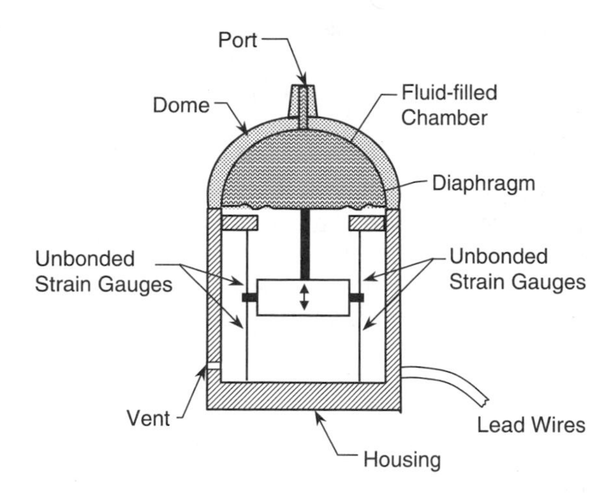

FIGURE 8.1 Unbonded strain gauge pressure sensor.

stretch by a small amount while the other two wires contract by the same amount. The electrical resistance of the wires that are stretched increases while that of the wires that contract decreases. By connecting these wires, or more correctly these unbonded strain gauges, into a Wheatstone bridge circuit, a voltage proportional to the deflection of the diaphragm can be obtained.

In recent years semiconductor technology has been applied to the design of pressure transducers resulting in smaller, less expensive devices. Silicon strain gauges that are much more sensitive than their wire counterparts are formed on a silicon chip, and micromachining technology is used to form this portion of the chip into a diaphragm with the strain gauges integrated into its surface. This structure is then incorporated into a plastic housing and dome assembly as illustrated in Figure 8.2. The entire sensor can be fabricated and sold inexpensively so that disposable, single-use devices can be made. These have the advantage that they are only used on one patient and they do not have to be cleaned and sterilized between patients. By using them only once, the risk of transmitting blood-borne infections is eliminated.

In biomedical applications pressure is generally referenced to atmospheric pressure, i.e., gauge pressure. Therefore, one side of the diaphragm of the pressure transducer must be maintained at atmospheric pressure while the other side of the diaphragm is at the pressure being measured. This is done by means of a vent in the pressure sensor wall or a fine-bore, flexible capillary tube that couples one side of the diaphragm to the atmosphere. This tube is usually included in the electrical cable connecting the pressure transducer to the external instrumentation such that the tube is open to the atmosphere at the cable connecter.

The pressure sensor is used to measure blood pressure by coupling the measurement side of the diaphragm to a flexible plastic tube, known as a catheter, and the sensor and tube are filled with a physiological saline solution. As described by Pascal's law, the pressure in the sensor against the diaphragm will be the same as that at the tip of the tube provided the tip of the tube is at the same horizontal level as the sensor. Thus, by threading the tube into a blood vessel, an invasive procedure, the blood pressure in that vessel can be transmitted to the diaphragm of the pressure sensor. The pressure sensor will, therefore, measure the pressure in the vessel. This technique is known as external direct blood pressure measurement. It is important to remember that the horizontal level of the blood pressure transducer diaphragm must be the same as that of

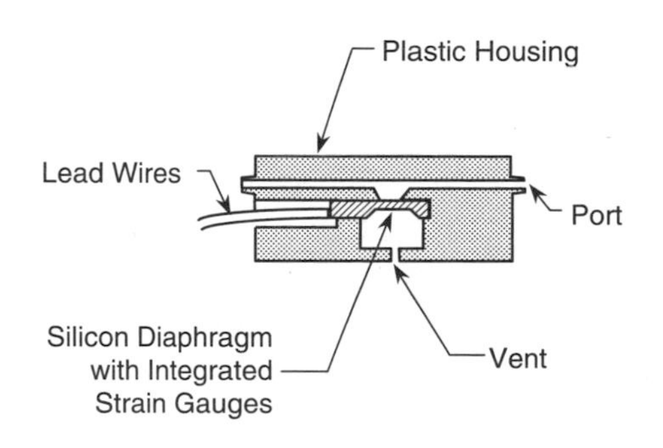

FIGURE 8.2 Silicon-based disposable pressure sensor.

the tip of the catheter in the blood vessel to accurately measure the pressure in that vessel without adding an error due to the hydrostatic pressure in the catheter.

Pressure errors can also be introduced as a result of the dynamic and material properties of the catheter, fluid, sensor volume, and diaphragm. These properties, as well as air bubbles in the catheter or obstructions due to clotted blood or other materials, can introduce resonances and damping. These problems can be minimized by utilizing miniature pressure transducers that are located at the tip of a catheter rather than at the end that is external to the body. A general arrangement for such a pressure transducer is shown in Figure 8.3. As with the disposable sensors, strain gauges are integrated into the diaphragm of the transducer such that they detect very small deflections of this diaphragm. Because of the small size, small diaphragm displacement, and lack of a catheter with a fluid column, these sensors have a broad frequency response, give a clearer signal, and do not have any hydrostatic pressure error.

Although the indwelling catheter tip pressure sensor appears to solve many of the problems associated with the external pressure sensor, there are still important problems in pressure sensor design that need to be addressed. Long-term stability of pressure sensors is not very good. This is especially problematic for venous or intracranial pressure measurements that are carried out at relatively low pressure. Long-term changes in baseline pressure require pressure sensors to be frequently adjusted to be certain of zero pressure. While this can be done relatively easily for external and indwelling pressure sensors, there is no way to carry out this procedure for implanted sensors, since there is no way to establish zero pressure at the sensor. Thus, devices that have very low long-term baseline drift are essential for implantable applications.

The packaging of the pressure sensor also represents a problem that needs to be addressed. Packaging must both protect the sensor and not affect the pressure being measured. In other words, it must be biocompatible. The package must also allow the appropriate pressure to be transmitted from the biological fluid to the sensor diaphragm. The amount of packaging material required should be kept at a minimum so as not to substantially increase the size of implantable or indwelling sensors. Furthermore, the material must be mechanically stable so that it does not swell or contract, since this could change the baseline pressure seen by the sensor. These problems need to be overcome before miniature pressure transducers can be used reliably in implantable applications.

Indwelling and external pressure sensors are used in medicine in many ways. Not only can they measure blood pressure in the arterial and venous systems, but they are also used to measure pressures within the heart itself. This is done by threading a fluid-filled catheter or catheter-tip pressure transducer into the heart through a peripheral vein or artery. Pressures in other organs are measured in similar ways. Table 8.3 gives examples of common biological pressures that can be measured using direct or indirect pressure instrumentation.

Flow is the other physical variable that is difficult to measure in biological systems. Blood flow is a particularly important variable in that it can be used to determine cardiac output when measured at the heart. Various methods have been developed to measure the flow of blood and other biological fluids, and the principal ones are listed in Table 8.4. As can be seen from the table, most of these are invasive measurements and require surgical intervention to make the measurement. This limits their clinical usefulness. Of the

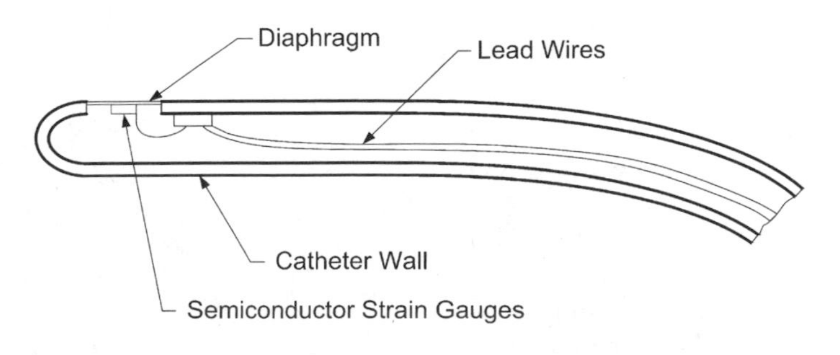

FIGURE 8.3 Catheter tip pressure sensor.

TABLE 8.3 Biologic Pressures that Can Be Measured Using Direct or Indirect Pressure Sensors

Anatomic Structure	Pressure Signal	Direct Sensor	Indirect Sensor
Artery	Arterial blood pressure	Fluid-filled catheter with external pressure sensor Catheter tip sensor	Sphygmomanometer Tonometer
Vein	Venous blood pressure	Fluid-filled catheter with external pressure sensor	No method
Heart	Intracardiac pressure	Fluid-filled catheter with external pressure sensor	No method
Urinary bladder	Cystometric pressure	Catheter tip sensor	No method
Eye	Intraocular pressure	Intraocular sensor	Tonometer
Stomach	Intragastric pressure	Balloon-tipped catheter Catheter tip sensor	No method
Brain	Intracranial pressure	Fluid-filled catheter with external pressure sensor Intracranial sensor	Tonometer (newborn infants only)
Spinal cord	Cerebral–spinal fluid pressure	Fluid-filled catheter with external pressure sensor	No method

invasive blood flow sensors, some must be placed around an artery or vein to make a measurement, and this requires significant surgical intervention and subject recovery. Other sensors placed on a catheter can be introduced into the body by accessing a peripheral artery or vein and threading in the catheter to get the sensor to the point in the vessel where the measurement is to be made. This still involves an invasive surgical procedure, but the trauma can be minimized, and this can reduce the effect that the surgical procedure has on the variable being measured.

The most commonly used types of invasive blood flow sensors are the electromagnetic flowmeter and the Doppler ultrasonic flowmeter. The fundamental principles of each are based on a characteristic property of the blood. In the former case, the fact that blood contains ions, among other components, and in the latter case that the blood contains cells that are large enough to scatter and reflect ultrasonic waves. The basic form of an electromagnetic flowmeter is illustrated in Figure 8.4. Because the blood flowing in the vessel contains ions, they will be moving with the blood at a velocity corresponding to the flow. When they pass the region of the vessel where the magnetic field from the external (to the vessel) magnet is situated, positive ions will experience a deflecting force perpendicular to both the direction of the ion movement and the direction of the magnetic field. Negative ions in the blood will experience a deflecting force in the opposite direction. In both

TABLE 8.4 Methods to Measure Fluid Flow in the Body

Flow Measurement Method	Example Biomedical Application	Degree of Invasion	Type of Measurement
Fick principle	Cardiac output	Non- or minimally invasive	Sampled
Indicator dilution	Cardiac output	Minimally invasive	Sampled
Electromagnetic flowmeter	Arterial or venous blood flow	Invasive	Continuous
Ultrasonic Doppler flowmeter	Arterial or venous blood flow	Invasive	Continuous
Pulsed Doppler ultrasound	Arterial or venous blood flow combined with imaging	Noninvasive	Rapid sampled, essentially continuous
Magnetic resonance imaging	Tissue perfusion combined with imaging	Noninvasive	Rapid sampled, essentially continuous

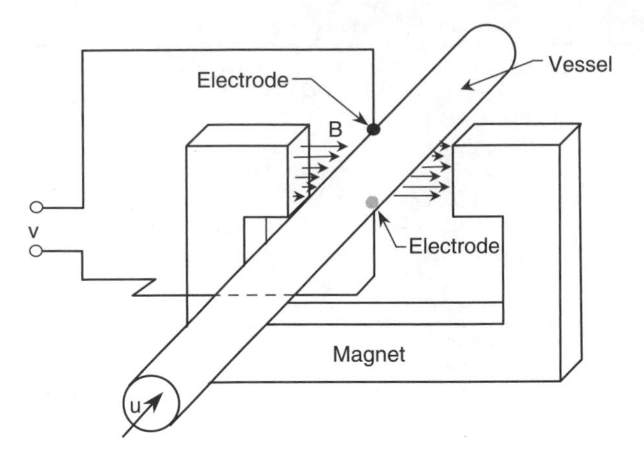

FIGURE 8.4 Basic structure of an electromagnetic flow sensor.

cases the magnitude of the deflecting force will be proportional to the magnetic field strength and the velocity of the blood, and so the actual deflection of these ions will be proportional to the blood velocity when the magnetic field is uniform and of constant magnitude. Thus, if we put a pair of electrodes on the vessel wall along the axis of these deflecting forces, we should see a potential difference due to the deflection of these ions. This potential difference will be proportional to the blood velocity. Blood volume flow can be determined from this by knowing the cross-sectional area of the flowing column of blood either by measuring the vessel inner diameter or by constraining the vessel to have a fixed inner diameter by putting a fixed cuff around it.

Ultrasonic flowmeters are based on the interaction of ultrasonic waves with the flowing blood. Ultrasonic energy in the megahertz range is readily scattered and reflected by the blood cells. Thus, if the cells reflecting the ultrasonic energy are moving, the reflected energy will be shifted in frequency in proportion to the velocity of these cells according to the Doppler effect. By measuring this frequency shift, one can determine the relative velocity of the cells and, hence, the velocity of the blood. If the angle of the ultrasonic wave propagation direction with respect to the direction of the blood cells' velocity vector is known, one can quantitatively determine the blood velocity from the Doppler frequency shift. It is then possible to use the same approach as described for the electromagnetic blood flowmeter to determine the volume blood flow from the blood velocity.

Ultrasound is also used to estimate blood flow noninvasively. An ultrasonic beam can be introduced into the body from a transducer on its surface, and the same transducer can receive the reflected signal from the flowing blood. The extent of the Doppler shift will be proportional to the blood velocity of the vessel being illuminated by the ultrasonic beam. Clinical instruments combine this mode of operation with ultrasonic imaging to show images of the anatomic structures surrounding the vessels being studied, with a color display within the vessel where the color represents the velocity of the blood. This technique is especially useful in observing partial obstruction and turbulence within blood vessels.

8.3 Chemical Sensors

There are many biomedical situations where it is necessary to know the concentration or chemical activity of a particular substance in a biological sample. Chemical sensors provide the interface between an instrument and the specimen to allow one to determine these quantities. These sensors can be used on a biological specimen taken from the host and tested in a laboratory, or they can be used for *in vivo* measurements either as noninvasive or invasive sensors. There are many types of chemical sensors used in biomedical instrumentation. Table 8.5 lists some general categories of sensors. Electrochemical and optical sensors are most frequently used for biomedical measurements both *in vivo* and *in vitro.* An example of an

TABLE 8.5 Classifications of Chemical Biomedical Sensors

1. Electrochemical
   a. Amperometric
   b. Potentiometric
   c. Coulometric
2. Optical
   a. Colorimetric
   b. Emission and absorption spectroscopy
   c. Fluorescence
   d. Chemiluminescence
3. Thermal methods
   a. Calorimetry
   b. Thermoconductivity
4. Nuclear magnetic resonance

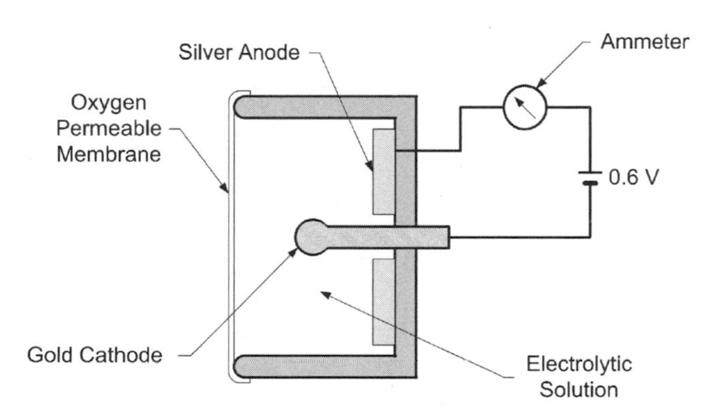

FIGURE 8.5 A Clark amperometric electrode for sensing oxygen.

electrochemical sensor is the Clark electrode illustrated in Figure 8.5. It consists of an electrochemical cell separated from the specimen being measured by an oxygen-permeable membrane. The cell is biased at a fixed potential of 600 mV, and under these conditions the following reaction occurs at the noble metal cathode:

$$O_2 + 2H_2O = 4e^- \rightarrow 4OH^-$$

This reaction involves the reduction of molecular oxygen that diffuses into the cell through the oxygen-permeable membrane. Since the other components of the reaction are in abundance, the rate of the reaction is limited by the amount of oxygen available. Thus, the rate of electrons used at the cathode is directly related to the available oxygen. In other words, the cathode current is proportional to the partial pressure of oxygen in the specimen being measured.

The electrochemical cell is completed by the silver anode. The reaction at the anode involves forming the low-solubility salt, silver-chloride, from the anode material itself and the chloride ion contained in the electrolytic solution. The cell is designed with these materials in abundance so that their activity does not affect the sensor performance. This type of sensor is an example of an **amperometric** electrochemical sensor, that is the current in the cell is proportional to the concentration of the analyte; in this case, oxygen.

Another type of electrochemical sensor that is frequently used in biomedical laboratories is the glass pH electrode illustrated in Figure 8.6. The acidity or alkalinity of a solution is characterized by its pH. This quantity is defined as

$$\text{pH} = -\log_{10}[H^+]$$

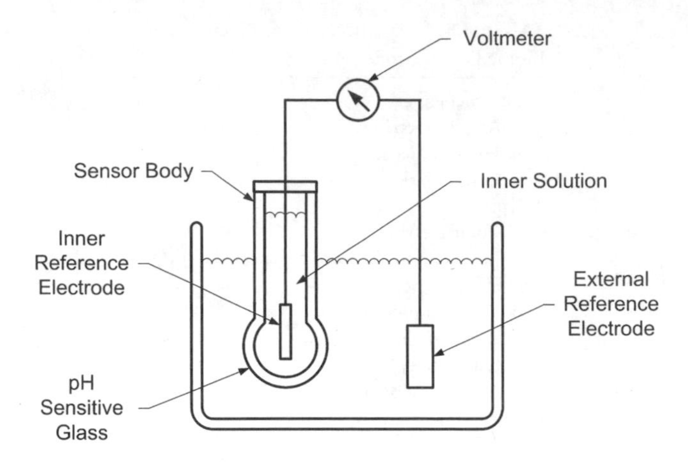

FIGURE 8.6 A glass electrode pH sensor.

where $[H^+]$ is the activity of the hydrogen ions in solution, a quantity that is related to the concentration of the hydrogen ions. This sensor only works in an aqueous environment. It consists of an inner chamber containing an electrolytic solution of known pH and an outer solution with an unknown pH that is to be measured. The membrane consists of a specially formulated glass that appears to allow hydrogen ions to pass in either direction but will not pass other chemical species. In practice, the processes in this glass membrane and on its surfaces are much more complicated, but the above description is adequate to understand the fundamental operation of a glass pH electrode. If the concentration of hydrogen ions in the external solution is greater than that in the internal solution, there will be a gradient that appears to force hydrogen ions to diffuse through the membrane into the internal solution. This will cause the internal solution side of the membrane to have a greater positive charge than the external solution side, so that an electrical potential and, hence, an electric field will exist across the membrane. This field will counteract the diffusion of hydrogen ions due to the concentration difference and equilibrium will eventually be established. The potential across the membrane at this equilibrium condition will be related to the hydrogen ion concentration difference (or more accurately, the activity difference) between the inner and outer solutions. This potential is given by the Nernst equation:

$$E = -\frac{RT}{nF}\ln\left(\frac{a_1}{a_2}\right)$$

where E is the potential measured, R is the universal gas constant, T is the absolute temperature, n is the valence of the ion, and a_1 and a_2 are the activities of the ions on each side of the membrane. Thus, the potential measured across the glass membrane will be proportional to the pH of the solution being studied. At room temperature the sensitivity of the electrode is approximately 60 mV/pH. It is not practical to measure the potential across the membrane directly, so reference electrodes, sensors that can be used to measure electrical potential of an electrolytic solution, are used to contact the solution on either side of the membrane to measure the potential difference across it. The reference electrodes and the glass membrane are incorporated into the structure shown in Figure 8.6 which is known as a glass pH electrode. This is an example of a **potentiometric** measurement made using an ion-selective membrane because the sensor potential is proportional to the logarithm of the activity difference of the analyte across the analyte-selective membrane.

There are other types of ion-selective membrane potentiometric chemical sensors that are used for biomedical applications. The membranes of these sensors determine the ion being sensed. The membrane can be based upon glass or a highly plasticized polymeric material such as polyvinyl chloride, but the key component is the substance that is added to the membrane that allows it to appear to selectively pass a single ion.

Important problems in the development of chemical biomedical sensors are similar to those discussed above for the pressure sensor. Issues of long-term stability and packaging are critical to the success of a chemical sensor. The package is even more critical in chemical sensors than it was in pressure sensors in that the package must protect portions of the sensor that require isolation from the solution being measured while it provides direct contact of the chemically sensitive portions of the sensor to the solution. The maintenance of a window through the package for this contact represents a critical aspect of sensor development. Frequent calibration is also necessary for chemical sensors. Just about every type of chemical sensor requires some sort of calibration using a standard solution with known concentration of the analyte being sensed. Although this might be an inconvenience in the clinical laboratory, it is readily achieved and important for quality control. When a sensor is implanted in the body, it is not accessible for calibration, and this is one of the principal reasons that sensors of the types mentioned in this section are usually unsuitable for chronic implantation.

8.4 Bioanalytical Sensors

A special class of sensors of biological molecules has evolved in recent years. These bioanalytical sensors take advantage of one of the following biochemical reactions: (1) enzyme–substrate, (2) antigen–antibody, or (3) ligand–receptor. The advantage of using these reactions in a sensor is that they are highly specific to a particular biological molecule, and sensors with high sensitivity and selectivity can be developed based upon these reactions. The basic structure of a bioanalytical sensor is shown in Figure 8.7. There are two principal regions of the sensor. The first contains one component of the biological sensing reaction such as the enzyme or the antibody, and the second region involves a means of detecting whether the biological reaction has taken place. This second portion of a bioanalytical sensor is made up of either a physical or chemical sensor that serves as the detector of the biological reaction. As illustrated in Figure 8.7, this detector can consist of an electrical sensor such as used in electrochemical sensors, a thermal sensor, a sensor of changes in capacitance, a sensor of changes in mass, or a sensor of optical properties.

One example of a bioanalytical sensor is a glucose sensor. The first portion of the sensor contains the enzyme glucose oxidase. This enzyme promotes the oxidation of glucose to glucuronic acid and hydrogen peroxide while consuming oxygen in the process. Thus, by placing a hydrogen peroxide or an oxygen sensor along with the glucose oxidase in the bioanalytical sensor, one can determine the amount of glucose oxidized by measuring the amount of hydrogen peroxide produced or oxygen consumed.

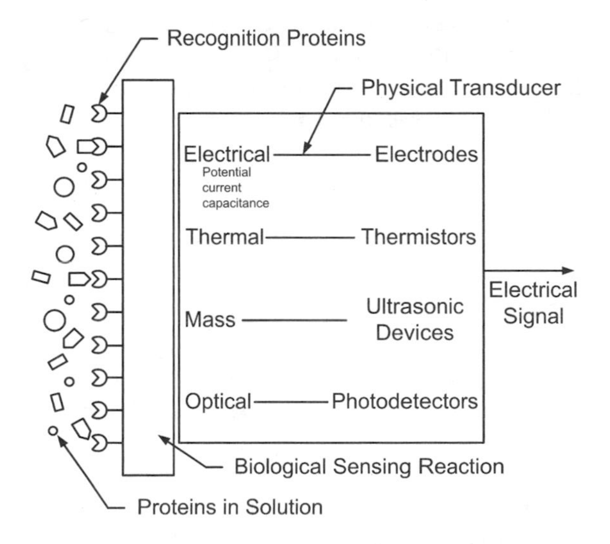

FIGURE 8.7 Schematic view of a bioanalytical sensor.

Stability is important for bioanalytical sensors, especially those that are used for long-term measurements. Not only are the stability issues the same as for the physical and chemical sensors, but they are also related to preservation of the biological molecules used in the first portion of the sensor. These molecules can often be degraded or destroyed by heat or exposure to light. Even aging can degrade some of these molecules. Thus, an important issue in dealing with bioanalytical sensors is the preservation of the biochemical components of the sensor.

8.5 Applications

Biomedical sensors and instrumentation are used in biomedical research and patient care applications. In terms of patient care, sensors are used as a part of instruments that carry out patient screening by making measurements such as blood pressure using automated or manually operated apparatus. Specimen analysis is another important application of biomedical sensors in patient care. This can include analyses that can be carried out by the patients themselves in their homes such as is done with home blood glucose analyzers. Instrumentation based upon biomedical sensors also can be used in the physician's office for carrying out some chemical analyses of patient specimens such as urinalysis or elementary blood chemistries such as serum glucose and electrolytes. Sensors also are a part of large, multi-component, automatic blood analyzers used in the central clinical laboratories of medical centers. Another application for biomedical sensors is in patient monitoring. Sensors represent the front end of critical care monitors used in the intensive care unit and in the operating and recovery rooms. Measurements cover a wide range of biomedical variables such as continuous recordings of blood pressure and oxygen saturation of the arterial blood. The performance of these instruments is strongly dependent on biomedical sensors. Patient monitoring can also be carried out in the various clinical units of the hospital. Devices such as ambulatory cardiac monitors that allow patients to be observed while they are free to move around on the ward are becoming important for clinical care in "step-down" units for patients who have completed their stay in the intensive care unit. Patient monitoring has even made its way into the home. Home cardiorespiratory monitors have been used with patients immediately after discharge from the hospital to follow them in the critical first few days at home. The availability of this technology makes it possible to discharge patients earlier, thereby helping to reduce healthcare costs while still maintaining high quality medical care.

Summary

Sensors serve an important function in biomedical instrumentation systems in that they provide the interface between the electronic instrument and the biological system being measured. Very often the quality of the instrument is based upon the quality of the sensor at the instrument's front end. Although electronic signal processing has been developed to a high level, the signals are no better than the quality of the sensors that provide them. Even though there have been many advances in biomedical sensor technology, many problems remain to be overcome. Biomedical sensors will continue to be an important area for research and development in biomedical engineering.

Defining Terms

Amperometric sensor: An electrochemical sensor that determines the amount of a substance by means of an oxidation-reduction reaction involving that substance. Electrons are transferred as a part of the reaction, so that the electrical current through the sensor is related to the amount of the substance seen by the sensor.

Analyte: The substance being measured by a chemical or bioanalytical sensor and instrumentation system.

Bioanalytical sensor: A special case of a chemical sensor that determines the amount of a biochemical substance. This type of sensor usually makes use of one of the following types of biochemical reactions: enzyme–substrate, antigen–antibody, or ligand–receptor.

Biomedical sensor: A device for interfacing an instrumentation system with a biological system such as a biological specimen or an entire organism. The device serves the function of detecting and measuring in a quantitative fashion a physiological property of the biologic system.

Chemical sensor: The interface device for an instrumentation system that determines the concentration of a chemical substance.

Noninvasive sensor: The interface device of an instrumentation system that measures a physiologic variable from an organism without interrupting the integrity of that organism. This device can be in direct contact with the surface of the organism or it can measure the physiologic quantity while remaining remote from the organism.

Physical sensor: An interface device at the input of an instrumentation system that quantitatively measures a physical quantity such as pressure or temperature.

Potentiometric sensor: A chemical sensor that measures the concentration or activity of a substance by determining an electrical potential.

References

R.S.C. Cobbold, *Transducers for Biomedical Measurements: Principles and Applications,* New York: Wiley, 1974.

D.G. Fleming, W.H. Ko, and M.R. Neuman, Eds., *Indwelling and Implantable Pressure Transducers,* Cleveland, OH: CRC Press, 1977.

L.A. Geddes, *The Direct and Indirect Measurement of Blood Pressure,* Chicago, IL: Year Book Medical Publishers, 1970.

Jacob Fraden, *Handbook of Modern Sensors: Physics, Designs, and Applications*, 3rd ed., Berlin: Springer, 2004.

W. Gopel, J. Hesse, and J.N. Zemel, *Sensors; A Comprehensive Survey,* Weinheim, Germany: VCH Verlagsgesellschaft, 1989.

J. Janata, *Principles of Chemical Sensors,* New York: Plenum Press, 1989.

R. Pallas-Areny and J.G. Webster, *Sensors and Signal Conditioning,* 2nd ed., New York: Wiley, 2001.

Tatsuo Togawa; Toshiyo Tamura; P. Ake Oberg, *Biomedical Transducers and Instruments*, Boca Raton, FL: CRC Press, 1997.

B.R. Eggins, *Chemical Sensors and Biosensors (Analytical Techniques in the Sciences)*, New York: Wiley, 2002.

J.G. Webster, Ed., *Encyclopedia of Medical Devices and Instrumentation*, New York: Wiley, 1988.

A. Heller, "Implanted electrochemical glucose sensors for the management of diabetes," *Annu. Rev. Biomed. Eng.*, vol. 1, pp. 153–75, 1999.

R.B. Northrup, *Noninvasive Instrumentation and Measurement in Medical Diagnosis*, Boca Raton, FL: CRC Press, 2001.

J.G. Webster, Ed., *Bioinstrumentation*, New York: Wiley, 2004.

Further Information

Research reports on biomedical sensors appear in many different journals ranging from those that are concerned with clinical medicine through those that are engineering and chemistry oriented. The journals and other sources listed below, however, represent major sources of biomedical sensor papers:

The journal *Physiological Measurement* sponsored by the Institute of Physicists and Engineers in Medicine of the United Kingdom and published by the Institute of Physics Publishing, Bristol, U.K., is devoted to biomedical instrumentation and measurement. It often has papers on biomedical sensors. More information can be found on their web site: http://www.iop.org/pm.

The *IEEE Sensors Journal* (http://www.IEEE.org/sensors) has original research reports on sensors for many different applications, and some of these are in the biomedical area.

Another journal devoted to all types of sensors is *Sensors and Actuators* published by Elsevier. This journal is divided into two sections that are published separately. Part A is devoted to physical sensors and Part B is concerned with chemical sensors.

The *IEEE Transactions on Biomedical Engineering* is a monthly journal devoted to research papers on biomedical engineering. Papers on biomedical sensors frequently are published. For more information or subscriptions, contact IEEE Service Center, 445 Hoes Lane, P.O. Box 1331, Piscataway, NJ 08855-1331.

The international journal *Medical and Biological Engineering and Computing* is published bimonthly by the International Federation for Medical and Biological Engineering. This journal frequently contains reports on biomedical sensors and related topics. Subscription information can be obtained from Peter Peregrinus Ltd., P.O. Box 96, Stevenage, Herts SG12SD, U.K.

The journal *Biomedical Instrumentation and Technology* is published by the Association for the Advancement of Medical Instrumentation. This bimonthly journal has reports on biomedical instrumentation for clinical applications, including papers on biomedical sensors. Subscription information can be obtained from Hanley and Belfus, 210 S. 13th Street, Philadelphia, PA 19107.

There are also several scientific meetings that include biomedical sensors. The major meetings in the area include the international conference of the IEEE Engineering in Medicine and Biology Society and the Annual Meeting of the Biomedical Engineering Society. Extended abstracts for these meetings are published on CD-ROM each year.

9

Bioelectronics and Instruments

Joseph D. Bronzino
Trinity College

Edward J. Berbari
Indiana University/Purdue University

9.1 The Electro-encephalogram **9**-1
The Language of the Brain • Historical Perspective • EEG Recording Techniques • Frequency Analysis of the EEG • Nonlinear Analysis of the EEG • Topographic Mapping

9.2 The Electrocardiograph **9**-14
Physiology • Instrumentation • Conclusions

9.1 The Electro-encephalogram

Joseph D. Bronzino

Electro-encephalograms (EEGs) are recordings of the minute (generally less than 300 μV) electrical potentials produced by the brain. Since 1924, when Hans Berger reported the measurements of rhythmic electrical activity on the human scalp, it has been suggested that these patterns of bioelectrical origin may provide clues regarding the neuronal bases for specific behaviors and has offered great promise to reveal correlations between pathological processes and the electrical activity of specific regions of the brain.

Over the years, EEG analyses have been conducted primarily in clinical settings, to detect gross organic pathologies and epilepsies, and in research facilities to quantify the central effect of new pharmacological agents. As a result of these efforts, cortical EEG patterns have been shown to be modified by a wide variety of variables including biochemical, metabolic, circulatory, hormonal, neuroelectric, and behavioral factors. In the past, interpretation of the EEG was limited to visual inspection by a trained electroencephalographer capable of distinguishing normal activity from localized or generalized abnormalities of particular types from relatively long EEG records. This approach has left clinicians and researchers alike lost in a sea of EEG paper records. Computer technology permits the application of a host of methods to quantify EEG changes. With this in mind, this section provides an introduction to some of the basic concepts underlying the generation of the EEG, a review of the basic approaches used in quantifying alterations in the EEG, and some insights regarding quantitative electrophysiological techniques.

The Language of the Brain

The mass of brain tissue is composed of bundles of nerve cells (neurons), which constitute the fundamental building blocks of the nervous system. Figure 9.1 is a schematic drawing of just such a cell. It consists of three major components: the cell body (or soma), the receptor zone (or dendrites), and the axon, which carries electrical signals from the soma to target sites such as muscles, glands, or other neurons. Numbering approximately 20 billion in each human being, these tiny cells come in a variety of sizes and shapes. Although neurons are anatomically distinct units having no physical continuity between their processes, the axon ends on the soma and the dendrites of other cells in what is called a synapse. Under the microscope this often stands out as a spherical enlargement at the end of the axon to which various names have been given, for example, boutons, end-plate, or synaptic terminals. This ending does not actually make physical contact with the soma or dendrite, but is separated by a narrow cleft (gap) approximately 100 to 200 Å wide. This is known as the synaptic cleft. Each of these synaptic endings contains a large number of submicroscopic spherical structures (synaptic vesicles) that can be detected only by using an electron microscope. These synaptic vesicles, in turn, are essentially "chemical carriers" containing transmitter substance that is released into the synaptic cleft on excitation (Kandel et al., 2000).

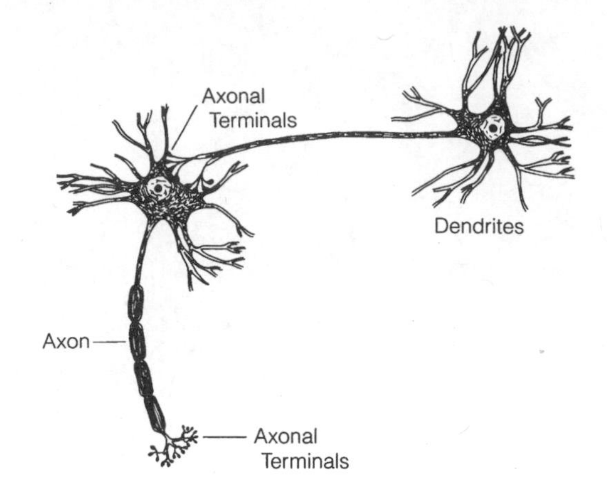

FIGURE 9.1 Basic structure of the neuron.

When an individual neuron is excited, an electrical signal is transmitted along its axon to many tiny branching, diverging fibers near its far end. These axonal terminals end as synapse on a large number of other neurons. When an electrical pulse arrives at the synapse, it triggers the release of a tiny amount of transmitter substance, which crosses the synaptic cleft thereby altering the membrane potential of the receiving neuron. If the change is above a certain threshold value, the neuron is activated and generates an action potential of its own which is propagated along its axon, and the process is repeated.

Neurons are involved in every conceivable action taken by the body, whether it is to control their own internal environment or to respond to changes in the external world. As a result, they are responsible for such essential functions as:

- Accepting and converting sensory information into a form that can be processed within the nervous system by other neurons
- Processing and analyzing this information so that an "integrated portrait" of the incoming data can be obtained
- Translating the final outcome or "decision" of this analysis process into appropriate electrical or chemical form needed to stimulate glands or activate muscles

Evolution has played a significant role in the development of these unique neurons and in the arrangement and development of interconnections between nerve cells in the various parts of the brain. Since the brain is a most complex organ, it contains numerous regions designed for specific tasks. One might, in fact, consider it to be a collection of organs arranged together to act in the harmony of activity we recognize as the individual's state of consciousness or as life itself. Over the years, anatomists and physiologists have identified and named most pathways (tracts), most groups of neurons (nuclei), and most of the major parts of the human brain. Such attention to detail is certainly not necessary here. It will serve our purpose to simply provide a broad overview of the organization of the brain and speak of three general regions: the brainstem, the cerebellum, and the cerebral cortex.

The brainstem, or old brain, is really an extension and elaboration of the spinal chord. This section of the brain evolved first and is the location of all the centers that control the regulatory systems, such as respiration, necessary for physical survival of the organism. In addition, all sensory pathways find their way into the brainstem, thereby permitting the integration of complex input patterns to take place within its domain.

Above the brainstem is a spherical mass of neuronal tissue called the cerebellum. This remarkable structure is a complex monitor and modifier of body movements. The cerebellum does not initiate movements, but only modifies motor control activated in other areas. Cerebellar operation is not only dependent on evolutionary

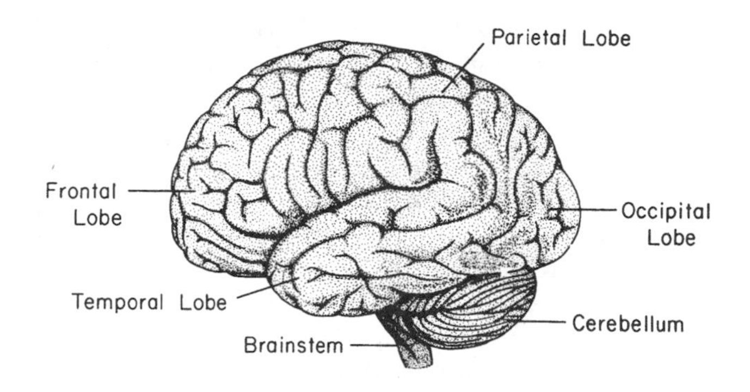

FIGURE 9.2 Major divisions of the cerebral cortex.

development, but relies heavily on actual use and patterns of learned motor behavior acquired throughout life. It is for this reason that the movements of a gymnast are smooth and seemingly effortless.

The most conspicuous part of all in the human brain is the cerebral cortex. Compared to most mammals, it is so large in man that it becomes a covering that surrounds and hides most of the other regions of the brain. Wrinkled and folded, the cerebral tissue is literally pressed into the limited space allocated to it. Although it has been possible to ascertain that certain cortical areas such as the visual cortex, the sensory projection area, and the motor strip are associated with specific functions, the overall operation of this complex structure is still not completely understood. However, for the sake of convenience, it has been arbitrarily divided (based primarily on anatomical considerations) into the following areas: frontal lobe, parietal lobe, temporal lobe, and occipital lobe (Figure 9.2). Each of these segments of the cortex, which is the source of intellectual and imaginative capacities, includes millions of neurons and a host of interconnections.

It is generally agreed that brain function is based on the organization of the activity of large numbers of neurons into coherent patterns. Since the primary mode of activity of these nerve cells is electrical in nature, it is not surprising that a composite of this activity can be detected in the form of electrical signals. Of extreme interest, then, are the actual oscillations, rhythms, and patterns seen in the cryptic flow of electrical energy coming from the brain itself, i.e., in the EEG.

Historical Perspective

In 1875, Caton published the initial account of the recording of the spontaneous electrical activity of the brain from the cerebral cortex of an experimental animal. The amplitude of these electrical oscillations was so low, that is, on the order of microvolts, that Caton's discovery is all the more amazing because it was made 50 years before suitable electronic amplifiers became available. In 1924, Hans Berger, of the University of Jena in Austria, carried out the first human EEG recordings using electrical metal strips pasted to the scalps of his subjects as electrodes and a sensitive galvanometer as the recording instrument. Berger was able to measure the irregular, relatively small electrical potentials (i.e., 50 to 100 μV) coming from the brain. By studying the successive positions of the moving element of the galvanometer recorded on a continuous roll of paper, he was able to observe the resultant patterns in these brain waves as they varied with time. From 1924 to 1938, Berger laid the foundation for many of the present applications of electroencephalography. He was the first to use the word *electroencephalogram* in describing these brain potentials in man. Berger noted that these brain waves were not entirely random, but instead displayed certain periodicities and regularities. For example, he observed that although these brain waves were slow (i.e., exhibited a synchronized patter of high amplitude and low frequency, $<$3 Hz) in sleep and states of depressed function, they were faster (i.e., exhibited a desynchronized pattern of low amplitude and high frequency, 15 to 25 Hz) during waking behavior. He suggested, quite correctly, that the brain's activity changed in a consistent and recognizable fashion when the general status of the subject changed, as from relaxation to alertness. Berger also concluded that these brain waves could be greatly affected by certain pathological conditions after noting the marked increase in the amplitude of these brain waves brought about by convulsive seizures. However, despite the insights provided by these studies, Berger's original paper published in 1929 did not invite much attention. In essence, the efforts of this most remarkable pioneer were largely ignored until similar investigations were carried out and verified by British investigators.

It was not until 1934 when Adrian and Matthews published their classic paper verifying Berger's findings that the reality of human brain waves was accepted and EEG studies were put on a firmly established basis. One of their primary contributions was the identification of certain rhythms in the EEG, regular oscillations at approximately 10 to 12 Hz in the occipital lobes of the cerebral cortex. They found that this alpha rhythm in the EEG would disappear when the brain displayed any type of attention or alertness or focused on objects in the visual field. The physiological basis for these results, the "arousing influence" of external stimuli on the cortex, was not formulated until 1949 when Moruzzi and Magoun demonstrated the existence of widely spread pathways through the central reticular core of the brainstem capable of exerting a diffuse activating influence on the cerebral cortex. This reticular activating system has been called the brain's response selector because it alerts the cortex to focus on certain incoming information while ignoring other. It is for this reason that a sleeping mother will immediately be awakened by her crying baby or the smell of smoke, and yet ignores the traffic outside her window or the television still playing in the next room. An in-depth discussion of these early studies is beyond the scope of this presentation; however, for the interested reader an excellent historical review of this early era in brain research has been recorded in a fascinating text by Brazier (1968).

EEG Recording Techniques

Scalp recordings of spontaneous neuronal activity in the brain, identified as the EEG, allow measurement of potential changes over time between a signal electrode and a reference electrode (Kondraski, 1986). Compared to other biopotentials, such as the electrocardiogram, the EEG is extremely difficult for an untrained observer to interpret. As might be expected, partially as a result of the spatial mapping of functions onto different regions of the brain, correspondingly different waveforms are visible, depending on electrode placement. Recognizing that some standardization was necessary for comparison of research as well as clinical EEG records, the International Federation in Electroencephalography and Clinical Neurophysiology adopted the 10 to 20 electrode placement system (Jasper, 1958). Additional electrodes to monitor extracerebral contaminants of the EEG such as eye movement, EKG, and muscle activity are essential. The acquisition of EEG for quantitative analysis should also require the ability to view the EEG during collection on a polygraph or high-resolution video display.

Since amplification, filtering, and digitization determine the frequency characteristics of the EEG and the source of potential artifacts, the acquisition parameters must be chosen with an understanding of their effects on signal acquisition and subsequent analysis. Amplification, for example, increases the amplitude range (volts) of the analog-to-digital converter (ADC). The resolution of the ADC is determined by the smallest amplitude of steps that can be sampled. This is calculated by dividing the voltage range of the ADC by 2 to the power of the number of bits of the ADC. For example, an ADC with a range of ± 5 V with 12-bit resolution can resolve samples as small as ± 2.4 mV. Appropriate matching of amplification and ADC sensitivity permits resolution of the smallest signal while preventing clipping of the largest signal amplitudes.

The bandwidth of the filters and the rate of digitization determine the frequency components of interest that are passed, while other frequencies outside the band of interest that may represent potential artifacts, such as aliasing, are rejected. A filter's characteristics are determined by the rate of the amplitude decrease at the bandwidth's upper and lower edges. Proper digital representation of the analog signal depends on the rate of data sampling, which is governed by the Nyquist theorem that states that data sampling should be at least twice the highest frequency of interest.

In addition to the information available from spontaneous electrical activity of the EEG, the brain's electrical response to sensory stimulation can contribute data as to the status of cortical and subcortical regions activated by sensory input. Because of the relatively small amplitude of a stimulus-evoked potential as compared to the spontaneous EEG potentials, the technique of signal averaging is used to enhance the stimulus-evoked response. Stimulus averaging takes advantage of the fact that the brain's electrical response is time-locked to the onset of the stimulus and the nonevoked background potentials are randomly distributed in time. Consequently, the average of multiple stimulus responses will result in the enhancement of time-locked activity, while the averaged random background activity will approach zero. The result is an evoked response that consists of a number of discrete and replicable peaks that occur, depending upon the stimulus and the recording parameters, at predicted latencies from the onset of stimulation. The spatial localization of maximum peak amplitudes has been associated with cortical generators in primary sensory cortex.

Instrumentation required for EEG recordings can be simple or elaborate (Kondraski, 1986). (Note: Although the discussion presented in this section is for a single-channel system it can be extended to simultaneous multichannel recordings simply by multiplying the hardware by the number of channels required. In cases that do not require true simultaneous recordings, special electrode selector panels can minimize hardware requirements.) Any EEG system consists of electrodes, amplifiers (with appropriate filters) and a recording device.

Commonly used scalp electrodes consist of Ag-AgCl disks, 1 to 3 mm in diameter, with a very flexible long lead that can be plugged into an amplifier. Although it is desirable to obtain a low-impedance contact at the electrode–skin interface (less than 10 kΩ), this objective is confounded by hair and the difficulty of mechanically stabilizing the electrodes. Conductive electrode paste helps obtain low impedance and keep the electrodes in place. A type of cement (collodion) is used to fix small patches of gauze over electrodes for mechanical stability, and leads are usually taped to the subject to provide some strain relief. Slight abrasion of the skin is sometimes used to obtain better electrode impedances, but this can cause irritation and sometimes infection (as well as pain in sensitive subjects).

For long-term recordings, as in seizure monitoring, electrodes present major problems. Needle electrodes, which must be inserted into the tissue between the surface of the scalp and skull, are sometimes useful. However, the danger of infection increases significantly. Electrodes with self-contained miniature amplifiers are somewhat more tolerant because they provide a low-impedance source to interconnecting leads, but they are expensive. Despite numerous attempts to simplify the electrode application process and to guarantee long-term stability, none has been widely accepted.

Instruments are available for measuring impedance between electrode pairs. The procedure is recommended strongly as good practice, since high impedance leads to distortions that may be difficult to separate from actual EEG signals. In fact, electrode impedance monitors are built into some commercial devices for recording EEGs. Standard dc ohmmeters should not be used, since they apply a polarizing current that causes build-up of noisy electrode potential at the skin–electrode interface. Commercial devices apply a known-amplitude sinusoidal voltage (typically 1 kHz) to an electrode pair circuit and measure root mean square (rms) current, which is directly related to the magnitude of the impedance.

From carefully applied electrodes, signal amplitudes of 1 to 10 μV can be obtained. Considerable amplification (gain $= 10^6$) is required to bring these levels up to an acceptable level for input to recording devices. Because of long electrode leads and the common electrically noisy environment where recordings take place, differential amplifiers with inherently high input impedance and high common mode rejection ratios are essential for high-quality EEG recordings.

In some facilities, special electrically shielded rooms minimize environmental electrical noise, particularly 60-Hz alternating current (ac) line noise. Since much of the information of interest in the EEG lies in the frequency bands less than 40 Hz, low-pass filters in the amplifier can be switched into attenuate 60-Hz noise sharply.

For attenuating ac noise when the low-pass cutoff is greater than 60 Hz, many EEG amplifiers have notch filters that attenuate only frequencies in a narrow band centered around 60 Hz. Since important signal information may also be attenuated, notch filtering should be used as a last resort; one should try to identify and eliminate the source of interference instead.

In trying to identify 60-Hz sources to eliminate or minimize their effect, it is sometimes useful to use a dummy source, such as a fixed 100-kΩ resistor attached to the electrodes. An amplifier output represents only contributions from interfering sources. If noise can be reduced to an acceptable level (at least by a factor of ten less than EEG signals) under this condition, one is likely to obtain uncontaminated EEG records.

Different types of recording instruments obtain a temporary or permanent record of the EEG. The most common recording device is a pen or chart recorder (usually multichannel) that is an integral part of most commercially available EEG instruments. The bandwidth of clinical EEGs is relatively low (less than 40 Hz) and therefore within the frequency response capabilities of these devices. Recordings are on a long sheet of continuous paper (from a folded stack), fed past the moving pen at one of several selectable constant speeds. The paper speed translates into distance per unit time or cycles per unit time, to allow EEG interpreters to identify different frequency components or patterns within the EEG. Paper speed is selected according to the monitoring situation at hand: slow speeds (10 mm/sec) for observing the spiking characteristically associated with seizures and faster speeds (up to 120 mm/sec) for the presence of individual frequency bands in the EEG.

In addition to (or instead of) a pen recorder, the EEG may be recorded on a multichannel frequency modulated (FM) analog tape recorder. During such recordings, a visual output device such as an oscilloscope or video display is necessary to allow visual monitoring of signals, so that corrective action (reapplying the electrodes and so on) can take place immediately if necessary.

Sophisticated FM cassette recording and playback systems allow clinicians to review long EEG recordings over a greatly reduced time, compared to that required to flip through stacks of paper or observe recordings as they occur in real time. Such systems take advantage of time compensation schemes, whereby a signal recorded at one speed (speed of the tape moving past the recording head of the cassette drive) is played back at a different, faster speed. The ratio of playback to recording speed is known, so the appropriate correction factor can be applied to played-back data to generate a properly scaled video display. A standard ratio of 60:1 is often used. Thus, a trained clinician can review each minute of real-time EEG in 1 sec. The display appears to be scrolled at a high rate horizontally across the display screen. Features of these instruments allow the clinician to freeze a segment of EEG on the display and to slow down or accelerate tape speed from the standard playback as needed. A time mark channel is usually displayed as one of the traces as a convenient reference (vertical "tick" mark displayed at periodic intervals across the screen).

Computers can also be recording devices, digitizing (converting to digital form) one or several amplified EEG channels at a fixed rate. In such sampled data systems, each channel is repeatedly sampled at a fixed time interval (sample interval), and this sample is converted into a binary number representation by an ADC. The ADC is interfaced to a computer system so that each sample can be saved in the computer's memory. A set of such samples, acquired at a sufficient sampling rate (at least two times the highest frequency component in the sampled signal), is sufficient to represent all the information in the waveform. To ensure that the signal is band-limited, a low-pass filter with a cutoff frequency equal to the highest frequency of interest is used. Since physically realizable filters do not have the ideal characteristics, the sampling rate is usually greater than two times the filter's cutoff frequency. Furthermore, once converted to a digital format, digital filtering techniques can be used.

On-line computer recordings are only practical for short-term recordings, or for situations in which the EEG is immediately processed. This limitation is primarily due to storage requirements. For example, a typical sampling rate of 128 Hz yields 128 new samples per second that require storage. For an eight-channel recording, 1024 samples are acquired per second. A 10-minute recording period yields 614,400 data points. Assuming 8-bit resolution per sample, over 0.5 megabyte (MB) of storage is required to save the 10-minute recording.

Processing can consist of compression for more efficient storage (with associated loss of total information content), as in data record or epoch averaging associated with evoked responses, or feature extraction and subsequent pattern recognition, as in automated spike detection in seizure monitoring.

Frequency Analysis of the EEG

In general, the EEG contains information regarding changes in the electrical potential of the brain obtained from a given set of recording electrodes. These data include the characteristic waveform with its variation in amplitude, frequency, phase, etc. and the occurrence of brief electrical patterns, such as spindles. Any analysis procedure cannot simultaneously provide information regarding all of these variables. Consequently, the selection of any analytic technique will emphasize changes in one particular variable at the expense of the others. This observation is extremely important if one is to properly interpret the results obtained by any analytic technique. In this chapter, special attention is given to frequency analysis of the EEG.

In early attempts to correlate the EEG with behavior, analog frequency analyzers were used to examine single channels of EEG data. Although disappointing, these initial efforts did introduce the utilization of frequency analysis to study gross brain wave activity. Although, *power spectral analysis*, i.e., the magnitude square of Fourier transform, provides a quantitative measure of the frequency distribution of the EEG, it does so as mentioned above, at the expense of other details in the EEG such as the amplitude distribution, as well as the presence of specific patterns in the EEG.

The first systematic application of power spectral analysis by general-purpose computers was reported in 1963 by Walter; however, it was not until the introduction of the *fast Fourier transform (FFT)* by Cooley and Tukey in the early 1970s that machine computation of the EEG became commonplace. Although an individual FFT is ordinarily calculated for a short section of EEG data (e.g., from 1 to 8 sec epoch), such segmentation of a signal with subsequent averaging over individual modified periodograms has been shown to provide a consistent estimator of the power spectrum, and an extension of this technique, the compressed spectral array, has been particularly useful for computing EEG spectra over long periods of time. A detailed review of the development and use of various methods to analyze the EEG is provided by Givens and Redmond (1987).

Figure 9.3 provides an overview of the computational processes involved in performing spectral analysis of the EEG, i.e., including computation of auto and *cross-spectra* (Bronzino, 1984). It is to be noted that the power spectrum is the autocorrellogram, i.e., the correlation of the signal with itself. As a result, the power

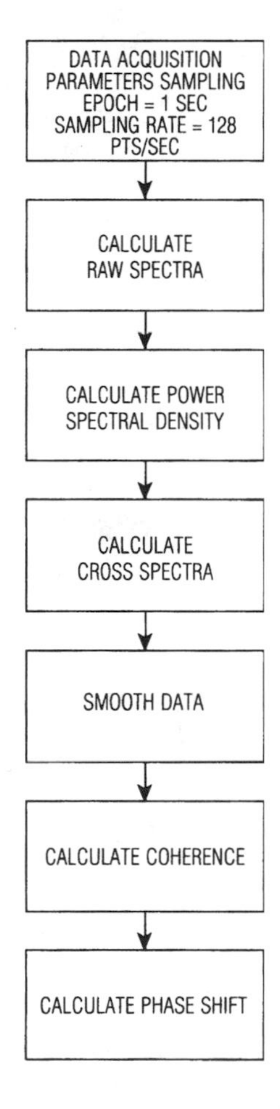

FIGURE 9.3 Block diagram of measures determined from spectral analysis.

spectrum provides only magnitude information in the frequency domain; it does not provide any data regarding phase. The power spectrum is computed by:

$$P(f) = \mathrm{Re}^2[X(f)] + \mathrm{Im}^2[X(f)] \tag{9.1}$$

where $X(f)$ is the Fourier transform of the EEG.

Power spectral analysis not only provides a summary of the EEG in a convenient graphic form, but also facilitates statistical analysis of EEG changes, which may not be evident on simple inspection of the records. In addition to absolute power derived directly from the power spectrum, other measures calculated from absolute power have been demonstrated to be of value in quantifying various aspects of the EEG. Relative power expresses the percent contribution of each frequency band to the total power and is calculated by dividing the power within a band by the total power across all bands. Relative power has the benefit of reducing the intersubject variance associated with absolute power that arises from intersubject differences in skull and scalp conductance. The disadvantage of relative power is that an increase in one frequency band will be reflected in the calculation by a decrease in other bands; for example, it has been reported that directional shifts between high and low frequencies are associated with changes in cerebral blood flow and metabolism. Power ratios between low (0 to 7 Hz) and high (10 to 20 Hz) frequency bands have been demonstrated to be an accurate estimator of changes in cerebral activity during these metabolic changes.

Although the power spectrum quantifies activity at each electrode, other variables derivable from FFT offer a measure of the relationship between activity recorded at distinct electrode sites. Coherence (which is a complex number), calculated from the cross-spectrum analysis of two signals, is similar to cross-correlation in the time domain. The *magnitude squared coherence* (*MSC*) values range from 1 to 0, indicating maximum or no synchrony, respectively, and are independent of power. The temporal relationship between two signals is expressed by phase, which is a measure of the lag between two signals for common frequency components or bands. Phase is expressed in units of degrees, 0° indicating no time lag between signals and 180° if the signals are of opposite polarity. Phase can also be transformed into the time domain, giving a measure of the time difference between two frequencies.

Cross-spectrum is computed by:

$$\text{cross-spectrum} = X(f)Y^*(f) \tag{9.2}$$

where $X(f)$, $Y(f)$ are Fourier transforms and * indicates complex conjugates and coherence is calculated by

$$\text{coherence} = \frac{\text{cross-spectrum}}{\sqrt{PX(f) - PY(f)}} \tag{9.3}$$

Since coherence is a complex number, the phase is simply the angle associated with the polar expression of that number. MSC and phase represent measures that can be employed to investigate the cortical interactions of cerebral activity. For example, short (intracortical) and long (cortico-cortical) pathways have been proposed as the anatomic substrate underlying the spatial frequency and patterns of coherence. Therefore, discrete cortical regions linked by such fiber systems should demonstrate a relatively high degree of synchrony, whereas the time lag between signals, as represented by phase, quantifies the extent to which one signal leads another.

Nonlinear Analysis of the EEG

As mentioned earlier, the EEG has been studied extensively using signal-processing schemes, most of which are based on the assumption that the EEG is a linear, Gaussian process. Although linear analysis schemes are computationally efficient and useful, they only utilize information retained in the autocorrelation function (i.e., the second-order cumulant). Additional information stored in higher-order cumulants is therefore ignored by linear analysis of the EEG. Thus, while the power spectrum provides the energy distribution of a stationary process in the frequency domain, it cannot distinguish nonlinearly coupled frequencies from spontaneously generated signals with the same resonance condition (Nikias and Raghvveer, 1987).

There is evidence showing that the amplitude distribution of the EEG often deviates from Gaussian behavior. It has been reported, for example, that the EEGs of humans involved in the performance of mental arithmetic tasks exhibit significant non-Gaussian behavior. In addition, the degree of deviation from Gaussian behavior of the EEG has been shown to depend to the behavioral state, with the state of slow-wave sleep showing less Gaussian behavior than quiet waking, which is less Gaussian than rapid eye movement (REM) sleep (Ning and Bronzino, 1989; Ferri et al., 2002, 2003). Nonlinear signal-processing algorithms such as bispectral analysis are therefore necessary to address non-Gaussian and nonlinear behavior of the EEG in order to better describe it in the frequency domain.

What exactly is the bispectrum? For a zero-mean, stationary process $\{X(k)\}$, the bispectrum, by definition, is the Fourier transform of its third-order cumulant (TOC) sequence:

$$B(\omega_1, \omega_2) = \sum_{m=-\alpha}^{a} \sum_{n=-\alpha}^{a} C(m, n) e^{-j(w_1 m + w_2 n)} \tag{9.4}$$

The TOC sequence $\{C(m, n)\}$ is defined as the expected value of the triple product:

$$C(m, n) = E\{X(k)X(k+m)X(k+n)\} \tag{9.5}$$

If process $X(k)$ is purely Gaussian, then its third-order cumulant $C(m, n)$ is zero for each (m, n), and consequently, its Fourier transform, the bispectrum, $B(\omega_1, \omega_2)$ is also zero. This property makes the estimated bispectrum an immediate measure describing the degree of deviation from Gaussian behavior. In our studies (Ning and Bronzino, 1989), the sum of magnitude of the estimated bispectrum was used as a measure to describe the EEG's deviation from Gaussian behavior, that is:

$$D = \sum_{(\omega_1, \omega_2)} |B(\omega_1, \omega_2)|$$

Using bispectral analysis, the existence of significant *quadratic phase coupling* (*QPC*) in the hippocampal EEG obtained during REM sleep in the adult rat was demonstrated (Ning and Bronzino, 1989, 1990). The result of this nonlinear coupling is the appearance, in the frequency spectrum, of a small peak centered at approximately 13 to 14 Hz (beta range) that reflects the summation of the two theta frequency (i.e., in the 6- to 7-Hz range) waves. Conventional power spectral (linear) approaches are incapable of distinguishing the fact that this peak results from the interaction of these two generators and is not intrinsic to either.

To examine the phase relationship between nonlinear signals collected at different sites, the cross-bispectrum is also a useful tool. For example, given three zero-mean, stationary processes $x_j(n)j = 1, 2, 3\}$, there are two conventional methods for determining the cross-bispectral relationship, direct and indirect. Both methods first divide these three processes into M segments of shorter but equal length. The direct method computes the Fourier transform of each segment for all three processes and then estimates the cross-bispectrum by taking the average of triple products of Fourier coefficients over M segments, that is:

$$B_{x_1 x_2 x_3}(\omega_1, \omega_2) = \frac{1}{M} \sum_{m=1}^{M} X_1^m(\omega_1) X_2^m(\omega_2) X_3^{m^*}(\omega_1 + \omega_2) \tag{9.7}$$

where $X_j^m(\omega)$ is the Fourier transform of the mth segment of $\{x_j(n)\}$, and * indicates the complex conjugate.

The indirect method computes the third-order cross-cumulant sequence for all segments:

$$C^m_{x_1x_2x_3}(k,l) = \sum_{n\in\tau} x_1^m(n)x_2^m(n+k)x_3^m(n+l) \tag{9.8}$$

where τ is the admissible set for argument n. The cross-cumulant sequences of all segments will be averaged to give a resultant estimate:

$$C_{x_1x_2x_3}(k,l) = \frac{1}{M}\sum_{m=1}^{M} C^m_{x_1x_2x_3}(k,l) \tag{9.9}$$

The cross-bispectrum is then estimated by taking the Fourier transform of the third-order cross-cumulant sequence:

$$B_{x_1x_2x_3}(\omega_1,\omega_2) = \sum_{k=-\alpha}^{\alpha}\sum_{l=-\alpha}^{\alpha} C_{x_1x_2x_3}(k,l)^{-j(\omega_1 k+\omega_2 l)} \tag{9.10}$$

Since the variance of the estimated cross-bispectrum is inversely proportional to the length of each segment, computation of the cross-bispectrum for processes of finite data length requires careful consideration of both the length of individual segments and the total number of segments to be used.

The cross-bispectrum can be applied to determine the level of cross-QPC occurring between $\{x_1(n)\}$ and $\{x_2(n)\}$ and its effects on $\{x_3(n)\}$. For example, a peak at $Bx_1x_2x_3(\omega_1, \omega_2)$ suggests that the energy component at frequency $\omega_1 + \omega_2$ of $\{x_3(n)\}$ is generated due to the QPC between frequency ω_1 of $\{x_1(n)\}$ and frequency ω_2 of $\{x_2(n)\}$. In theory, the absence of QPC will generate a flat cross-bispectrum. However, due to the finite data length encountered in practice, peaks may appear in the cross-bispectrum at locations where there is no significant cross-QPC. To avoid improper interpretation, the cross-bicoherence index, which indicates the significance level of cross-QPC, can be computed as follows:

$$\mathrm{bic}_{x_1x_2x_3}(\omega_1,\omega_2) = \frac{B_{x_1x_2x_3}(\omega_1,\omega_2)}{\sqrt{P_{x_1}(\omega_1)P_{x_2}(\omega_2)P_{x_3}(\omega_1+\omega_2)}} \tag{9.11}$$

where $P_{xj}(\omega)$ is the power spectrum of process $\{x_j(n)\}$. The theoretical value of the bicoherence index ranges between 0 and 1, i.e., from nonsignificant to highly significant.

In situations where the interest is the presence of QPC and its effects on $\{x(n)\}$, the cross-bispectrum equations can be modified by replacing $\{x_1(n)\}$ and $\{x_3(n)\}$ with $\{x(n)\}$ and $\{x_2(n)\}$ with $\{y(n)\}$, that is:

$$B_{xyz}(\omega_1,\omega_2) = \frac{1}{M}\sum_{m=1}^{M} X^m(\omega_1)Y^m(\omega_2)X^{m^*}(\omega_1+\omega_2) \tag{9.12}$$

In theory, both methods will lead to the same cross-bispectrum when data length is infinite. However, with finite data records, direct and indirect methods generally lead to cross-bispectrum estimates with different shapes (Figure 9.4). Therefore, like power spectrum estimation, users have to choose an appropriate method to extract the information desired.

Topographic Mapping

Computerized tomography (CT) and magnetic resonance imaging (MRI) have demonstrated the impact of spatial displays on data interpretation and analysis. Similarly, mapping techniques have been applied to electrophysiologic data to depict the spatial information available from multi-electrode recordings. This effort has been assisted by the development and implementation of low-cost, high-resolution graphic displays on

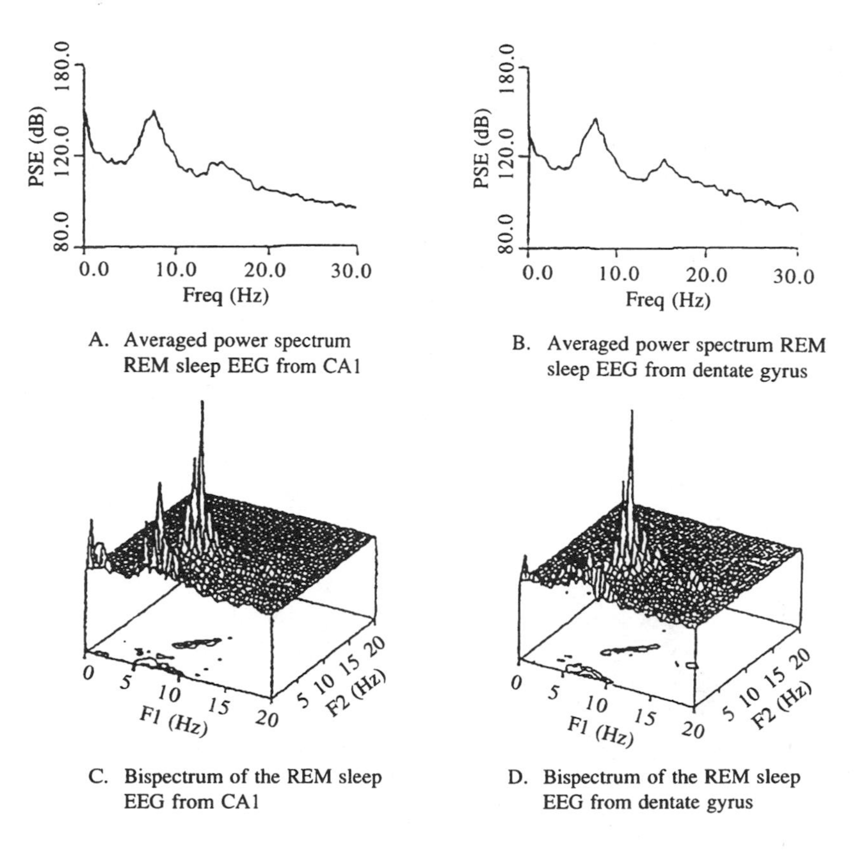

A. Averaged power spectrum REM sleep EEG from CA1

B. Averaged power spectrum REM sleep EEG from dentate gyrus

C. Bispectrum of the REM sleep EEG from CA1

D. Bispectrum of the REM sleep EEG from dentate gyrus

FIGURE 9.4 A and B represent the averaged power spectra of 80 4-sec epochs of REM sleep (sampling rate = 128 Hz) obtained from hippocampal CA1 and the dentate gyrus, respectively. Note that both spectra exhibit clear power peaks at 7-Hz (theta) and 14-Hz (beta) frequencies. C and D represent the bispectrum of these same epochs from CA1 and the dentate gyrus, respectively. Computation of the bicoherence index at 7 Hz shows significant quadratic phase coupling at this frequency, indicating that the 14-Hz peak is not spontaneously generated, but results from quadratic phase coupling.

microcomputer systems. The data are frequently presented as two-dimensional topographic color maps (Zappulla, 1991). In the time domain, color values depict the changes in potential across the scalp at each time point. This is exemplified by mapping peaks of an evoked potential or the spatial distribution of an epileptic spike. Temporal changes in the spatial distribution of voltage can be presented graphically as a series of maps constructed at adjacent time points or by cartooning the topographic maps over the time interval of interest. In the frequency domain, color coding can be used to spatially map power, covariance, and phase values. These maps may be constructed for the broadband activity or for selective frequency components.

Unlike CT and MRI displays where each picture element or pixel value represents real data, most of the pixels comprising an EEG and ER topographic map consist of interpolated values. This is because the activity from a finite number of electrodes represents a sampling of the spatial activity over the scalp. Consequently, the remaining values of the map located outside the electrode positions must be estimated from this sampled activity. One technique for deriving these values is linear interpolation. In the case of a four-point interpolation, the map is divided into boxes whose corners are defined by real data. The interpolated points within the boxes are calculated by the weighted sum of the four real data points, based on their distance from the interpolated point. Although linear interpolation is the most popular technique, polynomial regression and surface spline interpolation have been employed as alternative procedures. These methods reduce the discontinuities inherent in linear interpolation and offer better estimates of extreme values. Polynomial regression has the additional advantage of permitting quantitative comparisons between maps by taking into account the topographic information represented in the map.

Maps can be presented in any of several projections to assist in interpretation (Zappulla, 1991). The most common projection is the top view which presents the spatial distribution of variables from all leads simultaneously. Lateral, posterior, and anterior projections highlight focal areas of interest. Although mapping presents a method by which spatial information can be efficiently communicated, it is important to be alert to the artifacts that can arise from map construction and manipulation. Topographic spatial artifacts that can lead to misinterpretation include ring enhancement around a spike using source-derivation references, spatial aliasing arising from linear interpolation which causes maximal activity to be mapped at electrode sites, the enhancement of activity away from the midline, and the attenuation of midline activity on amplitude asymmetry maps (centrifugal effect).

The quality of the spatial information derivable from EEG recordings depends upon the number of recording electrodes, the choice of the reference electrode, and the conductive properties of intracranial and extracranial structures. The localization of cortical activity from scalp recordings assumes that the potentials recorded from the scalp reflect cortical activity generated in proximity to the recording electrode. Therefore, the greater the density of recording electrodes, the more accurate the estimate of the spatial distribution of scalp potentials and the localization of cortical generators. However, since the distance between the cortical source and recording electrode, as well as the low conductivity of the skull, results in a selective attenuation of small dipole fields, most available EEG information can be obtained with an average scalp–electrode spacing of 2 cm.

Topographic maps are constructed from monopolar electrodes referenced to a common cephalic (linked ears or mandible, chin and nose) or noncephalic (linked clavicles or a balanced sternum-vertebra) electrode. Although the reference electrode should be free of any EEG activity, in practice most cephalic electrodes contain some EEG activity, while noncephalic electrodes are a potential source of EKG or muscle activity. Differential amplification of an EEG-contaminated reference electrode can decrease or cancel similar activity in neighboring electrodes, while at electrodes distant from the reference, the injected activity will be present as a potential of opposite polarity. Similarly, noncerebral potentials can be injected into scalp electrodes and misinterpreted as cerebral activity. Therefore, a nonneutral reference electrode can result in misleading map configurations. Several techniques have been applied to circumvent this problem. The construction of multiple maps using several different references can sometimes assist in differentiating active and reference electrode activity. This can be accomplished by acquiring serial EEG records using different references. Alternatively, various references can be acquired simultaneously during acquisition, and various montages can be digitally reconstructed, post hoc.

A more computationally intensive method for localizing a source at an electrode involves calculating the local source activity at any one electrode based on the average activity of its neighbors, weighted by their distance from the source. The technique has the advantage of suppressing potentials that originate outside the measurement area and weighing factors for implementing source deviation techniques for each of the electrodes in the 10 to 20 system are available.

Another reference technique, the average head reference, uses the average activity of all active electrodes as the common reference. In this approach, the activity at any one electrode will vary depending upon the activity at the site of the reference electrode, which can be anywhere on the recording montage. Therefore, for N number of recording electrodes, each being a potential reference, there are $N - 1$ possible voltage measurements at each instant of time for each electrode. Maps constructed using the average head reference represent a unique solution to the problem of active reference electrodes in that the average reference produces an amplitude-weighted reference-free map of maximal and minimal field potentials. Power maps constructed from the average reference best depict the spatial orientation of the generating field, and the areas with extreme values are closest to the generating processes (Zappulla, 1991).

Topographical maps represent an efficient format for displaying the extensive amount of data generated by quantitative analysis. However, for reasons discussed above, the researcher and clinician must be cautious in deriving spatial and functional conclusions from mapped data. Although the replicability of map configurations across subjects or experimental conditions may represent a useful basis for experimental and diagnostic classification, judgments concerning the localization of cortical generators or functional localization of cerebral activity are less certain and more controversial. Research continues on defining models and validating assumptions that relate scalp potentials to cortical generators in an attempt to arrive at accurate mathematical solutions that can be applied to mapping functions.

Defining Terms

Bispectra: Computation of the frequency distribution of the EEG exhibiting nonlinear behavior.

Cross spectra: Computation of the energy in the frequency distribution of two different electrical signals.

Electroencephalogram (EEG): Recordings of the electrical potentials produced by the brain.

Fast Fourier transform (FFT): Algorithms that permit rapid computation of the Fourier transform of an electrical signal, thereby representing it in the frequency domain.

Magnitude squared coherence (MSC): A measure of the degree of synchrony between two electrical signals at specific frequencies.

Power spectral analysis: Computation of the energy in the frequency distribution of an electrical signal.

Quadratic phase coupling: A measure of the degree to which specific frequencies interact to produce a third frequency.

References

M. Brazier, *Electrical Activity of the Nervous System*, 3rd ed., Baltimore, MD: Williams and Wilkins, 1968.

J.D. Bronzino, M. Kelly, and C. Cordova, "Utilization of amplitude histograms to quantify the EEG: effects of systemic administration of morphine in the chronically implanted rat," *IEEE Trans. Biomed. Eng.*, vol. 28, no. 10, p. 673, 1981.

J.D. Bronzino, "Quantitative analysis of the EEG: general concepts and animal studies," *IEEE Trans. Biomed. Eng.*, vol. 31, no. 12, p. 850, 1984.

J.W. Cooley and J.S. Tukey, "An algorithm for the machine calculation of complex Fourier series," *Math. Comput.*, vol. 19, p. 267, 1965.

R. Ferri, L. Parrino, A. Smerieri, M.G. Terzano, M. Elia, S.A. Musumeci, S. Pettinato, and C.J. Stam, "Nonlinear EEG measures during sleep: effects of the different sleep stages and cyclic alternating pattern," *Int. J. Psychophysiol.*, vol. 43, no. 3, pp. 273–286, 2002.

R. Ferri, R. Chiaramonti, M. Elia, S.A. Musumeci, A. Ragazzoni, and C.J. Stam, "Nonlinear EEG analysis in premature and full-term newborns," *Clin. Neurophysiol.*, vol. 114, no. 7, pp. 1176–1180, 2003.

A.S. Givens and A. Remond, Eds., "Methods of analysis of brain electrical and magnetic signals," in *EEG Handbook*, vol. 1, Amsterdam: Elsevier, 1987.

S.M. Kay and S.L. Maple, "Spectrum analysis—a modern perspective," *Proc. IEEE.*, vol. 69, p. 1380, 1981.

E.R. Kandel, J.H. Schwartz, and T.M. Jessel, *Principles of Neural Science*, 4th ed., New York: McGraw-Hill, 2000.

G.V. Kondraski, "Neurophysiological measurements," in *Biomedical Engineering and Instrumentation*, J.D. Bronzino, Ed., Boston, MA: PWS Publishing, pp. 138–179, 1986.

C.L. Nikias and M.R. Raghuveer, "Bispectrum estimation: a digital signal processing framework," *Proc. IEEE*, vol. 75, p. 869, 1987.

T. Ning and J.D. Bronzino, "Bispectral analysis of the rat EEG during different vigilance states," *IEEE Trans. Biomed. Eng.*, vol. 36, no. 4, p. 497, 1989

T. Ning and J.D. Bronzino, "Autoregressive and bispectral analysis techniques: EEG applications, Special Issue on Biomedical Signal Processing," *IEEE Eng. Med. Biol. Mag.*, vol. 9, p. 47, 1990.

J.R. Smith, "Automated analysis of sleep EEG data," in *Clinical Applications of Computer Analysis of EEG and Other Neurophysiological Signals*, EEG Handbook, revised series, vol. 2, Amsterdam: Elsevier, 1986, pp. 93–130.

Further Information

The Biomedical Engineering Handbook, J.D. Bronzino, Ed., Boca Raton, FL: CRC Press, 1st ed. 1995, 2nd ed. 2000.

See also the journals, *Annals of Biomedical Engineering: IEEE Transactions in Biomedical Engineering* and *Electroencephalography and Clinical Neurophysiology.*

9.2 The Electrocardiograph

Edward J. Berbari

An electrocardiogram (ECG) is the recording on the body surface of the electrical activity generated by the heart. It was originally observed by Waller in 1889 using his pet bulldog as the signal source and the capillary electrometer as the recording device. In 1903, Einthoven enhanced the technology by using the string galvanometer as the recording device and using human subjects with a variety of cardiac abnormalities. Einthoven is chiefly responsible for introducing some concepts still in use today including the labeling of the various waves, defining some of the standard recording sites using the arms and legs, and developing the first theoretical construct whereby the heart is modeled as a single time-varying dipole. We also owe the "EKG" acronym to Einthoven's native Dutch language where the root word "cardio" is spelled with a "k."

In order to record an ECG waveform, a differential recording between two points on the body is made. Traditionally, each differential recording is referred to as a lead. Einthoven defined three leads numbered with the Roman numerals I, II, and III. They are defined as:

$$\mathrm{I} = V_{\mathrm{LA}} - V_{\mathrm{RA}}$$

$$\mathrm{II} = V_{\mathrm{LL}} - V_{\mathrm{RA}}$$

$$\mathrm{III} = V_{\mathrm{LL}} - V_{\mathrm{LA}}$$

where RA = right arm, LA = left arm, and LL = left leg. Because the body is assumed to be purely resistive at ECG frequencies, the four limbs can be thought of as wires attached to the torso. Hence, lead I could be recorded from the respective shoulders without a significant loss of cardiac information. Note that these three leads are not independent and the following relationship holds:

$$\mathrm{II} = \mathrm{I} + \mathrm{III}$$

In the 30 years following Einthoven's work, several additions were made complementing his work and evolving into the standard ECG still used today. F. N. Wilson (1934) added concepts of a "unipolar" recording. He created a reference point by tying the three limbs together and averaging their potentials so that individual recording sites on the limbs or chest surface would be differentially recorded with the same reference point. Investigators in this era incorrectly deduced that the average of these three time-varying potentials would be zero. This so-called physiological zero, while not correct, continues to serve as a reference point for the so-called unipolar leads. Wilson extended the biophysical models to include the concept of the cardiac source enclosed within the volume conductor of the body. However, from the mid-1930s until today the 12 leads composed of the three limb leads, three leads in which the limb potentials are referenced to a modified Wilson terminal, the augmented leads (Goldberger, 1942), and six leads placed across the front of the chest and referenced to the Wilson terminal form the basis of the standard 12-lead ECG, summarized in Figure 9.5. These sites are historically based, have a built-in redundancy, and are not optimal for all cardiac events. The voltage difference from any two sites will record an ECG, but it is these standardized sites with the massive 100-year collection of empirical observations that has firmly established their role as the standard.

Figure 9.6 is a stylized ECG recording from lead II. Einthoven chose the letters of the alphabet from P to U to label the waves and to avoid conflict with other physiologic waves being studied at the turn of the century. The ECG signals are typically in the range of ± 2 mV and require a recording bandwidth of 0.05 to 150 Hz. Full technical specification for ECG equipment has been proposed by both the American Heart Association (1984) and the Association for the Advancement of Medical Instrumentation (Bailey et al., 1990).

There have been several attempts to change the approach for recording the ECG. The vectorcardiogram used a weighted set of recording sites to form an orthogonal *XYZ* lead set. The advantage here was a

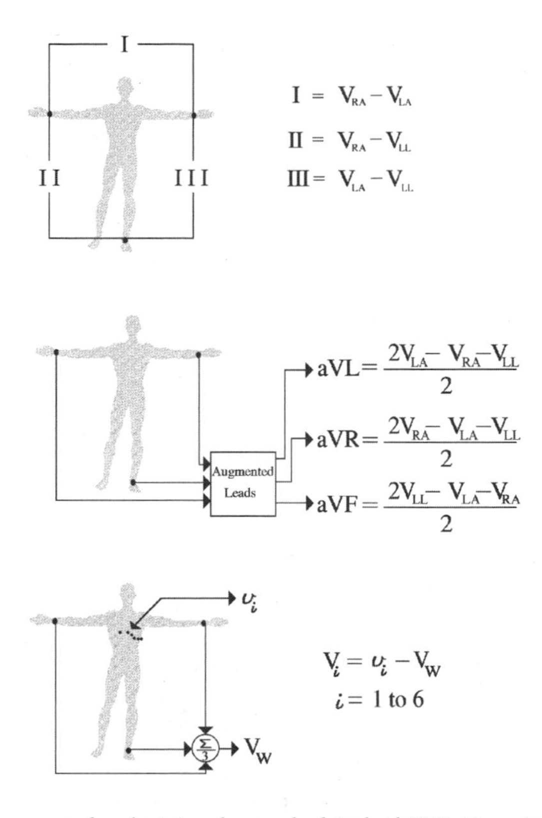

FIGURE 9.5 Lead placements for obtaining the standard 12-lead ECG. V_W = Wilson Central Terminal.

minimum lead set, but in practice it gained only a moderate degree of enthusiasm among physicians. Body-surface mapping refers to the use of many recording sites (>64) arranged on the body so that isopotential surfaces could be computed and analyzed over time. This approach still has a role in research investigations. Other subsets of the 12-lead ECG are used in limited mode recording situations such as the tape recorded ambulatory ECG (usually two leads), or in intensive care monitoring at the bedside (usually one or two leads), or telemetered within regions of the hospital from patients who are not confined to bed (one lead). Another approach is to use a few leads and, using a transform matrix, convert it to the standard 12-lead ECG

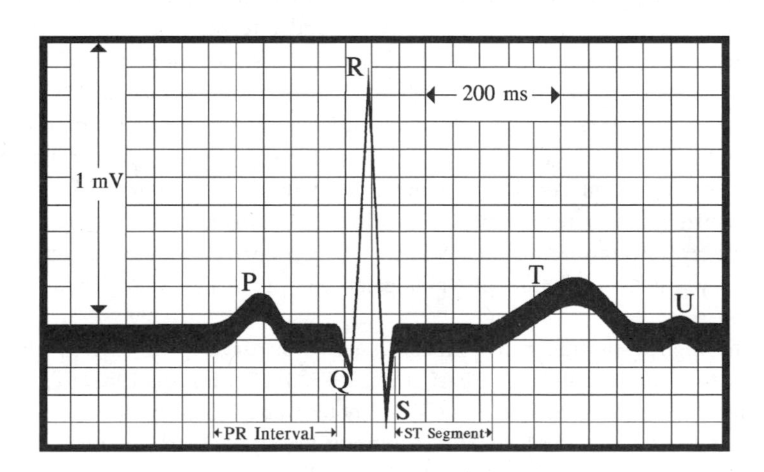

FIGURE 9.6 Schematic of a lead II ECG showing the standard waves and intervals.

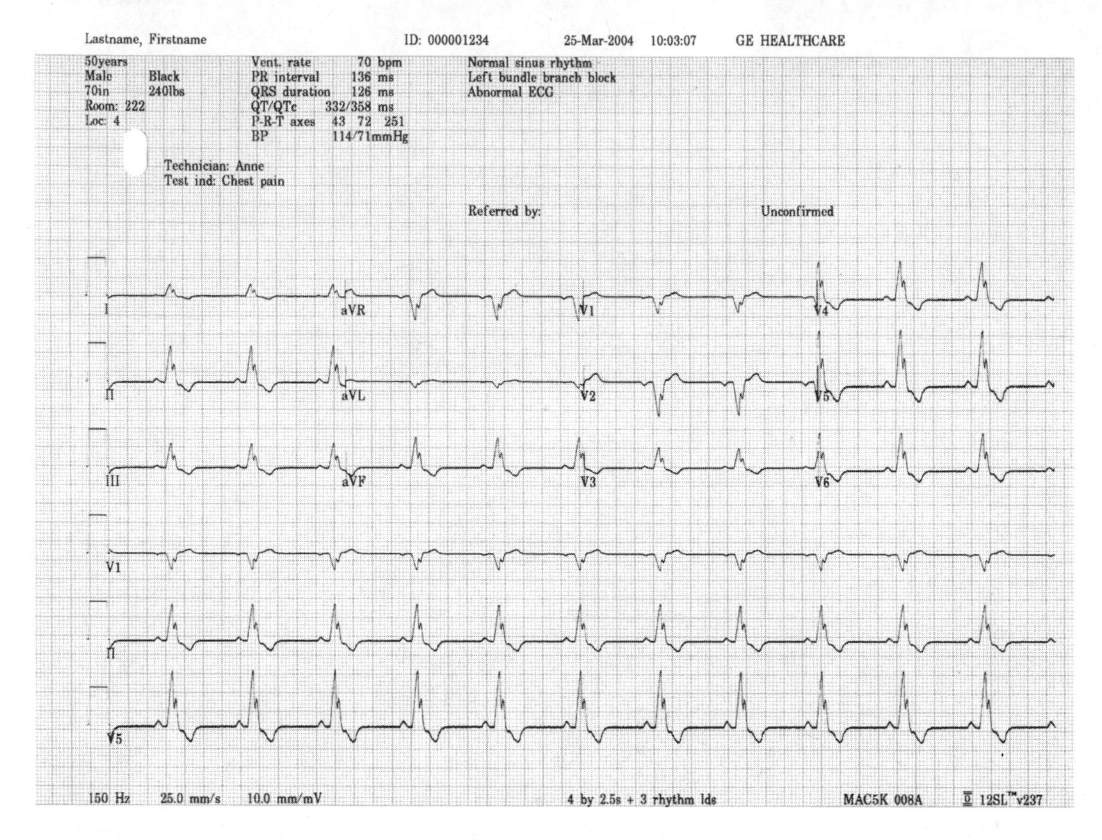

FIGURE 9.7 An example of a 12-lead ECG recording obtained with a computer based, interpretive electrocardiograph. The measurements and diagnostic statements were obtained automatically via software programs. (Diagram courtesy of GE Healthcare Technologies, Waukesha, WI.)

(Dower et al., 1988). The recording electronics of these ECG systems have followed the typical evolution of modern instrumentation, e.g., vacuum tubes, transistors, ICs, and microprocessors.

Application of computers to the ECG for machine interpretation was one of the earliest uses of computers in medicine (Jenkins, 1981). Of primary interest in computer-based systems was the replacement of the human reader and the elucidation of the standard waves and intervals. Originally, this was performed by linking the ECG machine to a centralized computer via phone lines. The modern ECG machine is completely integrated with an analog front end, a 12- to 16-bit A/D converter, a computational microprocessor, and dedicated I/O processors. These systems compute a measurement matrix derived from the 12-lead signals and analyze this matrix with a set of rules to obtain the final set of interpretive statements. The depiction of the 12 analog signals and this set of interpretive statements form the final output, with an example shown in Figure 9.7. The physician will over-read each ECG and modify or correct those statements which are deemed inappropriate. The larger hospital-based system will record these corrections and maintain a large database of all ECGs accessible by any combination of parameters, e.g., all males, older than 50, with an inferior myocardial infarction.

More recently, the high-resolution ECG (HRECG) has been developed whereby the digitized ECG is signal averaged to reduce random noise (Berbari et al., 1973, 1977; Simson, 1981). This approach, coupled with post averaging high-pass filtering, is used to detect and quantify low-level signals ($\sim$1.0 μV) not detectable with standard approaches. This computer-based approach has enabled the recording of events which are predictive of future life-threatening cardiac events (Simson et al., 1981; Berbari and Steinberg, 2000).

Physiology

The heart has four chambers: the upper two chambers are called the atria and the lower two chambers are called the ventricles. The atria are thin-walled, low-pressure pumps, that receive blood from venous circulation. Located in the top right atrium is a group of cells that act as the primary pacemaker of the heart. Through a complex change of ionic concentration across the cell membranes (the current source), an extracellular potential field is established, which then excites neighboring cells and a cell-to-cell propagation of electrical events occurs. Because the body acts as a purely resistive medium, these potential fields extend to the body surface (Geselowitz, 1989). The character of the body-surface waves depends upon the amount of tissue activating at one time and the relative speed and direction of the activation wavefront. Therefore, the pacemaker potentials, which are generated by a small tissue mass, are not seen on the ECG. As the activation wavefront encounters the increased mass of atrial muscle, the initiation of electrical activity is observed on the body surface, and the first ECG wave of the cardiac cycle is seen. This is the P wave and it represents activation of the atria. Conduction of the cardiac impulse proceeds from the atria through a series of specialized cardiac cells (the AN node and the His-Purkinje system), which again are too small in total mass to generate a signal large enough to be seen on the standard ECG. There is a short, relatively isoelectric segment following the P wave. Once the large muscle mass of the ventricles is excited, a rapid and large deflection is seen on the body surface. The excitation of the ventricles causes them to contract and provides the main force for circulating blood to the organs of the body. This large wave appears to have several components. The initial downward deflection is called the Q wave, the initial upward deflection is the R wave, and the second downward deflection is the S wave. The polarity and actual presence of these three components depends upon the position of the leads on the body as well as a multitude of abnormalities that may exist. In several pathologies there are sequential waves named as R′ or S′, but in general, the large ventricular waveform is generically called the QRS complex regardless of its makeup. Following the QRS complex is another short, relatively isoelectric segment. After this short segment, the ventricles return to their electrical resting state, and a wave of repolarization is seen as a low-frequency signal called the T wave. In some individuals, a small peak occurs at the end or after the T wave and is called the U wave. Its origin has never been fully established but is believed to be a repolarization potential.

Instrumentation

The general instrumentation requirements for the ECG have been addressed by professional societies through the years (American Heart Association, 1984; Bailey et al., 1990). Briefly, they recommend a system bandwidth 0.05 to 150 Hz. Of great importance in ECG diagnosis is the low-frequency response of the system because shifts in some of the low-frequency regions, e.g., the ST segment, have critical diagnostic value. While the heart rate may only have a 1-Hz fundamental frequency, the phase response of typical analog high-pass filters is such that the system corner frequency must be much smaller than the 3-dB corner frequency where only the amplitude response is considered. The system gain depends upon the total system design. The typical ECG amplitude is ± 2 mV, and if A/D conversion is used in a digital system, then enough gain to span the only 20% of the ADC's dynamic range is needed. This margin allows for recording abnormally large signals as well as accommodating baseline drift if present and not corrected.

To first obtain an ECG, the patient must be physically connected to the amplifier front end. The patient–amplifier interface is formed by a special bioelectrode that converts the ionic current flow of the body to the electron flow of the metallic wire. These electrodes typically rely on a chemical paste or gel with a high ionic concentration. This acts as the transducer at the tissue–electrode interface. For short-term applications, silver-coated suction electrodes or "sticky" metallic foil electrodes are used. Long-term recordings, such as the case for the monitored patient, require a stable electrode–tissue interface and special adhesive tape material surrounds the gel and an Ag^+/AgCl electrode.

At any given time, the patient can be connected to a variety of devices, e.g., respirator, blood pressure monitor, temporary pacemaker, etc., some of which will invade the body and provide a low-resistance pathway to the heart. It is essential that the device not act as a current source and inject the patient with enough current to stimulate the heart and cause it to fibrillate. Some bias currents are unavoidable for the system input stage, and recommendations are that these leakage currents be less than 10 μA per device. In recent years, there has been some controversy regarding the level of allowable leakage current. The Association for the Advancement of Medical Instrumentation (1993) has written its standards to allow leakage currents as high as 50 μA. Recent studies (Swerdlow et al., 1999; Malkin et al., 2001) have shown that there may be complex and lethal physiological response to 60 Hz currents as low as 32 μA. In light of the reduced standards, these research results were commented on by members of the American Heart Association Committee on Electrocardiography (Laks et al., 2000).

There is also a 10-μA maximum current limitation due to a fault condition if a patient comes in contact with the high voltage side of the ac power lines. In this case, the isolation must be adequate to prevent 10 μA of fault current as well. This mandates that the ECG reference ground not be connected physically to the low side of the ac power line or its third wire ground. For ECG machines, the solution has typically been to AM modulate a medium-frequency carrier signal (400 kHz) and use an isolation transformer with subsequent demodulation. Other methods of signal isolation can be used, but the primary reason for the isolation is to keep the patient from being part of the ac circuit in the case of a patient to power line fault. In addition, with many devices connected in a patient monitoring situation, it is possible that ground loop currents will be generated. To obviate this potential hazard, a low-impedance ground buss is often installed in these rooms and each device chassis will have an external ground wire connected to the buss. Another unique feature of these amplifiers is that they must be able to withstand the high-energy discharge of a cardiac defibrillator.

A typical ECG amplifier is based on the three op-amp instrumentation amplifier. The patient is dc coupled to the two high impedance inputs of the instrumentation amplifier. The first stage of gain is relatively low ($\sim$100), because there can be a significant signal drift due to a high static charge on the body or low-frequency offset potentials generated by the electrolyte in the tissue/electrode interface. In this particular amplifier the signal is bandpass filtered prior to the isolation stage. To further limit the high floating potential of the patient

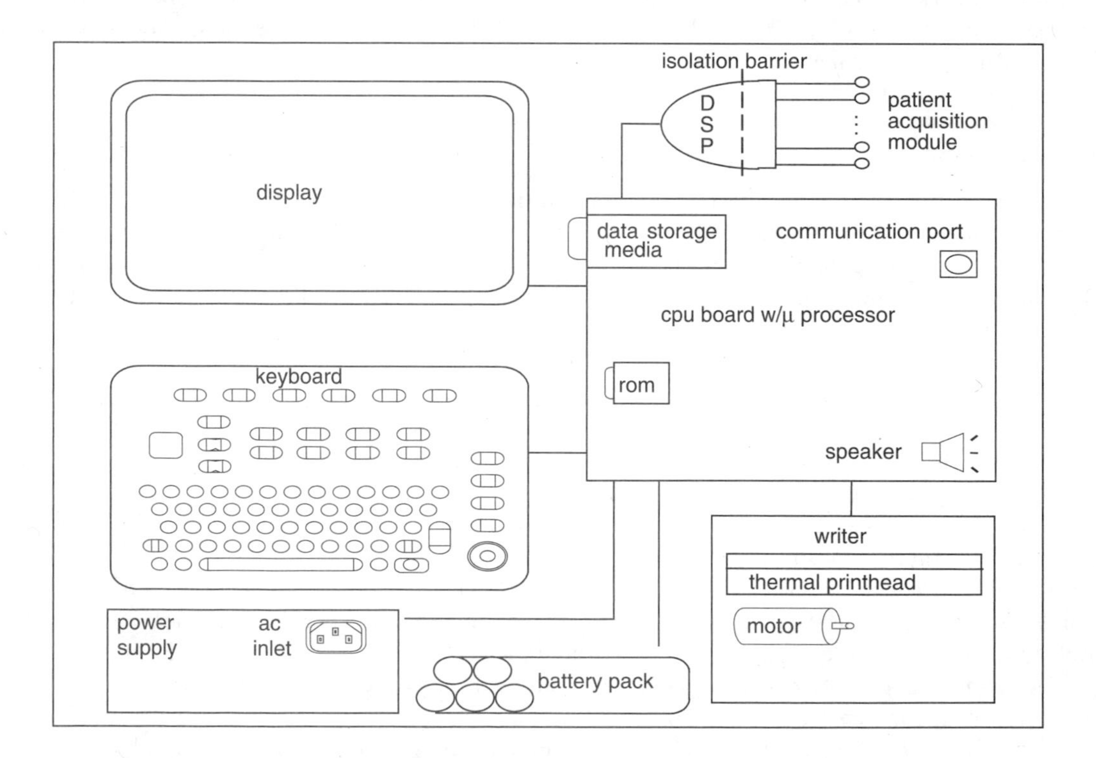

FIGURE 9.8 Block diagram of a modern computer-based electrocardiograph. (Diagram courtesy of GE Healthcare Technologies, Waukesha, WI.)

and to improve the system common mode rejection a driven ground is usually used. This ground is simply an average of the limb potentials inverted by a single amplifier and connected to the right leg.

Older-style ECG machines recorded one lead at a time, then evolved to three simultaneous leads. This necessitated the use of switching circuits as well as analog weighting circuits to generate the various 12 leads. This is usually eliminated in modern digital systems by using an individual single-ended amplifier for each electrode on the body. Each potential signal is then digitally converted and all of the ECG leads can be formed mathematically in software. This would necessitate a nine-amplifier system. By performing some of the lead calculations with the analog differential amplifiers, this can be reduced to an eight-channel system. Thus, only the individual chest leads V_I to V_6 and any two of the limb leads, e.g., I and III, are needed to calculate the full 12-lead ECG. Figure 9.8 is a block diagram of a modern digital-based ECG system and represents a fully integrated multi-microprocessor based data acquisition and display system. This system uses up to 13 single-ended amplifiers and a 16-bit ADC, all within a small lead wire manifold or amplifier lead stage. The digital signals are optically isolated and sent via a high-speed serial link to the main ECG instrument. Here the 32-bit CPU and DSP chip perform all of the calculations, and a hard copy report is generated as shown in Figure 9.8. Notice that each functional block has its own controller and the system requires a real-time, multi-tasking operating system to coordinate all system functions. Concomitant with data acquisition is the automatic interpretation of the ECG. These programs are quite sophisticated and are continually evolving. It is still a medical/legal requirement that these ECGs be over-read by the physician.

High-resolution capability is now a standard feature on most digitally based ECG systems or as a stand-alone microprocessor-based unit (Berbari, 1988). The most common application of the HRECG is to record

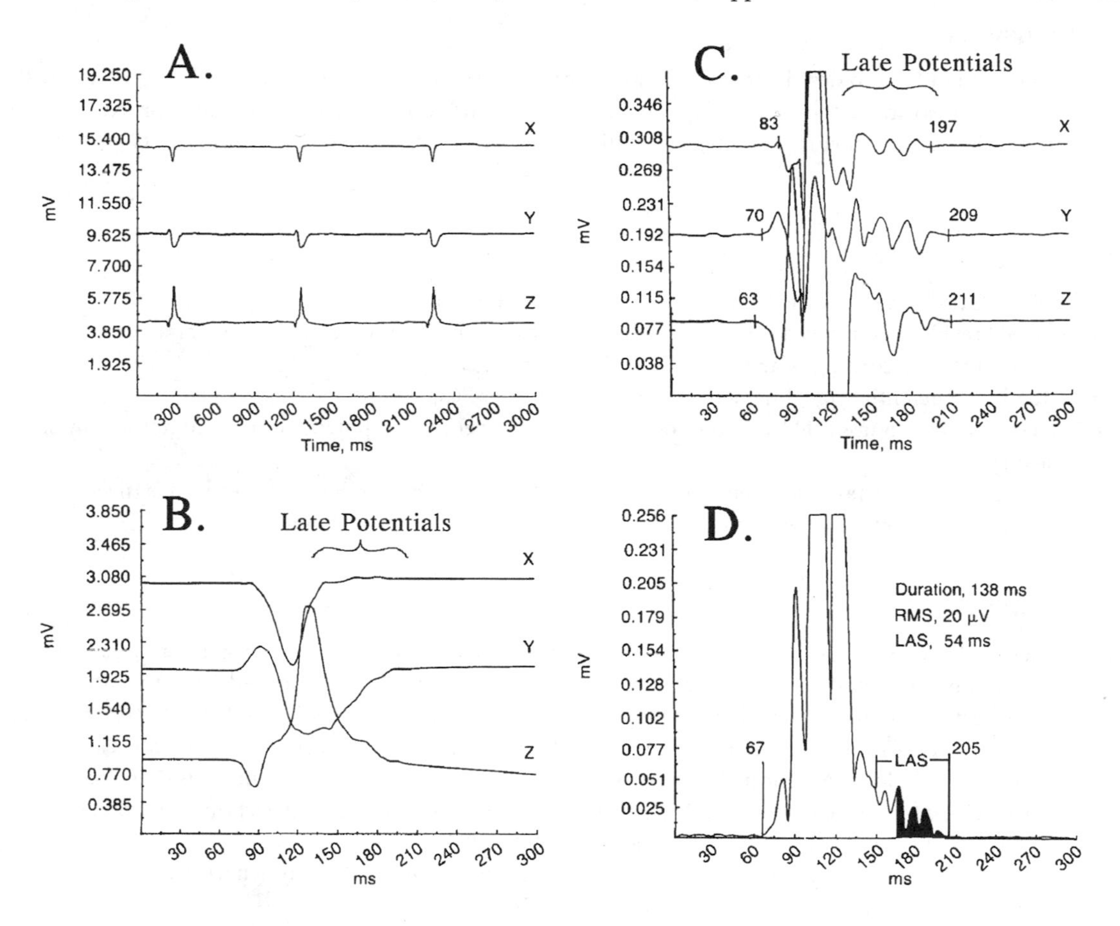

FIGURE 9.9 The processing steps (see text) used to measure cardiac late potentials via a high-resolution electrocardiograph (HRECG).

very low-level ($<1.0\ \mu V$) signals, which occur after the QRS complex, but are not evident on the standard ECG. These "late potentials" are generated from abnormal regions of the ventricles and have been strongly associated with the substrate responsible for a life-threatening rapid heart rate (ventricular tachycardia). The typical HRECG is derived from three bipolar leads configured in an anatomic *XYZ* coordinate system. These three ECG signals are then digitized at a rate of 1000 to 2000 Hz/channel, time aligned via a real-time QRS correlator, and summated in the form of a signal average. Signal averaging will theoretically improve the signal-to-noise ratio by the square root of the number of beats averaged. The underlying assumptions are that the signals of interest do not vary, on a beat-to-beat basis, and that the noise is random. Figure 9.9 has four panels depicting the most common sequence for processing the HRECG to measure the late potentials. Panel A depicts a 3-sec recording of the *XYZ* leads close to normal resolution. Panel B was obtained after averaging 200 beats and with a sampling frequency of ten times that shown in panel A. The gain is also 5 times greater. Panel C is the high-pass filtered signal using a partially time reversed digital filter having a second-order Butterworth response and a 3-dB corner frequency of 40 Hz (Simson, 1981). Note the appearance of the signals at the terminal portion of the QRS complex. A common method of analysis, but necessarily optimal, is to combine the filtered *XYZ* leads into a vector magnitude $(X^2 + Y^2 + Z^2)^{1/2}$. This waveform is shown in panel D. From this waveform, several parameters have been derived such as total QRS duration, including late potentials, the rms voltage value of the terminal 40 ms, and the low-amplitude signal (LAS) duration from the 40-μV level to the end of the late potentials. Abnormal values for these parameters are used to identify patients at high risk of ventricular tachycardia following a heart attack.

Conclusions

The ECG is one of the oldest instrument-bound measurements in medicine. It has faithfully followed the progression of instrumentation technology. Its most recent evolutionary step, to the microprocessor-based system, has allowed for an enhanced, high-resolution ECG, which has opened new vistas of ECG analysis and interpretation.

Defining Terms

12-lead ECG: Twelve traditional ECG leads comprising the standard set.

ECG: Abbreviation for the device (electrocardiograph) or the output (electrocardiogram) depicting the body surface recording of the electrical activity of the heart.

ECG lead: Differential signal depicting one channel of the ECG record.

HRECG: High-resolution ECG used to detect microvolt-level cardiac potentials most commonly by signal averaging.

Wilson central terminal: Reference point for forming most of the standard ECG leads. It is the average of the right arm, left arm, and left leg potentials. It is a time-varying reference.

References

J.J. Bailey, A.S. Berson, A. Carson, L.G. Horan, P.W. Macfarlane, D.W. Mortara, and C. Zywietz, "Recommendations for standardization and specifications in automated electrocardiography: bandwidth and digital signal processing," A report for health professionals by an ad hoc writing group of the Committee on Electrocardiography and Cardiac Electrophysiology of the Council on Clinical Cardiology, American Heart Association, *Circulation*, vol. 81, no. 2, pp. 730–739, 1990.

E.J. Berbari, R. Lazzara, P. Samet, and B.J. Scherlag, "Noninvasive technique for detection of electrical activity during the PR segment," *Circulation*, vol. 48, p. 1006, 1973.

E.]. Berbari, R. Lazzara, and B.J. Scherlag, "A computerized technique to record new components of the electrocardiogram," *Proc. IEEE*, vol. 65, p. 799, 1977.

E.J. Berbari, B.J. Scherlag, R.R. Hope, and R. Lazzara, "Recording from the body surface of arrhythmogenic ventricular activity during the ST segment," *Am. J. Cardiol.*, vol. 41, p. 697, 1978.

G.E. Dower, A. Yakush, S.B. Nazzal, R.V. Jutzy, and C.E. Ruiz, "Deriving the 12-lead electrocardiogram from four (EASI) electrodes," *J. Electrocardiol.*, vol. 21, Suppl. S182-7, 1988.

W. Einthoven, "Die galvanometrische Registrirung des menschlichen Elektrokardiogramms, zugleich eine Beurtheilung der Anwendung des Capillar-Elecktrometers in der Physiologic," *Pflugers Arch. Gas. Physiol.*, vol. 99, p. 472, 1903.

D.B. Geselowitz, "On the theory of the electrocardiogram," *Proc. IEEE*, vol. 77, p. 857, 1989.

E. Goldberger, "A simple, indifferent, electrocardiographic electrode of zero potential and a technique of obtaining augmented, unipolar, extremity leads," *Am. Heart J.*, vol. 23, p. 483, 1942.

J.M. Jenkins, "Computerized electrocardiography," *CRC Crit. Rev. Bioeng.*, vol. 6, p. 307, 1981.

R.A. Malkin and B.K. Hoffmeister, "Mechanisms by which AC leakage currents cause complete hemodynamic collapse without inducing fibrillation. [see comment]," *J. Cardiovasc. Electrophysiol.*, vol. 12, no. 10, pp. 1154–1161, 2001.

M.M. Laks, R. Arzbaecher, D. Geselowitz, J.J Bailey, and A. Berson, "Revisiting the question: will relaxing safe current limits for electromedical equipment increase hazards to patients?," *Circulation* vol. 102, no. 8, 823–825, 2000 Aug 22

M.B. Simson, "Use of signals in the terminal QRS complex to identify patients with ventricular tachycardia after myocardial infarction," *Circulation*, vol. 64, p. 235, 1981.

C.D. Swerdlow, W.H. Olson, M.E. O'Connor, et al., "Cardiovascular collapse caused by electrocardiographically silent 60 Hz intracardiac leakage current: implications for electrical safety," *Circulation*, vol. 99, pp. 2559–2564, 1999.

Safe Current Limits for Electromedical Apparatus: American National Standard, ANSI/AAMI ES1–1993. Arlington, VA: Association for the Advancement of Medical Instrumentation; 1993.

A.D. Waller, "On the electromotive changes connected with the beat of the mammalian heart, and the human heart in particular," *Phil. Trans. B.*, vol. 180, p. 169, 1889.

E.N. Wilson, F.S. Johnston, and I.G.W. Hill, "The interpretation of the galvanometric curves obtained when one electrode is distant from the heart and the other near or in contact with the ventricular surface," *Am. Heart J.*, vol. 10, p. 176, 1934.

Further Information

P.W. Macfarlanc and T.D. Veitch Lawrie, Eds., *Comprehensive Electrocardiology: Theory and Practice in Health and Disease,* Volumes 1–3, Oxford: Pergamon Press, 1989.

E.J. Berbari and J.S. Steinberg, *A Practical Guide to High Resolution Electrocardiography*, Armonk, NY: Futura Publishers, 2000.

Webter, J.G., Ed., *Medical Instrumentation: Application and Design*, 3rd ed., Boston, MA: Houghton Mifflin, 1998.

10

Tomography

10.1 Computerized Tomography 10-1
10.2 Positron Emission Tomography 10-3
10.3 Single Photon Emission Computed Tomography 10-4
10.4 Magnetic Resonance Imaging 10-4
10.5 Imaging 10-5

Martin D. Fox
University of Connecticut

The term **tomography** derives from the Greek *tomos* (cutting) and *grapho* (to write). Originally the term was applied to sectional radiography achieved by a synchronous motion of the x-ray source and detector in order to blur undesired data while creating a sharp image of the selected plane. The term *tomography* was used to distinguish between such slices and the more conventional plain film radiograph, which represents a two-dimensional shadowgraphic superposition of all x-ray absorbing structures within a volumetric body.

Computerized tomography, also known as **computerized axial tomography,** was introduced by EMI Ltd. in 1973 and transformed medical imaging by obviating the superposition of intervening structures present in conventional radiographic images. Initially, the clinical application was for imaging the head, but soon the technique found wide application in body imaging.

As medical imaging has evolved into a multimodality field, the meaning of tomography has broadened to include any images of thin cross-sectional slices, regardless of the modality utilized to produce them. Thus, tomographic images can be generated by **magnetic resonance imaging** (MRI), ultrasound (US), computerized tomography (CT), or such nuclear medicine techniques as **positron emission tomography** (PET) or **single photon emission computerized tomography** (SPECT). For the purposes of this discussion we will cover all of the foregoing modalities with the exception of ultrasound, which will be treated separately.

Since the power of such computerized techniques was recognized, the practice of radiology has been revolutionized by making possible much more precise diagnosis of a wide range of conditions. In this necessarily brief discussion we will describe the basic physical principles of the major tomographic modalities as well as their key clinical applications.

10.1 Computerized Tomography

The basic concept of computerized tomography can be described by consideration of Figure 10.1. An x-ray source is passed through an aperture to produce a fan-shaped beam that passes through the body of interest with absorption along approximately parallel lines. The natural logarithm of the detected intensity will be the integral of the linear attenuation coefficient of the object along the ray directed from the source to the detector element. If the source and the detector array are synchronously rotated about a point within the object, a number of lines of data can be collected, each representing the projected density of the object as a function of lateral position and angle.

A number of mathematical techniques can and have been used to recover the two-dimensional distribution of the linear attenuation coefficient from this array of measurements. These include iterative solution of a set of simultaneous linear equations, Fourier transform approaches, and techniques utilizing back-projection

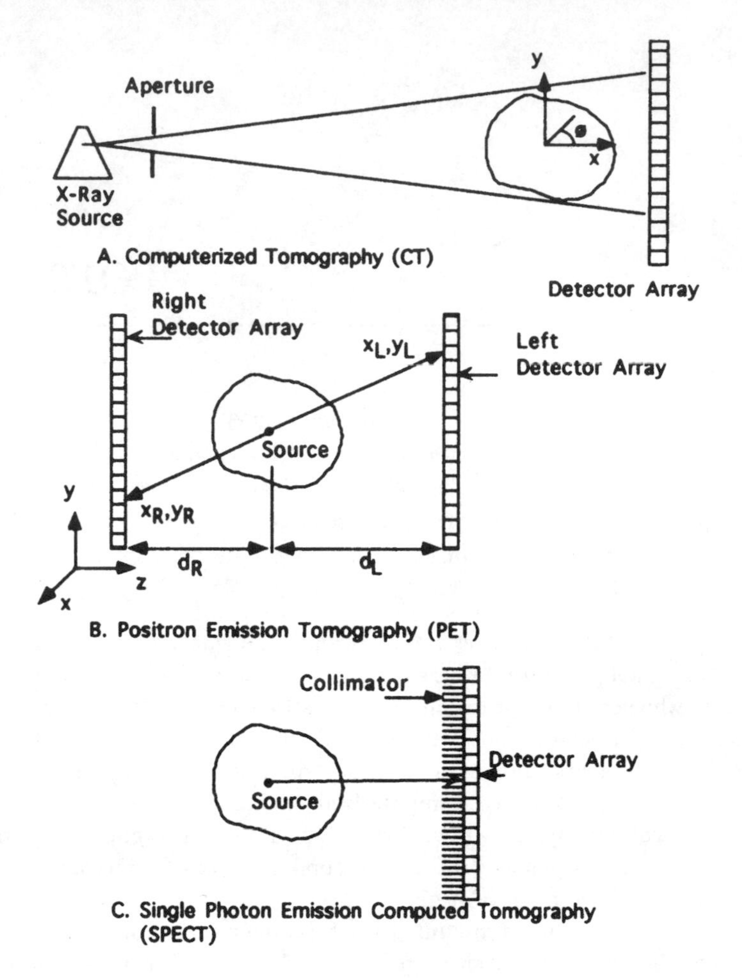

FIGURE 10.1 Comparison of three photon-based tomographic imaging modalities.

followed by deconvolution (Macovski, 1983). Conceptually, the Fourier transform approach is perhaps the most straightforward, so we will describe it in some detail.

Using the coordinate system of Figure 10.1(A) and assuming parallel rays, the intensity picked up by the detector array can be expressed as

$$I_{\mathrm{d}}(y) = I_0 \exp\left[-\int a(x,y)\mathrm{d}x\right]$$

where $a(x, y)$ represents the linear attenuation coefficient to x-ray photons within the body as a function of x, y position, and I_0 is the source intensity. Rearranging, we see that

$$a_{\mathrm{p}}(y) = \int_{-\infty}^{\infty} a(x,y)\mathrm{d}x = \ln[I_{\mathrm{d}}(y)/I_0]$$

where $a_{\mathrm{p}}(y)$ is the projected attenuation function. Taking a one-dimensional Fourier transform of this projected density function we see that

$$F[a_p(y)] = A_p(f_y) = \int_{-\infty}^{\infty}\int_{-\infty}^{\infty} a(x,y)\mathrm{d}x\, e^{-j2\pi f_y y}\mathrm{d}y$$

where $A_p(f_y)$ is the Fourier transform of a single line of detected data. However, this can also be written:

$$A_p(0, f_y) = \int_{-\infty}^{\infty}\int_{-\infty}^{\infty} a(x,y)\mathrm{d}x\, e^{-j2\pi(0x+f_y y)}\mathrm{d}y$$

Thus, the one-dimensional Fourier transform of the projection of the linear attenuation function, $a_p(y)$, is equal to the two-dimensional Fourier transform of the original attenuation function evaluated along a line in the frequency domain (in this case the $f_x = 0$ line).

It can readily be demonstrated that if we rotate a function $a(x, y)$ through an angle ϕ in the x, y plane, its transform will be similarly rotated through an angle ϕ (Castleman, 1979). Thus as we rotate the source and detector around the object, each projected density function detected $a_p(\rho, \phi_i)$ can be Fourier transformed to provide one radial line of the two-dimensional Fourier transform of the desired reconstructed image, $A(\rho, \phi_i)$, where ρ is a radial spatial frequency. The set of all $A(\rho, \phi_i)$ for small angular displacements ϕ_i form a set of spokes in the transform domain which can be interpolated to estimate $A(f_x, f_y)$, the two-dimensional Fourier transform of the image in rectangular coordinates. The image can then be recovered by inverse transformation of $A(f_x, f_y)$, which can readily be carried out digitally using fast Fourier transform algorithms, i.e.:

$$a(x,y) = F^{-1}[A(f_x, f_y)]$$

While the Fourier transform approach is mathematically straightforward, many commercial scanners utilize the equivalent but more easily implemented back-projection/deconvolution approach, where each ray is traced back along its propagation axis. When all rays have been back-projected and the result summed, one obtains an approximate (blurred) image of that plane. This image can then be sharpened (deblurred) through the use of an appropriate filter, which is usually implemented by convolving with an appropriate two-dimensional deblurring function. Refer to Macovski (1983) for the details of this process.

Clinically, the impact of computerized tomography was dramatic due to the vastly increased density resolution, coupled with the elimination of the superposition of overlying structures, allowing enhanced differentiation of tissues with similar x-ray transmittance, such as blood, muscle, and organ parenchyma. CT scans of the head are useful for evaluation of head injury and detection of tumor, stroke, or infection. In the body, CT is also excellent in detecting and characterizing focal lesions, such as tumors and abscesses, and for the evaluation of the skeletal system (Axel et al., 1983). In recent years the advent of magnetic resonance systems has provided even greater soft tissue contrast, and thus the role of CT has been constrained by this at times competing modality.

10.2 Positron Emission Tomography

Unlike CT, which relies on photons produced by an external source, in the modalities of PET and SPECT, the source of radiation is a radioisotope that is distributed within the body, and thus these modalities are sometimes referred to as forms of emission computed tomography (ECT). While conventional CT can produce images based upon anatomy of organs, emission CT techniques can quantitate the distribution of tracer materials that can potentially elucidate physiologic function.

The positron or positive electron is a positively charged particle that can be emitted from the nucleus of a radionuclide. The positron travels at most a few millimeters before being annihilated by interaction with a negative electron from the surrounding tissue. The product of this event is the emission of 511-keV gamma-ray photons which travel in almost exactly opposite directions. The detectors themselves can be either discrete detectors or a modified Anger camera like those used in conventional nuclear imaging. A coincidence detector is employed to limit recorded outputs to cases in which events are detected simultaneously in both detector arrays, thus reducing the pickup of noise or scattering.

A possible detection scheme is illustrated in Figure 10.1(B). The detector arrays shown can be made energy selective to eliminate lower energy scattered gamma rays. While the distribution of radioactivity can be reconstructed using the reconstruction from projection techniques described in the section on CT (Hurculak, 1987), the x, y source position of an event can be determined directly from the detection geometry as follows (Macovski, 1983):

$$x \approx x_L d_R/(d_R + d_L) + x_R d_L/(d_R + d_L)$$

$$y \approx y_L d_R/(d_R + d_L) + y_R d_L/(d_R + d_L)$$

Typically a single plane is studied, and no collimators are required. A drawback of PET has been that because of the short half-lives of positron-producing radioisotopes, the use of this modality has required the presence of an expensive cyclotron facility located near the hospital.

One important radionuclide commonly used in PET is oxygen 15 with a half-life of 2.07 min, which can be bonded to water for measurement of cerebral blood flow or to O_2/CO_2 to assess cerebral oxygen utilization. Another is carbon 11 with a half-life of 20.4 min, which can be bonded to glucose to trace glucose utilization. F-18 fluorodeoxyglucose (FDG) has been used to demonstrate the degree of malignancy of primary brain tumors, to distinguish necrosis from tumor, and to predict outcome (Coleman, 1991). Perhaps the most unusual feature of this modality is the ability to quantitate the regional metabolism of the human heart (Schelbert, 1990).

10.3 Single Photon Emission Computed Tomography

In contrast to PET, SPECT can be utilized with any radioisotope that emits gamma rays, including such common radioisotopes as Tc-99m, I-125, and I-131 which have been utilized in conventional nuclear imaging for the last 30 to 35 years and which due to their relatively long half-lives are available at reasonable cost at nearly every modern hospital. Because of the need for direction sensitivity of the detector, a collimator must be used to eliminate gamma rays from other than the prescribed direction, thus resulting in a 1 to 2 order of magnitude decrease in quantum efficiency as compared with PET scanning (Knoll, 1983).

The basic concept of SPECT is illustrated in Figure 10.1(C). A gamma ray photon from a radionuclide with energy above 100 keV will typically escape from the body without further interaction, and thus the body can be regarded as a transparent object with luminosity proportional to the concentration of the radionuclide at each point. The reconstruction mathematics are similar to those derived for absorption CT, with the exception that the variable reconstructed is a source distribution rather than an attenuation coefficient. Some errors can be introduced in the reconstruction because of the inevitable interaction of gamma rays with overlying tissue, even at energies above 100 keV, although this can be compensated for to some extent. Detection of scattered radiation can be reduced through the use of an energy acceptance window in the detector.

Technetium 99m can be used to tag red blood cells for blood pool measurements, human serum albumin for blood pool and protein distribution, or monoclonal antibodies for potential detection of individual tumors or blood cells. ECT techniques such as PET and SPECT follow the recent trend toward imaging techniques that image physiologic processes as opposed to anatomic imaging of organ systems. The relatively low cost of SPECT systems has led to a recent resurgence of interest in this modality.

10.4 Magnetic Resonance Imaging

The basic magnetic resonance concept has been used as a tool in chemistry and physics since its discovery by Bloch in 1946, but its use expanded tremendously in the 1980s with the development of means to represent magnetic resonance signals in the form of tomographic images. MRI is based on the magnetic properties of atomic nuclei with odd numbers of protons or neutrons, which exhibit magnetic properties because of their spin. The predominant source of magnetic resonance signals in the human body is hydrogen nuclei or protons. In the presence of an external magnetic field, these hydrogen nuclei align along the axis of the field and can precess or wobble around that field direction at a definite frequency known as the Larmour frequency. This can be expressed:

$$f_0 = \gamma H$$

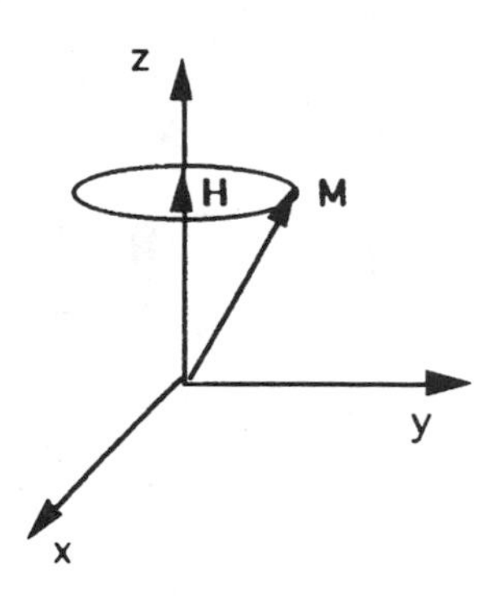

FIGURE 10.2 Geometry of precessing proton in a static magnetic field oriented in the *z* direction.

where f_0 is the Larmour frequency, γ is the gyromagnetic ratio which is a property of the atomic element, and H is the magnitude of the external magnetic field. For example, given a gyromagnetic ratio of 42.7 MHz/tesla for hydrogen and a field strength of 1 tesla (10 kilogauss), the Larmour frequency would be 42.7 MHz, which falls into the radio frequency range.

The magnetic resonance effect occurs when nuclei in a static magnetic field H are excited by a rotating magnetic field H_1 in the x, y plane, resulting in a total vector field **M** given by

$$\mathbf{M} = H\mathbf{z} + H_1(\mathbf{x}\cos\omega_0 t + \mathbf{y}\sin\omega_0 t)$$

Upon cessation of excitation, the magnetic field decays back to its original alignment with the static field H, emitting electromagnetic radiation at the Larmour frequency, which can be detected by the same coil that produced the excitation (Macovski, 1983).

10.5 Imaging

As shown in Figure 10.3, one method for imaging utilizes a transmit/receive coil to emit a magnetic field at frequency f_0 which is the Larmour frequency of plane *P*. Subsequently, magnetic gradients are applied in the y and x directions. The detected signal during the data collection window can be expressed as

$$S(t_x, t_{yi}) = \int_{-\infty}^{\infty}\int_{-\infty}^{\infty} s(x, y)\exp[-\mathrm{i}\gamma(G_x x t_x + G_y y t_{yi})]\mathrm{d}x\,\mathrm{d}y$$

where $s(x, y)$ represents the magnetic resonance signal at position (x, y) (G_x, G_y) are the x and y gradients, t_x is time within the data collection window, t_{yi} is the y direction gradient application times, and γ is the gyromagnetic ratio. The two-dimensional spatial integration is obtained by appropriate geometry of the detection coil. Collecting a number of such signals for a range of t_{yi}, we can obtain the two-dimensional function $S(t_x, t_y)$. Comparing this to the two-dimensional Fourier transform relation:

$$F(u, v) = \int_{-\infty}^{\infty}\int_{-\infty}^{\infty} f(x, y)\exp[-\mathrm{i}2\pi(ux + vy)]\mathrm{d}x\,\mathrm{d}y$$

we see that the detected signal $S(t_x, t_y)$ is the two-dimensional Fourier transform of the magnetic resonance signal $s(x, y)$ with $u = \gamma G_x t_x/2\pi$, $v = \gamma G_y t_y/2\pi$. The magnetic resonance signal $s(x, y)$ depends on the

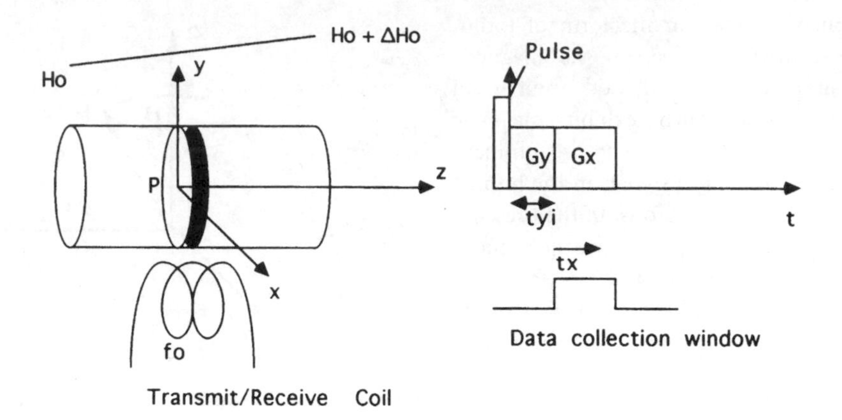

FIGURE 10.3 Concept of magnetic resonance imaging. The static magnetic field H_0 has a gradient such that excitation at frequency f_0 excites only the plane *P*. Gradient G_y in the *y* direction is applied for time t_{yi}, causing a phase shift along the *y* direction. Gradient G_x in the *x* direction is applied for time t_x, causing a frequency shift along the *x* direction. Repetition of this process for different t_{yi} allows the receive coil to pick up a signal which is the two-dimensional Fourier transform of the magnetic resonance effect within the slice.

precise sequence of pulses of magnetic energy used to perturb the nuclei. For a typical sequence known as spin-echo consisting of a 90° pulse followed by a 180° pulse spaced at time τ with the data collection at $t_e = 2\tau$, and t_r being the repetition time between 90° pulses, the detected magnetic resonance signal can be expressed:

$$s(x, y) = \rho(1 - e^{-tr}/T_1)(e^{-te}/T_2)$$

where ρ is the proton density, and T_1 (the spin-lattice decay time) and T_2 (the spin-spin decay time) are constants of the material related to the bonding of water in cells (Wolf and Popp, 1984). Typically T_1 ranges from 0.2 to 1.2 sec, while T_2 ranges from 0.05 to 0.15 sec.

By modification of the repetition and orientation of excitation pulses, an image can be made T_1, T_2, or proton density dominated. A proton density image shows static blood and fat as white and bone as black, while a T_1 weighted image shows fat as white, blood as gray, and cerebrospinal fluid as black. T_2 weighted images tend to highlight pathology since pathologic tissue tends to have longer T_2 than normal.

In general, magnetic resonance imaging has greater intrinsic ability to distinguish between soft tissues than computerized tomography. It also has some ability to visualize moving blood. As the preceding discussion indicates, magnetic resonance is a richer and more complex modality than CT. Typically MRI has been more expensive than CT. Both MRI and CT have been used primarily for anatomic imaging, but MRI has the potential through spectroscopy (visualization of other nuclei than hydrogen) to become a factor in physiologic imaging. Thus, it can be anticipated that magnetic resonance imaging will continue to increase and become an even more important modality in the next decade.

Defining Terms

Computerized axial tomography (CATscan, CT): A form of medical imaging based upon the linear attenuation coefficient of x-rays in which a tomographic image is reconstructed from computer-based analysis of a multiplicity of x-ray projections taken at different angles around the body.

Magnetic resonance imaging (MRI, NMR): A form of medical imaging with tomographic display which represents the density and bonding of protons (primarily in water) in the tissues of the body, based upon the ability of certain atomic nuclei in a magnetic field to absorb and reemit electromagnetic radiation at specific frequencies.

Positron emission tomography (PET scan): A form of tomographic medical imaging based upon the density of positron-emitting radionuclides in an object.

Single photon emission computed tomography (SPECT): A form of tomographic medical imaging based upon the density of gamma ray-emitting radionuclides in the body.

Tomography: A method of image presentation in which the data is displayed in the form of individual slices that represent planar sections of the object.

References

L. Axel, P.H. Arger, and R. Zimmerman, "Applications of computerized tomography to diagnostic radiology," in *Proc. IEEE*, vol. 71, no. 3, p. 293, 1983.

K.R. Castleman, *Digital Image Processing*, Englewood Cliffs, NJ: Prentice-Hall, 1979.

R.E. Coleman, "Single photon emission computed tomography and positron emission tomography," *Cancer*, vol. 67 (4 Suppl.), pp. 1261–1270, 1991.

P.M. Hurculak, "Positron emission tomography," *Can. J. Med. Radiat. Technol.*, vol. 18, no. 1, 1987.

G.F. Knoll, "Single-photon emission computed tomography," *Proc. IEEE*, vol. 71, no. 3, p. 320, 1983.

A. Macovski, *Medical Imaging Systems*, Englewood Cliffs, NJ: Prentice-Hall, 1983.

H.R. Schelbert, "Future perspectives: Diagnostic possibilities with positron emission tomography," *Roentgen Blaetter*, vol. 43, no. 9, pp. 384–390, 1990.

G.L. Wolf and C. Popp, *NMR, A Primer for Medical Imaging*, Thorofare, NJ: Slack, Inc., 1984.

Further Information

The journal *IEEE Transactions on Medical Imaging* describes advances in imaging techniques and image processing. *Investigative Radiology*, published by the Association of University Radiologists, emphasizes research carried out by hospital-based physicists and engineers. *Radiology*, published by the North American Society of Radiologists, contains articles which emphasize clinical applications of imaging technology. *Diagnostic Imaging*, publishing by Miller Freeman, Inc., is a good source of review articles and information on the imaging marketplace

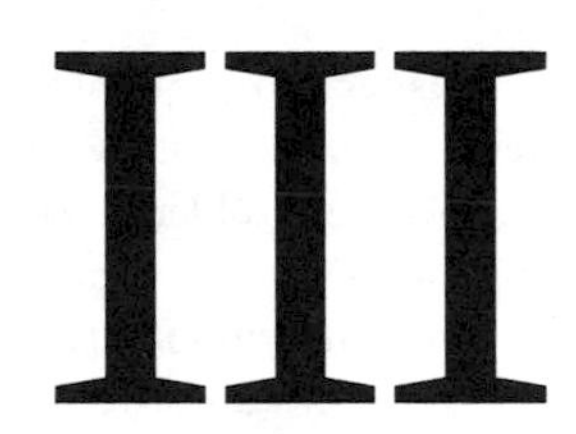

Mathematics, Symbols, and Physical Constants

Greek Alphabet III-3

International System of Units (SI) III-3
Definitions of SI Base Units • Names and Symbols for the SI Base Units • SI Derived Units with Special Names and Symbols • Units in Use Together with the SI

Conversion Constants and Multipliers III-6
Recommended Decimal Multiples and Submultiples • Conversion Factors—Metric to English • Conversion Factors—English to Metric • Conversion Factors—General • Temperature Factors • Conversion of Temperatures

Physical Constants III-8
General • π Constants • Constants Involving e • Numerical Constants

Symbols and Terminology for Physical and Chemical Quantities III-9
Classical Mechanics • Electricity and Magnetism • Electromagnetic Radiation • Solid State

Credits III-13

Probability for Electrical and Computer Engineers *Charles W. Therrien* III-14
The Algebra of Events • Probability • An Example • Conditional Probability and Bayes' Rule • Communication Example

Ronald J. Tallarida
Temple University

THE GREAT ACHIEVEMENTS in engineering deeply affect the lives of all of us and also serve to remind us of the importance of mathematics. Interest in mathematics has grown steadily with these engineering achievements and with concomitant advances in pure physical science. Whereas scholars in nonscientific fields, and even in such fields as botany, medicine, geology, etc., can communicate most of the problems and results in nonmathematical language, this is virtually impossible in present-day engineering and physics. Yet it is interesting to note that until the beginning of the twentieth century, engineers regarded calculus as something of a mystery. Modern students of engineering now study calculus, as well as differential equations, complex variables, vector analysis, orthogonal functions, and a variety of other topics in applied analysis. The study of systems has ushered in matrix algebra and, indeed, most engineering students now take linear algebra as a core topic early in their mathematical education.

This section contains concise summaries of relevant topics in applied engineering mathematics and certain key formulas, that is, those formulas that are most often needed in the formulation and solution of engineering problems. Whereas even inexpensive electronic calculators contain tabular material (e.g., tables of trigonometric and logarithmic functions) that used to be needed in this kind of handbook, most calculators do not give symbolic results. Hence, we have included formulas along with brief summaries that guide their use. In many cases we have added numerical examples, as in the discussions of matrices, their inverses, and their use in the solutions of linear systems. A table of derivatives is included, as well as key applications of the derivative in the solution of problems in maxima and minima, related rates, analysis of curvature, and finding approximate roots by numerical methods. A list of infinite series, along with the interval of convergence of each, is also included.

Of the two branches of calculus, integral calculus is richer in its applications, as well as in its theoretical content. Though the theory is not emphasized here, important applications such as finding areas, lengths, volumes, centroids, and the work done by a nonconstant force are included. Both cylindrical and spherical polar coordinates are discussed, and a table of integrals is included. Vector analysis is summarized in a separate section and includes a summary of the algebraic formulas involving dot and cross multiplication, frequently needed in the study of fields, as well as the important theorems of Stokes and Gauss. The part on special functions includes the gamma function, hyperbolic functions, Fourier series, orthogonal functions, and both Laplace and z-transforms. The Laplace transform provides a basis for the solution of differential equations and is fundamental to all concepts and definitions underlying analytical tools for describing feedback control systems. The z-transform, not discussed in most applied mathematics books, is most useful in the analysis of discrete signals as, for example, when a computer receives data sampled at some prespecified time interval. The Bessel functions, also called cylindrical functions, arise in many physical applications, such as the heat transfer in a “long” cylinder, whereas the other orthogonal functions discussed—Legendre, Hermite, and Laguerre polynomials—are needed in quantum mechanics and many other subjects (e.g., solid-state electronics) that use concepts of modern physics.

The world of mathematics, even applied mathematics, is vast. Even the best mathematicians cannot keep up with more than a small piece of this world. The topics included in this section, however, have withstood the test of time and, thus, are truly *core* for the modern engineer.

This section also incorporates tables of physical constants and symbols widely used by engineers. While not exhaustive, the constants, conversion factors, and symbols provided will enable the reader to accommodate a majority of the needs that arise in design, test, and manufacturing functions.

Mathematics, Symbols, and Physical Constants

Greek Alphabet

Greek Letter	Greek Name	English Equivalent	Greek Letter	Greek Name	English Equivalent
Α α	Alpha	a	Ν ν	Nu	n
Β β	Beta	b	Ξ ξ	Xi	x
Γ γ	Gamma	g	Ο ο	Omicron	ŏ
Δ δ	Delta	d	Π π	Pi	P
Ε ε	Epsilon	ĕ	Ρ ρ	Rho	r
Ζ ζ	Zeta	z	Σ σ	Sigma	s
Η η	Eta	ē	Τ τ	Tau	t
Θ θ ϑ	Theta	th	Υ υ	Upsilon	u
Ι ι	Iota	i	Φ ϕ φ	Phi	ph
Κ κ	Kappa	k	Χ χ	Chi	ch
Λ λ	Lambda	l	Ψ ψ	Psi	ps
Μ μ	Mu	m	Ω ω	Omega	ō

International System of Units (SI)

The International System of units (SI) was adopted by the 11th General Conference on Weights and Measures (CGPM) in 1960. It is a coherent system of units built form seven *SI base units,* one for each of the seven dimensionally independent base quantities: they are the meter, kilogram, second, ampere, kelvin, mole, and candela, for the dimensions length, mass, time, electric current, thermodynamic temperature, amount of substance, and luminous intensity, respectively. The definitions of the SI base units are given below. The *SI derived units* are expressed as products of powers of the base units, analogous to the corresponding relations between physical quantities but with numerical factors equal to unity.

In the International System there is only one SI unit for each physical quantity. This is either the appropriate SI base unit itself or the appropriate SI derived unit. However, any of the approved decimal prefixes, called *SI prefixes,* may be used to construct decimal multiples or submultiples of SI units.

It is recommended that only SI units be used in science and technology (with SI prefixes where appropriate). Where there are special reasons for making an exception to this rule, it is recommended always to define the units used in terms of SI units. This section is based on information supplied by IUPAC.

Definitions of SI Base Units

Meter: The meter is the length of path traveled by light in vacuum during a time interval of 1/299,792,458 of a second (17th CGPM, 1983).

Kilogram: The kilogram is the unit of mass; it is equal to the mass of the international prototype of the kilogram (3rd CGPM, 1901).

Second: The second is the duration of 9,192,631,770 periods of the radiation corresponding to the transition between the two hyperfine levels of the ground state of the cesium-133 atom (13th CGPM, 1967).

Ampere: The ampere is that constant current which, if maintained in two straight parallel conductors of infinite length, of negligible circular cross-section, and placed 1 m apart in vacuum, would produce between these conductors a force equal to 2×10^{-7} newton per meter of length (9th CGPM, 1948).

Kelvin: The kelvin, unit of thermodynamic temperature, is the fraction 1/273.16 of the thermodynamic temperature of the triple point of water (13th CGPM, 1967).

Mole: The mole is the amount of substance of a system which contains as many elementary entities as there are atoms in 0.012 kg of carbon-12. When the mole is used, the elementary entities must be specified and may be atoms, molecules, ions, electrons, or other particles or specified groups of such particles (14th CGPM, 1971).

Examples of the use of the mole:

1 mol of H_2 contains about 6.022×10^{23} H_2 molecules, or 12.044×10^{23} H atoms.
1 mol of HgCl has a mass of 236.04 g.
1 mol of Hg_2Cl_2 has a mass of 472.08 g.
1 mol of $Hg_2{}^{2+}$ has a mass of 401.18 g and a charge of 192.97 kC.
1 mol of $Fe_{0.91}S$ has a mass of 82.88 g.
1 mol of e^- has a mass of 548.60 μg and a charge of −96.49 kC.
1 mol of photons whose frequency is 10^{14} Hz has energy of about 39.90 kJ.

Candela: The candela is the luminous intensity in a given direction of a source that emits monochromatic radiation of frequency 540×10^{12} hertz and that has a radiant intensity in that direction of (1/683) watt per steradian (16th CGPM, 1979).

Names and Symbols for the SI Base Units

Physical Quantity	Name of SI Unit	Symbol for SI Unit
Length	meter	m
Mass	kilogram	kg
Time	second	s
Electric current	ampere	A
Thermodynamic temperature	kelvin	K
Amount of substance	mole	mol
Luminous intensity	candela	cd

SI Derived Units with Special Names and Symbols

Physical Quantity	Name of SI Unit	Symbol for SI Unit	Expression in Terms of SI Base Units	
Frequency[1]	hertz	Hz	s^{-1}	
Force	newton	N	$m\ kg\ s^{-2}$	
Pressure, stress	pascal	Pa	$N\ m^{-2}$	$= m^{-1}\ kg\ s^{-2}$
Energy, work, heat	joule	J	N m	$= m^2\ kg\ s^{-2}$
Power, radiant flux	watt	W	$J\ s^{-1}$	$= m^2\ kg\ s^{-3}$
Electric charge	coulomb	C	A s	
Electric potential, electromotive force	volt	V	$J\ C^{-1}$	$= m^2\ kg\ s^{-3}\ A^{-1}$
Electric resistance	ohm	Ω	$V\ A^{-1}$	$= m^2\ kg\ s^{-3}\ A^{-2}$
Electric conductance	siemens	S	Ω^{-1}	$= m^{-2}\ kg^{-1}\ s^3\ A^2$
Electric capacitance	farad	F	$C\ V^{-1}$	$= m^{-2}\ kg^{-1}\ s^4\ A^2$
Magnetic flux density	tesla	T	$V\ s\ m^{-2}$	$= kg\ s^{-2}\ A^{-1}$
Magnetic flux	weber	Wb	V s	$= m^2\ kg\ s^{-2}\ A^{-1}$
Inductance	henry	H	$V\ A^{-1}\ s$	$= m^2\ kg\ s^{-2}\ A^{-2}$
Celsius temperature[2]	degree Celsius	°C	K	

(continued)

SI Derived Units with Special Names and Symbols (continued)

Physical Quantity	Name of SI Unit	Symbol for SI Unit	Expression in Terms of SI Base Units	
Luminous flux	lumen	lm	cd sr	
Illuminance	lux	lx	cd sr m^{-2}	
Activity (radioactive)	becquerel	Bq	s^{-1}	
Absorbed dose (of radiation)	gray	Gy	J kg^{-1}	$= m^2\ s^{-2}$
Dose equivalent (dose equivalent index)	sievert	Sv	J kg^{-1}	$= m^2\ s^{-2}$
Plane angle	radian	rad	1	$= m\ m^{-1}$
Solid angle	steradian	sr	1	$= m^2\ m^{-2}$

[1]For radial (circular) frequency and for angular velocity the unit rad s^{-1}, or simply s^{-1}, should be used, and this may not be simplified to Hz. The unit Hz should be used only for frequency in the sense of cycles per second.

[2]The Celsius temperature θ is defined by the equation:

$$\theta/°\mathrm{C} = T/K - 273.15$$

The SI unit of Celsius temperature interval is the degree Celsius, °C, which is equal to the kelvin, K. °C should be treated as a single symbol, with no space between the ° sign and the letter C. (The symbol °K and the symbol ° should no longer be used.)

Units in Use Together with the SI

These units are not part of the SI, but it is recognized that they will continue to be used in appropriate contexts. SI prefixes may be attached to some of these units, such as milliliter, ml; millibar, mbar; megaelectronvolt, MeV; kilotonne, ktonne.

Physical Quantity	Name of Unit	Symbol for Unit	Value in SI Units
Time	minute	min	60 s
Time	hour	h	3600 s
Time	day	d	86,400 s
Plane angle	degree	°	(π/180) rad
Plane angle	minute	′	(π/10,800) rad
Plane angle	second	″	(π/648,000) rad
Length	ångstrom[1]	Å	10^{-10} m
Area	barn	b	$10^{-28}\ m^2$
Volume	liter	l, L	$dm^3 = 10^{-3}\ m^3$
Mass	tonne	t	$Mg = 10^3$ kg
Pressure	bar[1]	bar	10^5 Pa $= 10^5\ N\ m^{-2}$
Energy	electronvolt[2]	eV ($= e \times V$)	$\approx 1.60218 \times 10^{-19}$ J
Mass	unified atomic mass unit[2,3]	u ($= m_a(^{12}C)/12$)	$\approx 1.66054 \times 10^{-27}$ kg

[1]The ångstrom and the bar are approved by CIPM for "temporary use with SI units," until CIPM makes a further recommendation. However, they should not be introduced where they are not used at present.

[2]The values of these units in terms of the corresponding SI units are not exact, since they depend on the values of the physical constants e (for the electronvolt) and N_a (for the unified atomic mass unit), which are determined by experiment.

[3]The unified atomic mass unit is also sometimes called the dalton, with symbol Da, although the name and symbol have not been approved by CGPM.

Conversion Constants and Multipliers

Recommended Decimal Multiples and Submultiples

Multiples and Submultiples	Prefixes	Symbols	Multiples and Submultiples	Prefixes	Symbols
10^{18}	exa	E	10^{-1}	deci	d
10^{15}	peta	P	10^{-2}	centi	c
10^{12}	tera	T	10^{-3}	milli	m
10^{9}	giga	G	10^{-6}	micro	μ (Greek mu)
10^{6}	mega	M	10^{-9}	nano	n
10^{3}	kilo	k	10^{-12}	pico	p
10^{2}	hecto	h	10^{-15}	femto	f
10	deca	da	10^{-18}	atto	a

Conversion Factors—Metric to English

To Obtain	Multiply	By
Inches	centimeters	0.3937007874
Feet	meters	3.280839895
Yards	meters	1.093613298
Miles	kilometers	0.6213711922
Ounces	grams	$3.527396195 \times 10^{-2}$
Pounds	kilogram	2.204622622
Gallons (U.S. liquid)	liters	0.2641720524
Fluid ounces	milliliters (cc)	$3.381402270 \times 10^{-2}$
Square inches	square centimeters	0.155003100
Square feet	square meters	10.76391042
Square yards	square meters	1.195990046
Cubic inches	milliliters (cc)	$6.102374409 \times 10^{-2}$
Cubic feet	cubic meters	35.31466672
Cubic yards	cubic meters	1.307950619

Conversion Factors—English to Metric*

To Obtain	Multiply	By
Microns	mils	**25.4**
Centimeters	inches	**2.54**
Meters	feet	**0.3048**
Meters	yards	**0.9144**
Kilometers	miles	**1.609344**
Grams	ounces	28.34952313
Kilograms	pounds	**0.45359237**
Liters	gallons (U.S. liquid)	**3.785411784**
Millimeters (cc)	fluid ounces	29.57352956
Square centimeters	square inches	**6.4516**
Square meters	square feet	**0.09290304**
Square meters	square yards	**0.83612736**
Milliliters (cc)	cubic inches	**16.387064**
Cubic meters	cubic feet	$2.831684659 \times 10^{-2}$
Cubic meters	cubic yards	0.764554858

*Boldface numbers are exact; others are given to ten significant figures where so indicated by the multiplier factor.

Conversion Factors—General*

To Obtain	Multiply	By
Atmospheres	feet of water @ 4°C	2.950×10^{-2}
Atmospheres	inches of mercury @ 0°C	3.342×10^{-2}
Atmospheres	pounds per square inch	6.804×10^{-2}
BTU	foot-pounds	1.285×10^{-3}
BTU	joules	9.480×10^{-4}
Cubic feet	cords	**128**
Degree (angle)	radians	57.2958
Ergs	foot-pounds	1.356×10^{7}
Feet	miles	**5280**
Feet of water @ 4°C	atmospheres	33.90
Foot-pounds	horsepower-hours	1.98×10^{6}
Foot-pounds	kilowatt-hours	2.655×10^{6}
Foot-pounds per min	horsepower	3.3×10^{4}
Horsepower	foot-pounds per sec	1.818×10^{-3}
Inches of mercury @ 0°C	pounds per square inch	2.036
Joules	BTU	1054.8
Joules	foot-pounds	1.35582
Kilowatts	BTU per min	1.758×10^{-2}
Kilowatts	foot-pounds per min	2.26×10^{-5}
Kilowatts	horsepower	0.745712
Knots	miles per hour	0.86897624
Miles	feet	1.894×10^{-4}
Nautical miles	miles	0.86897624
Radians	degrees	1.745×10^{-2}
Square feet	acres	**43,560**
Watts	BTU per min	17.5796

*Boldface numbers are exact; others are given to ten significant figures where so indicated by the multiplier factor.

Temperature Factors

$$°F = 9/5\,(°C) + 32$$

$$\text{Fahrenheit temperature} = 1.8\,(\text{temperature in kelvins}) - 459.67$$

$$°C = 5/9\,[(°F) - 32)]$$

$$\text{Celsius temperature} = \text{temperature in kelvins} - 273.15$$

$$\text{Fahrenheit temperature} = 1.8\,(\text{Celsius temperature}) + 32$$

Conversion of Temperatures

From	To	
°Celsius	°Fahrenheit	$t_F = (t_C \times 1.8) + 32$
	Kelvin	$T_K = t_C + 273.15$
	°Rankine	$T_R = (t_C + 273.15) \times 18$
°Fahrenheit	°Celsius	$t_C = \frac{t_F - 32}{1.8}$
	Kelvin	$T_k = \frac{t_F - 32}{1.8} + 273.15$
	°Rankine	$T_R = t_F + 459.67$
Kelvin	°Celsius	$t_C = T_K - 273.15$
	°Rankine	$T_R = T_K \times 1.8$
°Rankine	Kelvin	$T_K = \frac{T_R}{1.8}$
	°Fahrenheit	$t_F = T_R - 459.67$

Physical Constants

General

Equatorial radius of the Earth = 6378.388 km = 3963.34 miles (statute)
Polar radius of the Earth, 6356.912 km = 3949.99 miles (statute)
1 degree of latitude at 40° = 69 miles
1 international nautical mile = 1.15078 miles (statute) = 1852 m = 6076.115 ft
Mean density of the earth = 5.522 g/cm^3 = 344.7 lb/ft^3
Constant of gravitation $(6.673 \pm 0.003) \times 10^{-8}$ cm^3 gm^{-1} s^{-2}
Acceleration due to gravity at sea level, latitude 45° = 980.6194 cm/s^2 = 32.1726 ft/s^2
Length of seconds pendulum at sea level, latitude 45° = 99.3575 cm = 39.1171 in.
1 knot (international) = 101.269 ft/min = 1.6878 ft/s = 1.1508 miles (statute)/h
1 micron = 10^{-4} cm
1 ångstrom = 10^{-8} cm
Mass of hydrogen atom = $(1.67339 \pm 0.0031) \times 10^{-24}$ g
Density of mercury at 0°C = 13.5955 g/ml
Density of water at 3.98°C = 1.000000 g/ml
Density, maximum, of water, at 3.98°C = 0.999973 g/cm^3
Density of dry air at 0°C, 760 mm = 1.2929 g/l
Velocity of sound in dry air at 0°C = 331.36 m/s – 1087.1 ft/s
Velocity of light in vacuum = $(2.997925 \pm 0.000002) \times 10^{10}$ cm/s
Heat of fusion of water 0°C = 79.71 cal/g
Heat of vaporization of water 100°C = 539.55 cal/g
Electrochemical equivalent of silver 0.001118 g/s international amp
Absolute wavelength of red cadmium light in air at 15°C, 760 mm pressure = 6438.4696 Å
Wavelength of orange-red line of krypton 86 = 6057.802 Å

π Constants

π = 3.14159 26535 89793 23846 26433 83279 50288 41971 69399 37511
$1/\pi$ = 0.31830 98861 83790 67153 77675 26745 02872 40689 19291 48091
π^2 = 9.8690 44010 89358 61883 44909 99876 15113 53136 99407 24079
$\log_e \pi$ = 1.14472 98858 49400 17414 34273 51353 05871 16472 94812 91531
$\log_{10} \pi$ = 0.49714 98726 94133 85435 12682 88290 89887 36516 78324 38044
$\log_{10} \sqrt{2\pi}$ = 0.39908 99341 79057 52478 25035 91507 69595 02099 34102 92128

Constants Involving *e*

e = 2.71828 18284 59045 23536 02874 71352 66249 77572 47093 69996
$1/e$ = 0.36787 94411 71442 32159 55237 70161 46086 74458 11131 03177
e^2 = 7.38905 60989 30650 22723 04274 60575 00781 31803 15570 55185
$M = \log_{10} e$ = 0.43429 44819 03251 82765 11289 18916 60508 22943 97005 80367
$1/M = \log_e 10$ = 2.30258 50929 94045 68401 79914 54684 36420 67011 01488 62877
$\log_{10} M$ = 9.63778 43113 00536 78912 29674 98645 –10

Numerical Constants

$\sqrt{2}$ = 1.41421 35623 73095 04880 16887 24209 69807 85696 71875 37695
$3\sqrt{2}$ = 1.25992 10498 94873 16476 72106 07278 22835 05702 51464 70151
$\log_e 2$ = 0.69314 71805 59945 30941 72321 21458 17656 80755 00134 36026
$\log_{10} 2$ = 0.30102 99956 63981 19521 37388 94724 49302 67881 89881 46211

$$\sqrt{3} = 1.73205\ 08075\ 68877\ 29352\ 74463\ 41505\ 87236\ 69428\ 05253\ 81039$$
$$\sqrt[3]{3} = 1.44224\ 95703\ 07408\ 38232\ 16383\ 10780\ 10958\ 83918\ 69253\ 49935$$
$$\log_e 3 = 1.09861\ 22886\ 68109\ 69139\ 52452\ 36922\ 52570\ 46474\ 90557\ 82275$$
$$\log_{10} 3 = 0.47712\ 12547\ 19662\ 43729\ 50279\ 03255\ 11530\ 92001\ 28864\ 19070$$

Symbols and Terminology for Physical and Chemical Quantities

Name	*Symbol*	*Definition*	*SI Unit*
		Classical Mechanics	
Mass	m		kg
Reduced mass	μ	$\mu = m_1m_2/(m_1 + m_2)$	kg
Density, mass density	ρ	$\rho = M/V$	kg m^{-3}
Relative density	d	$d = \rho/\rho^\theta$	1
Surface density	ρ_A, ρ_S	$\rho_A = m/A$	kg m^{-2}
Momentum	p	$p = mv$	kg m s^{-1}
Angular momentum, action	L	$l = r$ ¥ p	J s
Moment of inertia	I, J	$I = \Sigma m_i r_i^2$	kg m^2
Force	F	$F = d\mathbf{p}/dt = ma$	N
Torque, moment of a force	T, (M)	$T = r \times \mathbf{F}$	N m
Energy	E		J
Potential energy	E_p, V, Φ	$E_p = Fds$	J
Kinetic energy	E_k, T, K	$e_k = (1/2)mv^2$	J
Work	W, w	$w = Fds$	J
Hamilton function	H	$H(q, p) = T(q, p) + V(q)$	J
Lagrange function	L	$L(q, \dot{q})T(q, \dot{q}) - V(q)$	J
Pressure	p, P	$p = F/A$	Pa, N m^{-2}
Surface tension	γ, σ	$\gamma = dW/dA$	N m^{-1}, J m^{-2}
Weight	G, (W, P)	$G = mg$	N
Gravitational constant	G	$F = Gm_1m_2/r^2$	N m^2 kg^{-2}
Normal stress	σ	$\sigma = F/A$	Pa
Shear stress	τ	$\tau = F/A$	Pa
Linear strain, relative elongation	ε, e	$\varepsilon = \Delta l/l$	1
Modulus of elasticity, Young's modulus	E	$E = \sigma/\varepsilon$	Pa
Shear strain	γ	$\gamma = \Delta x/d$	1
Shear modulus	G	$G = \tau/\gamma$	Pa
Volume strain, bulk strain	θ	$\theta = \Delta V/V_0$	1
Bulk modulus,	K	$K = -V_0(dp/dV)$	Pa
compression modulus	η, μ	$\tau_{x,z} = \eta(dv_x/dz)$	Pa s
Viscosity, dynamic viscosity			
Fluidity	ϕ	$\phi = 1/\eta$	m kg^{-1} s
Kinematic viscosity	v	$v = \eta/\rho$	m^2 s^{-1}
Friction coefficient	μ, (f)	$F_{frict} = \mu F_{norm}$	1
Power	P	$P = dW/dt$	W
Sound energy flux	P, P_a	$P = dE/dt$	W
Acoustic factors			
Reflection factor	ρ	$\rho = P_t/P_0$	1
Acoustic absorption factor	α_a, (α)	$\alpha_a = 1 - \rho$	1
Transmission factor	τ	$\tau = P_{tr}/P_0$	1
Dissipation factor	δ	$\delta = \alpha_a - \tau$	1

(continued)

Symbols and Terminology for Physical and Chemical Quantities (continued)

Name	*Symbol*	*Definition*	*SI Unit*
Electricity and Magnetism			
Quantity of electricity, electric charge	Q		C
Charge density	ρ	$\rho = Q/V$	$C\ m^{-3}$
Surface charge density	σ	$\sigma = Q/A$	$C\ m^{-2}$
Electric potential	V, ϕ	$V = dW/dQ$	$V, J\ C^{-1}$
Electric potential difference	$U, \Delta V, \Delta\phi$	$U = V_2 - V_1$	V
Electromotive force	E	$E = (F/Q)ds$	V
Electric field strength	$\mathbf{E}$	$\mathbf{E} = \mathbf{F}/Q = -\text{grad } V$	$V\ m^{-1}$
Electric flux	Ψ	$\Psi = \mathbf{D}d\mathbf{A}$	C
Electric displacement	$\mathbf{D}$	$\mathbf{D} = \varepsilon\mathbf{E}$	$C\ m^{-2}$
Capacitance	C	$C = Q/U$	$F, C\ V^{-1}$
Permittivity	ε	$D = \varepsilon E$	$F\ m^{-1}$
Permittivity of vacuum	ε_0	$\varepsilon_0 = \mu_0^{-1} c_0^{-2}$	$F\ m^{-1}$
Relative permittivity	ε_r	$\varepsilon_r = \varepsilon/\varepsilon_0$	1
Dielectric polarization (dipole moment per volume)	$\mathbf{P}$	$\mathbf{P} = \mathbf{D} - \varepsilon_0\mathbf{E}$	$C\ m^{-2}$
Electric susceptibility	χ_e	$\chi_e = \varepsilon_r - 1$	1
Electric dipole moment	$\mathbf{p}, \mu$	$\mathbf{p} = Q\mathbf{r}$	C m
Electric current	I	$I = dQ/dt$	A
Electric current density	$\mathbf{j}, \mathbf{J}$	$I = \mathbf{j}dx\mathbf{A}$	$A\ m^{-2}$
Magnetic flux density, magnetic induction	$\mathbf{B}$	$\mathbf{F} = Qv \times \mathbf{B}$	T
Magnetic flux	Φ	$\Phi = \mathbf{B}dA$	Wb
Magnetic field strength	$\mathbf{H}$	$\mathbf{B} = \mu\mathbf{H}$	$A\ M^{-1}$
Permeability	μ	$\mathbf{B} = \mu\mathbf{H}$	$N\ A^{-2}, H\ m^{-1}$
Permeability of vacuum	μ_0		$H\ m^{-1}$
Relative permeability	μ_r	$\mu_r = \mu/\mu_0$	1
Magnetization (magnetic dipole moment per volume)	$\mathbf{M}$	$\mathbf{M} = \mathbf{B}/\mu_0 - \mathbf{H}$	$A\ m^{-1}$
Magnetic susceptibility	$\chi, \kappa, (\chi_m)$	$\chi = \mu_r - 1$	1
Molar magnetic susceptibility	χ_m	$\chi_m = V_m\chi$	$m^3\ mol^{-1}$
Magnetic dipole moment	$\mathbf{m}, \mu$	$E_p = -\mathbf{m} \cdot \mathbf{B}$	$A\ m^2, J\ T^{-1}$
Electrical resistance	R	$\mathbf{P} = \mathbf{Y}/\mathbf{I}$	Ω
Conductance	G	$G = 1/R$	S
Loss angle	δ	$\delta = (\pi/2) + \phi_I - \phi_U$	1, rad
Reactance	X	$X = (U/I)\sin \delta$	Ω
Impedance (complex impedance)	Z	$Z = R + iX$	Ω
Admittance (complex admittance)	Y	$Y = 1/Z$	S
Susceptance	B	$Y = G + iB$	S
Resistivity	ρ	$\rho = E/j$	Ω m
Conductivity	κ, γ, σ	$\kappa = 1/\rho$	$S\ m^{-1}$
Self-inductance	L	$E = -L(dI/dt)$	H
Mutual inductance	M, L_{12}	$E_1 = L_{12}(Di_2/dt)$	H
Magnetic vector potential	$\mathbf{A}$	$\mathbf{B} = \mathbf{V} \times \mathbf{A}$	$Wb\ m^{-1}$
Poynting vector	$\mathbf{S}$	$\mathbf{S} = \mathbf{E} \times \mathbf{H}$	$W\ m^{-2}$
Electromagnetic Radiation			
Wavelength	λ		m
Speed of light			$m\ s^{-1}$
in vacuum	c_0		
in a medium	c	$c = c_0/n$	

(continued)

Symbols and Terminology for Physical and Chemical Quantities (continued)

Name	*Symbol*	*Definition*	*SI Unit*
Electromagnetic Radiation			
Wavenumber in vacuum	V	$V = V/c_0 = 1/n\lambda$	m^{-1}
Wavenumber (in a medium)	σ	$\sigma = 1/\lambda$	m^{-1}
Frequency	v	$v = c/\lambda$	Hz
Circular frequency, pulsatance	ω	$\omega = 2\pi v$	s^{-1}, rad s^{-1}
Refractive index	n	$n = c_0/c$	1
Planck constant	h		J s
Planck constant/2π	$\hbar$	$\hbar = h/2\pi$	J s
Radiant energy	Q, W		J
Radiant energy density	ρ, w	$\rho = Q/V$	J m^{-3}
Spectral radiant energy density			
in terms of frequency	ρ_v, w_v	$\rho_v = \delta\rho/dv$	J m^{-3} Hz^{-1}
in terms of wavenumber	$\rho_{\bar{v}}$, $w_{\bar{v}}$	$\rho_{\bar{v}} = d\rho/d\bar{v}$	J m^{-2}
in terms of wavelength	ρ_λ, w_λ	$\rho_\lambda = \delta\rho/d\lambda$	J m^{-4}
Einstein transition probabilities			
Spontaneous emission	A_{nm}	$dN_n/dt = -A_{nm}N_n$	s^{-1}
Stimulated emission	B_{nm}	$dn_n/dt = -\rho\bar{v}(\bar{V}_{nm}) \times B_{nm}N_n$	s kg^{-1}
Radiant power, radiant energy per time	Φ, P	$\Phi = dQ/dt$	W
Radiant intensity	I	$I = d\Phi/d\Omega$	W sr^{-1}
Radiant exitance (emitted radiant flux)	M	$M = d\Phi/dA_{source}$	W m^{-2}
Irradiance (radiant flux received)	E, (I)	$E = d\Phi/\delta A$	W m^{-2}
Emittance	ε	$\varepsilon = M/M_{bb}$	1
Stefan–Boltzmann constant	σ	$M_{bb} = \sigma T^4$	W m^{-2} K^{-4}
First radiation constant	c_1	$c_1 = 2\pi hc_0{}^2$	W m^2
Second radiation constant	c_2	$c_2 = hc_0/k$	K m
Transmittance, transmission factor	τ, T	$\tau = \Phi_{tr}/\Phi_0$	1
Absorptance, absorption factor	α	$\alpha = \phi_{abs}/\phi_0$	1
Reflectance, reflection factor	ρ	$\rho = \phi_{refl}/\Phi_0$	1
(Decadic) absorbance	A	$A = \lg(1 - \alpha_i)$	1
Napierian absorbance	B	$B = \ln(1 - \alpha_i)$	1
Absorption coefficient			
(Linear) decadic	a, K	$a = A/l$	m^{-1}
(Linear) napierian	α	$\alpha = B/l$	m^{-1}
Molar (decadic)	ε	$\varepsilon = a/c = A/cl$	m^2 mol^{-1}
Molar napierian	κ	$\kappa = \alpha/c = B/cl$	m^2 mol^{-1}
Absorption index	k	$k = \alpha/4\pi\bar{v}$	1
Complex refractive index	$\hat{n}$	$\hat{n} = n + ik$	1
Molar refraction	R, R_m	$R = \frac{(n^2-1)}{(n^2+2)} V_m$	m^3 mol^{-1}
Angle of optical rotation	α		1, rad
Solid State			
Lattice vector	$\mathbf{R}$, $\mathbf{R_0}$		m
Fundamental translation vectors for the crystal lattice	$\mathbf{a}_1$; $\mathbf{a}_2$; $\mathbf{a}_3$, $\mathbf{a}$; $\mathbf{b}$; $\mathbf{c}$	$R = n_1\mathbf{a}_1 + n_2\mathbf{a}_2 + n_3\mathbf{a}_3$	m
(Circular) reciprocal lattice vector	$\mathbf{G}$	$G \cdot R = 2\pi m$	m^{-1}

(continued)

Symbols and Terminology for Physical and Chemical Quantities (continued)

Name	Symbol	Definition	SI Unit
	Solid State		
(Circular) fundamental translation vectors for the reciprocal lattice	$\mathbf{b}_1; \mathbf{b}_2; \mathbf{b}_3, \mathbf{a}^*; \mathbf{b}^*; \mathbf{c}^*$	$\mathbf{a}_i \cdot \mathbf{b}_k = 2\pi\delta_{ik}$	m^{-1}
Lattice plane spacing	d		m
Bragg angle	θ	$n\lambda = 2d \sin \theta$	l, rad
Order of reflection	n		l
Order parameters			
Short range	σ		l
Long range	s		l
Burgers vector	b		m
Particle position vector	r, R_j		m
Equilibrium position vector of an ion	R_o		m
Displacement vector of an ion	$\mathbf{u}$	$\mathbf{u} = \mathbf{R} - \mathbf{R}_0$	m
Debye–Waller factor	B, D		l
Debye circular wavenumber	q_D		m^{-1}
Debye circular frequency	ω_D		s^{-1}
Grüneisen parameter	γ, Γ	$\gamma = \alpha V/\kappa C_V$	l
Madelung constant	$\alpha, \mathcal{M}$	$E_{coul} = \frac{\alpha N_A z_+ z_- e^2}{4\pi\varepsilon_0 R_0}$	l
Density of states	N_E	$N_E = dN(E)/dE$	$J^{-1}\ m^{-3}$
(Spectral) density of vibrational modes	N_ω, g	$N_\omega = dN(\omega)/d\omega$	$s\ m^{-3}$
Resistivity tensor	ρ_{ik}	$E = \rho \cdot j$	Ω m
Conductivity tensor	σ_{ik}	$\sigma = \rho^{-1}$	$S\ m^{-1}$
Thermal conductivity tensor	λ_{ik}	$J_q = -\lambda \cdot \text{grad}\ T$	$W\ m^{-1}\ K^{-1}$
Residual resistivity	ρ_R		Ω m
Relaxation time	τ	$\tau = l/v_F$	s
Lorenz coefficient	L	$L = \lambda/\sigma T$	$V^2\ K^{-2}$
Hall coefficient	A_H, R_H	$\mathbf{E} = \rho \cdot \mathbf{j} + R_H(\mathbf{B} \times \mathbf{j})$	$m^3\ C^{-1}$
Thermoelectric force	E		V
Peltier coefficient	Π		V
Thomson coefficient	$\mu,(\tau)$		$V\ K^{-1}$
Work function	Φ	$\Phi = E_\infty - E_F$	J
Number density, number concentration	$n, (p)$		m^{-3}
Gap energy	E_γ		J
Donor ionization energy	E_δ		J
Acceptor ionization energy	E_α		J
Fermi energy	E_Φ, ε_F		J
Circular wave vector, propagation vector	$\boldsymbol{k}, \boldsymbol{q}$	$k = 2\pi/\lambda$	m^{-1}
Bloch function	$u_k(\boldsymbol{r})$	$\psi(\boldsymbol{r}) = u_k(\boldsymbol{r}) \exp(i\mathbf{k} \cdot \mathbf{r})$	$m^{-3/2}$
Charge density of electrons	ρ	$\rho(\boldsymbol{r}) = -e\psi^*(\mathbf{r})\psi(\mathbf{r})$	$C\ m^{-3}$
Effective mass	m^*		kg
Mobility	μ	$\mu = v_{drift}/E$	$m^2\ V^{-1}\ s^{-1}$
Mobility ratio	b	$b = \mu_n/\mu_p$	l
Diffusion coefficient	D	$dN/dt = -DA(dn/dx)$	$m^2\ s^{-1}$
Diffusion length	L	$L = \sqrt{D\tau}$	m
Characteristic (Weiss) temperature	ϕ, ϕ_W		K
Curie temperature	T_C		K
Néel temperature	T_N		K

Credits

Material in Section III was reprinted from the following sources:

D. R. Lide, Ed., *CRC Handbook of Chemistry and Physics,* 76th ed., Boca Raton, FL: CRC Press, 1992: International System of Units (SI), conversion constants and multipliers (conversion of temperatures), symbols and terminology for physical and chemical quantities, fundamental physical constants, classification of electromagnetic radiation.

D. Zwillinger, Ed., *CRC Standard Mathematical Tables and Formulae,* 30th ed., Boca Raton, FL: CRC Press, 1996: Greek alphabet, conversion constants and multipliers (recommended decimal multiples and submultiples, metric to English, English to metric, general, temperature factors), physical constants, series expansion.

Probability for Electrical and Computer Engineers

Charles W. Therrien

The Algebra of Events

The study of probability is based upon experiments that have uncertain outcomes. Collections of these outcomes comprise *events* and the collection of all possible outcomes of the experiment comprise what is called the *sample space*, denoted by S. Outcomes are members of the sample space and events of interest are represented as *sets* of outcomes (see Figure III.1).

The algebra $\mathcal{A}$ that deals with representing events is the usual set algebra. If A is an event, then A^c (the *complement* of A) represents the event that "A did not occur." The complement of the sample space is the *null event*, $\varnothing = S^c$. The event that *both* event A_1 and event A_2 have occurred is the intersection, written as "$A_1 \cdot A_2$" or "A_1A_2" while the event that *either* A_1 or A_2 *or both* have occurred is the union, written as "$A_1 + A_2$."[1]

Table III.1 lists the two postulates that define the algebra $\mathcal{A}$, while Table III.2 lists seven axioms that define properties of its operations. Together these tables can be used to show all of the properties of the algebra of events. Table III.3 lists some additional useful relations that can be derived from the axioms and the postulates.

Since the events "$A_1 + A_2$" and "A_1A_2" are included in the algebra, it follows by induction that for any finite number of events $A_1 + A_2 + \cdots + A_N$ and $A_1 \cdot A_2 \cdots A_N$ are also included in the algebra. Since problems often involve the union or intersection of an *infinite* number of events, however, the algebra of events must be defined to include these infinite intersections and unions. This extension to infinite unions and intersections is known as a sigma algebra.

A set of events that satisfies the two conditions:

1. $A_iA_j = \varnothing \neq$ for $\neq i \neq j$
2. $A_1 + A_2 + A_3 + \cdots = S$

is known as a *partition* and is important for the solution of problems in probability. The events of a partition are said to be *mutually exclusive* and *collectively exhaustive*. The most fundamental partition is the set outcomes defining the random experiment, which comprise the sample space by definition.

Probability

Probability measures the likelihood of occurrence of events represented on a scale of 0 to 1. We often estimate probability by measuring the *relative frequency* of an event, which is defined as

$$\text{relative frequency} = \frac{\text{number of occurrences of the event}}{\text{number of repetitions of the experiment}}$$

(for a large number of repetitions). Probability can be defined formally by the following axioms:

(I) The probability of any event is nonnegative:

$$\Pr[A] \geqslant 0 \tag{III.1}$$

(II) The probability of the universal event (i.e., the entire sample space) is 1:

$$\Pr[S] = 1 \tag{III.2}$$

[1]Some authors use $\cap$ and $\cup$ rather than $\cdot$ and $+$, respectively.

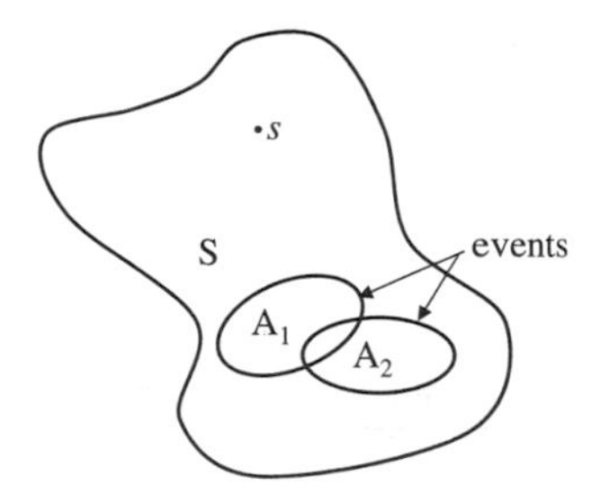

FIGURE III.1 Abstract representation of the sample space S with outcome s and sets A_1 and A_2 representing events.

(III) If A_1 and A_2 are mutually exclusive, i.e., $A_1A_2 = \varnothing$, then

$$\Pr[A_1 + A_2] = \Pr[A_1] + \Pr[A_2] \tag{III.3}$$

(IV) If $\{A_i\}$ represent a countably infinite set of mutually exclusive events, then

$$\Pr[A_1 + A_2 + A_3 + \cdot\cdot\cdot] = \sum_{i=1}^{\infty} \Pr[A_i] \quad (\text{if } A_iA_j = \varnothing \quad i \neq j) \tag{III.4}$$

Note that although the additivity of probability for any finite set of disjoint events follows from (III), the property has to be stated explicitly for an infinite set in (IV). These axioms and the algebra of events can be used to show a number of other important properties which are summarized in Table III.4. The last item in the table is an especially important formula since it uses probabilistic information about

TABLE III.1 Postulates for an Algebra of Events

1.	*If* $A \in \mathcal{A}$ *then* $A^c \in \mathcal{A}$
2.	*If* $A_1 \in \mathcal{A}$ *and* $A_2 \in \mathcal{A}$ *then* $A_1 + A_2 \in \mathcal{A}$

TABLE III.2 Axioms of Operations on Events

$A_1A_1^c = \varnothing$	Mutual exclusion
$A_1S = A_1$	Inclusion
$(A_1^c)^c = A_1$	Double complement
$A_1 + A_2 = A_2 + A_1$	Commutative law
$A_1 + (A_2 + A_3) = (A_1 + A_2) + A_3$	Associative law
$A_1(A_2 + A_3) = A_1A_2 + A_1A_3$	Distributive law
$(A_1A_2)^c = A_1^c + A_2^c$	DeMorgan's law

TABLE III.3 Additional Identities in the Algebra of Events

$S^c = \varnothing$	
$A_1 + \varnothing = A_1$	Inclusion
$A_1A_2 = A_2A_1$	Commutative law
$A_1(A_2A_3) = (A_1A_2)A_3$	Associative law
$A_1 + (A_2A_3) = (A_1 + A_2)(A_1 + A_3)$	Distributive law
$(A_1 + A_2)^c = A_1^c A_2^c$	DeMorgan's law

TABLE III.4 Some Corollaries Derived from the Axioms of Probability

$\Pr[A^c] = 1 - \Pr[A]$
$0 \leq \Pr[A] \leq 1$
If $A_1 \subseteq A_2$ then $\Pr[A_1] \leq \Pr[A_2]$
$\Pr[\varnothing] = 0$
If $A_1A_2 = \varnothing$ – then = $\Pr[A_1A_2] = 0$
$\Pr[A_1 + A_2] = \Pr[A_1] + \Pr[A_2] - \Pr[A_1A_2]$

individual events to compute the probability of the union of two events. The term $\Pr[A_1A_2]$ is referred to as the *joint probability* of the two events. This last equation shows that the probabilities of two events add as in Equation (III.3) only if their joint probability is 0. The joint probability is 0 when the two events have no intersection ($A_1A_2 = \varnothing$).

Two events are said to be statistically *independent* if and only if

$$\Pr[A_1A_2] = \Pr[A_1]\cdot\Pr[A_2] \quad \text{(independent events)} \tag{III.5}$$

This definition is not derived from the earlier properties of probability. An argument to give this definition intuitive meaning can be found in Ref. [1]. Independence occurs in problems where two events are not influenced by one another and Equation (III.5) simplifies such problems considerably.

A final important result deals with partitions. A *partition* is a finite or countably infinite set of events $A_1, A_2, A_3, \ldots$ that satisfy the two conditions:

$$A_iA_j = \varnothing \text{ for } i \neq j$$

$$A_1 + A_2 + A_3 + \cdots = S$$

The events in a partition satisfy the relation:

$$\sum_i \Pr[A_i] = 1 \tag{III.6}$$

Further, if B is *any* other event, then

$$\Pr[B] = \sum_i \Pr[A_iB] \tag{III.7}$$

The latter result is referred to as the *principle of total probability* and is frequently used in solving problems. The principle is illustrated by a Venn diagram in Figure III.2. The rectangle represents the sample space and other events are defined therein. The event B is seen to be comprised of all of the pieces

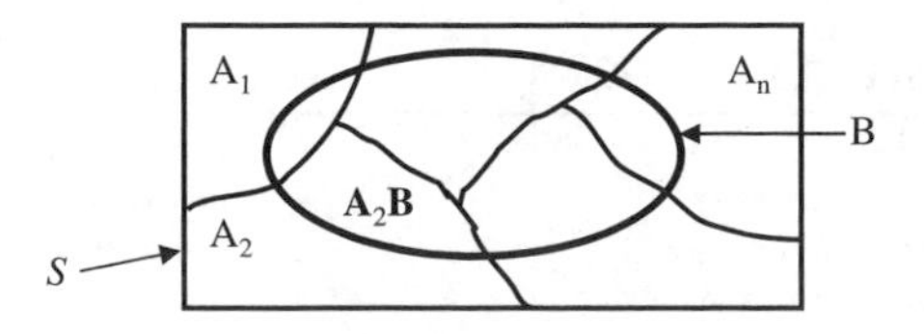

FIGURE III.2 Venn diagram illustrating the principle of total probability.

that represent intersections or overlap of event B with the events A_i. This is the graphical interpretation of Equation (III.7).

An Example

Simon's Surplus Warehouse has large barrels of mixed electronic components (parts) that you can buy by the handful or by the pound. You are not allowed to select parts individually. Based on your previous experience, you have determined that in one barrel, 29% of the parts are bad (faulted), 3% are bad resistors, 12% are good resistors, 5% are bad capacitors, and 32% are diodes. You decide to assign probabilities based on these percentages. Let us define the following events:

Event	Symbol
Bad (faulted) component	B
Good component	G
Resistor	R
Capacitor	C
Diode	D

A Venn diagram representing this situation is shown below along with probabilities of various events as given:

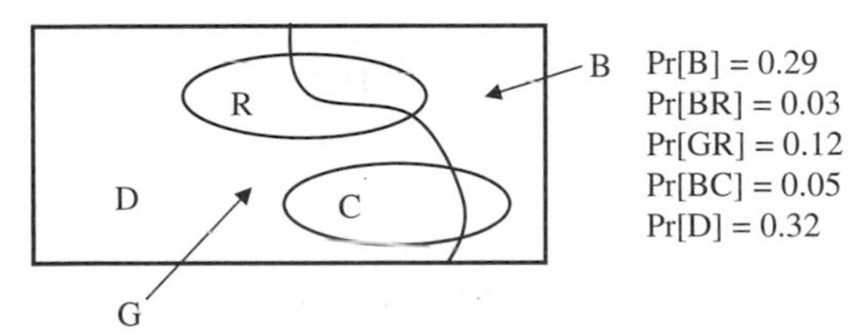

Note that since any component must be a resistor, capacitor, or diode, the region labeled D in the diagram represents everything in the sample space which is not included in R or C.

We can answer a number of questions.

1. What is the probability that a component is a resistor (either good *or* bad)?
   Since the events B and G form a partition of the sample space, we can use the principle of total probability Equation (III.7) to write:

$$\Pr[R] = \Pr[GR] + \Pr[BR] = 0.12 + 0.03 = 0.15$$

2. Are bad parts and resistors independent?
   We know that $\Pr[BR] = 0.03$ and we can compute:

$$\Pr[B] \cdot \Pr[R] = (0.29)(0.15) = 0.0435$$

   Since $\Pr[BR] \neq \Pr[B] \cdot \Pr[R]$, the events are *not* independent.
3. You have no use for either bad parts or resistors. What is the probability that a part is either bad and/or a resistor?

Using the formula from Table III.4 and the previous result we can write:

$$\Pr[B+R] = \Pr[B] + \Pr[R] - \Pr[BR] = 0.29 + 0.15 - 0.03 = 0.41$$

4. What is the probability that a part is useful to you?
   Let U represent the event that the part is useful. Then (see Table III.4):

$$\Pr[U] = 1 - \Pr[U^c] = 1 - 0.41 = 0.59$$

5. What is the probability of a bad diode?
   Observe that the events R, C, and D form a partition, since a component has to be one and only one type of part. Then using Equation (III.7) we write:

$$\Pr[B] = \Pr[BR] + \Pr[BC] + \Pr[BD]$$

   Substituting the known numerical values and solving yields

$$0.29 = 0.03 + 0.05 + \Pr[BD] \text{ or } \Pr[BD] = 0.21$$

Conditional Probability and Bayes' Rule

The *conditional* probability of an event A_1 given that an event A_2 has occurred is defined by

$$\Pr[A_1|A_2] = \frac{\Pr[A_1A_2]}{\Pr[A_2]} \qquad \text{(III.8)}$$

($\Pr[A_1|A_2]$ is read "probability of A_1 *given* A_2.") As an illustration, let us compute the probability that a component in the previous example is bad given that it is a resistor:

$$\Pr[B|R] = \frac{\Pr[BR]}{\Pr[R]} = \frac{0.03}{0.15} = 0.2$$

(The value for $\Pr[R]$ was computed in question 1 of the example.) Frequently the statement of a problem is in terms of conditional probability rather than joint probability, so Equation (III.8) is used in the form:

$$\Pr[A_1A_2] = \Pr[A_1|A_2] \cdot \Pr[A_2] = \Pr[A_2|A_1] \cdot \Pr[A_1] \qquad \text{(III.9)}$$

(The last expression follows because $\Pr[A_1A_2]$ and $\Pr[A_2A_1]$ are the same thing.) Using this result, the principle of total probability Equation (III.7) can be rewritten as

$$\Pr[B] = \sum_j \Pr[B|A_j]\,\Pr[A_j] \qquad \text{(III.10)}$$

where B is any event and $\{A_j\}$ is a set of events that forms a partition.

Now, consider any one of the events A_i in the partition. It follows from Equation (III.9) that

$$\Pr[A_i|B] = \frac{\Pr[B|A_i] \cdot \Pr[A_i]}{\Pr[B]}$$

Then substituting in Equation (III.10) yields:

$$\Pr[A_i|B] = \frac{\Pr[B|A_i] \cdot \Pr[A_i]}{\sum_j \Pr[B|A_j]\Pr[A_j]} \tag{III.11}$$

This result is known as *Bayes' theorem* or *Bayes' rule.* It is used in a number of problems that commonly arise in electrical engineering. We illustrate and end this section with an example from the field of communications.

Communication Example

The transmission of bits over a binary communication channel is represented in the drawing below:

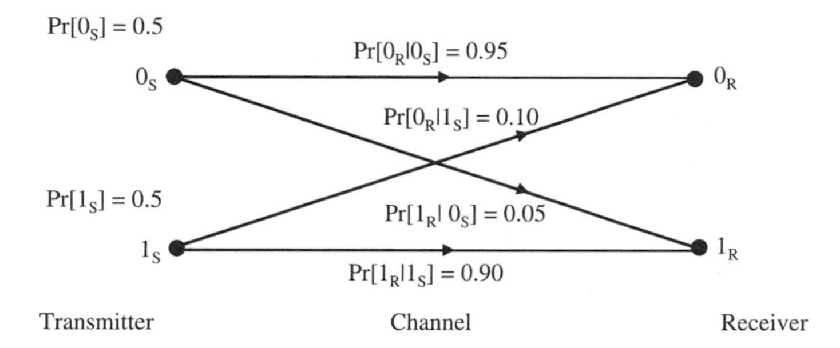

where we use notation like 0_S, 0_R ... to denote events "0 sent," "0 received," etc. When a 0 is transmitted, it is correctly received with probability 0.95 or incorrectly received with probability 0.05. That is, $\Pr[0_R|0_S] = 0.95$ and $\Pr[1_R|0_S] = 0.05$. When a 1 is transmitted, it is correctly received with probability 0.90 and incorrectly received with probability 0.10. The probabilities of sending a 0 or a 1 are denoted by $\Pr[0_S]$ and $\Pr[1_S]$. It is desired to compute the *probability of error* for the system.

This is an application of the principle of total probability. The two events 0_S and 1_S are mutually exclusive and collectively exhaustive and thus form a partition. Take the event B to be the event that an error occurs. It follows from Equation (III.10) that

$$\begin{aligned}\Pr[\text{error}] &= \Pr[\text{error}|0_S]\Pr[0_S] + \Pr[\text{error}|1_S]\Pr[1_S] \\ &= \Pr[1_R|0_S]\Pr[0_S] + \Pr[0_R|1_S]\Pr[1_S] \\ &= (0.05)(0.5) + (0.10)(0.5) = 0.075\end{aligned}$$

Next, given that an error has occurred, let us compute the probability that a 1 was sent or a 0 was sent. This is an application of Bayes' rule. For a 1, Equation (III.11) becomes

$$\Pr[1_S|\text{error}] = \frac{\Pr[\text{error}|1_S]\Pr[1_S]}{\Pr[\text{error}|1_S]\Pr[1_S] + \Pr[\text{error}|0_S]\Pr[0_S]}$$

Substituting the numerical values then yields:

$$\Pr[1_S|\text{error}] = \frac{(0.10)(0.5)}{(0.10)(0.5) + (0.05)(0.5)} \approx 0.667$$

For a 0, a similar analysis applies:

$$\Pr[0_S|\text{error}] = \frac{\Pr[\text{error}|0_S]\Pr[0_S]}{\Pr[\text{error}|1_S]\Pr[1_S] + \Pr[\text{error}|0_S]\Pr[0_S]}$$
$$= \frac{(0.05)(0.5)}{(0.10)(0.5) + (0.05)(0.5)} \approx 0.333$$

The two resulting probabilities sum to 1 because 0_S and 1_S form a partition for the experiment.

Reference

1. C. W. Therrien and M. Tummala, *Probability for Electrical and Computer Engineers.* Boca Raton, FL: CRC Press, 2004.

Indexes

Author Index A-1
Subject Index S-1

Author Index

A

Arif, Ronald, *Semiconductor Nano-Electroncis and Nano-Optoelectronics*, Materials and Nanoscience, **4**-68 to **4**-89

B

Barnes, Frank, *Biological Effects and Electromagnetic Fields*, Bioelectricity, **7**-33 to **7**-54
Barr, R. C., *Bioelectric Events*, Bioelectricity, **7**-13 to **7**-33
Berbari, Edward J., *The Electrocardiograph*, Bioelectronics and Instruments, **9**-14 to **9**-21
Bond, Robert A., *Embedded Signal Processing*, Bioelectricity, **7**-55 to **7**-75
Bronzino, Joseph D., *The Electro-encephalogram*, Bioelectronics and Instruments, **9**-1 to **9**-13

D

Dhillon, B. S., *Reliability Engineering*, **6**-1 to **6**-19
Dorval II, Alan D., *Neuroelectric Principles*, Bioelectricity, **7**-1 to **7**-12

E

Eren, Halit, *Portable Instruments and Systems*, Instruments and Measurements, **5**-27 to **5**-35

F

Fox, Martin D., *Tomography*, **10**-1 to **10**-7

G

Geddes, L. A., *Bioelectric Events*, Bioelectricity, **7**-13 to **7**-33
Giurgiutiu, Victor, *Micromechatronics*, Materials and Nanoscience, **4**-20 to **4**-42

H

Hall, David L., *An Introduction to Multi-Sensor Data Fusion*, **2**-1 to **2**-14
Hobbs, Bryan Stewart, *Electrochemical Sensors*, Sensors, **1**-11 to **1**-17

J

Jin, Zhian, *Semiconductor Nano-Electroncis and Nano-Optoelectronics*, Materials and Nanoscience, **4**-68 to **4**-89

K

Khalilieh, Sam S., *Electrical Equipment in Hazardous Areas*, Instruments and Measurements, **5**-1 to **5**-27

L

Llinas, James, *An Introduction to Multi-Sensor Data Fusion*, **2**-1 to **2**-14
Lyshevski, Sergey Edward *Micromechatronics*, Materials and Nanoscience, **4**-20 to **4**-42
Nanocomputers, Nano-Architectronics, and Nano-ICs, Materials and Nanoscience, **4**-42 to **4**-68

M

Martinez, David R., *Embedded Signal Processing*, Bioelectricity, **7**-55 to **7**-75
Meyyappan, M., *Carbon Nanotubes*, Materials and Nanoscience, **4**-1 to **4**-8

N

Neuman, Michael R., *Biomedical Sensors*, **8**-1 to **8**-12

P

Pelasko, John, *Modeling MEMS and NEMS*, Materials and Nanoscience, **4**-9 to **4**-20
Pu, Yuan, *Magneto-optics*, **3**-1 to **3**-10

R

Relf, Christopher G., *G (LabVIEW®) Software Engineering*, Instruments and Measurements, **5**-36 to **5**-54

S

Slaten, Bonnie Keillor, *Biological Effects and Electromagnetic Fields*, Bioelectricity, **7**-33 to **7**-54

Smith, Rosemary L., *Introduction*, Sensors, **1**-1 to **1**-10

T

Tallarida, Ronald J., *Mathematics, Symbols, and Physical Constants*, **III**-1 to **III**-20
Tansu, Nelson, *Semiconductor Nano-Electroncis and Nano-Optoelectronics*, Materials and Nanoscience, **4**-68 to **4**-89
Therrien, Charles W., *Probability for Electrical and Computer Engineers*, Mathematics, Symbols, and Physical Constants, **III**-14 to **III**-20

V

Vai, M. Michael, *Embedded Signal Processing*, Bioelectricity, **7**-55 to **7**-75

W

Watson, Joseph, *The Stannic Oxide Semiconductor Gas Sensor*, Sensors, **1**-18 to **1**-24
White, John A., *Neuroelectric Principles*, Bioelectricity, **7**-1 to **7**-12

Y

Young, David, *Magneto-optics*, **3**-1 to **3**-10

Subject Index

A

Action potential, **7-1**, **7-11**; *see also* Neuroelectric principles
Activating function, **7-11**
Activation, **7-11**
Air current and ventilation, **5-4**
Amperometric sensor, **8-10**
Analyte, **8-10**
Atrophy, **7-32**
Autonomic, **7-32**
Availability, **6-2**

B

Babbage, Charles, **4**-44
Bioanalytical sensors, **8-2**, **8-10**; *see also* Biosensors
Bioelectric events, **7**-13, **7**-31 to **7**-32
  electro-encephalography (EEG), **7**-23 to **7**-24
    clinical EEG, **7**-26 to **7**-27
    evoked potentials, **7**-27 to **7**-29
    instrumentation, **7**-27
    normal EEG, **7**-25 to **7**-26
    recording technique, **7**-24 to **7**-25
  electrocardiogram (ECG)
    clinical signal, **7**-17 to **7**-19
    ECG leads, **7**-19
    instrumentation, **7**-19 to **7**-720
    origin, **7**-15 to **7**-17
    recordings taken directly from the heart, **7**-21
  electrograms, **7**-21
  electromyography (EMG), **7**-21
    clinical EMG, **7**-22 to **7**-23
    contraction of skeletal muscle, **7**-21 to **7**-22
    instrumentation, **7**-23
  law of stimulation, **7**-14
  magnetic (Eddy-Current) stimulation, **7**-29 to **7**-30
  recording action potentials, **7**-14 to **7**-15
  terminology, **7**-32
Bioelectrical nanocomputers, **4**-43 to **4**-44
Bioelectricity, origins, **7**-13 to **7**-14; *see also* Bioelectric events; Biological effects and electromagnetic fields; Embedded signal processing; Neuroelectric principles
Bioelectronics and instruments. *See* Electrocardiograph; Electro-encephalogram
Biological effects and electromagnetic fields, **7**-33, **7**-52
  biological effects of electric shock, **7**-34, **7**-34
  electromagnetic fields from cell phones and base stations, **7**-41
    animal studies (*in vivo*), **7**-44 to **7**-45
    cellular studies, **7**-45 to **7**-46
    epidemiological studies, **7**-42 to **7**-43
    exposures, **7**-42
  low-level/time-varying electromagnetic fields from power lines, **7**-36
    animal studies, **7**-38 to **7**-40
    cellular studies, **7**-40 to **7**-41
    epidemiological studies, **7**-37 to **7**-38
    exposures, **7**-36 to **7**-37
  other adverse effects of electricity, electrical arc flash, **7**-36
  risk, **7**-50 to **7**-52
  shock from household voltage, **7**-35
  standards/guidelines, **7**-46 to **7**-48
Biomedical sensors, **8**-1 to **8**-2, **8**-10, **8-11**
  applications, **8**-10
  bioanalytical sensors, **8**-9 to **8**-10
  chemical sensors, **8**-6 to **8**-9
  physical sensors, **8**-2 to **8**-6
Biosensors, **1-7**, **8**-2
  enzyme sensor, **1**-8
  immunosensor, **1**-7 to **1**-8
Bispectra, **9-13**
Block (wiring) diagram, **5-53**
"Buckeyball structure", **4**-17

C

Carbon nanotubes (CNTs), **4**-1, **4**-8
  atomic force microscopy (AFT) and CNT probes, **4**-6 to **4**-7
  field emission, **4**-8
  growth, **4**-2 to **4**-5
    arc synthesis, **4**-2 to **4**-3
    CVD (chemical vapor deposition), **4**-3
    PECVD (plasma enhanced CVD), **4**-3
    plasma sources, **4**-4
  nano-electronics, **4**-5 to **4**-6
  sensors, **4**-7 to **4**-8
  structure and properties, **4**-2

Page on which a term is defined is indicated in bold.

Chemical sensors, **1**-5 to **1**-6, **8-11**
gas chromatograph, **1**-7
ion-selective electrode (ISE), **1**-6 to **1**-7
Chronaxie, **7-11**
CMOS (complementary metal oxide semiconductor), **4**-25
CMOS transistors, **4**-55
Combustible liquids, **5-3**
Compton, Arthur H., scattering experiment, **4**-70
Constituitive relation, **4-18**
Continuum hypothesis, **4**-12, **4-18**
Continuum mechanics, **4-18**
Conversion constants and multipliers, **III**-6 to **III**-7
Cotton—Mouton effect/magnetic linear birefringence, **3**-3 to **3**-4, **3-10**
Coulomb blockade, **4-79**
Coupled domain problem, **4-18**
Cross spectra, **9-13**
Current clamp, **7-11**

D

Dasarathy's Functional Model (data fusion process model), **2**-11
Data fusion; *see also* Multi-sensor data fusion
applications, **2**-5
condition-based monitoring (CBM) of complex systems, **2**-6
environmental monitoring, **2**-6
medical applications, **2**-7
military applications, **2**-7
nondestructive evaluation (NDE), **2**-7
limitations of systems, to **2**-13, **2**-12
process models, **2**-7 to **2**-8
Bedworth and O'Brien's Omnibus Model, **2**-11
Boyd's Decision Loop Model, **2**-11
Dasarathy's Functional Model, **2**-11
Joint Directors of Laboratories (JDL) model, **2**-8 to **2**-11
similarities to human cognitive processes, **2**-1 to **2**-2
techniques, **2**-3
a priori knowledge about input data/estimation processes, **2**-5
data fusion architecture, **2**-5
decision level fusion, **2**-3
nature/heterogeneity of input data, **2**-3, **2**-5
Data type, **5-53**
de Broglie's hypothesis, **4**-70 to **4**-71
Decision Loop Model (Boyd), **2**-11
Dynamic clamp, **7-11**

E

ECG lead, **9-20**
Ectopic beat, **7-32**
Electrical equipment/hazardous areas, **5**-1; *see also* Explosion protection
certification and approval, **5**-17 to **5**-19
enclosure types/requirements, **5**-10
equipment use and hierarchy, **5**-26 to **5**-27
hazardous areas classification, **5**-4 to **5**-5
hazardous areas classification/methods, **5**-5
hazardous areas division classification (NEC method), **5**-6 to **5**-7
ignition curves, **5**-14 to **5**-17
IS ground rules, **5**-20
combustible gas detection system, **5**-25 to **5**-26
dust-ignition proof, **5**-20 to **5**-22
encapsulation, **5**-24 to **5**-25
explosion proof design, **5**-20
hermetically sealed, **5**-25
increased safety, **5**-25
non sparking (nonincendive), **5**-24
nonincendive circuit, **5**-24
nonincendive component, **5**-24
oil immersion, **5**-24
powder filled, **5**-23 to **5**-24
purging and pressurization methodology, **5**-22 to **5**-23
making field devices intrinsically safe, **5**-13 to **5**-14
protection methodologies, **5**-11
intrinsic safety (IS), **5**-11 to **5**-13
terminology, **5**-3 to **5**-4, **5**-27
zone classification, **5**-7 to **5**-10
Electro-encephalogram (EEG), **9**-1, **9-13**
frequency analysis, **9**-6 to **9**-8
historical perspective, **9**-3 to **9**-4
language of the brain, **9**-1 to **9**-3
nonlinear analysis, **9**-8 to **9**-10
recording techniques, **9**-4 to **9**-6
topographic mapping, **9**-10 to **9**-12
Electrocardiograph (ECG), **9**-14 to **9**-16, **9-20**
instrumentation, **9**-17 to **9**-20
physiology, **9**-17
Electrochemical sensors
advantages, **1**-11
amperometric sensors, **1**-13, **1**-15 to **1**-17
potentiomatic sensors, **1**-11 to **1**-12
Electron tunneling, **4-78**
Embedded digital signal processor (DSP), **7**-60
programmable
advantages of, **7**-60 to **7**-61
challenges of, **7**-61 to **7**-62
DSP hardware, **7**-62 to **7**-65
benchmarking, **7**-66
technology trends, **7**-69 to **7**-70
software/runtime and development environment, **7**-67 to **7**-69
Embedded signal processing, **7**-55 to **7**-56, **7-55**, **7**-75
active electronically steered array (AESA)-based sensor systems, **7**-55
application-specific hardware, **7**-70 to **7**-71
FPGA (field programmable gate arrays) design, **7**-73 to **7**-74
full-custom ASIC (application-specific integrated circuits), **7**-72 to **7**-73
intellectual property (IP) core approach, **7**-74 to **7**-75
and semiconductor technology, **7**-71 to **7**-72
standard-cell ASIC (application-specific integrated circuits), **7**-73
structured ASIC, **7**-74
generic architecture, **7**-56 to **7**-60
Error cluster, **5-54**
Explosion protection
avoidance techniques, **5**-2 to **5**-3
basic reaction, **5**-2
hazardous area terminology, **5**-3 to **5**-4

F

Failure, **6-2**
Farraday rotation/magnetic circular birefringence, **3**-2 to **3**-3, **3-10**
Fast Fourier transform (FFT), **9-13**
Feynman, Richard, **4-9**
Flammable limits (FL), **5-3**
Flammable liquids, **5-3**
Flash point (FP), **5-3**
Front panel, **5-54**
Fuels, **5-4**

G

G, **5-54**; *see also* LabVIEW development system
Gas sensors, "solid state", **1**-18; *see also* Stannic oxide semiconductor gas sensor
Greek alphabet, **III**-3
Ground, **5-27**

H

Hazard rate, **6-2**
Heat equation, **4-18**
HRECG, **9-20**

Human error, **6-2**
Hypocapnia, **7-32**
Hypoxia, **7-32**

I

Ignition temperature, **5-3**
Inactivation, **7-12**
Inductance, **5-27**
Installer, **5-54**
Intel Pentium processor/Microburst microarchitecture, **4**-44
International Electrotechnical Commission (IEC)/Zone Classification method, **5**-5
International System of Units (SI)
  definitions, **III**-3 to **III**-4
  names and symbols for SI base units, **III**-4
  SI derived units with special names and symbols, **III**-4 to **III**-5
  units in use with SI, **III**-5

J

Joint Directors of Laboratories (JDL) model, **2**-8 to **2**-11

K

Kerr effects, **3**-4 to **3**-5, **3-10**

L

LabVIEW development system, **5**-36, **5-54**
  application building (creating executables), **5**-50
    installers, **5**-52
    reverse engineering built executables, **5**-51
    runtime engine (RTE), **5**-51
    runtime licenses (RTLs), **5**-51 to **5**-52
  code distribution, **5**-48
    application distribution library, **5**-49
    development distribution library, **5**-49
    diagram access, 550t, **5**-49 to **5**-50
    VI library (*.llb), **5**-49
  data coerceion, **5**-40 to **5**-41
  data types, **5**-36 to **5**-37
  error handling, **5**-41
    custom error codes, **5**-44 to **5**-46
    default error codes, **5**-44
    error cluster, **5**-41
    usage, **5**-41 to **5**-43
    wiring errors/subVI connector pane, **5**-43
  G programming language, **5**-36, **5-54**
  GOOP (graphical object-oriented programming), **5**-47 to **5**-49
  open source G/distributed development, **5**-52 to **5**-53
  polymorphism, **5**-38 to **5**-39
  shortcuts, **5**-47
    front panel and block diagram, **5**-47
    keyboard, **5**-46
    tool palette, **5**-46 to **5**-47
  terminology, **5**-53 to **5**-54
  units, **5**-39 to **5**-40
LIGA/LIGA-like high-aspect-ratio, **4**-25
Ligand-gated ion channels, **7-12**
Linear thermoelasticity, **4-18**
Lower explosive limit (LEL), **5-3**
Lower flammable limit (LFL), **5-3**

M

Magnetic stimulation, **7-32**
Magneto-optics, **3**-1 to **3**-2
  applications
    magneto-optic recording, **3**-9 to **3**-10, **3-10**
    MSW-based guided-wave magneto-optic Bragg cell, **3**-8 to **3**-9, **3-10**
    optical isolator and circulator, **3**-5 to **3**-8, **3-10**
  classification of effects
    Cotton—Mouton effect/magnetic linear birefringence, **3**-3 to **3**-4
    Farraday rotation/magnetic circular birefringence, **3**-2 to **3**-3
    Kerr effects, **3**-4 to **3**-5
Magnitude squared coherence (MSC), **9-13**
Mathematical modeling, **4**-10, **4-18**
Mathematics, **III**-1 to **III**-2; *see also* Symbols and physical constants
Maximum surface temperature, **5-3**
Maxwell's equations, **4-18**
Mean time to failure (exponential distribution), **6-2**
Measuring instruments, **5**-27
Measuring instruments (portable), **5**-35
  applications, **5**-33 to **5**-35
  communicating and networking of, **5**-31 to **5**-32
  digital portable instruments, **5**-29 to **5**-30
  features, **5**-28
  main groups, **5**-28
  power requirements, **5**-28 to **5**-29
  sensor for, **5**-30 to **5**-31
  wireless portable instruments and networks, **5**-32 to **5**-33
Membrane potential, **7-12**
MEMS and NEMS modeling, **4**-9, **4-18**, **4-19**
  approaches, **4**-12
    continuum mechanics, **4**-12 to **4**-17
    coupled domains, **4**-17
  history of, **4**-9 to **4**-10
  other tools, **4**-17 to **4**-18
    "Buckeyball structure", **4**-17
    self-assembly, **4**-17 to **4**-18
  and resonant gate transistor development, **4**-10
  science of scale, **4**-10 to **4**-12
  self-assembly (SA) and self-organization (SO) study, **4**-18
Metabolic process, **7-32**
Micro-electrical modeling systems (MEMS). *See* MEMS and NEMS modeling
Micromatching, **1-8** to **1-9**, **1-10**
Micromechatronics, **4**-20; *see also* Piezoelectric wafer active sensors (PWAS)
  electroactive and magnetoactive materials, **4**-26
    electroactive materials, **4**-26 to **4**-27
    magnetoactive materials, **4**-27 to **4**-28
  fabrication aspects, **4**-25 to **4**-26
  induced-strain actuators, **4**-28
    design with, **4**-20
  linearized electromechanical behavior of induced-strain actuators, **4**-29 to **4**-31
  microcontrollers sensing/actuation/ process control, **4**-40 to **4**-42
  synchronous micromachines, **4**-22 to **4**-25
  systems introduction, **4**-20 to **4**-21
Microsensors, **1-8** to **1-9**
Molecular dynamics, **4-18**
Moore's laws, **4**-44
Multi-sensor data fusion, **2**-1 to **2**-2, **2**-13 to **2**-14; *see also* Data fusion
Muscular dystrophy, **7**-23
Myasthenia gravis, **7**-23
Myocardial infarction, **7-32**
Myotonia, **7**-23

N

Nano-architectronics. *See* Nanocomputers/ nano-architectronics/nano-ICs
Nano-electromechanical modeling systems (NEMS). *See* MEMS and NEMS modeling
Nano-ICs. *See* Nanocomputers/ nano-architectronics/nano-ICs

Nanocompensator synthesis and design aspects, **4**-66 to **4**-67
Nanocomputers/nano-architectronics/nano-ICs, **4**-42 to **4**-44
 applied and experimental results, **4**-43
 architecture (nanocomputers), **4**-54 to **4**-59
 benchmarking opportunities, **4**-42 to **4**-43
 classification of nanocomputers, **4**-47
 fundamentals (nanoelectronics and nanocomputers), **4**-45 to **4**-54
  memory management, **4**-46
  memory—processor interface, **4**-48 to **4**-50
  multiprocessors, **4**-51 to **4**-52
  nanocomputer architectronics, **4**-52 to **4**-53
  parallel memories, **4**-50 to **4**-51
  pipelining, **4**-51
  processor and memory hierarchy, **4**-47
  two-/three-dimensional topology aggregation, **4**-53 to **4**-54
 hierarchical finite-state machines/use in hardware and software design, **4**-59 to **4**-63
  steps in heuristic synthesis, **4**-60
 mathematical models (nanocomputers)
  with parameters set, **4**-66
  sixtuple nanocomputer model, **4**-65
 and Moore's laws, **4**-44
 nanocompensator synthesis and design aspects, **4**-66 to **4**-67
 reconfigurable nanocomputers, **4**-63 to **4**-65
 three-dimensional nano-ICs, **4**-44
 types of nanocomputers, **4**-43
  bioelectrical, **4**-43 to **4**-44
  mechanical, **4**-44
  reversible/irreversible, **4**-45
Nanoscience materials. *See* Carbon nanotubes; MEMS and NEMS modeling; Micromechatronics; Nanocomputers, nano-architectronics, and nano-ICs; Semiconductor nano-electronics and nano-optoelectronics
Navier equations, **4-18**
Navier—Stokes equations, **4-18**
NEC Division Classification method, **5**-5
Nernst potential, **1-6**
Neuroelectric principles, **7**-1 to **7**-2
 action potentials, **7-1**, **7**-3 to **7**-6
 application/deep brain stimulation, **7**-10 to **7**-11
 dynamic clamp, **7**-6 to **7**-8
 electrochemical potential, **7**-2 to **7**-3
 extracellular stimulation models, **7**-8 to **7**-10
  activating function, **7-8**
  chronaxie, **7-8**
  rheobase, **7-8**
 synaptic transmission, **7**-6
Noninvasive sensor, **8-11**
Normal Operation, **5-27**

O

Occipital, **7-32**
Omnibus Model (Bedworth and O'Brien), **2**-11
Optical fiber telecommunications applications. *See* Semiconductor nano-optoelectronics
Oxidation, **5-27**

P

Parietal, **7-32**
Pellistor sensor, **1**-18
pH glass electrode, **1**-6
Physical constants. *See* Symbols and physical constants
Physical sensor, **8-11**
Physical sensors, **1**-2, **1**-4
 displacement and force, **1**-5
 optical radiation, **1**-5
 temperature, **1**-4
Piezoelectric wafer active sensors (PWAS), **4**-32
 PWAS modal sensor and electromechanical impedance method, **4**-38 to **4**-40
 PWAS phased array, **4**-37 to **4**-38
 PWAS resonators, **4**-32
  circular, **4**-33 to **4**-34
  rectangular, **4**-32 to **4**-33
 PWAS transmitters and receivers of elastic waves, **4**-34, **4**-36
Piezoresistor, **1**-2
Planck's Law, **4**-69
Pn-junction photodiode, **1**-5
Polymorphic virtual instruments (VIs), **5-38**, **5-54**
Portable instruments. *See* Measuring instruments (portable)
Potentiomatic sensors, **1**-11 to **1**-12
Potentiometric sensor, **8-11**
Potentiometric measurement, **8-8**
Power spectral analysis, **9-13**

Q

Quadratic phase coupling, **9-13**

R

Random failure, **6-2**
Redundancy, **6-2**
Refractory period, **7-12**
Reliability, **6-2**
Reliability engineering, **6**-1
 bathtub hazard-rate concept, **6**-2 to **6**-3
 formulas, **6**-3 to **6**-5
 human reliability, **6**-13
  classification and causes of human errors, **6**-13
  measures, **6**-13 to **6**-14
  modeling human operation in a fluctuating environment, **6**-14 to **6**-16
 reliability evaluation methods, **6**-8
  failure modes and effect analysis, **6**-8 to **6**-9
  fault-tree analysis, **6**-9
  Markov method, **6**-11 to **6**-13
  probability evaluation, **6**-10 to **6**-11
 reliability networks, **6**-5
  k-out-of-*m* network, **6**-7 to **6**-8
  parallel network, **6**-6 to **6**-7
  series network, **6**-5 to **6**-6
 robot reliability, **6**-16
  measures, **6**-16 to **6**-18
  robot failure classification and causes, **6**-16
 terms/definitions, **6**-2
Reliability formula, **6**-3
Repair rate, **6-2**
Repeatability, **1-10**
Resistance thermometer, **1**-4
Resonant gate transistor development, **4**-10
RTD, **5-27**
Runtime engine (RTE), **5-54**
Runtime license (RTL), **5-54**

S

Seebeck effect, **1**-4
Self-assembly, **4-19**
Semiconductor nano-optoelectronics
 gain media for telecom lasers/InGaAsN and InAs QDs, **4**-85 to **4**-86
 implementation/epitaxy of gain media into devices, **4**-82
 quantum dots lasers, **4**-84
 quantum-effects based gain media/laser applications, 4, 80 to **4**-82
 quantum intersubband lasers, **4**-87 to **4**-88
 strained quantum well lasers, **4**-83 to **4**-84
 Type-II quantum well lasers, **4**-86 to **4**-87

Semiconductor nanoelectronics/resonant tunneling diode
application, **4**-77 to **4**-78
nanoelectronics and tunneling phenomenon, **4**-72 to **4**-73
particle tunneling through a potential barrier, **4**-75
quantum tunneling phenomenon, **4**-73 to **4**-74
resonant tunneling—double barrier potential, **4**-75 to **4**-77
Semiconductor nanotechnology, **4**-68 to **4**-69
fundamental physics of/quantum physics
duality of particle and wave/ electron as a wave, **4**-70 to **4**-71
duality of particle and wave/light as a particle, **4**-69 to **4**-70
and quantum effects, **4**-71 to **4**-72
future directions, **4**-88 to **4**-89
Semiconductor nanoelectronics/single electron transistors
operation, **4**-80
theoretical basis, **4**-78 to **4**-79
Sensitivity, **1-10**
Sensors, **1-1**, **1-10**; *See also* Biosensors; Chemical sensors; Electrochemical sensors; Multi-sensor data fusion; Physical sensors; Stannic oxide semiconductor gas sensor
block diagram, **1**-1 to **1**-2
demand for, **1**-1
direct/indirect, **1**-1
factors in choice for applications, **1**-2
SET. *See* Semiconductor nanoelectronics/ single electron transistors
Space clamp, **7-12**
Stability, **1-10**
Stannic oxide semiconductor gas sensor, **1**-18
basic electric parameters and operation, **1**-18 to **1**-20
electrical operating parameters, **1**-23
future directions, **1**-23
operating temperature, **1**-21
substrate materials, **1**-22
Steady-state condition (statistical), **6-2**
Strain gage, **1**-5
Surface micromachining technologies, **4**-25
Symbols and physical constants; *See also* Conversion constants and multipliers; International System of Units (SI)
Greek alphabet, **III**-3
physical constants, **III**-8 to **III**-9

T

Thermistors, **1**-4
Thermocouple, **1**-4
Tomography, **10-1**, **10-7**
computerized, **10**-1 to **10**-3
axial tomography (CAT/CATscan), **10-1**, **10-6**
tomography (CT), **10-1**
imaging, **10**-5 to **10**-6
magnetic resonance imaging (MRI), **10-1**, **10**-4 to **10**-5, **10-6**
positron emission tomography (PET), **10-1**, **10**-3 to **10**-4, **10-7**
single photon emission computed tomography (SPECT), **10-1**, **10**-4, **10-7**
Transducer, **1-1**
auto-generators, **1**-2
mechanisms, **1**-2
modulators, **1**-2
Twelve-lead ECG, **9-20**

U

Unit, **5-54**
Upper explosive limit (UEL), **5-3**

V

Vapor density, **5-3**
Vapor dispersion, **5-4**
Voltage clamp, **7-12**
Voltage-gated ion channels, **7-12**

W

Wilson central terminal, **9-20**

Z

Zener diode, **5-27**